HANDBOOK OF PEDIATRIC PSYCHOLOGY AND PSYCHIATRY

Volume I

HANDBOOK OF PEDIATRIC PSYCHOLOGY AND PSYCHIATRY

Volume I

Psychological and Psychiatric Issues in the Pediatric Setting

Edited by

Robert T. Ammerman

Allegheny University of the Health Sciences
Pittsburgh, Pennsylvania

John V. Campo

University of Pittsburgh School of Medicine

Allyn and Bacon

Boston   London   Toronto   Sydney   Tokyo   Singapore

Series editor: Carla F. Daves
Series editorial assistant: Susan Hutchinson
Manufacturing buyer: Suzanne Lareau

Library of Congress Cataloging-in-Publication Data

Handbook of pediatric psychology and psychiatry / edited by Robert T. Ammerman and John V. Campo.
    p.   cm.
    Includes bibliographical references and indexes.
    Contents: v. 1: Psychological and psychiatric issues in the pediatric setting — v. 2: Disease, injury, and illness.
    ISBN 0–205–16560–5 (v. 1). — ISBN 0–205–27601–6 (v. 2).
    1. Child psychiatry—Handbooks, manuals, etc. 2. Child psychology—Handbooks, manuals, etc. I. Ammerman, Robert T.
II. Campo, John V.
    [DNLM: 1. Child Psychiatry. 2. Mental Disorders—in infancy & childhood. 3. Child Development Disorders, Pervasive. WS 350
H23595   1998]
RJ499.3.H364   1998
618.92′89—dc21
DNLM/DLC
for Library of Congress   97–42736
                                   CIP

Printed in the United States of America

10 9 8 7 6 5 4 3 2 1   02 01 00 99 98

To Caroline, Patrick, and Evan

—RTA

To my parents, my wife, and my children

—JVC

CONTENTS

FOREWORD

The reader may wonder, and rightfully so, why the editors would request a pediatrician to write the foreword to these excellent volumes dealing with pediatric psychology and psychiatry. A colleague of similar discipline or specialty is usually honored in this way. I, therefore, feel both honored and privileged to do so.

Although not usual, it is certainly most fitting that a pediatrician be given the opportunity to comment upon a book addressing the broad range of developmental, psychiatric, behavioral, and medical conditions in which pediatricians are, or should be, involved.

The relationship between pediatrics and the behavioral sciences, psychology, and psychiatry continues to be a special one. Consider that child growth and psychological development is the basic science of pediatrics and recall that child psychiatry developed independently, not as an offspring of adult psychiatry, but more as a cousin of pediatrics. Almost 70 years ago, the first child psychiatry clinic was established in an academic pediatric department, and child psychology and psychiatry has become strengthened, as evidenced by increased collaboration in practice and educational settings, and among our professional organizations.

Primary care physicians, especially pediatricians, play a major role in the provision of mental health services. A high percentage of problems encountered in pediatric practice are psychosocial in nature. Pediatricians have known that 85 percent or more of their time practicing pediatrics is spent giving advice, guidance, and counseling for psychological or development problems. Such activities constitute the art of pediatrics based on science. The early diagnosis of psychiatric illness with appropriate and timely referral is also the art and science of psychiatry and clinical psychology.

The title, *Handbook of Pediatric Psychology and Psychiatry*, may erroneously imply that the work is relatively superficial and entirely clinically oriented. Not so! Each chapter is a complete review of a subject or condition, providing current research findings and references. A case illustration is included in each chapter; a very helpful feature bridging current knowledge and understanding of diagnosis and treatment with a clinical example.

Current knowledge and understanding of the psychopathology of mental illness is certainly a prerequisite for good diagnosis and management; without clinical application the patient and family are unlikely to be helped. The late Dr. Dennis Cantwell (1990) expressed this so well:

> The scientifically minded artist (thinks) scientifically and empirically but will acquire and use clinical skills effectively. The scientifically minded artist accepts the fact that the same time one is searching for ultimate truth, one must frequently take therapeutic action based on data that are known to be inadequate. (pp. xv–xvi).

There is also a place for pediatricians working together with mental health professionals. I have had the great privilege and opportunity to work in a psychiatric setting shoulder to shoulder with a wide variety of mental health professionals. Such ideal arrangements are currently being threatened by the economic environment of medicine. It is an ideal that we should continue to strive to achieve.

I am pleased to have been given the opportunity to introduce these outstanding books edited by two outstanding teachers and practitioners. This comprehensive and in-depth, yet practical, treatise should be in the libraries of pediatric generalists, and all behavioral pediatricians and child mental health providers.

The conditions presented and explored in these texts affect the most vulnerable of the vulnerable, those children and adolescents who suffer from psychological conditions and serious mental illness. The care and nurturing of such children is among our most important human activities. The editors and contributors are dedicated to this activity, and the questions they raise that are still unanswered will be left to our younger colleagues. They, students, residents, fellows, and faculty, will be helped by these books in their pursuit of answers.

I take this opportunity to thank my many colleagues in child and adolescent psychology and psychiatry who have made invaluable contributions to the education of pediatricians in training and in practice, and to my own career development—and for their patience.

REFERENCE

Cantwell, D. P. (1990). Foreword. In B. D. Garfinkel, G. A. Carlson, & E. B. Weller (Eds.), *Psychiatric disorders in children and adolescents*. Philadelphia: W.B. Saunders.

GEORGE D. COMERCI, M.D., F.A.A.P.
Former President of the American Academy
    of Pediatrics
Clinical Professor of Pediatrics and
Past Professor of Pediatrics and of
    Family and Community Medicine
University of Arizona College of Medicine

PREFACE

The idea for this book grew out of our sometimes heated, but always collegial, discussions about various issues in psychology and psychiatry, which began during our years in training, and continued as our careers developed. Several observations emerged from our discussions, which eventually became the focal point for a book.

First, both psychology and psychiatry have become partners of primary care physicians in pediatrics and family medicine, as well as a variety of sub-specialists. The pediatric primary care provider has been increasingly recognized as the "gatekeeper" for behavioral health services for children and adolescents, and the primary care setting appears to be the place where such intervention is most likely to take place. Most children are seen by their primary care medical provider within a given year, and there appears to be considerable overlap between so-called mental health problems and physical problems, with relevant examples including accidents and injury prevention, maltreatment, chronic physical illness, somatization, and psychophysiologically reactive disorders such as migraine.

A variety of psychiatric disorders occur concurrently with health problems. Emotional and behavioral disorders quite commonly first present in pediatric medical settings, often with medically unexplained somatic symptoms, and children and adolescents with psychiatric disorders may be higher utilizers of medical services. It is also relevant that psychiatric symptoms may be closely associated with or caused by physical disease. Psychiatric symptoms or disorders can negatively impact the course of physical disease as a result of influences on the behavior of children and families, and sometimes a direct physiologic effect on the disease process itself. The ex-

citing developments of the past several years in behavioral medicine, psychopharmacology, and the psychobiology of illness have stimulated research and highlighted the richness and complexity of conceptualizations of mind and body.

The biomedical model of illness and disease has been responsible for many of the major achievements of modern Western medicine, though it soon became clear that many individuals experience subjective distress or illness in the absence of the clear-cut physical pathology or physical signs generally associated with disease. This resulted in a psychological model of illness developing alongside the biomedical model and the development of parallel systems of care delivery, one based on the biomedical model and focused on "legitimate" illness and its treatment, and another based on a presumed psychological model and focused on "mental illness," which has been considered somehow "illegitimate," a result of some sort of sociomoral failure on the part of the patient and family, and a source of great stigma and potential embarrassment. While it is true that much has changed in our views of psychiatric illness, much has stayed the same, and stigma remains with us. The practical and theoretical problems and inconsistencies of modern practices such as mental health "carve-outs" regarding health care insurance appear to be derivative of the false dichotomy that has been perpetuated in the traditional health care delivery system. It is clear that we are living in exciting times, which have presented both challenges and opportunities for psychology and psychiatry, and it appears to be somewhat ironic that the economics of modern health care may actually provide the impetus for successfully addressing the issue of stigma and integrating the various disciplines that function in medical settings, regardless of their supposed orientation regarding the mind-body split that has been pervasive in Western medicine.

Another consequence of our discussions over the years has been the shared conviction that the traditional distinctions between pediatric psychology and psychiatry are unrealistic and largely in error. Pediatric psychology and psychiatry appear to be complementary disciplines, each with its own unique strengths and areas of emphasis, but disciplines with extensive areas of overlap and much in common. We share much of the same literature, have a commitment to the comprehensive care of children and adolescents, and utilize an ecological perspective in which it is recognized that biological, psychological, and social variables interact in complex ways to bring about the clinical presentation of children in both medical and mental health settings. Dramatic shifts in the way health care is provided, driven primarily by financial imperatives, require partnerships between pediatric psychology and psychiatry and call for new models of pediatric health care, such as truly integrated medical and mental health services. The future demands a new collegiality and sense of collaboration across the disciplines engaged in the care of children and adolescents, as well as flexibility and a shared sense of purpose.

The two volumes of *Handbook of Pediatric Psychology and Psychiatry* reflect the interdigitation of pediatrics, psychiatry, and psychology. Unlike most volumes on this topic, in which each discipline has its own reference books written by similarly trained professionals primarily using their own literatures, this book established bridges connecting psychology, psychiatry, and pediatrics. This is evident in the chapter topics, which are comprehensive and broad in scope. Separate chapters are included on psychiatric disorders (Volume I) which frequently present in pediatric settings, in addition to chapters on pediatric illnesses and conditions (Volume II) which have psychological and psychiatric components. Sections on general issues (e.g., consultation and liaison, cultural issues) and special topics (e.g., child maltreatment, pain) are also included. Most of the chapters are coauthored by both psychologists and psychiatrists, and many also include pediatricians. Lastly, most of the chapters follow a standardized format within each section, which ensures that pediatric medical, psychological, and psychiatric issues and perspectives are addressed. Case illustrations are included to highlight multidisciplinary assessment and treatment. In sum, we have striven

to compile a handbook that is state of the art clinically, has a strong empirical foundation, and is relevant and useful to pediatricians, psychologists, psychiatrists, and other professionals who care for children and adolescents.

We are especially saddened by the untimely death of Dr. Marla Hooks, the coauthor with Dr. Elizabeth McCauley of the chapter, "Affective Disorders." It is clear that she was an extraordinary person. She was trained in both pediatrics and psychiatry, and had been the recipient of many honors, including a fellowship with the Health Services Research Institute for Minority Faculty through the Association of American Medical Colleges. In addition to her many strengths as a wife and mother, she showed great promise professionally, both clinically and academically. We extend our condolences and deepest sympathy to her husband, her children, and other family members, as well as to her many friends and colleagues. Dr. Hooks will be greatly missed, and we are proud that her contribution is appearing in this book.

We would like to acknowledge the help, assistance, and encouragement that we have received from numerous individuals in putting together this book. First and foremost, we thank the contributors for sharing with us their experience and expertise. Their enthusiasm for assembling writing teams across disciplines was both gratifying and inspiring. We extend our appreciation to Mylan Jaixen and Carla Daves, our editors at Allyn and Bacon, who from the beginning have understood and supported our efforts to create a multidisciplinary text for pediatric psychology and psychiatry. Their unswerving patience and understanding in the face of inevitable delays are especially noteworthy. We gratefully acknowledge the administrative support provided by Nancy Simpson, Cindy DeLuca, Roberta Farren, Patricia O'Donnell, Maryann Ruffing, Ann Huber, Stuart McKenna, and Sue Hutchinson (at Allyn and Bacon). Our appreciation also goes to the following reviewers for their comments on the manuscript: Karla Doepke, Auburn University; Kevin J. Armstrong, Western Michigan University; and Jennifer Johnson, University of California, Irvine. Finally, we are thankful for our friendship, and especially grateful for the love, support, and patience of our respective wives and families, the figurative glue which has served to hold this project together.

Robert T. Ammerman
John V. Campo

Pittsburgh, Pennsylvania

ABOUT THE EDITORS
AND CONTRIBUTORS

Robert T. Ammerman (Ph.D., University of Pittsburgh, 1986) is Associate Professor of Psychiatry, Allegheny University of the Health Sciences, Allegheny Campus, and Director, Mental Health Services in Childhood Disabilities, Department of Psychiatry and Allegheny Neuropsychiatric Institute, Allegheny General Hospital (Pittsburgh, PA). He is a Diplomate in Behavioral Psychology from the American Board of Professional Psychology. He is the recipient of grants from the National Institute on Disabilities and Rehabilitation Research, Vira I. Heinz Foundation, Children's Trust Fund of Pennsylvania, National Institute on Drug Abuse, National Institute on Alcoholism and Alcohol Abuse, and the Staunton Farm Foundation. His research interests are child abuse and neglect, psychopathology in children and youth with disabilities, psychosocial impact of congenital neurological syndromes, and adolescent substance abuse.

John V. Campo (M.D., University of Pennsylvania, 1982) is Assistant Professor of Psychiatry and Pediatrics at the University of Pittsburgh School of Medicine. He is Director of the Center for Pediatric Psychiatry and Medicine Module at the Western Psychiatric Institute and Clinic, and Director of the Behavioral Science Division at the Children's Hospital of Pittsburgh. He is board certified in pediatrics, psychiatry, and child and adolescent psychiatry. His interests include medically unexplained physical symptoms in children and adolescents, the association between psychopathology and physical disease, and models of delivering pediatric behavioral health care within medical settings.

Michael Aman (Ph.D., University of Auckland, New Zealand, 1979) is Professor of Psychology and Psychiatry at the Ohio State University. He is co-developer of the Aberrant Behavior Checklist, an instrument for assessing treatment effects and behavior in people with developmental disabilities. He has done extensive research on psychotropic drugs in children with ADHD and with epilepsy and in individuals (both children and adults) with mental retardation. He has also done substantial research assessing rating instruments used in these clinical populations.

Ronald E. Dahl (M.D., University of Pittsburgh, 1984) is Associate Professor of Psychiatry and Pediatrics at the University of Pittsburgh School of Medicine where he directs a clinical program in Child and Adolescent Sleep Disorders, and co-directs a research program in the Psychobiology of Early Onset Affective Disorders. His primary research interest is the regulation of sleep and arousal in relation to the development of psychobiology in children and adolescents.

Ann M. DiGirolamo (Ph.D., Indiana University, 1994) is a Clinical Psychologist at St. Louis Children's Hospital in St. Louis, Missouri. Her clinical specialty is pediatric psychology. Her primary research interests focus on stress and coping processes among children with chronic illnesses and their families.

Gloria D. Eldridge (Ph.D., University of Manitoba, 1991) is a Project Director in the Community Health Program, Jackson State University, Jackson, MS. She was behavioral science consultant on a Government of Kenya/Government of Canada project to strengthen STD and HIV control in Kenya. She worked with a multidisciplinary group from Canada, the United States, Belgium, and several African countries to develop training programs for STD/HIV counseling for primary care service providers. Her current research interests are in HIV-risk-reduction interventions for low-income African-American women, for male and female crack cocaine users in drug treatment, and for incarcerated women.

Judy Garber (Ph.D., University of Minnesota, 1987) is Associate Professor of Psychology and Human Development and Co-Director of the Development Psychopathology Training Program at Vanderbilt University. She is currently conducting a longitudinal study of adolescents at risk for the development of mood disorders. This study examines the role of social-cognitions, stress, and family interactions in the prediction of adolescent depression. In collaboration with Lynn Walker, Ph.D., she is conducting another longitudinal study exploring factors predicting the maintenance of illness behavior among children with a history of recurrent abdominal pain.

Heather Geis (M.D., University of Oklahoma, 1985) is in private practice with Psychiatric Associates, Inc. in Oklahoma City, Oklahoma. Her positions include Medical Director of Child and Adolescent Psychiatric Services at CPC Southwinds and Saint Anthony's Hospitals.

Marla Hooks (M.D., Northwestern University, 1980) was Acting Assistant Professor in the Department of Psychiatry and Behavioral Sciences, University of Washington, and Director of Psychiatric Services, King County Juvenile Detention. Dr. Hooks initiated an innovative preventive intervention for youth already involved in the juvenile justice system and after some early research in the area of autism had turned her focus to research on youth with externalizing disorders and psychiatrically impaired youth within the juvenile system.

John B. Jolly (Psy.D., Baylor University, 1987) is Associate Professor in the Department of Psychology at Mississippi College. He is a Diplomate in Clinical Psychology from the American Board of Professional Psychology (ABPP). He conducts research in cognitive models of depression and anxiety across the life span and serves on the editorial board of *Cognitive Therapy and Research*. He maintains a private practice in Jackson, MS.

Yifrah Kaminer (M.D., University of Tel Aviv, 1976) is Associate Professor of Psychiatry at the Alcohol Research Center, University of Connecticut Health Center in Farmington. He is currently the recipient of a clinician scientist award, and a principal investigator or co-investigator on several federally/state funded grants, evaluating psychosocial and psychopharmacological treatment of adolescent substance abuse. Dr. Kaminer is also interested in typology and patient treatment matching of adolescent substance abuse.

Cynthia J. Kapphahn (M.D., Yale University School of Medicine, 1987) is Clinical Assistant Professor with the Division of Adolescent Medicine at Stanford University School of Medicine. She serves as medical attending for adolescents on the inpatient med/psych unit, in the partial hospitalization program, and the outpatient eating disorders and youth clinics at the Lucile Salter Packard Children's Hospital at Stanford. She is Assistant Editor of the *Journal of Adolescent Health*. Dr. Kapphahn has a Masters in Public Health from the Johns Hopkins School of Hygiene and Public Health and is also interested in adolescent health policy, particularly access to care.

Richard A. Kern (M.D., Ohio State University, 1982) is Clinical Associate Professor of Pediatrics at the Ohio State University College of Medicine and Medical Director of the Nisonger Center UAP. Dr. Kern works with a wide variety of pediatric developmental and behavioral problems, including autism, mental retardation, learning disabilities, and sleep disorders. He also pursues research in the pharmacologic treatment of attentional and conduct problems.

Sally A. Kush (Ph.D., Arizona State University, 1986) is a school psychologist with Shaler Area School District in Pittsburgh, PA. She has worked extensively in educational settings as well as in medical settings involving both psychiatry and pediatric mental health services. Dr. Kush has co-authored a book on children's psychological testing. Current areas of interest include the adjustment and management in the educational setting of children with somatization disorders and children with chronic illnesses.

Judith A. Libow (Ph.D., State University of New York at Albany, 1978) is Management Coordinator of Psychology and Director of Training in the Department of Psychiatry at Children's Hospital Oakland. She has authored and co-authored numerous journal articles and chapters on Munchausen by Proxy Syndrome, as well as the first published book on this disorder. Her interests and writings also include gender issues in family therapy, adolescent chronic illness, and the effects of media exposure on traumatized children.

Richard Livingston (M.D., University of Arkansas, 1978) is Professor and Director of Child and Adolescent Psychiatry at the New Jersey Medical School. His academic interests include anxiety, learning disorders, abuse and violence, somatization, and cultural issues. He is a fellow of the American Academy of Child and Adolescent Psychiatry and author of numerous papers and chapters.

Elizabeth McCauley (Ph.D., State University of New York at Buffalo, 1973) is Associate Professor in the Department of Psychiatry and Behavioral Sciences, University of Washington, and the Clinical Director of the Inpatient and Partial Hospitalization programs at Children's Hospital and Medical Center. Dr. McCauley has been involved in a program of research aimed at articulating the course, correlates, and contributors to mood disorders in children and adolescents.

Michael W. Mellon (Ph.D., University of Memphis, 1993) is Assistant Professor of Pediatrics in the Section of Behavioral pediatrics at the University of Arkansas for Medical Sciences and Arkansas Children's Hospital. He is Co-Director of the Elimination Disorders Clinic at Arkansas Children's Hospital. He is a pediatric psychologist whose research interests include behavioral treatments for enuresis and encopresis, the investigation of the mechanism of action for the enuresis alarm, and wellness promotion in a local Boys' and Girls' Club.

Jodi A. Mindell (Ph.D., State University of New York at Albany, 1989) is Associate Professor of Psychology at St. Joseph's University and Clinical Associate Professor of Neurology at MCP Hahnemann School of Medicine, Allegheny University of the Health Sciences. She specializes in pediatric sleep disorders and maintains a broad-scale clinical research program investigating the assessment and treatment of sleep problems in children and adolescents. She is the author of over 25 empirical articles and book chapters in the area of pediatric sleep.

Betty Pfefferbaum (M.D., University of California, San Francisco, 1972) is Professor and Chief of the Child Section in the Department of Psychiatry and Behavioral Sciences at the University of Oklahoma College of Medicine and Adjunct Professor at the Oklahoma

City University School of Law. She has authored over 100 professional abstracts, articles, and book chapters on medical, psychiatric, and legal issues related to children. Her research interests include deviant behavior, the effects of man-made trauma, and mental health law.

Johannes Rojahn (Ph.D., University of Vienna, 1976) is Professor of Psychology and Psychiatry at The Ohio State University. His research has focused on assessment and treatment of severe behavior disorders and other forms of psychopathology in mental retardation. Currently, Dr. Rojahn is conducting research on emotion recognition by individuals with mental retardation and its relationship to psychopathology.

Eileen P. Ryan (D.O., Chicago College of Osteopathic Medicine, 1984) is Assistant Professor of Clinical Psychiatric Medicine, University of Virginia, School of Medicine and an inpatient child and adolescent psychiatrist at DeJarnette Center in Staunton, Virginia. She was previously Medical Director of the Psychiatric Emergency Department, the Diagnostic and Evaluation Center of the Western Psychiatric Institute and Clinic, University of Pittsburgh. Her clinical interests include suicide and self-mutilation, and affective and psychotic disorders in children and adolescents.

Janet S. St. Lawrence (Ph.D., Nova University, 1980) is Chief of the Behavioral Interventions and Research Branch, National Center for HIV, STD, TB Prevention, Division of STD, at the Centers for Disease Control in Atlanta. Her research interest are in developing and evaluating the effectiveness of interventions in applied community settings to reduce transmission of sexually-transmitted diseases, including HIV-infection, and working with underserved populations. She is currently principal investigator on several NIH grants examining the efficacy of cognitive-behavioral interventions with low-income minority women, substance-dependent adolescents, and prisoners.

Mary J. Sanders (Ph.D., Memphis State University, 1985) is Director of Psychological Services and Clinical Instructor in the Division of Child Psychiatry and Development in the Department of Psychiatry at Stanford University School of Medicine and Behavioral Sciences. Since 1986, she has been at Lucile Salter Packard Children's Hospital at Stanford where she has worked predominantly with children and families dealing with eating disorders. Her other interests include child abuse and family therapy training.

Herbert A. Schreier (M.D., Albert Einstein College of Medicine, 1968) is Chief of Psychiatry at Children's Hospital Oakland in Oakland, California. He trained in child psychiatry at Albert Einstein College of Medicine, and was a Commonwealth Foundation Instructor in the Department of Psychiatry at Harvard Medical School. His current clinical and research interests include community response to disasters, socially inept children, and the genetics and treatment of Tourette's syndrome and bipolar disorders in childhood.

Gregory T. Slomka (Ph.D., University of Pittsburgh, 1986) is Assistant Professor of Psychiatry at Western Psychiatric Institute and Clinic, University of Pittsburgh School of Medicine. His research interests are focused on functional implications of specific developmental disorders with an emphasis on congenital conditions.

Hans Steiner (Dr. med. Univ., University of Vienna, Austria, 1973) is Professor of Psychiatry and Behavioral Sciences at the Stanford University School of Medicine, where he is the Training Director of Child Psychiatry and Child Development and the Chief of Psychiatry at the Lucile Salter Packard Children's Hospital. He is the author of over 100 publications, among them his recent volume *Treating Adolescents*. His research focuses on the development of stress and coping responses in relationship to psychopathology.

H. Patrick Stern (M.D., Case Western Reserve University, 1974) is Associate Professor of Pediatrics and Assistant Professor of Psychiatry and Behavioral Sciences at the University of Arkansas for Medical Sciences. He is the Chief of the Section of Behavioral Pediatrics at Arkansas Children's Hospital. He has authored or co-authored multiple articles on encopresis, and children of divorce. Research interests include encopresis, enuresis, wellness, children's sports, and children of divorce.

Marc J. Tassé (Ph.D., Université du Québec à Montréal, 1994) completed a postdoctoral fellowship at the Nisonger Center UAP at the Ohio State University. He is currently Assistant Professor in the Department of Psychology at the Université du Québec à Montréal. His research interests are in the area of mental retardation/development disabilities. He is currently involved in research in the areas of assessment and intervention of adaptive skills, severe behavior disorders, and the co-occurrence of mental retardation and psychopathology.

Gary Vallano (M.D., University of Pittsburgh, 1985) is Clinical Assistant Professor of Psychiatry at the University of Pittsburgh and is also a private practice child and adolescent psychiatrist with Penn Group Medical Associates in Pittsburgh, PA. His interests have included previous involvement in several research projects on ADHD and he has co-authored several articles and several book chapters in the area of ADHD. Current interests include inpatient and outpatient clinical treatment of children and adolescents in the context of the evolving managed care systems.

Eric F. Wagner (Ph.D., University of Pittsburgh, 1992) is director of the Teen Intervention Center for Psychological Studies at Nova Southeastern University and works in the area of adolescent substance abuse.

C. Eugene Walker (Ph.D., Purdue University, 1965) obtained his B.S. degree, summa cum laude with special honors in psychology at Geneva College in 1960. He completed his M.S. in 1963 and his Ph.D. with a major in clinical psychology and minors in experimental psychology and sociology. He moved to the University of Oklahoma Medical School in 1974 where he was Professor of Psychology, Director of Pediatric Psychology Training, and Co-Chief of Mental Health Services at Children's Hospital of Oklahoma. He is currently Professor Emeritus.

CHAPTER 1

DEVELOPMENTAL ISSUES

Ann M. DiGirolamo
Heather K. Geis
C. Eugene Walker

INTRODUCTION

For researchers and clinicians in the growing fields of pediatric psychology and psychiatry, it is important to integrate information derived from both the clinical and developmental literature. As we place more emphasis on prevention and intervention, knowledge of both normal expectations and behaviors that deviate from the norm is necessary to fully understand the processes involved in clinical problems. Clinicians and researchers often must address factors that may impede or interfere with the normal developmental process (e.g., chronic childhood illness). Knowledge of developmental milestones, normal variations in the developmental process, and when behaviors warrant further attention is crucial to understanding whether these factors are in fact interfering and for providing early intervention.

A growing field in psychology is the discipline of developmental psychopathology. Developmental psychopathology, which emerged in the 1980s, advocates a developmental focus for the study of maladaptive behavior, and has been described as "an integration of the developmental and clinical sciences" (Garmezy, 1993, p. 95). It has further been defined as "the study of the origins and course of individual patterns of behavioral maladaptation, whatever the age of onset, whatever the causes, whatever the transformations in behavioral manifestation, and however complex the course of the developmental pattern may be" (Sroufe & Rutter, 1984, p. 18).

One of the main goals of developmental psychopathology is to examine the time course of clinical problems and to observe the different behavioral changes that occur at different points in development (Attie, Brooks-Gunn, & Petersen, 1990). Knowing what constitutes normative behavior, comparing typical and atypical behavior, and identifying those children "at risk" for clinical problems, along with the factors associated with being "at risk," are all crucial to the understanding of maladaptive behavior and are of prime interest to those in the field of developmental psychopathology (Garmezy, 1993).

In order to fully understand the recent advances in child developmental and clinical research and to effectively work in a pediatric setting, it is critical to be aware of the normal expectations for children of different ages in several areas of development (i.e., physical/motor, cognitive/language, personality/socioemotional). The purpose of this chapter is to give an overview of the various developmental stages, normative behavior at these stages, and "red flags" that may signify the development of maladaptive behavior or developmental delay.

Development has been characterized as a continuous process that begins at the moment of conception (Billingham, 1982; Mussen, 1963). Researchers have proposed that each phase of development has certain characteristic traits, and that growth and changes in behavior usually occur in predictable sequences (Murray & Zentner, 1989; Mussen, 1963). However, despite the patterned and continuous nature of development, the rate of growth tends to be variable. Periods of very rapid physical and psychological growth, often described as "growth spurts," occur during several different developmental phases. Examples include sudden increases in height and weight during early adolescence, and large increases in vocabulary during the preschool years (Mussen, 1963). Furthermore, there may be certain "critical periods" of development, during which certain events assume a major role in influencing the developmental process. For example, feeding experiences are critical during the first year of life, socialization training during the second and third years, and school entrance and peer relationships during the fifth year. Interference with normal development during these periods may result in deficits or delays which are difficult to overcome (Mussen, 1963; Mussen, Conger, & Kagan, 1963).

Developmental delay occurs when a child has not reached specific developmental milestones by a certain age, even after taking into account the great variation that occurs among children. The criterion often used is a discrepancy from the expected rate of development of 25 percent or more (Simeonsson & Sharp, 1992). Drillien and colleagues found that approximately 9 percent to 10 percent of preschool children exhibited some type of developmental delay (Drillien, Pickering, & Drummond, 1988). Simeonsson and Sharp (1992) suggest that 5 percent to 10 percent of children in a typical pediatric practice are developmentally delayed. It should be noted, however, that early identification of these problems is difficult, with most speech impairments, hyperactivity, and emotional disorders not identified before three or four years of age (Palfrey, Singer, Walker, & Butler, 1987). The wide variation in normal development makes it easy to miss subtle findings. Furthermore, reluctance to admit that delay may exist can lead to an overreliance on the explanation of normal variation for certain behaviors, as well as an unwarranted expectation that the child will "grow out of it" (First & Palfrey, 1994).

Several methods of assessment can aid in the early diagnosis of developmental delay and clinical problems. These include a thorough history taking, a physical examination, continuous developmental observations, and more formal assessments when indicated (First & Palfrey, 1994). Risk factors that may become apparent during the history taking include prenatal maternal factors such as chronic illness, the use of drugs or alcohol, or previous miscarriage; perinatal factors such as obstetrical complications, prematurity, or low birth weight; neonatal factors such as seizures, sepsis, meningitis, or hypoxia due to respiratory problems; postnatal factors such as seizures, meningitis, otitis media, poor feeding and growth, or exposure to certain toxins (e.g., lead); factors in the family history such as developmental delay, deafness, blindness, or chromosomal abnormalities; and factors in the social history such as a history of abuse or neglect, financial problems, being a teenage or single parent, and other stressful life events (e.g., divorce) (First & Palfrey, 1994).

Risk factors for developmental delay can also be detected during a physical examination. Several of the risk factors that might be identified include abnormal growth, major congenital anomalies (e.g., spina bifida), neurocutaneous skin lesions (e.g., neurofibromas), abnormal optical or auditory findings, skeletal abnormalities, and neurologic abnormalities (e.g., lack of alertness) (First & Palfrey, 1994). Possible delay and clinical problems can also be identified through developmental observations conducted by both parents and professionals. Awareness of what is normal and what may signify a clinical problem is crucial for the early detection of and intervention for these problems.

The remainder of this chapter will focus on delineating the normal developmental tasks and expectations for children in various stages, as well as outlining certain "red flags" that should alert parents and professionals to possible deficits or developmental delay. This chapter will provide information on the following age groups and stages of development: prenatal development (conception to birth), infancy (birth to 12 months, including the neonatal period), early childhood (12 months to 5 years), middle childhood (6 to 12 years), adolescence (12 to 17 years), and early adulthood (18 to 30 years).

PRENATAL DEVELOPMENT

The main developmental goal of the prenatal period is to attain the level of physical development necessary prior to birth (Billingham, 1982). As mentioned earlier, development begins at conception, after which the cells divide and the newly formed cells assume highly specialized functions, a process called differentiation. The sequence of development during the prenatal period tends to be fairly fixed, with the head, eyes, trunk, arms, legs, genitals, and internal organs developing in a specific order (Billingham, 1982; Mussen, 1963). The upper end of the fetus develops faster than the lower end, with growth beginning at the head and then moving to the hands and feet. Furthermore, growth occurs in the central part of the body first and then moves to the extremities. Growth occurring on one side of the body is paralleled by growth that occurs simultaneously on the opposite side (Murray & Zentner, 1989).

Pregnancy lasts approximately 280 days (9 months) and is divided into three stages of development: germinal, embryonic, and fetal. During the germinal stage (lasting ten days to two weeks after fertilization), rapid cell division occurs, followed by implantation of the organism in the wall of the uterus. The complexity of the organism is also increasing at this time. The embryonic stage, which lasts from two to eight weeks, is characterized by rapid growth and differentiation of the major body organs and systems (Murray & Zentner, 1993). For example, by the fourth week, the embryo is approximately one-fifth of an inch long, with the head clearly visible. By the end of the eighth week, a face, arms, and legs are present, and all the major internal organs have begun to form. The nervous system is developing rapidly at this time as well, with some reflexes appearing during the eighth or ninth week (Baron, 1989). The embryonic stage is the critical period during which the embryo is most vulnerable to harmful prenatal influences, with birth defects occurring during the first three months of pregnancy (Murray & Zentner, 1993).

The final stage, the fetal stage, lasts from eight weeks until birth, and is characterized by growth and refinement of body tissues and organs. For example, hair and nails are evident by the end of the twentieth week. At the end of the twelfth week, the fetus is approximately three inches long and weighs three-fourths of an ounce; by the end of the twentieth week, the fetus is around twelve inches long and weighs close to twelve ounces. The fetus continues to grow rapidly during the last three months, gaining about eight ounces each week (Baron, 1989; Murray & Zentner, 1993).

The brain is also following a general pattern of development during this time, beginning as a neural tube and gradually developing the features of an adult brain. Cortical cell proliferation seems to be complete by the middle of pregnancy, although the cortex still does not look like that of an adult. Cell migration continues to occur, possibly even postnatally, and cortical lamination continues until after the child is born. Myelination, a rough index of cerebral maturation, occurs later than other aspects of cortical development. The primary sensory and motor areas begin to myelinate just before the end of gestation. The frontal and parietal association areas are among the last to myelinate; they begin to myelinate after the child is born and continue until age 15 or older (Kolb & Fantie, 1989).

Several risk factors for developmental complications have been identified during the prenatal period. Prenatal malnutrition has been shown to be associated with low birthweight, a greater risk of premature birth (Stechler & Halton, 1982), and possible immaturity in neuromotor functioning (Bhatia, Katiyar, & Agarwal, 1979). Characteristics of the mother such as age and number of previous pregnancies also can lead to increased risk of complications. For example, pregnancies occurring during adolescence often have been associated with premature birth, infant illness, and higher infant mortality (Dott & Fort, 1975; Murray & Zentner, 1989). Pregnancies occurring after age 35 have been associated with an increased risk of complications in labor and delivery, and problems with the neonate such as prematurity, low birth weight, Down Syndrome, birth defects, and higher rates of infant mortality. Furthermore, risk of complications has been shown to increase with the number of pregnancies, especially if the pregnancies closely follow one another (Murray & Zentner, 1989).

Preterm delivery has been associated with an increased risk for mortality and morbidity, and often requires mother-infant separation and aggressive medical care (Sostek & Magrab, 1992). Complications also may arise from low birth weight, defined as weight at birth less than 5 pounds, 8 ounces, regardless of gestational age (Tomchek & Lane, 1993). For example, studies have linked low birth weight to two-thirds of neonatal deaths, to child abuse, and to mental retardation (Petersen, Zink, & Farmer, 1992; Tomchek & Lane, 1993). Further potential problems include deficits in physical growth, speech and language delays, CNS abnormalities, deficits in intelligence and school performance, health problems, and deficits in motor and visual-motor behavior (Tomchek & Lane, 1993). Low birth weight has been associated with three major risk factors: cigarette smoking during pregnancy, low maternal weight gain, and low prepregnancy weight. Other risk factors for low birth weight include black race, first births, female sex, short maternal stature, maternal low birth weight, maternal illnesses, fetal infections, and several metabolic and genetic disorders (Shiono & Behrman, 1995). Less is known about the causes of preterm delivery, although there is some evidence that pre-term births have been associated with cigarette smoking during pregnancy, prior preterm birth, and low prepregnancy weight (Shiono & Behrman, 1995).

Another risk factor is exposure to teratogenic agents during pregnancy. Teratogenic agents include such substances as radiation, nicotine, caffeine, alcohol, and other drugs (Murray & Zentner, 1989; Sostek & Magrab, 1992). For example, heavy alcohol use during pregnancy has been associated with Fetal Alcohol Syndrome (FAS), which has a prevalence rate of approximately one to two cases per 1,000 live births in the United

States (Clarren & Smith, 1978). FAS is characterized by central nervous system dysfunctions (e.g., retardation, irritability in infancy), growth deficiency, abnormal facial appearance (e.g., thin upper lip, short nose), and several other major or minor defects (e.g., malformations of the eyes, cardiac murmurs) (Behnke & Eyler, 1993). The period when the child is most vulnerable to the effects of teratogens is during the embryonic stage (fourth to twelfth week of pregnancy), during the formation of all the major organs (Sostek & Magrab, 1992). As noted above, cigarette smoking during pregnancy also has been associated with several serious complications, including intrauterine growth retardation, obstetrical complications (Sostek & Magrab, 1992), spontaneous abortion, major congenital abnormalities (Himmelberger, Brown, & Cohen, 1978), and an increased perinatal death rate (Naeye, 1978).

There has been an increase in the use of cocaine among pregnant women over the past several years, with prevalence rates ranging from 8 percent to 17 percent (Matera, Warren, Moomjy, Fink, & Fox, 1990; Sostek & Magrab, 1992). Matera and colleagues found that in a sample from an urban hospital serving lower socioeconomic status women, cocaine use was reported in 10 percent of the population (Matera et al., 1990). The authors also reported that cocaine users were more likely than nonusers to have no prenatal care and to use cigarettes and alcohol. Problems associated with cocaine use during pregnancy include prematurity, poor fetal growth, persistent growth retardation (Sostek & Magrab, 1992), and possible neurological sequelae (Doberczak, Shanzer, Senie, & Kandall, 1988). One study found that cocaine exposure predicted poor verbal reasoning (Griffith, Azuma, & Chasnoff, 1994).

A final risk factor during the prenatal period is the mother's emotional state during pregnancy. Increased stress reactions during pregnancy can affect the fetus in several ways. Stress reactions (e.g., anxiety) can lead to changes in the mother's adrenocortical hormonal system, which in turn may contribute to hyperactivity of the fetus due to the secretion of increased maternal cortisol, which enters the blood, and crosses the placenta to the fetus (Murray & Zentner, 1989). An increase in adrenalin may also divert the mother's blood flow from the uterus to other organs in her body, thereby decreasing the amount of oxygen provided for the fetus (Stechler & Halton, 1982). Increased stress during pregnancy has been shown to be associated with Down Syndrome (Drillien & Wilkinson, 1964), infantile pyloric stenosis (i.e., a tightening of the stomach outlet due to an enlarged muscle; Revill & Dodge, 1978), and behavior problems in children (Stott & Latchford, 1976).

Conflicting evidence exists regarding the role of objective stressful life events in affecting reproductive outcomes (e.g., complications during pregnancy or at birth; deviant infant behavior). Wachs & Weizmann (1992) report that some studies have found a relation between stressful life events and future infant outcomes (e.g., Gorsuch & Key, 1974), while others have not (e.g., Aurelius, Radestad, Nylander, & Zetterstrom, 1987). The authors mention that some studies suggest that it is not the objective life events that are important, but rather more subjective variables such as maternal anxiety during pregnancy, which may influence outcomes such as premature labor (e.g., Omer, Elizur, Barnea, Friedlander, & Palti, 1986). Wachs and Weizmann (1992) further state that some studies have found that social support plays an important role in whether or not stress and psychological states affect reproductive outcomes (e.g., Klaus, Kennell, Robertson, & Sosa, 1986), while other studies have not supported this relationship (e.g., Magni, Rizzardo, & Andreoli, 1986).

INFANCY

Infancy is defined as the first 12 months after birth, with the neonatal period comprising the first four weeks of this period. Some of the major developmental tasks during this time include physiological stability after birth, awareness of what is familiar, a need for affection and response from others, development of new physical changes and motor skills, exploration to gain understanding and control of the physical environment, the use of emotional expression to indicate needs, and the development of preverbal communication (Billingham, 1982). These tasks encompass several different areas of development (e.g., cognitive, physical/motor). Each of these areas will be discussed within the context of the various normal expectations for development and the "red flags" indicating some type of developmental delay or abnormality.

Physical/Motor Development

During the neonatal period, the infant begins to become physiologically independent from the mother. At birth, the average weight for Caucasian males in America is 7.5 pounds, and 7 pounds for Caucasian females. Newborns of African American, Indian, and Oriental descent tend to be somewhat smaller. Shortly after birth, neonates lose up to 10 percent of their bodyweight due to water loss, followed by steady weight gain beginning one to two weeks after birth. An infant's birthweight doubles during the first six months and triples in the first year (Murray & Zentner, 1989; Mussen, 1963).

A baby may be small at birth because it was born too soon, because of impaired fetal growth, or because of some combination of these two factors. When identifying infants with low birthweight, it is important to distinguish between infants who are small due to *preterm delivery*, whose weight is appropriate for their actual gestational age, and infants who are *small for gestational age (SGA)*, with impaired fetal growth and weight below that expected for their age. This distinction facilitates the assessment of possible reasons for the low birthweight and the determination of appropriate interventions. Much more is known about the causes of impaired fetal growth than about the causes of preterm delivery. Furthermore, there is evidence that in developed nations, preterm delivery is more strongly linked to infant mortality. Although there are many possible harmful effects of impaired fetal growth on an infant, the association with infant mortality is not as strong (Paneth, 1995).

Neonates have a well developed sensory system, enabling them to see, hear, smell, and respond to the touch of others. By two weeks, neonates should be able to differentiate between sweet- and sour-tasting substances (Billingham, 1982), with some researchers suggesting that taste may be well developed even before birth (Acredolo & Hake, 1982). Mixed information exists on the development of visual coordination and convergence (e.g., depth-perception), with some authors suggesting that this sense is well established by the seventh or eighth week after birth (Mussen, 1963), and others suggesting that while some degree is probably present at birth, consistency and precision increase greatly over the first six months of age (Acredolo & Hake, 1982; Shalowitz & Gorski, 1990). Auditory development begins in utero, with studies showing that a variety of auditory stimuli will elicit movement and heartrate acceleration before birth (Acredolo & Hake, 1982). At birth, hearing is blurred for the first few days of life because fluid is retained in the middle ear. However, the neonate can respond to voice pitch changes and to sound direction, with differentiation of sounds and perception of their source developing over time (Murray & Zentner, 1989). Studies have shown that neonates are able to detect the presence of odors. For example, Steiner (1974, 1977) demonstrated that neonates will exhibit well-defined facial reflexes (e.g., facial relaxation, initiation of sucking, depression of the corners of the mouth, spitting) to pleasant and aversive odors. Finally, newborns are sensitive to touch, as indicated by reflexes such as an infant turning its head when touched on the cheek (Acredolo & Hake, 1982).

Several different types of reflexes are present during the neonatal period. Consummatory reflexes such as rooting and sucking influence feeding and promote survival of the infant. Avoidant reflexes such as sneezing, blinking, or coughing allow the newborn to avoid potentially harmful stimuli. The neonate exhibits exploratory reflexes when awake and held upright. For example, a visual object held at eye level may elicit a grabbing or reaching reflex from the child. Examples of social reflexes include smiling, quieting in response to touch, and crying in response to painful stimuli. Finally, attentional reflexes include orienting and attending to the surrounding environment (Murray & Zentner, 1989). Nelson (1981 in Billingham, 1982) suggested that there are significant racial differences in the reflexes exhibited by neonates. For example, Asian babies have no stepping reflex and do not struggle when their airway is obstructed. Neonates of African American descent develop motor control faster than neonates of other races.

During infancy (the first 12 months), different parts of the body grow at different rates. As during the neonatal period, the head and upper parts of the body grow at a faster pace than the trunk and the legs, with brain size doubling during the first two years (Mussen, 1963). At about three to four months of age, a neurodevelopmental reorganization occurs, during which rapid qualitative and quantitative changes in both physiology and behavior occur (Billingham, 1982). Girls generally develop more rapidly than boys, although boys usually exhibit a higher activity level. Furthermore, research has shown that African American infants mature faster than Caucasian infants in motor skills and walking, apparently because of genetic factors (Murray & Zentner, 1989). Normative behaviors expected during infancy are listed in Table 1.1. Risk factors indicating possible developmental delay are listed in Table 1.2.

In addition to assessing gross motor functions such as rolling over, sitting, and standing, it is important to assess more subtle and fine motor movements during infancy. For example, First and Palfrey (1994) suggest that the early presence of unilateral handedness in a child who is less than 15 months old may indicate a hemiplegia of the opposite side. Furthermore, Blasco (1991) suggests that the failure of a three-month-old infant to unclench the fist voluntarily may be an indicator of cerebral palsy. A simple way to assess fine motor functioning at early ages is with a set of blocks or cubes. At 24 weeks, the infant should be able to hold one block in his hand and will

Table 1.1. Normative Behavior during Infancy

AGE	NORMAL BEHAVIOR
3 months	Visual and auditory attention (head turns to sound)
	Hands usually open (no grasp reflex)
	Can hold rattle if placed in hand
	Smiling
	Babbling/Vocalizes when spoken to
6 months	Sensory-motor coordination (e.g., reaching and grasping)
	When lying down, can spontaneously lift head
	Can sit supported in chair; can sit on floor with hands forward for support
	Can completely roll over
	Can differentiate between mother/family and strangers
	Babbling with gestures (e.g., "ba," "da")
	Begins to chew
9 months	Crawling
	Can stand holding onto furniture
	Able to pick up a small object between the thumb and forefinger
	Object permanence
	Vocalization and gestures
12 months	Standing; walking with one hand held or without support
	Speaking first words
	Cooperating in games
	Begins to throw objects deliberately on the floor

Sources: Billingham (1982); Illingworth & Kaufman (1984).

Table 1.2. Risk Factors Indicating Possible Developmental Delay or Clinical Problems in the Areas of Physical/Motor, Cognitive, Language, and Socioemotional Development during Infancy

AREA AND AGE	FINDINGS
Gross Motor:	
4 1/2 months	Does not pull up to sit
5 months	Does not roll over
7–8 months	Does not sit without support
9–10 months	Does not stand while holding on
Fine Motor:	
3 1/2 months	Persistence of grasp reflex
4–5 months	Unable to hold rattle
7 months	Unable to hold an object in each hand
10–11 months	Absence of pincer grasp
Cognitive:	
2–3 months	Not alert to mother
6–7 months	Not searching for dropped object
8–9 months	No interest in peek-a-boo
12 months	Does not search for hidden object
Language:	
5–6 months	Not babbling
8–9 months	Not saying "da" or "ba"
10–11 months	Not saying "dada" or "baba"
Socioemotional:	
3 months	Not smiling socially
6–8 months	Not laughing in playful situation
12 months	Hard to console, stiffens when approached

Note. Table adapted from "The Infant or Young Child with Developmental Delay," by L. R. First and J. S. Palfrey, 1994, *New England Journal of Medicine, 330*, p. 480. Copyright 1994 by Massachusetts Medical Society. All rights reserved.

drop it when a second one is offered. At 28 weeks, the infant retains the first cube when the second one is offered and puts all objects in the mouth. At eight months of age (32 to 36 weeks), the infant should be able to bring two blocks together (Illingworth & Kaufman, 1984).

Cognitive and Language Development

Due to the difficulty in directly assessing reasoning abilities in infants and toddlers, First and Palfrey (1994) suggest that the best proxy indicators for true cognitive assessments at this age may be motor and language milestones. Some information does exist, however, on the development of infant cognitive abilities. Although much of the behavior of the young infant is controlled by reflexive acts, there is evidence that the neonate and infant are perceiving the surrounding world and learning from it even during the first few days of life (Petersen, 1982). For example, Fagan (1982; 1984) administered a measure of attention to novel stimuli to infants five to seven

months of age, and found that this measure was fairly predictive of IQ scores at two to seven years of age.

According to the developmental theories of Piaget, the first stage of cognitive development, the sensorimotor period, lasts from birth to approximately 18 months of age, and is characterized by infants gradually learning that there is a relationship between their actions and the external world. Infants begin to know the world through their motor activities and sensory impressions, and to develop a basic understanding of cause and effect. Piaget suggests that infants must accommodate their innate reflexes to variations in the environment, thereby developing schemes that influence their behavior (Baron, 1989; Ginsburg & Opper, 1969). For example, over the first few weeks, infants show increasing efficiency in searching for their mother's nipple during breastfeeding, thus refining their scheme for suckable objects (Petersen, 1982).

According to Piaget, during the first month of life, most behavior is reflexive, with neonates beginning to show more intention, and to develop and coordinate sensorimotor schemes during the next three months of life. When an infant is four to eight months old, he learns to initiate and recognize new experiences, repeat pleasurable ones, and anticipate familiar events. From eight to 12 months, the infant exhibits goal-directed behavior, and begins to be more concerned with events occurring in the outside world, rather than just being self-focused. During this stage, the infant begins to acquire object permanence—the ability to recognize that objects and persons continue to exist even after they are out of sight, and to mentally represent an object, whether or not it is actually present. Finally, the stage from 12 to 18 months consists of active, purposeful, trial-and-error learning, with the infant constantly looking for new ways to interact with the environment and to achieve goals (Dworetzky, 1993; Flavell, Miller, & Miller, 1993). Even when children are as young as one to one and a half years of age, they should begin to show a basic understanding of cause and effect. Evidence of this may be the child throwing a toy down just so a parent can pick it up (First & Palfrey, 1994).

A red flag for possible delays in cognitive development during the infancy stage may come at nine months or later if a child does not exhibit an understanding of object permanence. This becomes even more of a risk factor if object permanence is not present at 12 months. First and Palfrey (1994) suggest that the child who is not able to recognize that a hidden object is still present may not be making the appropriate mental connections. A common way of testing for object permanence involves covering an object and observing the infant as he or she moves the cover to view or obtain the object (Billingham, 1982; First & Palfrey, 1994). See Table 1.2 for additional risk factors indicating possible delays in cognitive development during infancy.

Language development is both guided by and the result of cognitive development. Language acquisition is a function of both innate communication abilities and the child's environment, especially interactions with the mother. Therefore, it is important to assess not only the extent of the child's expressive and receptive language performance, but also the characteristics of the environment in which the child is learning (First & Palfrey, 1994; Molfese, Molfese, & Carrell, 1982). Documenting language skills in the infant by observation may be especially difficult; therefore, obtaining a detailed history of language milestones from the parent is important. First and Palfrey (1994) suggest employing the Early Language Milestone Scale (Coplan, 1983) as a tool to help identify receptive or expressive abnormalities that

may contribute to speech delay. This instrument has shown sensitivity and specificity when employed with children less than three years of age (Coplan & Gleason, 1990; Walker, Gugenheim, Downs, & Northern, 1989).

Language refers to the meaningful use of words, phrases, and gestures to communicate thoughts and feelings. Language acquisition begins with crying, followed by cooing and babbling (incoherent sounds) during the second or third month of life, with the number of babbling sounds reaching a peak at eight months. The development of language begins with these speechlike sounds, followed later by meaningful speech. In the beginning, these sounds are reflexive and not associated with meaning. In fact, there appears to be no difference between the vocalizations of hearing and hearing-impaired infants before six months of age. By two months of age, the child with normal hearing can "take turns" making sounds with the caregiver. After six months, these sounds take on more meaning and become self-rewarding. At all ages, children's receptive language is better than their expressive language. Words are first associated with visual, tactile, and other sensations in the environment. Then, between the ages of nine to 12 months, infants learn to recognize their names, the names of certain objects, and the meaning of the word "no" (Billingham, 1982; Shalowitz & Gorski, 1990). Language continues to develop more fully during the period of early childhood (one to five years of age).

Table 1.2 lists some of the identifiable risk factors for possible delays in language development. It is important to note that delays in cognitive or language development may be a result of innate factors such as mental retardation or neurological deficiency, but could also be a result of deprivation within the environment (Billingham, 1982; Klein, 1991). Both of these possibilities should be examined when any of the risk factors listed in Table 1.2 are identified.

Socioemotional Development

Socioemotional development in the infant can best be understood in the context of social relationships. Different theorists have emphasized different aspects of the social context; however, an emphasis on the relationship between the infant and primary caregiver (e.g., mother) is often a common factor. For example, Freud posited that the first stage of development is the oral stage, prominent during the first 12 months of life. During this stage, the infant responds to hunger and thirst by sucking, swallowing, crying, and oral-tactile stimulation. Infants derive a great deal of pleasure from chewing and sucking behaviors. Tactile stimulation between the mother and infant is considered important during this early age for further social and personality development (Billingham, 1982; Dworetzky, 1993; Hall, 1954).

Erikson (1963) also emphasized the importance of the relationship between the infant and caretaker. Erikson describes the developmental crisis of infancy as one of "trust versus mistrust" (see Table 1.3). Trust is defined as confidence in oneself and in the world to satisfy one's needs. Mistrust, on the other hand, is a sense of not feeling satisfied and of lacking confidence in oneself and in the world. Greenspan (1995) emphasizes the importance of the caregiver's sensitivity to the infant's behavioral cues and the goodness of fit between the caregiving style and the infant's level of socioemotional development. He suggests that examples of appropriate caregiving include the caregiver comforting the infant, especially when the infant is upset; finding appropriate levels of stimulation to interest the infant in the world; engaging the infant pleasurably in a relationship (e.g., vocalizing, gentle touching) rather than being preoccupied or withdrawn; reading and responding to the child's different emotional signals and needs; and encouraging the infant to move forward in development rather than overprotecting the child (Greenspan, 1995).

At four months of age, the child should be responding to the environment by brightening to sights and sounds, and by responding to others with some vocalization or a smile. The infant should calm down when comforted and enjoy being cuddled and held firmly (Greenspan, 1991). After six months, several social developments occur. The child appears to experience a sense of self by the end of the first year as a result of a series of conflicts between the infant and the caretaker (Hodapp & Mueller, 1982). Conflicts may occur when

an infant's wish is in conflict with what the parent allows. Children feel this conflict within, thereby separating themselves from their parents. Attachment becomes apparent somewhere between the sixth and eighth month, when the infant forms a strong affectional bond with the primary caretaker, often the mother. Attachment behaviors include staying close to the parent and becoming distressed at the parent's absence (Hodapp & Mueller, 1982; Schaffer & Emerson, 1964). Some studies indicate that the hours immediately after birth are important to the development of attachment feelings in the parents (Klaus & Kennell, 1976; 1982). Kennell and colleagues suggest that this early contact is associated with more interest in the child by parents, less child abuse, increased communication between mother and child, decreased crying, and more weight gain (Kennell, Voos, & Klaus, 1979). Early separation of the mother and infant due to hospitalization may interfere with early attachment and make the initial relationship more difficult (Klaus & Kennell, 1982).

At eight months, the infant should be initiating simple interactions (e.g., looking to the caregiver to respond to a facial expression), responding to gestures with gestures, initiating comforting behavior, responding to simple games like peek-a-boo with pleasure, and showing special interest in and cautiousness toward new people. By one year of age, the child should be initiating complex interactions (e.g., rolling a ball back and forth), using complex behavior to establish closeness (e.g., reaching to be picked up), responding to limits set by the parent's voice or gesture, and trying different ways to make the parent react (Greenspan, 1991).

Delay or problems in socioemotional development may be difficult to distinguish from the behavioral struggles which occur for most young children. However, the quantity, severity, nature, and duration of the episodes, as well as any sudden changes in behavior, are key factors in determining whether the difficulties warrant further attention (Phillips, Sarles, & Friedman, 1992). Examples of infant behaviors that should be referred for psychological or behavioral testing include refusal to eat, rumination (repeated regurgitation and rechewing of food), pica (eating substances that are not usually eaten such as paint or dirt), excessive or disrupted sleep, extreme difficulty in separating, overexcitability, anxiety, and apathy (Thompson, 1990). Other infant risk factors are listed in Table 1.2.

Infants with chronic medical conditions may be at risk for social and psychological problems due to the loss of stimulation from prolonged hospitalization, restricted physical activity, and delayed or interrupted parent-child attachment (Sostek & Magrab, 1992). Parents, siblings,

Table 1.3. Erik Erikson's Stages of Development for Infancy through Young Adulthood

AGE/DEVELOPMENTAL PERIOD	STAGE OR CRISIS
First Year/Infancy	Trust vs. Mistrust
Second Year/Toddlerhood	Autonomy vs. Shame and Doubt
Third Through Fifth Years/ Preschool	Initiative vs. Guilt
Sixth Year Through Puberty/ Middle Childhood	Industry vs. Inferiority
Adolescence	Identity vs. Role Confusion
Early Adulthood	Intimacy vs. Isolation

Sources: Gardner (1982); Noam, Higgins, & Goethals (1982).

and extended family can greatly influence how children adjust to having a chronic illness. When possible, regular monitoring of the emotional and social adaptation of the child, parents, and siblings can aid in the early identification of problems and in making appropriate referrals when indicated (Perrin, 1995).

EARLY CHILDHOOD

Early childhood comprises the years between infancy and elementary school, from one to five years of age. Children, ages two and three, are often called toddlers; children, ages four and five are often referred to as preschoolers. As in the infancy stage, children during the early childhood stage are continuing to experience many changes in the areas of physical, cognitive, language, and psychosocial development. Again, both the normal expectations for development in these areas, as well as "red flags" to which one should pay attention will be discussed below.

Physical Development

The rate of physical growth during early childhood is slower than that occurring during infancy, but occurs in the same orderly manner. Between the first and second years, the average height increase is four to five inches, and the average weight gain is five pounds. The average two-year-old is approximately 32 to 33 inches tall and weighs about 26 to 28 pounds. Birth weight has quadrupled by this time. By age five, the average child is about 43 to 52 inches tall and weighs from 40 to 50 pounds. Growth of the upper body slows down (e.g., head), while growth of the trunk and limbs continues, with the result being that the child begins to acquire the body proportions of an adult. The "chubby toddler" turns into a much taller and thinner child (Murray & Zentner, 1989; Mussen, 1963).

Gross and fine motor skills also continue to emerge during these years. The emergence of these skills is made possible by the maturation of the neuromuscular system and the cortical and subcortical regions of the brain (Billingham, 1982). Billingham (1982) provides a quote from Freiberg (1979, p. 141) which nicely demonstrates the expectations for motor development during the early childhood years:

At age two, children walk upstairs holding onto a hand, rail, or wall. They place both feet on each step before proceeding to the next. By age three, they begin to alternate their feet, one to a step. By age four,

they have usually ceased to hold on to anything and alternate steps going both down and up. By age five, they may well run up the stairs. For many two-year-olds, holding a glass of liquid and drinking without spilling is a feat. By age three, children can drink well and feed themselves complete meals with very little assistance. At age three, children undress (quite successfully) and attempt to dress (less successfully). By age five, children dress without assistance, including washing faces, hands, and brushing teeth. Five-year-olds may even be able to tie the laces of their shoes in neat bows. Three-year-olds learn to jump over or off objects and maintain their balance. Five-year-olds learn to jump rope in rhythm.

Fine motor skills can also be measured through play with blocks or cubes. By 18 months, a child may build a short tower of about three cubes, and should be able to build a tower of six or seven cubes by age two. A three-year-old should be able to make a tower of about nine cubes, and a four-year-old should be able to build a tower of ten cubes. A five-year-old child should be able to build a complex building or staircase with blocks or cubes (First & Palfrey, 1994; Illingworth & Kaufman, 1984). "Red flags" indicating possible developmental delay in the areas of gross and fine motor development are listed in Table 1.4.

Cognitive and Language Development

During early childhood, children develop the cognitive skills that enable them to communicate better and participate more in symbolic thinking than during the infancy years. According to Piaget, the preoperational stage characterizes this period, and lasts from approximately 18 months to seven years of age. In contrast to the sensorimotor period when all thinking revolves around objects that are present in the immediate environment, children during the preoperational stage begin to use words and symbols to represent objects that are not immediately present (Baron, 1989; Ginsburg & Opper, 1969). Development of these symbolic-representational skills is illustrated by an explosive increase in language, the ability to use numbers to represent quantities, the acquisition of drawing skills, and the ability to engage in pretend play (Flavell et al., 1993). Flavell and colleagues also suggest that the cognitive systems of young children are not as different from those of older children as was once believed. They posit that young children are thinking in the same manner as older children just not as often, fully, or consistently.

Table 1.4. Risk Factors Indicating Possible Developmental Delay or Clinical Problems in the Areas of Physical/Motor, Cognitive, Language, and Socioemotional Development during Early Childhood

AREA AND AGE	FINDINGS
Gross Motor:	
15 months	Not walking
2 years	Not climbing up or down stairs
2 1/2 years	Not jumping with both feet
3 years	Unable to stand on one foot momentarily
4 years	Not hopping
5 years	Unable to walk a straight line back and forth or balance on one foot for 5 to 10 seconds
Fine Motor:	
15 months	Unable to put in or take out
20 months	Unable to remove socks or gloves by self
2 years	Unable to stack 5 blocks; not scribbling
2 1/2 years	Not turning a single page of a book
3 years	Unable to stack 8 blocks or draw a straight line
4 years	Unable to stack 10 blocks or copy a circle
4 1/2 years	Unable to copy a square
5 years	Unable to build a staircase of blocks or copy a cross
Cognitive:	
15–18 months	No interest in cause-and-effect games
2 years	Does not categorize similarities (e.g., animals vs. vehicles)
3 years	Does not know own full name
4 years	Cannot pick shorter or longer of two lines
4 1/2 years	Cannot count sequentially
5 years	Does not know colors or any letters
5 1/2 years	Does not know own birthday or address
Language:	
18 months	Has < 3 words with meaning
2 years	No two-word phrases or repetition of phrases
2 1/2 years	Not using at least one personal pronoun
3 1/2 years	Speech only half-understandable
4 years	Does not understand prepositions
5 years	Not using proper syntax in short sentences
Socioemotional:	
2 years	Kicks, bites, and screams easily and without provocation
	Rocks back and forth in crib
	No eye contact or engagement with other children or adults
3–5 years	In constant motion
	Resists discipline
	Does not play with other children

Note. Table adapted from "The Infant or Young Child with Developmental Delay," by L. R. First and J. S. Palfrey, 1994, *New England Journal of Medicine, 330*, p. 480. Copyright 1994 by Massachusetts Medical Society. All rights reserved. Adapted with permission.

Memory also continues to develop during this time. Recognition memory is well developed during early childhood, and the basic processing functions and storing capacity of memory are in place (Paris & Lindauer, 1982). Flavell and colleagues suggest that children's memory capacity, ability to use strategies, and knowledge all have a reciprocal relationship. For example, as children become older, they develop strategies and knowledge that enable them to expand their memory capacities (Flavell et al., 1993).

During early childhood, children often are unable to distinguish between their own point of view and someone else's point of view, a concept known as poor perspective taking or "egocentrism." They automatically attribute their own perspective to others (Flavell et al., 1993). Children also experience "magical thinking"; they think that objects are living and that things happen for a reason, and they exhibit little belief in accidents or coincidences (Billingham, 1982).

Children's cognitive development can also affect their conceptualization and understanding of illness. Bibace and Walsh (1980) described several stages of illness conceptualization that resemble Piaget's stages of cognitive development. During the early childhood years (ages 2 to 7), children develop "prelogical" explanations of illness. "Phenomenism" is the most developmentally immature explanation; it describes the cause of illness as an external concrete phenomenon that can occur simultaneously with the illness, but which is spatially and/or temporally remote. Children do not see their own actions as related to the cause of an illness. For example, a child in this stage may attribute the cause of a cold to the sun or the wind.

"Contagion" is the most common explanation offered by more mature children in the "prelogical" stage. Children attribute the cause of an illness to objects or people that are proximate to, but not touching the child. For example, they may say that they can get a cold when someone else gets near them. The link between the cause and the illness is due to mere proximity or to magic. Children in this stage may also perceive that they contracted an illness because of something they did that was idiosyncratic or unrelated to the illness (Bibace & Walsh, 1980; Eiser, 1985; Varni, 1983).

Early childhood is also a critical period for language development. Therefore, it is very important that the clinician be aware of normal expectations and be alert to problems in this area. It should be noted, however, that there is considerable variation in the rate and form of language development among children (Klein, 1991; Whitehurst, 1982). For example, many children begin to speak by 15 months, although others may wait until after two years (Billingham, 1982). Little evidence exists that suggests this variation has implications for adult language skill, if a child is normal in other areas (Whitehurst, 1982). Evidence exists for the influences of both innate processes and environmental stimuli on the development of language in the child. Klein (1991) suggests that the child's language environment, temperament, and cognitive potential all play a role in the progression of language development.

Despite the individual variation, some guidelines do exist for the development of both receptive and expressive language. As noted in an earlier section, children during infancy begin by babbling and imitating certain sounds. During this time, infants are also responding differently to some sounds and understanding a few words (e.g., obeys when hears the word "no") (Brocken, 1981 in Billingham, 1982; Gardner & Winner, 1982). At around one to one and a half years of age, children begin to utter single words, called holophrases (e.g., "ball"), which may contain a variety of meanings (Gardner & Winner, 1982; Whitehurst, 1982). Vocabulary size tends to be approximately 10 to 100 words, and children are able to attend to sounds in another room, point to a body part when named, and understand simple sentences (Brocken, 1981).

Between one and a half and two and a half years of age, children begin to emit two-word utterances called duos that reflect the child's sensorimotor understanding of the world. These duos represent some basic semantic relationships such as recurrence (e.g., "More ball"), nonexistence (e.g., "All gone ball"), and possession (e.g., "My ball") (Gardner & Winner, 1982; Whitehurst, 1982). By age two and a half, vocabulary size is between 200 to 400 words, children are able to refer to themselves by name, and there is some use of future tenses and plurals. In terms of receptive language, children obey simple commands, listen to brief picture stories, and respond to different forms of personal pronouns (Brocken, 1981).

From two and a half to three years of age, vocabulary size is between 400 to 850 words, and children begin to utter grammatical morphemes such as locative prepositions (e.g., "Ball in box"), plurals, possessives, and past tense (Brocken, 1981; Whitehurst, 1982). Children listen to stories or the television for approximately 15 to 20 minutes, and can understand direct versus indirect objects and negative word forms (Brocken, 1981). As children get older and more developed in their language, they may make more errors. For example, three-year-olds make more errors than two-year-olds. Although this does not seem like improvement, in reality, these errors signify a greater understanding of the underlying syntactic rules (Gardner & Winner, 1982).

Between the ages of three and four, vocabulary size is approximately 850 to 1,500 words, the child is using three-word sentences, and speech is about 90 percent intelligible (Brocken, 1981). Children begin using auxiliary verbs (e.g., "I am walking"), negative particles (e.g., "I didn't do it"), "Yes/No" questions, questions using words such as "what," "where," "why," and "how," and sentence clauses (Thompson, 1990; Whitehurst, 1982). In terms of receptive language development, children are able to carry out two commands (Brocken, 1981). Finally, by five years of age, vocabulary should be approximately 1,500 to 2,000 words, and the child should be using four-word sentences and complex sentences such as the conjunction of two sentences (e.g., "You think I can, but I can't"), be able to relate a long story accurately, and be using grammatical patterns similar to those of adults (Brocken, 1981; Thompson, 1990; Whitehurst, 1982). Children at this age can carry out three commands, understand different tenses, and acquire information from watching a children's program (Brocken, 1981).

As noted earlier, some variation is expected in language development. However, "red flags" do exist that signal the need for further evaluation of possible developmental delays. Clinicians may want to have a child imitate chewing movements, tongue thrusting, and repetition of syllables to identify any oral motor problems in phonation and expression (First & Palfrey, 1994). Brocken (1981) lists a number of age-related behaviors that signal the need for further evaluation. At age two, delay may exist if the child has not said a first word, if jargon continues, or if the child begins talking and then stops. At age three, a child should be evaluated if not using at least two-word combinations. Warning signs at age four include speech that is largely unintelligible, and at age five, sentence structure that is noticeably faulty.

A list of some of the risk factors for cognitive and language delays during early childhood can be found in Table 1.4. If some of these risk factors are present, more formal assessment of the child's cognitive and language abilities would be advised. It should be noted that children who are experiencing a physical illness and are often hospitalized, or children experiencing some other type of chronic outside stressor may perform more poorly on certain cognitive tasks (Gordon, 1981 in Billingham, 1982).

Socioemotional Development

During early childhood, social and emotional development occur in the context of interactions with family and with same-age peers. As mentioned in the section on infancy, different theorists tend to emphasize different aspects of development in this area. Freud focused on what he called the "anal stage" for toddlers and the "oedipal complex" during the preschool years (Hall, 1954). During the anal stage, children learn that they can control social interactions, make choices, and disobey what parents ask them to do. A major task during this period, according to Freud, is toilet training. With development of the oedipal complex, children become attached to the parent of the opposite sex and competitive with the parent of the same sex, continuing to develop notions of their sexual identity (Hall, 1954).

Erikson (1963), on the other hand, proposes that the toddler is involved in the conflict of "autonomy versus shame and doubt," and that the preschooler faces the issue of "initiative versus guilt" (see Table 1.3). According to Erikson, the toddler is mainly learning how to exercise choice and self-restraint, and is developing a sense of self-control. If these tasks are not achieved, then the child experiences shame and doubt (Erikson, 1963). Both Erikson and Freud emphasize the achievement of increased independence and competence during the toddler period. The preschool period involves contact with other people outside the family and emphasizes the development of sexual identity, superego, and relationships with peers. The preschooler attempts to develop a sense of purpose, to initiate activities, and to feel a sense of accomplishment. Children begin to reflect on and plan their behavior, and are more aware of the values and judgments of those around them (Billingham, 1982; Erikson, 1963).

Play tends to be an integral part of socioemotional development during early childhood. Toddlers tend to play independently with different toys, and often engage in conflictual behavior when interacting with one another. They begin to show intentional planning and exploration in their interactions and their play (e.g., finding their mother to play with them), and to engage in pretend play. Preschoolers become more involved with a play group, in which they develop an awareness of rules, social relationships, and traits or characteristics that are liked or disliked. They may compete with one another for an adult's attention (Billingham, 1982; Greenspan, 1991). Through play with peers and siblings, children are able to develop and practice social skills, and learn the skills necessary to adapt to their environment.

Greenspan (1991; 1995) provides some guidelines for socioemotional development during the early childhood years. At 18 months, the toddler should be communicating needs and feelings in gestures or words, balancing a desire for independence and closeness, recovering from being angry or upset within 15 minutes,

and using role playing as part of their play (e.g., washing dishes in a play sink). From two to two and a half years of age, the child uses words or gestures to express wants (e.g., to get someone to play with him), uses simple repetitive play to indicate interest in closeness, communicates anger with a gesture or a word, and recovers from anger after 10 minutes. From three to three and a half years of age, the child begins to know what is real and not real (e.g., that cartoons are not real), plays with another person and some toys to act out pretend dramas (e.g., nurturing, exploration, and aggression), realizes that behavior can be related to consequences, and interacts appropriately with peers and adults.

As early as age two, children begin to express their sexual awareness and to develop a sexual identity. This sexual awareness is coupled with information they receive from others about society's concept of gender (e.g., dolls given as a gift to girls and toy cars as a gift to boys), as well as imitation and observation of parents' behavior (Billingham, 1982). Maccoby and Jacklin (1974) suggest that there is a great deal of controversy over what constitutes valid differences between boys and girls. They provide a list of some of the most well-established differences among preschool children, as well as some of the unfounded beliefs about sex differences. In the area of social and play behavior, the following differences have been found: boys engage in more "gross motor" activity and more rough-and-tumble play; girls tend to be more obedient to adults, but not to peers; boys interact more positively with same-age peers; boys receive more pressure against behaving in a sex-inappropriate manner; boys receive more punishment than girls, but also receive more task-related praise and encouragement; and boys and girls prefer toys and activities that adults encourage as appropriate for their sex. In the area of emotional development, the following differences have been found: boys tend to have more negative outbursts in response to frustration than girls, with the frequency of these outbursts declining more quickly in girls than in boys; and girls may become afraid more quickly than boys in response to certain objects. Several of the unfounded differences between boys and girls in these areas include: girls being more "social" than boys; girls being more suggestible; girls having lower self-esteem; and girls lacking achievement motivation.

As with the other areas of development, there are some "red flags" in socioemotional development that merit our attention. Some problems are inevitable and do not represent the need for evaluation. For example, during the early years, it may be difficult to distinguish attentional difficulties and hyperactive behavior from normal rambunctious behavior. However, if there is a history of overactivity, impulsiveness, and oversensitivity to external stimuli (i.e., distractibility), then an evaluation for attention deficit-hyperactivity disorder may be warranted (Palfrey, Levine, Oberklaid, Lerner, & Aufseeser, 1981). Sleep problems such as refusing to go to bed and waking up in the middle of the night are common among two- to three-year-olds, as are fears among preschool children. However, if the problems become so severe that they are interfering with other areas of development, are exhausting for parents, or persist for a long period of time, then professional intervention may be necessary (Gordon, Schroeder, & Hawk, 1992). Signs of extreme aggressiveness or fearfulness, as well as persistent elimination or defecation problems not due to a physical disorder, should also be referred for further psychological or behavioral testing (Thompson, 1990). A list of possible risk factors for psychosocial problems warranting further attention can be found in Table 1.4.

MIDDLE CHILDHOOD

"Perhaps we have exaggerated the perturbation of adolescence and also the steadiness and stability of childhood. More goes on than frankly meets the eye between five and teens . . ." (Gesell & Ilg, 1946, p. 13).

The developmental stage from ages 6 to 12 has had many labels. It was called "latency" by Freud because he thought sexual issues were fairly dormant during this time (Freud, 1905). Similarly, Benson and Harrison (1991) describe this stage as "The Eye of the Hurricane." There is variation in the age range of this stage, illustrated by Shapiro and Perry's (1976) "Latency Revisited: The Age 7 Plus or Minus 1." Other descriptive labels include "school-age child," "grade school child," "childhood," and "late childhood."

Physical Development

Physical growth is generally recognized to be slow and steady in middle childhood, which contrasts with the dramatic cognitive changes associated with this developmental period (Benson & Harrison, 1991). Motor acquisitions include increased hand-eye coordination, resulting in such accomplishments as advanced throwing. Children at this stage also are able to stand on each foot alternately with their eyes closed, and to walk a line backwards, heel-to-toe (Lowery, 1986). Sense of body position and gross motor function develop to the point that participation in organized sports is possible (Levine, 1992a).

Cognitive Development

A hallmark of middle childhood is expanded cognitive ability. Attention, persistence, and goal-directedness improve to the point that it becomes possible for the child to participate in formal schooling. Related skills such as the ability to store, retain, and retrieve new information expand as well (Levine, 1992a).

Shapiro and Perry (1976) reviewed changes occurring within the central nervous system during this period. They considered these changes to be related to the above-mentioned capabilities. There are numerous changes in the microscopic structure of the frontal lobes, especially cell differentiation. Coyle and Harris (1987) discussed different maturation rates in rat neurotransmitter systems. It is possible that, in humans, expanded cognitive abilities could be related to maturation of neurotransmitter systems, although this research has not yet been accomplished. For example, maturation of dopaminergic pathways could be related to the increased attentional abilities attained in this period (Combrinck-Graham, 1991).

Piaget described the cognitive achievements of this stage as concrete operations, attained throughout the school-age period, and different than preoperational logic (Combrinck-Graham, 1991). A child with concrete operational skills is able to observe accurately, experiment, form complex classes, and make linked statements (Richmond, 1970). These abilities differ from the intuitive, magical, and idiosyncratic logic of the preoperational period. Limitations of the concrete operational period include the inability to interrelate classifications and the inability to think abstractly.

Piaget (1972) described operations as "some kind of action (the act of combining individuals or numeric units, displacing them, etc.) whose origin is always perceptual, intuitive (representational), or motoric" (p. 275).

The three concrete logical operations are listed below:

Composition	Red triangles + Blue triangles = Triangles	Combining elements leads to another class
Associativity	$A + B + C = C + B + A$	Combinations made in different orders have the same result

Reversibility	A < B	Being able to
	B < C	mentally
	A < C	return to an
		earlier
		point in the
		process

(Combrinck-Graham, 1991)

As noted earlier, the degree of cognitive development also can influence children's understanding of health and illness. During the stage of concrete logical reasoning, children are able to clearly distinguish between what is internal and external to the self (Varni, 1983). Bibace and Walsh (1980) described two explanations of illness causality common for children in this developmental stage. "Contamination" characterizes the explanations of the younger children in this stage. Illness causality is explained by the child's body coming into contact with a person or object external to the child which the child views as "harmful" or "bad." Children also believe they can become ill by physically engaging in a "harmful or bad action," and thus becoming contaminated. Curing the illness is described in terms of the child avoiding contact with the "bad" object or person, or by stopping the "harmful activity" (Bibace & Walsh, 1980; Varni, 1983). At this stage, children may be inclined to believe that non-contagious illnesses also are catching (Eiser, 1985).

The older children in the concrete logical stage tend to believe that illness is located inside the body, though the cause is external (usually a person or object). The illness comes inside the body through swallowing or inhaling a contaminant or harmful object, a process known as "internalization." The illness is still usually described in very vague and nonspecific terms. The explanation for curing an illness at this stage involves taking in an external agent that will affect the body in a positive way, such as taking medicine (Bibace & Walsh, 1980; Varni, 1983).

Socioemotional Development

Greenspan (1993) described three distinct periods in the emotional development of the school-age child. "The World is my Oyster" (ages 4½ to 7) is characterized by feelings of omnipotence, wonder, and a rich fantasy world. The next stage, "The World is Other Kids," is dominated by increasing identification with the peer group. Finally, the third stage, "The World Inside Me," occurs between ages 10 and 12, with the child developing a more consistent sense of self.

Table 1.5. Middle Childhood "Red Flags"

RED FLAGS

- Failing grades (or a dramatic drop in grades)
- Excessive fighting with peers
- Frequently in the principal's office
- Cries easily
- Tired much of the time
- No friends
- Temper outbursts
- Poor school attendance/school refusal
- Frequent complaints of illness
- Excessive preoccupation with fantasy world
- Strange questions
- Suicide attempts or suicidal ideation

Erikson (1963) noted several socioemotional changes during middle childhood, including children pulling away from their nuclear families, increasing identification with peer groups, and entrance into society. He describes the major struggle of this period as "industry versus inferiority." Industry is manifested as increased productivity, with inferiority being the result of repeated failures. Children of this age tend to associate with same sex-peers, with interest in opposite-sex peers beginning in early adolescence (Buhrmester & Furman, 1987).

Since Harry Stack Sullivan (1953) described middle childhood as the first opportunity society has to correct the influence of the family, perhaps it is not surprising that school-age children constitute a large proportion of cases referred and treated in mental health agencies (Furman, 1991). Characteristic issues include school achievement problems, peer relationship problems, and school phobias and homesickness. When the school-age child presents with problems, the evaluation should include educational and peer experiences, as well as intrapsychic and family factors. Equally essential is an evaluation of the child's cognitive level. "Red flags" signifying possible problems during middle childhood are listed in Table 1.5.

ADOLESCENCE

There has been a great deal of research on adolescence in recent years. Earlier in this century, adolescence was viewed as a tumultuous, problematic period, with psychopathology seen as the norm. More recently, Offer and Boxer (1991) reported that the majority (80 percent) of adolescents negotiate this period smoothly. The onset of adolescence is heralded by puberty, the period of rapid physical change that results in reproductive maturity. Adolescence ends when the identity is crystallized, and the youth is beginning to function more apart from the family of origin (Felice, 1992).

Adolescence is often divided into three substages. Early adolescence spans the years from approximately 12 to 14, and is characterized by much physical change (i.e., puberty). Mood swings are often present, presumably related to the vast physical changes (Golombek & Marton, 1992). Middle adolescence (15 to 16) seems to be a quieter time, bridging the period from puberty to late adolescence (Golombek & Marton, 1992). Late adolescence (17 to 19) is another change-filled period, as the adolescent is becoming more independent from the original family, and taking on more adult responsibilities. Adult forms of mental illness, such as schizophrenia and affective disorders, frequently appear for the first time during late adolescence (Golombek & Marton, 1992).

Physical Development

In contrast to the steady, gradual body changes of middle childhood, in adolescence the body shape changes from that of a child to that of an adult. In addition to rapid increases in body size, reproductive organs mature, and secondary sexual characteristics emerge. These adolescent changes are influenced by hormonal changes in the body (Tanner, 1971).

Pediatrician J. Tanner divided the physical changes of puberty into five stages (Marshall & Tanner, 1969). Stage one consists of the prepubescent form. Stage two consists of initial development (breast bud formation in the girl, and enlargement of the scrotum and testes in the boy). Stages three and four are intermediary stages, with stage five being complete maturation. There is considerable interindividual variation in the total time span encompassed during puberty, as well as the time of onset of puberty. Nottelmann and colleagues found that for boys, adolescent adjustment problems were more common for the later maturers. These authors found no real effect for girls (Nottelmann et al., 1987). However, others have suggested that early pubertal development may be disadvantageous for girls (Susman et al., 1985). Simmons and colleagues speculated that pubertal status was a problem when it placed the individual in a different or deviant position from peers (Simmons, Blyth, & McKinney, 1983).

Reproductive maturation includes an increase in testicular and penile size, and spermatogenesis in boys (Brook, 1981). Girls experience menarche, and later, ovulation. Anovulatory cycles are generally the rule in girls for approximately two years after menarche, but there are some exceptions (Brook, 1981). In addition, there is an increase in sexual urges concomitant with the maturation of the reproductive capacity. There is curiosity about sexual matters, masturbation, and sexual activity. A large percentage of teenagers become sexually active before age 19 (Hayes, 1987).

The secondary sex characteristics, anatomical features that differentiate between the sexes but do not have a direct reproductive function, emerge during this period as well (Offer & Boxer, 1991). Boys develop body and facial hair, and the voice changes. Girls develop broader hips, with fatty deposits in the breasts, hips, buttocks, and thighs. Boys develop a greater increase in muscle size and strength than girls (Tanner, 1971).

The adolescent growth spurt consists of a doubling in the growth velocity, which occurs for approximately one year (Tanner, 1971). There is an additional gain in height of 28 centimeters in boys and 25 centimeters in girls (Brook, 1981). Growth continues until epiphyseal closure, when the ends of the bones fuse with the bone shafts (Dubas & Peterson, 1993). Therefore, girls' total height will be less than that of boys, perhaps due to the earlier onset of puberty (Brook, 1981).

The adolescent must then integrate these vast morphological changes into a realistic body image. By-products of this process include children spending much time preening before mirrors, or feeling that all people are focusing on them (Felice, 1992).

Cognitive Development

Cognitive functioning in adolescence is characterized by the attainment of abstraction ability. Piaget called this stage formal operations. The adolescent becomes able to formulate and test hypotheses without actually manipulating concrete objects (Phillips, 1981). Thus, the youth is no longer bound by real-world possibilities. He can imagine what events might occur under imagined conditions. Metaphor, irony, satire, proverbs, parables, and analogies can now be understood (Phillips, 1981). However, not all individuals attain this level of cognitive achievement (Keating & Clark, 1980).

As with earlier stages of cognitive development, formal-logical thinking influences the way that adolescents and young adults conceptualize illness causality. Younger adolescents may rely on the "physiologic" explanation, the belief that the cause of the illness is triggered by external events, but actually lies in specific internal physiologic structures and functions which malfunction. The teenager begins to acknowledge individual vulnerability to illness and understands that mere exposure to illness does not cause illness in itself (Bibace & Walsh, 1980; Eiser, 1985; Varni, 1983). Older and more cognitively mature adolescents and young adults become aware of psychological causes of illness and of the relationship between stress and physical illness. These "psychophysiologic" explanations describe illness in terms of internal physiological processes, but also take into account that a person's thoughts and feelings can affect the way the body functions. Individuals at this stage also perceive themselves as having a reasonable amount of control over the onset and cure of an illness, and are better able to understand the long-term benefits of treatment (Bibace & Walsh, 1980; Eiser, 1985; Varni, 1983).

Socioemotional Development

Erik Erikson described the basic task during adolescence as the formation of the identity, with role confusion being the result if this task is not accomplished (Erikson, 1963). Ideally, the formed identity would be sex-appropriate and ego-syntonic (see Table 1.3).

Necessary for the formation of an identity is separation from one's parents. Blos (1967) describes adolescence as a second individuation process. Prior to adolescence, children identify strongly with their families, and look to one or both parents as their primary role model (Felice, 1992). During adolescence, teenagers may become adamantly opposed to parental value systems, in order to separate. They develop strong attachments to the peer group, or other adults outside of the family (Felice, 1992). Sometimes, the teenager accomplishes this by developing a "crush" on an adult, such as a rock star or teen idol (Felice, 1992).

In addition to the establishment of an identity, adolescents are also developing a sense of morality. Kohlberg and Gilligan (1972) described levels in the formation of morality. The level of morality associated with adolescence is called postconventional morality. Postconventional morality includes two stages, the first of which involves an emphasis on values agreed upon by society (including individual rights and rules for consensus). The second stage emphasizes values determined both by one's conscience and universal principles. Autonomous moral principles and a sense of universal justice are beginning to develop during this time, with youth ultimately moving toward a consistent value system (Dworetzky, 1993; Kohlberg & Gilligan, 1972).

As described earlier, most adolescents negotiate this stage without development of overt psychopathology; however there are many serious problems that can occur. Violence is a leading public health problem. During 1985–1991, annual homicide rates for males increased 154 percent, a dramatic change from the pattern during 1963–1984 (U.S. Department of Health and Human Services, 1994). Hutson, Anglin, and Pratts (1994) described characteristics of drive-by shooting victims in Los Angeles, and found that the majority of drive-by shootings occurred in areas with the most violent street gangs. Many of the child and adolescent victims were gang members. In addition, 10 percent to 20 percent of inner-city children in Los Angeles have witnessed a homicide (Groves, Zuckerman, Marans, & Cohen, 1993), and may suffer psychological sequelae such as post-traumatic stress disorder.

Other serious problems surface during the adolescent period. Teen pregnancy occurs, and is often linked to other psychiatric disorders (Kovacs, Krol, & Voti, 1994). Suicidal behavior is also common. Research findings have yielded various profiles of these youth. For example, Shaffer described three types of suicide victims: depressed, delinquent, and mixed depressed and delinquent (Shaffer, 1974). In general, however, adolescents expressing suicidal ideation or exhibiting suicidal behavior form a heterogeneous group. Drug use, AIDS, and other sexually transmitted diseases are additional serious problems of this age group. See Table 1.6 for a list of other possible "red flags" indicating a need for further evaluation.

While it is true that dangers lurk for the youth of today, nevertheless during adolescence many wonderful capabilities emerge that were not even possible in earlier developmental stages. An adult body is formed, opening up the possibility of adult gratifications, parenthood, and future generations. More advanced cognitive abilities are attained, leading to possibilities limited only by one's imagination. A new identity is formed—shaped by, but no longer dependent upon, previous generations.

EARLY ADULTHOOD

It becomes difficult to delineate when adolescence ends and adulthood begins in increasingly complex societies (Kaluger & Kaluger, 1976). It is also difficult to define when a human being reaches adulthood. Adulthood is generally defined as the stage of life when an individual accomplishes certain tasks, including the attainment of economic independence and vocational identity, as well as the formation of a family or a network of supportive individuals. Early adulthood spans the years from roughly 18 to 30, and is the time when these tasks are embarked upon. See Table 1.7 for a list of the developmental tasks of young adulthood.

Physical Development

Physical growth and maturation are completed during late adolescence and early adulthood (Turner & Helms,

Table 1.6. "Red Flags" Indicating Potential Clinical Problems during Adolescence

RED FLAGS

- Irresponsible behavior
- Argumentative behavior (beyond normal adolescent rebellion)
- Lack of motivation
- Solitary behavior (staying in room all day)
- Constant desire to be away from home/Nonparticipation in family activities
- New, unusual friends
- Forgetfulness
- Lying
- Changes in speaking patterns; rapid or slow speech
- Legal problems (drunk driving, coming home drunk/high)
- Drugs missing from medicine cabinet/Missing wine or liquor
- Falling grades/Truancy
- Car accidents
- Missing clothing or possessions
- Strange phone calls
- Obsession with loud music
- Fascination with flashing light displays
- Inability to account for allowance or wages
- Use of eye drops (clears redness from eyes)
- Use of incense (masks the odor of pot)
- Odd, small containers in pockets, purses, drawers
- White specks on nostrils or clothing (sniffing correction fluid)
- Appointments at odd hours
- Bloodshot eyes/Dull-looking eyes/Watering eyes
- Drowsiness
- Manic/Hyper behavior
- Runny nose
- Coughing
- Needle marks on arms
- Weight loss
- Constant desire for junk food
- Malnutrition

Note. Table adapted from *A Parent's Survival Guide: How to Cope When Your Kid is Using Drugs* (pp. 6–8), by Harriet W. Hodgson. Copyright 1986 by Hazelden Foundation, Center City, MN. Adapted with permission.

Table 1.7. Developmental Tasks of Young Adulthood

TASK

1. Courting and selecting a partner.
2. Learning to adjust to, and living harmoniously with, a partner.
3. Beginning a family and assimilating the new role of parent (if desired). (This may be delayed, however.)
4. If children are present, rearing them, and meeting their individual needs.
5. Learning to manage money and assuming household responsibilities.
6. Embarking on a career and/or continuing one's education.
7. Assuming some type of civic responsibility.
8. Searching for a congenial social group.

Note. Table adapted from *Developmental Tasks and Education* (pp. 85–93), by Robert J. Havighurst. Copyright 1972 by Longman Publishers. Adapted with permission.

1983). Peak physical strength usually is achieved between ages 25 and 30, with slow, but gradual declines after age 30 (Craig, 1986). Body shape and proportions reach their final state (Freiberg, 1983). Brain weight reaches its maximum during the early adult years, and electroencephalographic pattern stability occurs as well, although not until age 30 in some individuals (Turner & Helms, 1983). The last four molars, or wisdom teeth, also emerge during this time (Freiberg, 1983). The reproductive systems of both men and women are fully mature by the time they are in their twenties.

Cognitive Development

The ability to think abstractly (described as formal operational thought by Piaget) is often acquired during adolescence, but can be acquired in early adulthood as well (Freiberg, 1983). Young adults are in a position to learn much new information, be it new job skills "in vivo" or additional knowledge via higher education.

Socioemotional Development

Some of the major psychosocial tasks of young adulthood include becoming independent from the family of origin and the formation of a supportive network. These tasks have a variable course during this period, dependent upon the path chosen by the individual. Erik Erikson (1963) defined the task of this stage as intimacy, with the risk being isolation (see Table 1.3).

In this society, it is rather common for young adults to experience a period of "prolonged adolescence," during which they may still be economically dependent on their family of origin, and consider the family of origin to be "home base" (Freiberg, 1983). Attending college is an example of a situation which may lead to a period of "prolonged adolescence." However, young adults are generally more independent than adolescents.

The following vignette illustrates the conflicts of young adulthood:

I am absolutely exhausted today! It is my second week of Army Boot Camp. Up at 0430 to get ready for inspection, miles of walking with a heavy backpack, constant insults from the Drill Instructor.

I just think about only six months ago, I was a high school senior, on top of the world!!! I was living with my mother and step-father. Money was tight, so I always worked after school at the mall.

I had a nice boyfriend, but I just wasn't ready to get married and be saddled with a couple of children. My step-father thought I could support myself, earn money for college, and see the world if I joined the Army. I didn't realize that I would be totally exhausted and doing a bunch of disgusting things like scrubbing toilet bowls. YECH!!!

I always longed for my freedom, but I can barely believe how hard I have to work, and that it is really not that much fun. And, when I do finally get my first paycheck, I think that I have already spent it! I won't have any money left, after I pay off my car payment, car insurance, and the payment on my new stereo.

Gosh, I used to spend the money I made at my mall job on clothes and movies. Now, I won't even be able to afford stuff like that! I should probably just get a credit card, and then I could charge stuff I need, like new clothes.

About raising a family, I just don't know if I really even want that. I think about my mom and step-dad always working, and never having any fun. They said it was so they could have a home for us!

Sometimes I wonder if I even want to ever get married. It is hard to see the point of that—my parents divorced, and had a bunch of fights before that. It didn't seem like much fun at all. IF, and that is a big if, I do get married, I certainly will not get divorced.

Well, I had better stop daydreaming and get back to work. If I had known leaving home would be so rough, I might have stayed a while longer! NO—IT IS TIME TO BE ON MY OWN!

A possible pitfall associated with this age group is involvement with a cult, a group of people characterized by their devotion to a particular religious system or ritual. These groups provide belief and belonging to those who are having difficulty with the transition from adolescence into adulthood (Levine, 1992b). "The individual uses the group as a vehicle for separation from parents and achieving more autonomy and independence." (Levine, 1992b, pp. 71–72). Involvement with a cult can be detrimental to the young adult, especially with the large influence many of these groups have over attitudes and behavior. However, some authors suggest that many of the cults of today may be less harmful in general than the groups of the seventies (Levine, 1992b).

In summary, particularly in a complex society requiring much training beyond the traditional public school period, the time after adolescence is filled with diverse possibilities. Physical and cognitive maturation are, for the most part, complete. Some young adults have achieved autonomy from the family of origin, and have started their own family units, yet many have not. They may enter a period of "prolonged adolescence," comprised of pursuing additional training and/or experiences, while remaining largely tied to the family of origin.

SUMMARY

The goal of this chapter was to provide a general overview of normal human development from the prenatal period through young adulthood. "Red flags," or indications that a behavior should be referred for further evaluation, were identified for each developmental period. Professionals who work with children, adolescents, and young adults must have a good working knowledge of normal development in order to identify problems at the earliest point possible. Prompt identification and intervention provide the opportunity for optimal outcome and prevention of secondary complications.

Furthermore, due to the complex nature of the developmental process and to the involvement of many different systems which often interact (e.g., physical; cognitive), a multidisciplinary approach to addressing clinical problems and developmental delay appears to be ideal. Communication among clinicians, family members, and school systems, as well as between clinicians and researchers, seems crucial for obtaining an accurate assessment of the problem and for providing the most appropriate interventions. A common base of knowledge about human development should facilitate communication among these different professionals.

REFERENCES

Acredolo, L. P., & Hake, J. L. (1982). Infant perception. In B. B. Wolman (Ed.), *Handbook of developmental psychology* (pp. 244–283). Englewood Cliffs, NJ: Prentice-Hall.

Attie, I., Brooks-Gunn, J., & Petersen, A. (1990). A developmental perspective on eating disorders and eating problems. In M. Lewis & S. M. Miller (Eds.), *Handbook of developmental psychopathology* (pp. 409–420). New York: Plenum Press.

Aurelius, G., Radestad, A., Nylander, I., & Zetterstrom, R. (1987). Psychosocial factors and pregnancy outcome. *Scandinavian Journal of Society and Medicine, 15*, 79–85.

Baron, R. A. (1989). *Psychology: The essential science.* Boston: Allyn & Bacon.

Behnke, M., & Eyler, F. D. (1993). The consequences of prenatal substance use for the developing fetus, newborn, and young child. *The International Journal of the Addictions, 28*, 1341–1391.

Benson, R. M. & Harrison, S. I. (1991). The eye of the hurricane: From seven to ten. In S. I. Greenspan & G. H. Pollock (Eds.), *The course of life, Vol. III: Middle and late childhood* (pp. 137–144). Madison: International Universities Press.

Bhatia, V. P., Katiyar, G. P., & Agarwal, K. N. (1979). Effect of intrauterine nutritional deprivation on neuromotor behaviour of the newborn. *Acta Paediatra Scandinavia, 68*, 561–566.

Bibace, R., & Walsh, M. E. (1980). Development of children's concepts of illness *Pediatrics, 66*, 912–917.

Billingham, K. A. (1982). *Developmental psychology for the health care professions: Part 1—Prenatal through adolescent development.* Boulder, CO: Westview Press.

Blasco, P. A. (1991). Pitfalls in developmental diagnosis. *Pediatric Clinics of North America, 38*, 1425–1438.

Blos, P. (1967). The second individuation process of adolescence. *Psychoanalytic Study of the Child, 2*, 162–186.

Brocken, C. (1981). *Behavior through the life cycle: Early childhood development.* Unpublished manuscript, Rush Medical College, Chicago.

Brook, C. G. (1981). Endocrinological control of growth at puberty. *British Medical Bulletin, 37*, 281–285.

Buhrmester, D., & Furman, W. (1987). The development of companionship and intimacy. *Child Development, 58*, 1101–1113.

Clarren, S. K., & Smith, D. W. (1978). Medical progress: The fetal alcohol syndrome. *The New England Journal of Medicine, 298*, 1063–1067.

Combrinck-Graham, L. (1991). Development of school-age children. In M. Lewis (Ed.), *Child and adolescent psychiatry: A comprehensive textbook* (pp. 257–266). Baltimore: Williams & Wilkins.

Coplan, J. (1983). *ELM Scale (Early Language Milestone Scale).* Tulsa, OK: Modern Educational Corporation.

Coplan, J., & Gleason, J. R. (1990). Quantifying language development from birth to 3 years using the Early Language Milestone Scale. *Pediatrics, 86*, 963–971.

Coyle, J. T. & Harris, J. C. (1987). The development of neurotransmitters and neuropeptides. In J. Noshpitz (Ed.), *Textbook of child psychiatry, Vol. 7* (pp. 14–25). New York: Basic Books.

Craig, G. (1986). *Human development: An integrated study of the lifespan.* Englewood Cliffs, NJ: Prentice-Hall.

Doberczak, T. M., Shanzer, S., Senie, R. T., & Kandall, S. R. (1988). Neonatal neurologic and electroencephalographic effects of intrauterine cocaine exposure. *The Journal of Pediatrics, 113*, 354–358.

Dott, A. B., & Fort, A. T. (1975). The effect of maternal demographic factors on infant mortality rates: Summary of the findings of the Louisiana Infant Mortality Study. Part I. *American Journal of Obstetrics and Gynecology, 123*, 847–853.

Drillien, C. M., Pickering, R. M., & Drummond, M. B. (1988). Predictive value of screening for different areas of development. *Developmental Medicine & Child Neurology, 30*, 294–305.

Drillien, C. M., & Wilkinson, E. M. (1964). Emotional stress and mongoloid births. *Developmental Medicine and Child Neurology, 6*, 140–143.

Dubas, J. S. and Peterson, A. C. (1993). Female pubertal development. In M. Sugar (Ed.), *Female adolescent development* (pp. 3–26). New York: Brunner/Mazel.

Dworetzky, J. P. (1993). *Introduction to child development.* Minneapolis/St. Paul: West Publishing Company.

Eiser, C. (1985). Changes in understanding of illness as the child grows. *Archives of Disease in Childhood, 60*, 489–492.

Erikson, E. H. (1963). *Childhood and society* (2nd ed.). New York: W.W. Norton.

Fagan, J. F., III. (1982). A visual recognition test of infant intelligence. *Infant Behavior and Development, 5*, 75.

Fagan, J. F., III. (1984). A new look at infant intelligence. In D. K. Detterman (Ed.), *Current topics in human intelligence.* Norwood, NJ: Ablex.

Felice, M. E. (1992). Adolescence. In M. D. Levine, W. B. Carey, & A. C. Crocker (Eds.), *Developmental-behavioral pediatrics* (pp. 65–73). Philadelphia: W.B. Saunders Company.

First, L. R., & Palfrey, J. S. (1994). The infant or young child with developmental delay. *The New England Journal of Medicine, 330*, 478–483.

Flavell, J. H., Miller, P. H., & Miller, S. A. (1993). *Cognitive development* (3rd ed.) Englewood Cliffs, NJ: Prentice-Hall.

Freiberg, K. L. (1979). *Human development: A life-span approach.* Belmont, CA: Wadsworth.

Freiberg, K. L. (1983). *Human development: A life span approach.* Monterey, CA: Wadsworth Health Sciences Division.

Freud, S. (1905). Three essays on the theory of sexuality. In J. Strachey (Ed.), *The standard edition of the complete psychological works of Sigmund Freud, Vol. 7* (pp. 125–245). London: Hogarth Press.

Furman, E. (1991). Early latency: normal and pathological aspects. In S. I. Greenspan & G. H. Pollock (Eds.), *The course of life, Vol. III: Middle and late childhood* (pp. 161–203). Madison, WI: International Universities Press.

Gardner, H., & Winner, E. (1982). Language development. In H. Gardner, *Developmental psychology* (2nd edition) (pp. 157–198). Boston: Little, Brown.

Garmezy, N. (1993). Developmental psychopathology: Some historical and current perspectives. In D. Magnusson & P. Casaer (Eds.), *Longitudinal research on individual development: Present status and future per-*

spectives (pp. 95–126). Great Britain: Cambridge University Press.

Gesell, A., & Ilg, F. (1946). *The child from five to ten*. New York: Harper & Row.

Ginsburg, H., & Opper, S. (1969). *Piaget's theory of intellectual development: An introduction*. Englewood Cliffs, NJ: Prentice-Hall.

Golombek, H., & Marton, P. (1992). Adolescents over time: A longitudinal study of personality development. In S. C. Feinstein (Ed.), *Adolescent psychiatry (Vol. 18): Developmental and clinical studies* (pp. 213–284). Chicago: University of Chicago Press.

Gordon, B. N., Schroeder, C. S., & Hawk, B. (1992). Clinical problems of the preschool child. In C. E. Walker & M. C. Roberts (Eds.), *Handbook of clinical child psychology* (pp. 215–233). New York: John Wiley & Sons.

Gordon, L. B. (1981). *Behavior through the life cycle: Cognitive development*. Unpublished manuscript, Rush Medical College, Chicago.

Gorsuch, R. L., & Key, M. K. (1974). Abnormalities of pregnancy: A function of anxiety and life stress. *Psychosomatic Medicine, 36*, 352–362.

Greenspan, S. I. (1991). Clinical assessment of emotional milestones in infancy and early childhood. *Pediatric Clinics of North America, 38*, 1371–1385.

Greenspan, S. I. (1993). *Playground politics: Understanding the emotional life of your school-age child*. Reading, MA: Addison-Wesley.

Greenspan, S. I. (1995). Monitoring social and emotional development of young children. In S. Parker & B. Zuckerman (Eds.), *Behavioral and developmental pediatrics: A handbook for primary care* (pp. 35–40). Boston: Little, Brown.

Griffith, D. R., Azuma, S. D., & Chasnoff, I. J. (1994). Three year outcome of children exposed prenatally to drugs. *Journal of the American Academy of Child and Adolescent Psychiatry, 33*, 20–27.

Groves, B. M., Zuckerman, B., Marans, S., and Cohen, P. J. (1993). Silent victims: children who witness violence. *Journal of the American Medical Association, 269*(2), 262–264.

Hall, C. S. (1954). *A primer of Freudian psychology*. Cleveland: World Publishing Company.

Havighurst, R. J. (1972). *Developmental tasks and education*. New York: David McKay.

Hayes, C. D. (1987). *Risking the future: Adolescent sexuality, pregnancy, and childbearing (Vol.1)*. Washington, DC: National Academy Press.

Himmelberger, D. U., Brown, B. W., & Cohen, E. N. (1978). Cigarette smoking during pregnancy and the occurrence of spontaneous abortion and congenital abnormality. *American Journal of Epidemiology, 108*, 470–479.

Hodapp, R. M., & Mueller, E. (1982). Early social development. In B. B. Wolman (Ed.), *Handbook of developmental psychology* (pp. 284–300). Englewood Cliffs, NJ: Prentice-Hall.

Hutson, H. R., Anglin, D., and Pratts, M. J. (1994). Adolescents and children injured or killed in drive-by shootings in Los Angeles. *New England Journal of Medicine, 330*, 324–327.

Illingworth, R. S., & Kaufman, A. (1984). Psychomotor and intellectual development and developmental assessment. In J. O. Forfar & G. C. Arneil (Eds.), *Textbook of paediatrics* (3rd ed.) (pp. 331–365). Edinburgh: Churchill Livingstone.

Kaluger, G., & Kaluger, M. F. (1976). *Profiles in human development*. St. Louis: C.V. Mosby.

Keating, D. P. and Clark, L. V. (1980). Development of physical and social reasoning in adolescence. *Developmental Psychology, 23*, 23–30.

Kennell, J. H., Voos, D. K., & Klaus, M. H. (1979). Parent-infant bonding. In J. D. Osofsky (Ed.), *Handbook of infant development* (pp. 786–798). New York: John Wiley & Sons.

Klaus, M. H., & Kennell, J. H. (1976). *Maternal-infant bonding*. In M. H. Klaus & J. H. Kennell (Eds.), Maternal-infant bonding (pp. 1–15). St. Louis: C.V. Mosby.

Klaus, M. H., & Kennell, J. H. (1982). *Parent-infant bonding*. St. Louis: C.V. Mosby.

Klaus, M. H., Kennell, J. H., Robertson, S. S., & Sosa, R. (1986). Effects of social support during parturition on maternal and infant morbidity. *British Medical Journal, 293*, 585–587.

Klein, S. K. (1991). Evaluation for suspected language disorders in preschool children. *Pediatric Clinics of North America, 38*, 1455–1467.

Kohlberg, L., & Gilligan, C. (1972). The adolescent as a philosopher: The discovery of the self in a post-conventional world. In J. Kagan & R. Coles (Eds.), *12 to 16: Early adolescence* (pp. 144–179). New York: W.W. Norton.

Kolb, B., & Fantie, B. (1989). Development of the child's brain and behavior. In C. R. Reynolds & E. Fletcher-Janzen (Eds.), *Handbook of clinical child neuropsychology* (pp. 17–39). New York: Plenum Press.

Kovacs, M., Krol, R. S. M., & Voti, L. (1994). Early onset psychopathology and the risk for teenage pregnancy among clinically referred girls. *J. Am. Acad. Child Adolesc. Psychiatry, 33*, 106–113.

Levine, M. P. (1992a). Middle childhood. In M. D. Levine, W. B. Carey, & A. C. Crocker (Eds.), *Developmental-*

behavioral pediatrics (pp. 48–64). Philadelphia: W.B. Saunders Company.

Levine, S. (1992b). Cults revisited: Corporate and quasi-therapeutic co-optation. In S. C. Feinstein (Ed.), *Adolescent psychiatry (Vol.18): Developmental and clinical studies* (pp. 63–73). Chicago: University of Chicago Press.

Lowery, G. H. (1986). *Growth and development of children.* Chicago: Year Book Medical Publishers.

Maccoby, E., & Jacklin, C. N. (1974). *The psychology of sex differences.* Stanford, CA: Stanford University Press.

Magni, G., Rizzardo, R., & Andreoli, A. (1986). Psychosocial stress and obstetric complications. *Acta Obstetrica Gynecologia Scandinavia, 65,* 273–276.

Marshall, W. A. & Tanner, J. M. (1969). Variations on the pattern of pubertal changes in girls. *Archives of Diseases in Childhood, 14,* 291–303.

Matera, C., Warren, W. B., Moomjy, M., Fink, D. J., & Fox, H. E. (1990). Prevalence of use of cocaine and other substances in an obstetric population. *American Journal of Obstetrics and Gynecology, 163,* 797–801.

Molfese, D. L., Molfese, V. J., & Carrell, P. L. (1982). Early language development. In B. B. Wolman (Ed.), *Handbook of developmental psychology* (pp. 301–322). Englewood, NJ: Prentice-Hall.

Murray, R. B., & Zentner, J. P. (1989). *Nursing assessment and health promotion: Strategies through the life span* (4th ed.). Norwalk, CT: Appleton & Lange.

Murray, R. B., & Zentner, J. P. (1993). *Nursing assessment and health promotion: Strategies through the life span* (5th ed.). Norwalk, CT: Appleton & Lange.

Mussen, P. H. (1963). *The psychological development of the child.* Englewood Cliffs, NJ: Prentice-Hall.

Mussen, P. H., Conger, J. J., & Kagan, J. (1963). *Child development and personality* (2nd ed.). New York: Harper & Row.

Naeye, R. L. (1978). Relationship of cigarette smoking to congenital anomalies and perinatal death. *The American Journal of Pathology, 90,* 289–293.

Nelson, M. N. (1981). *Behavior in the life cycle: Syllabus for lectures on infancy.* Unpublished manuscript, Rush Medical College, Chicago.

Nottelmann, E. D., Susman, E. J., Inoff-Germain, G., Cutler, G. B., Loriaux, D. L., & Chrousos, G. P. (1987). Developmental processes in early adolescence: Relationships between adolescent adjustment problems and chronologic age, pubertal stage, and puberty-related serum hormone levels. *Journal of Pediatrics, 110,* 473–480.

Offer, P. and Boxer, A. M. (1991). Normal adolescent development: Empirical research findings. In M. Lewis (Ed.), *Child and adolescent psychiatry: A comprehensive textbook* (pp. 266–278). Baltimore: Williams & Wilkins.

Omer, H., Elizur, Y., Barnea, T., Friedlander, D., & Palti, Z. (1986). Psychological variables and premature labour: A possible solution for some methodological problems. *Journal of Psychosomatic Research, 30,* 559–565.

Palfrey, J. S., Levine, M. D., Oberklaid, F., Lerner, M., & Aufseeser, C. L. (1981). An analysis of observed attention and activity patterns in preschool children. *The Journal of Pediatrics, 98,* 1006–1011.

Palfrey, J. S., Singer, J. D., Walker, D. K., & Butler, J. A. (1987). Early identification of children's special needs: A study in five metropolitan communities. *The Journal of Pediatrics, 111,* 651–659.

Paneth, N. S. (1995). The problem of low birth weight. *The Future of Children, 5,* 19–34.

Paris, S. G., & Lindauer, B. K. (1982). The development of cognitive skills during childhood. In B. B. Wolman (Ed.), *Handbook of developmental psychology* (pp. 333–349). Englewood Cliffs, NJ: Prentice-Hall.

Perrin, E. C. (1995). Chronic conditions. In S. Parker & B. Zuckerman (Eds.), *Behavioral and developmental pediatrics: A handbook for primary care* (pp. 95–100). Boston: Little, Brown.

Petersen, G. A. (1982). Cognitive development in infancy. In B. B. Wolman (Ed.), *Handbook of developmental psychology* (pp. 323–332). Englewood Cliffs, NJ: Prentice-Hall.

Petersen, L., Zink, M., & Farmer, J. (1992). Prevention of disorders in children. In C. E. Walker & M. C. Roberts (Eds.), *Handbook of clinical child psychology* (pp. 951–966). New York: John Wiley & Sons.

Phillips, J. L. (1981). *Piaget's theory: A primer.* San Francisco: W.H. Freeman and Company.

Phillips, S., Sarles, R. M., & Friedman, S. B. (1992). Consultation and referral for behavioral and developmental problems. In R. A. Hoekelman, S. B. Friedman, N. M. Nelson, & H. M. Seidel (Eds.), *Primary pediatric care* (2nd ed.) (pp. 678–682). St. Louis: Mosby-Year Book.

Piaget, J. (1972). The mental development of the child. In I. B. Weiner & D. Elkind (Eds.), *Readings in child development* (pp. 271–279). New York: John Wiley & Sons.

Revill, S. I., & Dodge, J. A. (1978). Psychological determinants of infantile pyloric stenosis. *Archives of Disease in Childhood, 53,* 66–68.

Richmond, P. G. (1970). *An introduction to Piaget.* New York: Basic Books.

Schaffer, H. R., & Emerson, P. E. (1964). The development of social attachments in infancy. *Monographs of the Society for Research in Child Development, 29,* 3–77.

Shaffer, D. (1974). Suicide in childhood and early adolescence. *Journal of Child Psychology and Psychiatry, 15,* 275–191.

Shalowitz, M. U., & Gorski, P. A. (1990). Developmental assessment in the first year of life. In J. A.. Stockman (Ed.), *Difficult diagnosis in pediatrics* (pp. 3–14). Philadelphia: W.B. Saunders Company.

Shapiro, T., & Perry, R. (1976). Latency revisited: The age 7 plus or minus 1. *The Psychoanalytic Study of the Child, 31,* 79–105.

Shiono, P. H., & Behrman, R. E. (1995). Low birth weight: Analysis and recommendations. *The Future of Children, 5,* 4–18.

Simeonsson, R. J., & Sharp, M. C. (1992). Developmental delays. In R. A. Hoekelman, S. B. Friedman, N. M. Nelson, & H. M. Seidel (Eds.), *Primary pediatric care* (2nd ed.) (pp. 867–870). St. Louis: Mosby-Year Book.

Simmons, R. G., Blyth, D. A., & McKinney, K. L. (1983). The social and psychological effects of puberty on white females. In J. Brooks-Gunn & A. C. Peterson (Eds.), *Girls at puberty: Biological and psychosocial perspectives* (pp. 229–272). New York: Plenum Press.

Sostek, A. M., & Magrab, P. R. (1992). Clinical problems of birth, the neonate, and infant. In C. E. Walker & M. C. Roberts (Eds.), *Handbook of clinical child psychology* (pp. 199–214). New York: John Wiley & Sons.

Sroufe, L. A., & Rutter, M. (1984). The domain of developmental psychopathology. *Child Development, 55,* 17–29.

Stechler, G., & Halton, A. (1982). Prenatal influences on human development. In B. B. Wolman (Ed.), *Handbook of developmental psychology* (pp. 175–189). Englewood Cliffs, NJ: Prentice-Hall

Steiner, J. E. (1974). Discussion paper: Innate, discriminative human facial expressions to taste and smell stimulation. *Annals New York Academy of Sciences, 237,* 229–233.

Steiner, J. E. (1977). Facial expressions of the neonate infant indicating the hedonics of food-related chemical stimuli. In J. M. Weiffenbach (Ed.), *Taste and development: The genesis of sweet preference* (pp. 173–189). Bethesda, MD: U.S. Department of Health, Education, and Welfare.

Stott, D. H., & Latchford, S. A. (1976). Prenatal antecedents of child health, development, and behavior: An epidemiological report of incidence and association. *Journal of Child Psychiatry, 15,* 161–191.

Sullivan, H. S. (1953). *The interpersonal theory of psychiatry.* New York: W.W. Norton.

Susman, E. J., Nottelmann, E. D., Inoff-Germain, G., Dorn, L. D., Cutler, G. B., Jr., Loriaux, D. L., & Chrousos, G. P. (1985). The relation of relative hormonal levels and physical development and social-emotional behavior in young adolescents. *Journal of Youth and Adolescence, 14,* 245–264.

Tanner, J. M. (1971). Sequence, tempo, and individual variation in the growth and development of boys and girls age twelve to sixteen. *Daedalus, 100,* 907–930.

Thompson, M. G. G. (1990). Developmental assessment of the preschool child. In J. A. Stockman, III (Ed.), *Difficult diagnosis in pediatrics* (pp. 15–28). Philadelphia: W. B. Saunders Company.

Tomchek, S. D., & Lane, S. J. (1993). Full-term low birth weight infants: Etiology and developmental implications. *Physical & Occupational Therapy in Pediatrics, 13,* 43–65.

Turner, J. S. and Helms, D. B. (1983). *Lifespan development.* New York: CBS College Publishing.

U.S. Department of Health and Human Services/Public Health Service (1994). Homicides among 15–19 year old males—United States, 1963–1991. *MMWR, 43,* 725–727.

Varni, J. (1983). *Clinical behavioral pediatrics: An interdisciplinary biobehavioral approach.* Pergamon Press.

Wachs, T. D., & Weizmann, F. (1992). Prenatal and genetic influences upon behavior and development. In C. E. Walker & M. C. Roberts (Eds.), *Handbook of clinical child psychology* (pp. 183–198). New York: John Wiley & Sons.

Walker, D., Gugenheim, S., Downs, M. P., & Northern, J. L. (1989). Early Language Milestone Scale and language screening of young children. *Pediatrics, 83,* 284–288.

Whitehurst, G. J. (1982). Language development. In B. B. Wolman (Ed.), *Handbook of developmental psychology* (pp. 367–386). Englewood Cliffs, NJ: Prentice-Hall.

CHAPTER 2

CONSULTATION AND LIAISON IN THE PEDIATRIC SETTING

Sally A. Kush
John V. Campo

INTRODUCTION

Medical professionals who care for children may request help from colleagues in the mental health professions in the assessment or management of their patients. Such requests for help provide the basis for mental health consultation and liaison work in the pediatric setting. The request may be patient-centered, soliciting help with an individual patient or a particular group of patients, or it may be staff-centered, focusing on providing help with particular staff reactions or behaviors that have proven troublesome. In many cases, the thoughtful consultant may be required to shift between approaches, and a patient-centered consultation may, at times, require intervention on a systemic level, rather than on a purely individual level (Woolston, 1994). Indeed, consultation can focus on several different levels, including the subjective experience of the child; the relationship between child and family; the relationship between the child and family and the medical staff; the relationship of medical staff to one another; and the relationship of staff with outside agencies, such as the police or child protective services (Lewis, 1994).

Consultation may be requested for a variety of reasons (Lewis, 1994). These include emergency consultations, as in cases of attempted suicide or acute agitation and delirium. Consultation may also be requested for help in the assessment and management of patients with difficult to explain physical symptoms, as in cases of so-matoform disorders, malingering, or factitious disorder by proxy. Help may be requested in ameliorating the physical consequences of emotional or behavioral distress in patients with physical illnesses that appear to be sensitive to emotional arousal. Mental health consultation may also be requested regarding emotional and/or behavioral difficulties associated with physical illness and its treatment. Finally, the consultant may be asked to intervene in the event of serious psychological trauma, perhaps experienced by individuals who have suffered accidents, maltreatment, violence, loss, or overwhelmingly painful and frightening medical treatments or procedures.

The diversity of problems and requests places special demands on the pediatric psychologist or psychiatrist involved in consultation work (Lewis, 1994). The possibility of emergency consultation and the rapid pace of medical care require ready availability and appropriate clinical back-up. The contingencies of the medical setting also require a degree of flexibility and creativity, and a willingness to interact with a broad variety of patients, families, and professionals. Many mental health professionals fail to initially grasp the rapid pace of modern medical care and the expectations of pediatric personnel and can easily alienate medical referral sources by giving the impression that they are more interested in protecting the boxes in their own schedules than in the practical care of patients. Lastly, the consultant must be adept at communicating not only with patients and families, but also with other professionals. Both verbal and written communications should be practical, concise, problem focused, jargon-free, and action oriented.

Ideally, consultation in the pediatric setting is both challenging and rewarding. It also highlights the practical importance of multidisciplinary collaboration among pediatric medical professionals, psychiatrists, psychologists, nurses, social workers, child life specialists, and others. In our experience, the effective consultant is able to transcend the quite real but regrettable rivalries and conflicts that have plagued relations between the various relevant disciplines. Our goal throughout the chapter is to balance a focus on conceptual issues with the need for clinical practicality. Clearly, the importance of pediatrics as a discipline cannot be minimized and our focus on psychology and psychiatry is purely heuristic given the obvious importance of related disciplines, including social work, nursing, and child life.

Description of the Problem: Impediments to Multidisciplinary Collaboration

The use of the term *consultation* has generated a good deal of confusion. In an age when virtually everyone can call themselves a consultant, there exist boundless interpretations of consultation; there may be as many interpretations of the term as there are consultants. This is particularly true in mental health consultation where there exists an ever increasing array of individuals from all walks of professional life, and at all levels of training. Even in fields as seemingly similar as child psychology, child psychiatry, and pediatrics, consultation can be interpreted and practiced with widely divergent styles. Such differences in approach to consultation may develop in accordance with individual variations in experience and training background.

The concept "consultation and liaison in the pediatric setting" implies a consolidation of disciplines, as well as a technique, a practice, and even a conceptual framework of what it means to *do consultation*. What has long been heralded as the promise of collaboration among pediatricians and mental health professionals has in actuality failed to produce the anticipated expectations (Drotar, 1994; Drotar, 1993; Lask, 1994; Lewis & Vitulano, 1988; Steiner, Sanders, Canning, & Litt, 1994). While this failure has been a relatively recent frustration for the young field of pediatric psychology, child psychiatry has long

fought the battle for increased integration within pediatrics. For example, there is evidence that pediatricians as a group are more likely to refer to mental health professionals other than psychiatrists (Fritz & Bergman, 1985), perhaps because they perceive psychiatric referral as more stigmatizing (Bergman & Fritz, 1985). Brennemann's (1931) classic article that termed psychiatry's attempts at involvement with pediatrics as "the menace of psychiatry" highlights that the newer field of pediatric psychology is certainly not alone in its frustration, nor is this a newfound frustration.

Lest this appear to denigrate pediatricians, we quickly point out that psychiatry and psychology have unquestionably endured growing pains as both fields have simultaneously approached and avoided joint collaborative work over the years. Indeed, the history of child psychology and psychiatry is replete with turf battles. Sadly, given the impact of the rapidly changing political and economic climate in health care, and the resulting competition for reimbursement by managed health care providers, such long-standing turf issues are likely to remain unresolved for the immediate future. Despite the possibility of this potentially negative impact on the profession, high-quality patient care necessitates that pediatric professionals, regardless of theoretical orientation and political ideology, recognize the importance of collaboration in a true multidisciplinary fashion.

The rather dismal success rate of cross-discipline collaboration among pediatrics, psychology, and psychiatry is not entirely unexpected when one recognizes the considerable variations that exist among these disciplines in professional preparation and training. In this regard, four primary factors can be identified that account for most of the failures in cross-discipline consultation in pediatric psychology and psychiatry: (1) experiential differences during training, (2) philosophical differences in training philosophy and methodology, (3) evolutionary growth and maturity of consultative practice, and (4) barriers to collaboration in current practice settings.

Differences in Training

Despite their surface similarity of being child focused, pediatricians and pediatric psychologists/psychiatrists have unique and often independent training experiences that affect later collaborative efforts. In medicine, structured clinical rotations provide the resident education and familiarity with multiple medical specialties, typically including pediatrics and psychiatry. As a result, pediatricians and psychiatrists have at least some degree of shared experience via exposure to one another's specialties during training. While it is logical to assume that this will subsequently translate into increased utilization of psychiatric referrals by physicians, this has not proved to be the case. While psychiatrists are generally asked to consult when these are diagnoses such as depression and anorexia, other diagnoses such as hyperactivity, failure to thrive, abuse issues, and learning problems are more likely to be referred to psychologists and social workers (Fritz & Bergman, 1985). Thus, although physicians normally develop a preliminary knowledge of professional roles and clinical services that characterize each medical specialty, there remains a lack of continuing case collaboration that persists beyond training experiences (Davidson, 1988; Fritz & Bergman, 1985). This lack of shared experience between pediatricians and child psychiatrists has been cited as one reason for the rather polarized relationship that currently exists between these two medical specialties (Bergman & Fritz, 1985; Jellinek, 1982).

By comparison, psychological training curricula have provided even less exposure to cross-discipline consultation than medical training programs. In psychology, virtually all training is provided by other psychologists, with little to no structured training experience that involves psychiatrists or pediatricians. This method of training continues despite the inevitability of future cross-referral and case sharing among these disciplines. Thus, psychologists may have a much more limited understanding of the professional roles and clinical services of those very professionals with whom they desire future collaboration.

Differences in Philosophy and Conceptualization

In addition to differences in training experiences, the philosophy and conceptualization of the very nature of consultation differs between medicine and psychology. The traditional medical consultation model, so familiar to psychiatrists and pediatricians, is typically conceived of, and carried out as, a service performed at the request of an attending or primary physician. The purpose of this type of consultation is to render a specialty opinion about an aspect of the patient that is outside the boundaries of the requesting physician's expertise. This method of consultation is a standard part of medical practice with widespread and routine utilization. In most, if not all cases, medical consultation is characteristic of a direct model of service delivery; the consultant works directly with the patient.

In contrast to the medical consultation model, the central tenets of virtually all theories of psychological consultation are characterized by three underlying components: (a) an indirect model of service delivery; (b) a collegial rather than hierarchical relationship between consultant and consultee, and (c) an emphasis on longer-term skill facilitation and problem solving rather than instantaneous patient diagnosis (Brown, Pryzwansky, & Schulte, 1991). Traditionally, psychological consultation is designed to facilitate successful resolution of a presenting problem by providing the necessary problem-solving skills to the consultee, rather than working directly with the client. It is ultimately the consultee who, in turn, works with the client using a format that has been worked out in conjunction with the consultant. In this regard, the successful psychological consultant attempts to render obsolete any future need for his/her expertise by empowering the consultee.

Psychological consultation encompasses different conceptual models which then dictate the approach and techniques that are subsequently used. For example, behavioral consultation utilizes measurable objectives and sequenced steps of problem identification, intervention implementation, and evaluation, while organizational consultation utilizes action plans and management-by-objectives strategies for targeting system and subsystem level goals. Such diversity in frameworks is a function of the widespread application of psychological consultation beyond the medical setting. Current service delivery models of psychological consultation range from teaching conflict resolution in public schools to improving management and communication styles in business settings.

In many ways, the nature of psychological consultation is analogous to what is frequently described in the medical literature as psychiatric liaison work. While psychiatric consultation typically reflects a direct model of service delivery, psychiatric liaison reflects an indirect service function. As a liaison, the psychiatrist may utilize a consultee-centered or a system theory perspective to facilitate support and learning of professional staff and the associated health care delivery system. Identified models of liaison work include a case finding model that is based on structured, regular meetings with staff; an education and training component in which the psychiatrist provides expertise via participation in patient conferences and discussions; and a collaborative case model in which pediatric and psychiatric care continue concurrently for various pediatric illnesses with the pediatrician serving as the source of treatment (Lewis, 1994).

Lask (1994) has argued that distinctions between psychiatric *consultation* and *liaison* are arbitrary, artificial, and serve no useful purpose other than to increase semantic confusion. It is our belief that the same can apply to the differentiation of psychological consultation and psychiatric liaison, and at least at a semantic level, there is probably good common sense in such a viewpoint. Among professionals, however, differences usually run deeper than semantics, reflecting the process of professional identification and learning biases we all experience during training (Davidson, 1988). Nevertheless, in ordinary practice the thoughtful consultant in the pediatric setting must be capable of constantly shifting attention between the needs of the identified patient and family, the needs of the consultee, the interpersonal transactions between members of the clinical treatment team, and the broader social context of the problem (Lask, 1994).

The Evolution of Consultative Practice

The third factor, which further contributes to difficulties in collaboration among disciplines, is the growth and maturity of the consultative practice. The practice of psychological consultation is still very much evolving. This is true of consultative practice in all branches of applied psychology but is probably most acutely felt in the pediatric psychology field, due to the relative immaturity of the field. Thus, the growing pains pediatric consultation has endured on its way to becoming an established discipline have contributed to the difficulties of establishing collaborative ties with pediatricians and child psychiatrists.

Despite its relative infancy, the history of consultation-liaison (C-L) psychiatry is already rich in practice and teaching traditions. If indexed by the body of scientific literature that has accumulated, C-L psychiatry has grown and matured considerably in just the past few years, particularly as a result of the influx of federal funding (Steiner, Fritz, Mrazek, Gonzales, & Jensen, 1993). Further evidence of the stature of C-L psychiatry is found in the movement currently underway to have C-L recognized as a legitimate subspecialty in psychiatry. With the exception of child and adolescent specialties, psychiatric subspecialization is a relatively new alternative, with only a few areas of concentration having achieved specialty status (i.e., geriatrics, addictions, administrative and forensic psychiatry) (Ford, Fawzy, Frankel, & Noyes, 1994). Specialty recognition can be earned by successfully passing an additional Board and being granted a Certificate of Added Qualification. A second example of advanced specialty development is the Triple-Board Program in pediatrics, psychiatry, and child and adolescent psychiatry. Begun as a pilot in 1985, its goal is to produce pediatric psychiatrists trained in an integrated curriculum of pediatrics and general and child psychiatry (Fritz, 1990). Clearly, the state of consultative practice in psychology is in its infancy, by comparison, having no such specialty or subspecialty development and training standards.

Barriers to Multidisciplinary Collaboration in the Practice Setting

Finally, barriers in the practice setting must also be recognized as they contribute to difficulties in the development of integrated consultation across disciplines. To a large extent these barriers are reflective of logistical problems, engendered by interdisciplinary misunderstanding. Though issues such as timeliness of responses, work pace, and economics of practice may appear to be modest and manageable, they remain as consequential barriers to multidisciplinary collaboration that must be dealt with.

Many of these obstacles arise from a lack of direct understanding and knowledge of roles and services across disciplines that have been brought about by differences among the professions in training and experience. Consequently, many professionals are frequently left with only their personal beliefs and expectations of how another service ought to be performed. One specific area, timeliness of service, may be most reflective of this potential abeyance between disciplines. With the typical pediatric visit lasting approximately 11.5 minutes (D'Angelo & Delozier, 1986; Goldberg et al., 1983), and less than one minute of that visit being devoted to psychosocial concerns and the provision of guidance (National Center for Health Statistics, 1987), pediatricians may be surprised and perhaps dismayed to learn that a typical psychiatric consultation may last anywhere from one to upwards of four hours. Thus, expectations for prompt turnaround of diagnostic findings and recommendations can vary considerably.

Conversely, the fast-paced flow of patients through a busy pediatric practice may be overwhelming to psychiatrists and psychologists who subsequently begin to question the feasibility of traditional mental health services in a pediatric setting. Ultimately, of course, psychologists and psychiatrists must learn to adjust practice styles to suit their individual work setting without compromising standards of care. Economy-of-scale methods such as adjustment screening, and the ability to triage accurately and efficiently, take on increased importance for mental health practices based outside of traditional office settings.

Within the hospital setting, additional barriers to consultation abound, particularly for psychologists, including the privilege status of psychologists on hospital staffs, independence of practice within the medical community, and the long-standing medical hierarchy into which psychologists are forced to carve a place. Psychologists are relative newcomers to the hospital world where norms, both implicit and explicit, appear to be well entrenched and understood by the established members. While psychologists may look to other mental health professionals for guidance, the fact remains that psychiatrists and pediatricians not only understand this medical subspecialty hierarchy, they also hold established positions and may have a stake in maintaining the existing hierarchy. Psychologists who have been trained to function autonomously will no doubt be confused by questions such as: Who retains control? How are these boundaries defined and maintained? and How are such issues best managed and resolved? (Davidson, 1988).

In addition to obvious complexities that are familiar to both psychiatrists and psychologists, issues related to role definition, boundaries, and control are equally problematic for referring pediatricians. Does one refer select diagnoses to pediatric psychiatry and other diagnoses to pediatric psychology? Are the clinical services rendered by each discipline viewed as generally equivalent, or is psychology subsumed by psychiatry? Are psychologists relegated to traditional tasks of intellectual assessment and psychiatrists limited to prescribing medication simply because there is lack of knowledge of additional competencies held by individuals trained in either discipline? These are important questions that impact daily practice and require thoughtful solutions in order to be answered. In all likelihood, the development of accurate knowledge of the role and function of each discipline will require such questions being addressed in individual training programs, if collaborative relationships are to be developed and implemented (Davidson, 1988).

Obviously, the beliefs about consultation that are brought to the work setting are highly influenced by one's training and experience, and will not be changed overnight. The fact that collaborative relationships between pediatrics, psychiatry, and psychology have developed to any extent is more likely a function of perseverance and necessity than a clearly defined, well-established alliance. Indeed, despite the fact that there is much overlap in the skills possessed by pediatric psychologists and psychiatrists, it is our premise that the fields are quite complementary. Collaborative work is not just a "nice" thing to do, it adds to the quality of the service provided.

DEVELOPMENTAL PSYCHOPATHOLOGY IN PEDIATRICS

The rationale for attempting to establish consultation-liaison services in pediatrics stems from numerous empirical studies that cite high rates of developmental psychopathology in the pediatric population. These studies are generally consistent in their conclusion that the pediatric population has significant mental health needs with prevalence estimates ranging from 10 to 37 percent (Cundall, 1987; Fitzgerald, 1985; Garralda & Bailey, 1989). Although different definitions were employed across most studies, it is worthwhile considering the following statistics concerning prevalence rates of psychopathology in children and adolescents collected from pediatric ambulatory settings:

- American Academy of Pediatrics, 1978: 20 percent identified with biosocial or developmental problems.
- Costello et al., 1988: 24 percent with emotional and/or behavioral problems.
- Horwitz, Leaf, Leventhal, Forsyth, & Speechley, 1993: 27 percent identified with psychosocial problems.
- Lavigne, Binns, & Christoffel, 1993: 13 percent of preschoolers identified with behavioral concerns.
- McClelland et al., 1978: 37 percent of visits involved psychological concerns; another 19 percent involved academic concerns.
- Smithells, 1982: 50 percent with physical disorders thought to have psychological etiology.
- Starfield et al., 1980: 8–10 percent identified with psychosomatic symptoms; 5–10 percent with behavioral, educational, or social difficulties.

These statistics become even more pronounced when children with chronic physical illnesses are considered. Approximately 9–14 percent of children have a chronic condition (Cadman, Boyle, Szatman, & Offord, 1987). For these children, the risk of having or developing associated mental health problems appears to be increased. Significant functional impairment has been identified in 25 percent of children and adolescents with a chronic medical illness, which translates to 1–3 percent of the population (Garrison & McQuiston, 1989; Gortmaker et al., 1990). Chronic medical illness has also been implicated as a significant risk factor for psychological disorders and psychosocial morbidity (Gortmaker et al.,

1990; Rutter, Tizard, & Whitmore, 1970). As a group, chronically ill children are more likely than healthy controls to have psychobehavioral and educational problems (Newacheck & Stoddard, 1994) although there is wide variability in the prevalence of these problems, depending on the type of physical illness (Rutter et al., 1970). Disorders with central nervous system involvement such as epilepsy or cerebral palsy, for example, seem to present an especially high risk. Data derived from the Isle of Wight study (Rutter et al., 1970) indicated that 34 percent of children ages 9–11 with documented brain disease had a concurrent psychiatric disorder, compared to 12 percent of children with a chronic medical illness that did not involve the brain, and 7 percent of children with no physical disorder. Some studies have estimated that 12–13 percent of the chronically medically ill population have diagnosable psychological problems (Goldberg et al., 1979; Rutter et al., 1970), particularly internalizing diagnoses such as depression and anxiety (Bennett, 1994). Suspected depression and/or suicidal ideation is the most common psychiatric referral problem for chronically medically ill hospitalized children (Olson et al., 1988; Rait, Jacobsen, Lederberg, & Holland, 1988).

Case Identification

In spite of large numbers of both routine and chronically ill pediatric patients with mental health problems, the recognition of such patients in the primary care pediatric setting has proved troublesome. The literature is replete with findings on the poor detection rate of mental health problems by pediatricians. While prevalence rates of pediatric mental health problems generally range from 10–37 percent, pediatricians identify such problems in only 4–7 percent (Steiner et al., 1994). When compared with general population estimates, pediatricians are apt to miss approximately one-half of the amount of psychopathology (Costello, 1986). In one study, children age 7–11 years were rated by both pediatricians and by structured psychiatric interviews with parents for the presence of psychopathology (Costello et al., 1988). Pediatricians diagnosed problems in 5.6 percent of the group versus 11.8 percent diagnosed from structured interviews. More importantly, however, it was demonstrated that while pediatricians did not falsely identify non-disturbed children (specificity), they failed to detect pathology in 83 percent of the cases (sensitivity).

Findings such as these seem both surprising and unfortunate. Surprising because families may not be fully communicating their concerns, and/or pediatricians may not be effective at or interested in detecting psycholog-

ical problems, and similarly unfortunate, due to the potentially vast number of missed opportunities for early intervention, when recognition/referral may be most effective. Communication between parents and pediatricians is of obvious importance and can be positively influenced by physician characteristics such as warmth, caring, and responsiveness to parental concerns (Worchel et al., 1995). In a study examining various communication styles, it was found that sensitivity of the pediatrician, the communication of information to the parent, and the partnership between parent and pediatrician in which the pediatrician sought input from the parent were all related to decreased follow-up phone calls by the parent after a medical visit (Worchel et al., 1995). Additionally it was shown that physicians tended to underestimate the amount of interaction hoped for by parents. It is especially encouraging that pediatricians who are trained to recognize mental health problems in their patients and who have a close working relationship with mental health providers are able to detect behavioral problems in their patients at earlier stages than other medical providers (Finney, Riley, & Cataldo, 1991).

Pediatricians are often the very professionals with whom families have the most sustained contact. Most children in the United States make a medical visit at least annually (National Center for Health Statistics, 1990), although this rate gradually diminishes with increasing age. While it would seem logical that pediatricians typically become the sounding board for parents' concerns about their child's behavioral and mental health, this is not always the case.

In their review of maternal behavioral concerns in a pediatric office site, Hickson, Altemeier, and O'Conner (1983) pointed out that only slightly more than one-quarter of the 70 percent of mothers with psychosocial concerns raised these issues with the pediatrician. Mothers' perceptions of a lack of interest or ability on the part of the pediatrician, and the mothers' own lack of awareness of pediatricians' ability to help were cited as reasons for withholding their concerns.

Part of the difficulty in communication may also reside in the visit structure of the pediatric setting. A routine office visit for either well-child care or sick care may simply be too brief for what is bound to be a time-consuming discussion of behavioral/psychosocial concerns that may be reimbursed at a minimal level. In the study of Worchel et al. (1995), parents' expectations for time with their pediatrician for a medical visit ranged from 4 to 30 minutes with an average of 13 minutes. By contrast, visits for behavioral and emotional concerns would seem to be more time intensive. If a parent expectation versus a pediatrician expectation is for longer interaction time because of a higher intensity problem, the parent may leave the visit feeling rushed and inadequately served. Studies of communication between physicians and parents have also suggested that physicians may dominate the interaction, which may further impact a family's ability to raise psychosocial concerns (Pantell et al., 1982). Similarly, the fast-paced flow of patients through a busy pediatric practice does not lend itself to impromptu raising of behavioral concerns by a parent. The same is true for the busy pediatrician, who, faced with an overloaded schedule, may understandably be less likely to ask questions that might require a considerable amount of time to explore. These types of scheduling constraints may also be an impediment to pediatricians' ability to better identify mental health problems in their patients. The format does not allow for adequate observation of, or interaction with, the child on the part of the pediatrician. Unlike adult settings in which the patient can self-report psychological symptoms and distress, detection of psychological difficulties in children and adolescents is more cumbersome and time-consuming because of the need for both direct observation and parent report.

Perceptions of the pediatric office setting have also been considered a possible impediment to problem detection because families are more likely to focus on physical symptoms, not psychological symptoms. When there is a co-occurrence of physical and psychological problems, physicians may be more apt to concentrate on the physical given that this is their primary area of expertise. Children with emotional distress who also exhibited poor physical health were four times less likely to receive a psychiatric diagnosis than physically healthy, emotionally distressed children in a recent study (Riley et al., 1993). The majority of mental health diagnoses made by primary care physicians are listed as being secondary to physical health diagnoses, again highlighting a tendency to focus on the physical. One percent of all ambulatory pediatric medical visits are for mental health as the primary diagnosis while the figure increases to 3 percent when mental health is a secondary diagnosis (Starfield et al., 1980).

Interestingly, while pediatricians diagnose mental disorders in a relatively small proportion of their patients, it appears that pediatricians may recognize the need for psychological or psychiatric intervention without specifying a diagnosis, perhaps because of a lack of confidence in diagnosing mental disorders (Olfson, 1992). Further, there appears to be a discrepancy between diagnostic and therapeutic practices, with the majority of children receiving active psychological or psychopharmacologic treatment within the pediatrician's practice

being treated in the absence of a psychiatric diagnosis (Olfson, 1992).

Additional factors contributing to detection difficulties on the part of the pediatrician include a lack of awareness of standard psychiatric terminology, a lack of training in diagnosis and treatment of mental health conditions (Long, Starfield, & Kelleher, 1994), and financial disincentives for pediatricians to investigate mental health concerns because of the time-intensive nature of such investigations (Riley & Wissow, 1994). Additionally, concerns about stigmatizing children and their families also may interfere with detection. In an effort to avoid potentially uncomfortable and embarrassing situations, the pediatrician may adopt a "wait and see" approach, hoping the child outgrows the present difficulties.

Referral

Low detection rates of pediatric mental health problems by pediatricians naturally lead to a lowered rate of referral, even when considering that many pediatricians are comfortable in addressing psychological as well as medical issues (Fritz & Bergman, 1985). In fact, the majority of children with mental disorders are more likely to receive counseling from other primary care physicians such as family practitioners or nurses than from pediatricians, a situation not unlike adult medicine (Regier, Goldberg, & Taube, 1978; Tarnowski, 1991). A comparison of senior pediatricians versus medical residents supports this, showing that the pediatricians requested psychiatric consultation less often than did residents, leading the authors to postulate that seasoned pediatricians view themselves as better able and better equipped to deal with such problems without the consultation of mental health professionals (Burket & Hodgin, 1993).

Alternatively, low referral rates may reflect a general skepticism on the part of pediatricians and other nonmental health providers regarding the efficacy of mental health intervention (Olfson, 1992). Nonetheless, referral remains an important issue to mental health professionals who regard the referral rate for biopsychosocial/developmental problems as low. In Costello's (1986) study in which it was demonstrated that only approximately half of the children with mental health concerns were identified by pediatricians, it was additionally demonstrated that only half of the identified cases were further referred to mental health specialists. Even with chronically ill children, referral rates are still low (Gortmaker et al., 1990), and services available for these children are often described as fragmented (Sabbeth & Stein, 1990). Overall, less than 20 percent of chronically ill children receive any type of social or mental health services (Cadman, Boyle, & Offord, 1986; Walker, Gortmaker, & Weitzman, 1991).

Research studies have consistently shown that less than one-half of children with significant psychopathology seen in primary care settings receive a psychiatric diagnosis or mental health referral (Cadman et al., 1986; Costello, 1986; Costello et al., 1988; Riley et al., 1993). In a study of children and adolescents referred for mental health services, significant pathology of two forms, major depression symptoms and adjustment disorder symptoms, were experienced for an average of 32 and 25 weeks, respectively, prior to referral (Kovacs, 1987). In most of these cases, some psychosocial intervention had come from the primary care physician prior to making the referral. Other studies show prevalence rates of 1 to 11 percent of pediatric patients in which psychiatric consultation was requested (Monelly, Ianzito, & Stewart, 1973; Sack, Cohen, & Grout, 1977). Burket & Hodgin (1993) also found infrequent utilization of in-patient psychiatric consultations with only 15 percent of physicians requesting consultations "often."

Apart from psychiatric referrals, help is often sought from other professionals, although referral still occurs at a suboptimal rate. A national survey of members of the American Academy of Pediatrics found that 36 percent of pediatricians preferentially referred emotional and behavior problems to psychologists, 10 percent to social workers, and an additional 36 percent would refer to either profession (Fritz & Bergman, 1985). The clearest preference of pediatricians, however, was for referral to a behavioral pediatrician, perhaps reflecting the growth of this pediatric subspecialty as well as a desire to work within the discipline of pediatrics and with professionals who share a similar philosophy.

The advent of behavioral pediatrics was spawned by the American Academy of Pediatrics' call for a more comprehensive and inclusive definition of child health that included a biosocial/developmental framework of practice (AAP, 1978). While this request may reinforce pediatricians' preferences for including mental health services within their practice it also clearly established the need for a knowledge and service base within the specialty of pediatrics which encompassed pediatric behavior and development. As a result, behavioral pediatrics has increasingly come to be the first line of intervention for many early childhood problems (e.g., toileting, compliance, hyperactivity) that in the past were considered the purview of child psychiatrists and psychologists.

The availability of on-site, behaviorally oriented services within a general pediatric office setting also allows for better management of psychological factors that can interfere with a family's ability to follow through on a referral. Family follow-through on referrals to mental health specialists from the primary care provider average only 40–60 percent (Bergman, Corbin, & Haber, 1982). Seeing a family within the familiar pediatric office setting offers enormous advantages of simplicity and comfort, and may increase compliance with recommended interventions. Similarly, consultation with a behavioral psychologist or other mental health professional, working within the pediatrician's office, may be viewed by many parents as far less threatening, less embarrassing, and less severe than a visit to an unfamiliar office to see an unknown child psychiatrist or psychologist.

Integrated Services vs. Integral Health Services

Many of the problems associated with mental health referral may be addressed by more specialized mental health services becoming integrated into the ambulatory pediatric setting. Approximately one-third of pediatricians, most of whom are in a group practice, report having a psychologist or social worker available in the office setting for purposes of addressing psychosocial problems (Fritz & Bergman, 1985). This type of arrangement may lead to increased identification and referral for mental health diagnoses (Jacobsen et al., 1980). As a group, pediatricians employed by health maintenance organizations are less likely to refer to mental health providers (Kamerow, 1985), though it is far from clear that low referral rates will prove cost-effective over time.

The presence of a mental health professional within the ambulatory medical setting is also valuable in helping to reduce the stigma often associated with mental health services. First, it allows children and families to form a more realistic appraisal of the mental health professional and the services that can be provided, which may subsequently increase the comfort level for pediatricians in making a referral. Second, it sends a clear message to patients and families that such services are an integral part of balanced health care and may decrease the common concern of referred patients and families that they have been "written off." In addition, an important secondary message is communicated to the family that the mental health professional must be "OK" by being included in the pediatric practice and thereby sanctioned by the trusted primary care doctor. True integration also allows opportunities for educating primary care providers who may subsequently identify and refer appropriate children, particularly if they are able to witness the positive effects of psychological intervention themselves. As a result of more integrated mental health services, delicate diagnostic concerns including childhood depression, abuse, and post-traumatic stress disorder may be diagnosed and treated within the pediatric office or identified and referred to an appropriate provider.

Pediatric psychology, in particular, has made recent inroads by offering alternative service delivery within the primary care setting. Much of the success of modern pediatric consultation has been accomplished by effectively shifting away from traditional service delivery to one that better suits the demands of primary care pediatrics. Structurally, there tends to be less time spent per patient, greater numbers of patients seen, and decreased severity of presenting concerns when patients are seen in the primary care setting (Wright & Burns, 1986), even though the problems presented appear to be more complex than in the behavioral pediatrics population. In turn, difficulties presented in the ambulatory medical setting are balanced by significant gains in intangible yet powerful factors that influence compliance, including ease of follow-through, ability to immediately capitalize on a family's motivation, and lessened psychological threat.

Financial Issues

Presently, a growing number of office sites have begun to utilize an integrated pediatric–mental health model, although this is not the prevailing norm for either pediatrics or child psychiatry/psychology. Many pediatricians and mental health professionals question the economic viability of integrated models with impending health care reform on the horizon (Drotar, 1994). Economics, while obviously a reality of practice, have become a major focus in this era of managed care and health care cost containment. It should be remembered that what might not appear cost-effective in the short term may become so over time. Further, like many physical diseases with significant impact on the child's function and/or which cause suffering, cost-effectiveness is not the only consideration. Serious psychiatric illness should not be treated differently from other illness by being considered worthy of treatment only when cost-effectiveness of the service can be readily demonstrated. For example, one can argue that the medical treatment of many serious physical diseases may be life saving and effective in lessening suffering for the individual patient, despite the fact that the treatment may be extraordinarily expensive on an individual basis, and thus "not cost-effective." In any case, clinical services research in pediatric psychology and psychiatry may provide the guidance which is currently lacking (Gonzales, 1994).

Innovative approaches such as joint ventures between pediatrics and mental health or between family practice and mental health services seem to be receiving favorable reviews, in part because it is hoped that such arrangements will decrease overall medical cost and utilization. Children with concurrent medical and psychiatric diagnoses obviously require a more costly diagnostic work-up and increased utilization of medical resources over the course of treatment (Steiner et al., 1993). Studies in the adult C-L literature support the hypothesis that active mental health intervention in the medical setting may result in cost savings (Strain, Hammer, & Fulop, 1994). Research examining psychiatric overlay in medical and surgical patients reveals a strong relationship between mental health problems and increased length of hospital stay, as well as use of health care resources (Saravay & Lavin, 1994). Adult C-L psychiatry programs have been shown to decrease length of stay and days spent in rehabilitation following hospitalization, while at the same time increasing recognition of mental health problems (Strain et al., 1994).

While less data is available for the pediatric population, it is likely that similar trends would occur. Hospitalized pediatric patients, both chronically and acutely ill, experience psychological distress from multiple causes, such as the injury/illness itself, separation anxiety, and painful, invasive diagnostic procedures. Distress, whether manifested as anxiety, aggression, or non-compliance with treatment, can be a complicating variable in the course of care, and have a negative impact medically as well as financially. Appropriate management of the psychological distress in children may positively impact care in the pediatric setting in much the same way as has been shown in the adult population.

The question of cost savings associated with mental health treatment in the out-patient setting was examined with a pediatric population participating in an HMO plan (Kelleher & Starfield, 1990). Findings indicated that at least for specialty care utilization, there was decreased useage for those children aged 5 to 11 who had received mental health treatment. The authors noted, however, that results were mixed in that such a decrease was not observed for primary care useage. Despite this limitation, the potential for long-term savings appears evident. Interestingly, one factor shown to be predictive of primary care use for children of all ages was their comorbidity status. Those children with mental health needs and additional medical morbidity, of either an acute or chronic nature, required greater medical utilization for their multiple needs. This is not an altogether unexpected finding given the at-risk status of children with medical problems, especially chronic conditions, to develop mental health disorders. This trend becomes even more pronounced with the presence of additional chronic physical conditions, such that the rise in number of chronic conditions is commensurate with a rise in number of social-emotional/behavioral diagnoses, developmental delays, and learning disabilities (Newacheck & Stoddard, 1994). Indeed, one of the objectives for future joint pediatric-mental health service teams should be the prevention of such psychosocial morbidity and, accordingly, cost-effective use of resources (Steiner et al., 1993). Prime opportunities for reduction in health care costs (along with improved psychological outcomes) include (1) improving medical regimen compliance in chronic conditions, and (2) management of children with recurrent, medically unexplained, somatic complaints.

As important as medical compliance becomes for both immediate and longer-term consequences of disease, general findings on treatment compliance are rather abysmal. Cited figures vary widely (which may be a function of the problems of definition that plague the available literature), and range from approximately 50 percent for the majority of children and adolescents (Litt & Cuskey 1980) to as high as 89 percent (Eney & Goldstein, 1976). Particularly in the in-patient setting, consultation is often requested regarding children or adolescents who are perceived as "difficult to manage." Such patients may passively refuse to cooperate with diagnostic procedures, medications, or other treatments. Health care professionals are even more disturbed by patients who actively threaten or abuse professional staff, violate hospital rules, or actively disrupt their own treatment, as in the case of a patient who deliberately pulls out an intravenous line (King & Lewis, 1994). Standard approaches for treating non-compliance in chronic illness include patient education and multicomponent programs that are primarily behavioral in nature. It has been suggested that non-compliance should be anticipated as the "rule" rather than the exception if medical treatment regimens do not integrate systematic behavioral strategies (Varni & Wallander, 1984).

The presence of a pediatric psychiatrist or psychologist as a routine member of the multidisciplinary team provides an opportunity for cost-effective behavioral intervention early on in the process of medical diagnosis and treatment. Other advantages of a mental health presence on the team include decreasing stigma and reducing anxiety for the stressed families and children experiencing the psychological or behavioral problems commonly associated with chronic medical illness. Parents can gain indirect benefit from the experiences of a professional who has been involved with treatment of other such patients and families, in addition to the obvious and direct benefit of learning to properly manage

psychological problems associated with the individual's particular illness.

Children with recurrent medically unexplained physical symptoms and medically unexplained somatic complaints represent an additional population likely to benefit from improved utilization management. Recurrent somatic complaints, including recurrent abdominal pain (RAP), headache, limb pain, dizziness, nausea, fatigue and chest pain are relatively common occurrences in the pediatric population (Apley, 1975; Campo & Fritsch, 1994; Garber, Walker, & Zeman, 1991; Garralda, 1992). Approximately 2–4 percent of all pediatric visits surveyed in a one-year time period were for RAP, while another 1–2 percent were for headache complaints; this compares to only 1 percent of all ambulatory pediatric visits where the primary diagnosis is that of a mental health problem (Starfield et al., 1980). A review of in-patient pediatric consultation-liaison referrals showed that 12 percent of patients met criteria for diagnosis of a somatoform disorder (Mullins, Olson, & Chaney, 1992). Rarely, the consultant may assist the medical staff in the diagnosis and management of potentially costly and dangerous instances of factitious disorder by proxy (Munchausen syndrome by proxy), or in cases where malingering is identified. Smith (1994) has also found increased rates of polysymptomatic and chronic adult somatization in primary care health settings, which accounted for as many as 9 percent of patients, approximately three times higher than the rate found in the general population. It has also been demonstrated that psychiatric consultation is effective in improving physical function and reducing the cost of medical care in adult out-patients with somatization disorder (Smith, Monson, & Ray, 1986).

In addition to concerns of prevalence and cost, it is important to recognize that somatization complaints and symptoms often persist into adulthood; children do not appear to simply "outgrow it" (Apley & Hale, 1973; Billie, 1981; Orr, 1986; Spiering et al., 1990). Conversely, adults do not suddenly develop somatic complaints; many are able to trace the beginnings of somatization back to adolescence or childhood (Coryell & Norten, 1981). Thus, recognition and appropriate management of somatization early on in its course may be especially significant, with benefits potentially accruing across the life span. Recommendations for a *best practices* approach generally call for early involvement of a mental health professional, either as a direct provider of patient service or as a consultant with the primary care physician who guides management (Jones, 1994; Katon & Gonzales, 1994). This practice has significant ramifications for collaborative work in pediatrics given that it is estimated that pediatricians consult with mental health specialists in less than 20 percent of cases (Edwards, Mullins, Johnson, & Bernardy, 1994).

PRACTICAL CONSIDERATIONS IN ESTABLISHING PEDIATRIC CONSULTATION-LIAISON

Developmental Perspective

The mechanics of pediatric C-L work are to some degree setting specific, although there remain certain fundamentals of practice that transcend setting, with the most important reflecting the adoption of a developmental perspective. Although this might appear to be an assumed prerequisite given the nature of child work, an intimate understanding of development is required since pediatric psychiatry/psychology spans from very early childhood through adolescence. Thus, understanding the behavioral nuances of a 2-year-old compared to a 6-year-old becomes paramount. To a greater extent than in the adult world, developmental changes in children come rapidly and dramatically. Such rapid-fire change makes understanding pediatric illness and the patterns of illness-behavior relationships more complicated due to the subsequent potential to impact ongoing development.

As a part of the developmental framework, consultants move away from traditional patient-centered approaches, toward family-focused approaches of intervention and treatment. Again, unlike the adult world where the independent adult is able to be patient, informant, and behavioral observer, children are clearly dependent both psychologically and environmentally on adult caretakers. The consultant then must gather not only the child's self-report, but observations from adults familiar with the child and his/her life. Everything about the child has potential merit for consultative purposes, including factors as diverse as intellectual functioning, competence in completing daily care routines, ability to tolerate novel situations, and parental observations of distress and coping in the child. The major goal of this approach is to support the family in its caregiving role, by building on its unique array of strengths.

The practical implication of incorporating a family perspective is a significant increase in the amount of time necessary to do pediatric consultation work. While adult consultation may require 45–90 minutes, it is not unusual for a pediatric consultation to take 3 or 4 times longer. Despite the time-consuming nature of this process, family characteristics are simply too important to be overlooked. The family's acceptance of psychological intervention, its implicit messages to the child regarding the process, and its willingness to be the primary agents of behavior change in its children necessitate inclusion of adult caretakers in the consultative process (Gillman & Mullins, 1991).

Lask (1994) has advanced a systems model, identified as the illness network, as a way to conceptualize the interplay of multiple factors involved in pediatric illness. The network of child, family, illness, and environmental variables, is an interdependent system in which homeostasis can be affected by change in any one variable. Thus, the marital satisfaction of parents is an area of interest to the pediatric consultant because of its capacity to affect the child's emotional status and, in turn, illness condition. Similarly, a child's impaired intellectual functioning may affect the ability to understand illness concepts and cooperation with medical procedures, which may strain both the technical skills and empathic capabilities of the medical staff. By incorporating a broader family perspective, the management of pediatric illness and its treatment comes to involve much more than attention to medical symptoms. The consultant must recognize that there are multivariate influences on the child that must be considered in the context of consultation.

Theory and Pragmatics

Different theoretical and practical approaches to consultation have been widely explored as the field of pediatric mental health consultation has matured. Some of these approaches apply primarily to in-patient settings, some to out-patient settings, and some have general application across the board.

Regardless of specific setting, flexibility of approach has been touted as critical for meeting the needs of both patient and pediatrician (Roberts & Lyman, 1990). This includes not only flexibility in selecting an initial match of patient need with management approach, but in the ability to make adjustments in the ongoing course of the consultation process. Along with treatment flexibility, some advance agreement as to definition of role and function for each professional involved in the consultation helps to ensure a smooth venture. Equally important to pediatricians is the ease of accessibility of the consultant, timeliness of the consultant's response to the request, capability for completion of assessment versus ongoing assessment over time, and prompt turnaround of evaluation findings (Burket & Hodgin, 1993). Less emphasis is typically given to non-direct aspects such as liaison, participation in medical rounds, and familiarity with the medical floors.

Measurement Issues

Perhaps the most concrete aspect of consultative work which generalizes across settings is the role of assessment and screening. As discussed earlier, developmental psychopathology is well represented in pediatric populations, yet often poorly detected by the physician. For the pediatric mental health consultant, an important first step may be the establishment of screening procedures for use in out-patient and hospital clinic settings. The ability to have in place continuous screening procedures helps to improve upon poor detection rates and begin early identification and intervention. Examples of existing screening measures that enjoy popularity include the Parenting Stress Index (Abidin, 1983), the Child Behavior Checklist (Achenbach & Edelbrock, 1983), the Personality Inventory for Children (Lachar & Godowski, 1979), the Pediatric Symptom Checklist (Jellinek, Murphy, & Burns, 1986), and the Stony Brook Child Symptom Inventory (Gadow & Sprafkin, 1994). These paper-and-pencil tasks, completed by parents, attempt to identify clinically significant levels of pediatric psychopathology. Practical limitations of these scales include the length of time required for administration and scoring, and the extreme variability in developmental levels which may necessitate an infant, child, and adolescent version of the same instrument. Perhaps most important, many checklists and questionnaires are parent completed, which may be helpful for detecting externalizing behavioral problems, but less helpful for detecting internalizing problems.

The most common psychosocial problems cited by medical providers include family problems (7.2 percent), behavioral problems (6.7 percent), and language problems (5.5 percent) (Leaf et al., 1990). Physicians are less likely, however, to identify internalizing problems (Riley et al., 1993). It may prove to be true that there is no substitute for a thoughtful interview with the child to adequately detect internalizing disorders such as anxiety or depression.

In addition to concerns about how to best tailor screening instruments to the pediatric setting for maximum efficiency, simplicity, and early detection success, more global problems exist concerning the methodology of pediatric mental health assessment. Increasingly, concerns have been expressed about the validity and reliability of measuring psychological constructs in ill children, with and without mental health concerns, when these two specific populations did not serve as part of the normative group for most measures (La Greca, 1994; Steiner et al., 1993). In turn, generalizability is then significantly reduced as one moves away from a healthy group to an ill group of children. There is likely to be reduced generalizability even within an ill population, however, because of the wide age span in pediatrics and the lack of representation of age span in the norming process.

Available instruments may also lack sensitivity regarding the confound between medical and psychiatric symptoms, particularly with somatic symptoms such as fatigue, nausea, vomiting, headache, and dizziness. Thus, the presence of symptoms of physical disease may confound ratings of psychosocial adjustment, which may appear artificially worsened in select pediatric patients. Future efforts in pediatric assessment should examine disease-specific factors that help to mediate adjustment or predict compliance problems rather than to simply differentiate healthy controls from ill children (La Greca, 1994). As would be expected, there is an emphasis on developing new measures as well as adapting existing measures as much as possible in the interim. Such efforts may enhance the measurement match between patient and psychological construct and yield more useful findings.

STYLES OF CONSULTATION

Independent Functions Approach

Among the various "how-to" approaches of pediatric mental health consultation, perhaps the most traditional is the independent functions model (Roberts & Wright, 1982). In this model, the mental health consultant receives a referral from the pediatrician, independently conducts a work-up, and reports findings on the patient's medical chart as a means of communicating back to the referring pediatrician. This is closely akin to common medical practice, in which attending and consultant physicians interact with the patient but may have little interaction with one another. The central mission of the independent functions approach is the application of expert knowledge and judgment regarding a specific patient concern (Stabler, 1988). Various names have similarly been applied to this method including non-collaborative approach (Drotar, 1978) and resource consultation (Stabler, 1979).

Although this reflects a very popular way of treating pediatric mental health issues in a medical setting, this approach is not without its drawbacks (Roberts & Lyman, 1990). The model can be constraining as it tends to reinforce stereotypes of psychiatry and psychology practice (i.e., medication referrals for psychiatry and testing for psychologists) rather than allowing for more expansive roles to emerge. Another drawback of this model is the lack of opportunities for information sharing, education, and rapport building between professionals. To some extent, the in-patient setting offers several advantages over the out-patient setting, as it is easier to communicate directly with a referring colleague and subsequently provide a brief synopsis of the referral findings. With out-patient referrals, the customary communication tool is a letter to the pediatrician from the consultant, acknowledging the referral and outlining findings and treatment recommendations. The advantage of the independent functions model is independence—the independence of each professional to pursue his/her work-up with ease. Very specific questions such as continuation of medication while in the hospital or determination of developmental delay are usually best suited to an independent functions model (Roberts & Lyman, 1990).

Indirect Consultation Approach

Another approach to consultation, particularly when problems extend beyond a specific referral question, is the indirect consultation model (Roberts & Wright, 1982). In this model, there is little or no direct interaction with the patient on the part of the pediatric consultant. The primary emphasis is on providing professional guidance to the pediatrician who, in turn, works with the patient and family. This type of guidance may be provided via case conference attendance, or participation in check-in rounds, psychosocial rounds, or in medical clinics (Olson, Mullin, Chaney, & Gillman, 1994). This approach may also take on an informal air, such as the "hallway consult" or a quick phone call from the pediatrician for advice regarding a generic problem applicable to many patients.

A specific example of indirect consultation offered in the out-patient pediatric setting is provided by the development of disorder-specific treatment protocols (Roberts & Lyman, 1990). Common childhood problems that are frequently handled by the pediatrician (e.g., toileting, use of time-out, and behavioral compliance) lend themselves nicely to a checklist or "points to remember" type of format. Such recurring problems do not generally require the direct contact of a mental health professional with the patient in order to render generally effective interventions. Creating step-by-step behavioral management protocols for use by the pediatrician with the family on these common problems can be a valuable time saver for the pediatrician.

A broader but still indirect role that may be taken on by the consultant in the in-patient setting is that of a systems consultant. Here the mental health professional applies knowledge of systems theory to the various systems that impinge upon a patient, and subsequently designs multi-level interventions (Woolston, 1994). Systems may include family, staff, hospital, and patient, with each being targeted for intervention as indicated by evaluation. Quite possibly, the patient does not require direct intervention but may nonetheless benefit as a result of intervention with a medical system, with which the patient interacts.

A significant impediment to using indirect consultation, however, is the lack of reimbursement especially given the time commitment and effort involved in many instances. Because consultation may not be defined as a direct service provision, third-party billing may not be an option. And despite the value of such efforts to a busy pediatrician, non-revenue generating activities are rarely performed, particularly relative to the amount of professional time expended. The previously reported finding that liaison work is ranked by pediatricians as less important than more pragmatic, direct patient services, represents another disincentive to heavy use of liaison consultation.

Collaborative Approach

A model more geared toward joint care and collaborative efforts is the shared caregiving, or process collaboration model (Stabler, 1988), also called the collaborative team model (Roberts & Wright, 1990). Here, direct patient contact occurs, often provided equally by both the referring pediatrician and the consultant. A typical scenario in an in-patient setting requires the pediatric consultant to receive a consultation notice, speak with the referring pediatrician about concerns and past interactions with the patient and family, complete the consultation, and re-discuss findings with the pediatrician. This model, often regarded as a "best practices" model, offers close involvement and opportunities for cross-education between professionals as well as shared decision making about future treatment directions (Roberts & Lyman, 1990; Stabler, 1988). This type of close collaboration, as a routine practice, may be more prevalent in specialty clinics, such as burn units, hematology/oncology, or pediatric trauma. As noted previously, mental health services within the pediatric out-patient setting are gaining in popularity but still lag behind what is available in the in-patient setting.

Multidisciplinary Team Concept

The concept of a team approach that is multidisciplinary, interdisciplinary, transdisciplinary, or otherwise labeled, is frequently referenced in traditional models of pediatric mental health consultation. This is predominantly reflective of the in-patient setting because of the complexity of cases that present, as well as the pressing need for intervention in terms of both severity and timeliness. Also relevant team personnel, such as pediatricians, psychiatrists, social workers, psychologists/neuropsychologists, child life specialists, and pediatric nurses are often not available en masse in the pediatric out-patient setting.

Experts generally regard pediatric mental health consultation as best delivered from the infrastructure of a team (Lask, 1994; Lewis, 1994; Roberts & Lyman, 1990; Steiner et al., 1993; Steiner et al., 1994). The need for rapid and frequent communication, coordination across disciplines, and complexity of treatment planning for comorbid children are some of the factors considered critical for successful treatment outcomes. Multidisciplinary teams have become the central mechanism for service delivery in highly specialized medical- or pediatric-psychiatry units developed over the past 15 years (Wamboldt, 1994). Such specialty programs focus exclusively on patients whose medical needs are beyond the usual acuity of a purely psychiatric unit but whose mental health needs are greater than would typically be found on a purely pediatric unit. Some medical-psychiatry programs, such as the Lucile Packard Children's Hospital at Stanford University (Steiner et al., 1993) and that at the University of Pittsburgh (Campo & Raney, 1995), offer comprehensive services for the in-patient setting as well as for numerous out-patient clinics, all focusing on comorbidly ill children. Other programs such as the National Jewish Center for Immunology and Respiratory Medicine in Denver, Colorado offer a variety of inpatient units to service pediatric patients too complex for out-patient management.

In addition to furthering the development of multidisciplinary patient care, specialty programs also possess expertise in practical matters that are unique to this setting. These range from personnel matters (co-attending physician arrangements, role overlap of team members) to finance matters (program cost, payor mix, reimbursement patterns). Such logistics can be a roadblock to development or expansion of multidisciplinary pediatric–mental health ventures. This is particularly true when administrative concerns guide clinical initiatives, a not uncommon course in this fiscally minded era of health reform. Tapping into the experience and expertise available through specialty programs may help advance joint service ventures between pediatrics and mental health professionals.

SUMMARY

We have attempted to provide an overview of the significant issues in pediatric C-L psychology and psychiatry, trying to balance a discussion of the difficulties encountered by mental health professionals in the pediatric medical setting with attention to the numerous reasons why such consultative services are increasingly relevant in modern health care. Regarding problems, the failure of mental health professionals to arrive at mutually agreeable role definitions among themselves, coupled with the associated territoriality issues, have in our opinion, interfered with the rate of progress in clinical service delivery and research. A related problem has been the suspiciousness of pediatric medical providers regarding collaboration with mental health professionals. Such effective collaboration demands a willingness on the part of pediatric psychologists and psychiatrists to increase their familiarity with the medical setting and with physical disease and its treatment. Problems in the politics of effective collaboration may at times be driven by gaps in the experience or training of the relevant professionals. It appears that greater clinical experience and exposure to the various disciplines involved in the care of children increase the likelihood of effective collaboration among pediatricians, psychologists, psychiatrists, and other professionals.

Genuine collaboration is becoming increasingly tenable and important. More and more, the modern workplace demands efficiency and the use of cost-effective interventions. Creative approaches to the financing of pediatric health care appear worthy of exploration and experimentation, particularly integrated medical and mental health services where reimbursement may be "bundled." The primary care setting is rightly emerging as the focal point of modern health care, and thus demands the attention of mental health professionals. Access to patients and families in medical settings also presents unprecedented opportunities for preventive work, effective and cost-effective clinical interventions, research initiatives, the education of medical professionals, and for decreasing the stigma associated with mental health initiatives. Though impediments to effective work at the interface between pediatric health care, psychology, and psychiatry are considerable, with the issue of appropriate reimbursement for services being of special importance, we remain optimistic and convinced that the continued hard work of pediatric psychologists and psychiatrists to collaborate with pediatric medical professionals and with each other will pay handsome dividends in the future for the respective fields and, most importantly, for young persons and their families.

REFERENCES

Abidin, R. R. (1983). *Parenting Stress Index Manual (Form 6).* Charlottesville: Pediatric Psychology Press.

Achenbach, T. M., & Edelbrock, C. (1983). *Manual for the Child Behavior Checklist and Revised Child Behavior Profile.* Burlington: University of Vermont.

American Academy of Pediatrics. (1978). *A report by the task force on pediatric education: The future of pediatric education.* Elk Grove, IL: Author.

Apley, J. (1975). *The child with abdominal pain.* Oxford, UK: Blackwell.

Apley, J., & Hale, B. (1973). Children with recurrent abdominal pain: How do they grow up? *British Medical Journal, 3,* 79.

Bennett, D. S. (1994). Depression among children with chronic medical problems: A meta analysis. *Journal of Pediatric Psychology, 19,* 149–170.

Bergman, D. A., Corbin, S., & Haber, J. (1982). Analysis of a program for mental health referrals from a pediatric clinic. *Developmental and Behavioral Pediatrics, 3,* 232–235.

Bergman, A. S. & Fritz, G. K. (1985). Pediatricians and mental health professionals: Patterns of collaboration and utilization. *American Journal of Diseases of Children, 139,* 155–159.

Billie, B. (1981). Migraine in childhood and its prognosis. *Cephalalgia, 1,* 71–75.

Brennemann, J. (1931). The menace of psychiatry. *American Journal of Diseases of Children, 42,* 376–402.

Brown, D., Pryzwansky, W. B., & Schulte, A. C. (1991). *Psychological consultation: Introduction to theory and practice.* Boston: Allyn & Bacon.

Burket, R. C., & Hodgin, J. D. (1993). Pediatricians' perceptions of child psychiatry consultations. *Psychosomatics, 34,* 402–408.

Cadman, D., Boyle, M. A., & Offord, D. R. (1986). Chronic illnesses, medical conditions and limitations in Ontario children. *Canadian Medical Association Journal, 9,* 117–121.

Cadman, D., Boyle, M., Szatman, P., & Offord, D. R. (1987). Chronic illness, disability and mental and social well-being: Findings of the Ontario child health study. *Pediatrics, 79,* 805–813.

Campo, J. V., & Fritsch, S. L. (1994). Somatization in children and adolescents. *Journal of the American Academy of Child and Adolescent Psychiatry, 33,* 1223–1235.

Campo, J. V., & Raney, D. (1995). The pediatric medical-psychiatric unit in a psychiatric hospital. *Psychosomatics, 36,* 438–444.

Coryell, W., & Norten, S. G. (1981). Briquet's syndrome (somatization disorder) and primary depression: Comparisons of backgrounds and outcome. *Comprehensive Psychiatry, 22,* 249–256.

Costello, E. J. (1986). Primary care pediatrics and child psychopathology: A review of diagnostic, treatment, and referral practices. *Pediatrics, 78,* 1044–1051.

Costello, E. J., Edelbrock, C., Costello, A. J., Dulcan, M. K., Burns, B. J., & Brent, D. (1988). Psychopathology in pediatric primary care: The new hidden morbidity. *Pediatrics, 82,* 415–424.

Cundall, D. (1987). Children and mothers at clinics: Who is disturbed? *Archives of Disease in Childhood, 62,* 820–824.

D'Angelo, L. J., & Delozier, J. (1986). Who provides care for adolescents: A reappraisal of NAMCS. *Journal of Adolescent Health Care, 7,* 290–292.

Davidson, C. V. (1988). Training the pediatric psychologist and the developmental-behavioral pediatrician. In D. K. Routh (Ed.), *Handbook of pediatric psychology* (pp. 507–538). New York: Guilford Press.

Drotar, D. (1978). Training psychologists to consult with pediatricians: Problems and prospects. *Journal of Clinical Child Psychology, 7,* 57–60.

Drotar, D. (1993). Influences on collaborative activities among psychologists and pediatricians: Implications for practice, training and research. *Journal of Pediatric Psychology, 18,* 159–172.

Drotar, D. (1994). Psychological research with pediatric conditions: If we specialize, can we generalize? *Journal of Pediatric Psychology, 19,* 430–414.

Duff, R. S., Rowe, D. S., & Anderson, F. P. (1973). Patient care and student learning in a pediatric clinic. *Pediatrics, 50,* 839–846.

Edwards, M. C., Mullins. L. L., Johnson, J., & Bernardy, N. (1994). Survey of pediatricians' management practices for recurrent abdominal pain. *Journal of Pediatric Psychology, 19,* 241–255.

Eney, R. D., & Goldstein, E. O. (1976). Compliance of chronic asthmatics with oral administration of theophylline as measured by serum and salivary levels. *Pediatrics, 57,* 531–537.

Finney, J. W., Riley, A. W., & Cataldo, M. F. (1991). Psychology in primary health care: Effects of brief targeted therapy on children's medical care utilization. *Journal of Pediatric Psychology, 16*, 447–461.

Fitzgerald, M. (1985). Behavioural deviance and maternal depressive symptoms in outpatients. *Archives of Disease in Childhood, 60*, 560–562.

Ford, C. V., Fawzy, F. I., Frankel, B. L., & Noyes, Jr., R., (1994). Fellowship training in consultation-liaison psychiatry. *Psychosomatics, 35*, 118–129.

Fritz, G. K. (1990). Consultation-liaison in child psychiatry and the evolution of pediatric psychiatry. *Psychosomatics, 31*, 85–90.

Fritz, G. K., & Bergman, A. S. (1985). Child psychiatrists seen through pediatricians' eyes: Results of a national survey. *Journal of the American Academy of Child Psychiatry, 24*, 81–86.

Fritz, G. K., & Bergman, A. S. (1984). Consultation-liaison training for child psychiatrists: Results of a survey. *General Hospital Psychiatry, 6*, 25–29.

Gadow, K. D., & Sprafkin, J. (1994). *Manual for the Stony Brook Child Symptom Inventories*. Stony Brook, NY: Checkmate Plus, Ltd.

Garber, J., Walker, L. S., & Zeman, J. (1991). Somatization symptoms in a community sample of children and adolescents: Further validation of The Children's Somatization Inventory. *Psychological Assessment: A Journal of Consulting and Clinical Psychology, 3*, 588–595.

Garralda, M. E. (1992). A selective review of child psychiatric syndromes with a somatic presentation. *British Journal of Psychiatry, 161*, 759–773.

Garralda, E., & Bailey, D. (1989). Psychiatric disorders in general pediatric referrals. *Archives of Disease in Childhood, 64*, 1727–1733.

Garrison, W., & McQuiston, S. (1989). *Chronic illness during childhood and adolescence: Psychological aspects*. Newbury Park, CA: Sage.

Gillman, J., & Mullins, L. L. (1991). Professional and pragmatic issues in pediatric pain. In J. P. Bush & S. Harkins (Eds.), *Children in pain: Clinical and research issues from a developmental perspective*. New York: Springer/Verlag.

Goldberg, I. D., Regier, D. A., McInery, J. K., Pless, I. B., & Roghmann, K. J. (1979). The role of the pediatrician in the delivery of mental health services to children. *Pediatrics, 63*, 898–909.

Goldberg, I. D., Roghmann, K. J., McInerny, T. K., & Burke, Jr., J. D. (1983). Mental health problems among children seen in pediatric practice. *Pediatrics, 73*, 278–293.

Gonzales, J. J. (1994). Psychiatric problems in primary care: What are the problems, how will we recognize them, and how can we treat them? *Psychosomatic Medicine, 56*, 94–96.

Gortmaker, S. L., Walker, D. K., Weitzman, M., & Sobol, A. M. (1990). Chronic conditions, socioeconomic risks, and behavioral problems in children and adolescents. *Pediatrics, 85*, 267–276.

Hickson, G. B., Altemeier, W. A., & O'Conner, S. (1983). Concerns of mothers seeking care in private pediatric offices: Opportunities for expanding services. *Pediatrics, 72*, 619–624.

Horwitz, S. M., Leaf, P. J., Leventhal, J. M., Forsyth, B., & Speechley, K. N. (1992). Identification and management of psychosocial and developmental problems in community based, primary care pediatric practices. *Pediatrics, 89*, 480–485.

Jacobsen, A. M., Goldberg, I. D., Burns, B. J., Boeper, E. W., Hankin, J. R., & Hewitt, K. (1980). Diagnosed mental disorder in children and use of health services in four organized health care settings. *American Journal of Psychiatry, 137*, 559–565.

Jellinek, M. S. (1982). The present status of child psychiatry in pediatrics. *New England Journal of Medicine, 306*, 1227–1229.

Jellinek, M. S., Murphy, J. M., & Burns, B. (1986). Brief psychosocial screening in outpatient pediatric practice. *Journal of Pediatrics, 109*, 371–378.

Jones, J. (1994). Somatoform disorders: Medical issues. In R. A. Olson, L. L. Mullins, J. B. Gillman, & J. M. Chaney (Eds.), *The sourcebook of pediatric psychology*. Boston: Allyn & Bacon.

Kamerow, D. (1985). *Mental health problems among children seen in pediatric practice: Referral practices*. Unpublished manuscript.

Katon, W., & Gonzales, J. (1994). A review of randomized trials of psychiatric consultation-liaison studies in primary care. *Psychosomatics, 35*, 268–278.

Kelleher, K., & Starfield, B. (1990). Health care use by children receiving mental health services. *Pediatrics, 85*, 114–118.

King, R. A., & Lewis, M. (1994). The difficult child. *Child and Adolescent Psychiatric Clinics of North America, 3*, 531–543.

Kovacs, M. (1987). Diagnosis of depressive disorders in children. In G. L. Tischler (Ed.), *Diagnosis and classification in psychiatry, a critical appraisal of DSM III*. New York: Cambridge University Press.

Lachar, D., & Godowski, C. L. (1979). *Actuarial assessment of child and adolescent personality: An interpretative guide for the Personality Inventory for Children profile*. Los Angeles: Western Psychological Services.

La Greca, A. M. (1988). Adherence to prescribed medical

regimens. In D. K. Routh (Ed.), *Handbook of Pediatric Psychology* (pp. 299–321). New York: Guilford Press.

La Greca, A. M. (1994). Assessment in pediatric psychology: What's a researcher to do? *Journal of Pediatric Psychology, 19*, 283–290.

Lask, B. (1994). Pediatric liaison work. In M. Rutter, E. Taylor, & L. Hersov (Eds.), *Child and adolescent psychiatry modern approaches* (pp. 996–1005). London: Blackwell Scientific Publications.

Lavigne, J. V., Binns, H. J., & Christoffel, K. K. (1993). Behavioral and emotional problems among pre-school children in pediatric primary care: Prevalence and pediatrician's recognition. *Pediatrics, 91*, 649–657.

Leaf, P. J., Horwitz, S., Leventhal, J., Speechley, K., Forsyth, B., Schwab-Stone, M., & Pakes, J. (1990, October). *Primary care pediatrics: What is detected, what is done.* Paper presented at the American Academy of Child and Adolescent Psychiatry, Chicago.

Lewis, M. (1994). The consultation process in child and adolescent psychiatric consultation-liaison in pediatrics. *Child and Adolescent Psychiatric Clinics of North America, 3*, 439–449.

Lewis, M., & Vitulano, L. A. (1988). Child and adolescent psychiatry consultation-liaison services in pediatrics: What messages are being conveyed? *Developmental and Behavioral Pediatrics, 9*, 388–390.

Litt, I. F., & Cuskey, W. R. (1980). Compliance with medical regimens during adolescence. *Pediatric Clinics of North America, 27 C1*, 3–15.

Long, N., Starfield, B., & Kelleher, K. (1994). Co-occurrence of medical and mental disorders in pediatric primary care. In J. Miranda, A. H. Hohmann, C. C. Attkisson, & D. B. Larson (Eds.), *Mental disorders in primary care*. San Francisco: Jossey-Bass.

McClelland, C. Q., Staples, W. P., Weisberg, I., & Bergen, M. E. (1978). The practitioner's role in behavioral pediatrics. *Journal of Pediatrics, 82*, 325–331.

Monelly, E. P., Ianzito, B. M., & Stewart, M. A. (1973). Psychiatric consultations in a children's hospital. *American Journal of Psychiatry, 130*, 789–790.

Mullins, L. L., Olson, R. A., & Chaney, J. M. (1992). A social learning/family systems approach to the treatment of somatoform disorders in children and adolescents. *Family Systems Medicine, 10*, 1–5.

National Center for Health Statistics (1987). *Advance report of final mortality statistics, 1985. Monthly Vital Statistics Report*, 1–48. (DHHS Publication No. (PHS) 87-1120).

National Center for Health Statistics. (1990). *Health, United States, 1989* (DHHS Publication No. (PHS) 90-1232). Hyattsville, MD: Public Health Service.

Newacheck, P. W., & Stoddard, J. J. (1994). Prevalence and impact of multiple childhood chronic illnesses. *The Journal of Pediatrics, 124*, 40–47.

Olfson, M. (1992). Diagnosing mental disorders in office based pediatric practice. *Journal of Developmental & Behavioral Pediatrics, 13*, 363–365.

Olson, R. A., Holden, E. W., Friedman, A., Faust, J., Kenning, M., & Mason, P. J. (1988). Psychological consultation in a children's hospital: An evaluation of services. *Journal of Pediatric Psychology, 13*, 479–492.

Olson, R. A., Mullins, L. L., Chaney, J. M., & Gillman, J. B. (1994). The role of the pediatric psychologist in a consultation liaison service. In R. A. Olson, L. L. Mullins, J. B. Gillman, & J. M. Chaney (Eds.), *The sourcebook of pediatric psychology* (pp. 1–9). Boston: Allyn & Bacon.

Orr, D. (1986). Adolescence, stress and psychosomatic issues. *Journal of Adolescent Health Care, 7*, 97S–108S.

Pantell, R. H., Stewart, T. J., Dias, J. K., Wells, P., & Ross, A. W. (1982). Physician communication with children and parents. *Pediatrics, 70*, 396–402.

Rait, D. S., Jacobsen, P. B., Lederberg, M. S., & Holland, J. C. (1988). Characteristics of psychiatric consultations in a pediatric cancer center. *American Journal of Psychiatry, 145*, 363–364.

Regier, D. A., Goldberg, I. D., & Taube, C. A. (1978). The defacto U.S. mental health services system. *Archives of General Psychiatry, 35*, 685–693.

Riley, A. W., Finney, J. W., Mellitis, E. D., Starfield, B., Kidwell, S., Quaskey, S., Cataldo, M. F., Filipp, L., & Shematek, J. (1993). Determinants of children's health care use: An investigation of psychosocial factors. *Medical Care, 31*, 767–783.

Riley, A. W., & Wissow, L. S. (1994). Recognition of emotional and behavioral problems and family violence in pediatric primary care. In J. Miranda, A. H. Hohmann, C. C. Attkisson, & D. B. Larson (Eds.), *Mental disorders in primary care*. San Francisco: Jossey-Bass.

Roberts, M. C., & Lyman, R. D. (1990). The psychologist as a pediatric consultant. In A. M. Gross & R. S. Drabman (Eds.), *Handbook of clinical behavioral pediatrics* (pp. 11–28). New York: Plenum Press.

Roberts, M. C., & Wright, L. (1982). Role of the pediatric psychologist as consultant to pediatricians. In J. Tuma (Ed.), *Handbook for the Practice of Pediatric Psychology* (pp. 251–289). New York: Wiley-Interscience.

Rutter, M., Tizard, J., & Whitmore, K. (Eds.). (1970). *Education, health and behavior*. London: Longmans.

Sabbeth, B., & Stein, R. E. K. (1990). Mental h;ealth referral: A weak link in comprehensive care of children with chronic physical illness. *Journal of Developmental and Behavioral Pediatrics, 11*, 73–78.

Sack, W., Cohen, S., & Grout, C. (1977). One year's survey of child psychiatry consultations in a pediatric hospital.

Journal of the American Academy of Child Psychiatry, 16, 716–727.

Saravay, S. M., & Lavin, M. (1994). Psychiatric comorbidity and length of stay in the general hospital: A critical review of outcome studies. *Psychosomatics, 35*, 233–252.

Smith, G. R. (1994). The course of somatization and its effects on utilization of health care resources. *Psychosomatics, 35*, 263–267.

Smith, G. R., Monson, R. A., & Ray, D. C. (1986). Psychiatric consultation in somatization disorder. *New England Journal of Medicine, 314*, 1407–1413.

Smithells, R. (1982). In praise of outpatients: Partnerships in pediatrics. In J. Apley, & C. Cunstead (Eds.), *One Child* (pp. 135–146). London: Mackeith Press.

Spiering, C., Pels, P. J. E., Sijben, N., Gabreels, F. J. M., & Remier, W. O. (1990). Conversion disorders in childhood: A retrospective follow up of 84 inpatients. *Developmental Medicine and Child Neurology, 32*, 865–871.

Stabler, B. (1988). Pediatric consultation-liaison. In D. K. Routh (Ed.), *Handbook of pediatric psychology* (pp. 538–567). New York: Guilford Press.

Stabler, B. (1979). Emerging models of psychologist-pediatrician liaison. *Journal of Pediatric Psychology, 4*, 387–413.

Starfield, B., Gross, E., Wood, M., Pantell, R., Allen, C., Gordon, I. B., Moffatt, P., Drachman, R., & Fatz, H. (1980). Psychosocial and psychosomatic diagnoses in primary care of children. *Pediatrics, 66*, 159–167.

Steiner, H., Fritz, G. K., Mrazek, D., Gonzales, J., & Jensen, P. (1993). Pediatric and psychiatric comorbidity. Part one: The future of consultation-liaison psychiatry. *Psychosomatics, 34*, 107–111.

Steiner, H., Sanders, M., Canning, E., & Litt, I. (1994). A model for managing clinical and personnel issues in consultation-liaison psychiatry. *Psychosomatics, 35*, 73–79.

Strain, J. J., Hammer, J. S., & Fulop, G. (1994). Academy of Psychosomatic Medicine task force report on psychosocial interventions in the general hospital inpatient setting: A review of cost-offset studies. *Psychosomatics, 35*, 253–262.

Tarnowski, K. J. (1991). Disadvantaged children and families in pediatric primary care settings: 1. Broadening the scope of integrated mental health service. *Journal of Clinical Child Psychology, 20*, 351–359.

Varni, J. W., & Wallander, J. L. (1984). Adherence to health-related regimens in pediatric chronic disorders. *Clinical Psychology Review, 4*, 585–596.

Walker, D., Gortmaker, S., & Weitzman, M. (1991). *Chronic illness and psychosocial problems among children in Genesee County*. Boston: Harvard School of Public Health.

Wamboldt, M. Z. (1994). Current status of child and adolescent medical-psychiatry units. *Psychosomatics, 35*, 434–444.

Woolston, J. L. (1994). General systems issues in child and adolescent consultation and liaison psychiatry. *Child and Adolescent Psychiatric Clinics of North America, 3*, 427–439.

Worchel, F. F., Prevatt, B. C., Miner, J., Allen, M., Wagner, L., & Nation, P. (1995). Pediatrician's communication style: Relationship to parent's perceptions and behaviors. *Journal of Pediatric Psychology, 20*, 633–644.

Wright, L., & Burns, B. J. (1986). Primary mental health care: A "find" for psychology? *Professional Psychology—Research & Practice, 17*, 560–564.

CHAPTER 3

CULTURAL AND ETHNIC ISSUES AFFECTING PEDIATRIC SERVICE DELIVERY

Gloria D. Eldridge
Janet S. St. Lawrence

INTRODUCTION

By the year 2030, more than 40 percent of children in the United States will be children of color (Lynch & Hanson, 1993; Rounds, Weil, & Bishop, 1994). In many areas of the U.S., groups traditionally labeled as "minorities" now comprise more than half of the population. In California, for example, White school-aged children are already in the minority (Chan, 1990). Because minority children have higher health risks, health care providers in most areas of the country will find themselves providing care for increasing numbers of minority children in the foreseeable future (Lynch & Hanson, 1993).

Cultural and racial diversity among health care consumers is increasing rapidly. War, disaster, famine, global economic instability, and political unrest in many parts of the world have stimulated large-scale migrations and led to increased cultural and racial diversity within the U.S. (Berlin & Fowkes, 1983; Reiss, 1993; Rogler, 1993). Since 1975, nearly one million Southeast Asian refugees have immigrated into the U.S., with the majority being infants, children, and adolescents (Fox, Cowell, & Montgomery, 1994). Political turmoil in Central America, Cuba, and Haiti in recent years also brought large numbers of economic and political refugees to the U.S. Immigrants must cope with leaving a familiar sociocultural system, separating from family and social networks, and adapting to a new social system (Rogler, 1993; 1994). For many refugees, the effects of migration are compounded by pre-migration experiences of violence, trauma, starvation, limited health care, and lack of education. Multiple stressors place immigrants and refugees at risk for health problems. However, refugees and immigrants from other countries are not the only ones suffering the effects of dislocation. Economic hardship and social changes lead to within-country migrations, as rural dwellers move into cities in search of jobs and urban dwellers relocate into rural areas to escape urban violence. Both intra- and extra-country migrations bring people from different cultural, ethnic, and racial groups into closer contact.

Preparation of this chapter was supported, in part, by a grant from the National Institute of Child Health and Human Development (HD28842).

Another reason for the increasing cultural diversity in the U.S. is that many immigrant communities are younger, on average, than the majority American population, so a larger proportion of the population in minority groups is in their reproductive years. In addition, many minority groups have higher birth rates than the Anglo-American majority (Chan, 1990; Christensen, 1992). The combination of lower mean age and higher fecundity means that the rate of population increase in many minority groups is greater than that of the Anglo-American majority.

Erosion within traditional American cultures also contributes to increasing diversity among health care consumers. For example, the breakdown of traditional Native American culture in the U.S. and the lack of economic and educational opportunities for young people resulted in migrations away from traditional Native American communities. Fewer wage earners and fewer opportunities remained within these communities, gradually increasing poverty and social deprivation in those areas. Health problems such as substance abuse, disease, and injuries arising from poverty and isolation increased among those who remained behind (Reiss, 1993).

Paralleling increases in cultural diversity and ethnic minority populations, perceptions of cultural minorities, notably African-Americans and Native Americans, have begun to shift. Perceptions of minority group members change slowly. However, after decades in which cultural differences were viewed as pathological or deficient, academic and research communities have come to a growing appreciation that cultural differences do not necessarily reflect deficits in need of remediation. This changing viewpoint has provided an impetus for providers to increase their understanding of cultural differences and their impact on health care provision.

In the United States, most health care professionals are members of the majority Anglo-American culture. In years past, most providers could assume their careers would be spent providing services to patients from similar cultural backgrounds. However, increasing cultural diversity challenges health care practitioners to provide quality health care to patients from diverse cultural, ethnic, and racial groups, whose first language may not be English, and who may have markedly different beliefs about health, illness, and medical treatment. Cross-cultural health care, particularly for children, is a reality for many health care practitioners from all disciplines— physicians, nurses, psychologists, social workers, health educators, speech and occupational therapists (Clark, 1983). A recent survey of professionals practicing in early intervention programs for children in California showed that 60 percent of the providers served families and children from four or more ethnic groups. Although 73 percent of the professionals were White, 53 percent of the families served were from other racial groups (Christensen, 1992).

While cross-cultural health care is not synonymous with poor-quality care, there is greater potential for problems to arise when health care providers and patients come from different cultural or racial groups (Lynch & Hanson, 1993). There is little empirical evidence suggesting that medical treatment is less effective across cultures than within cultures. However, patients and their families often prefer providers from their own race or culture and feel that culturally dissimilar providers are less helpful. Practitioners also perceive themselves to be less comfortable and less effective with patients from other cultural or racial groups (Davis & Gelsomino, 1994).

A straightforward solution to the problem of providing quality health care for members of minority groups would be to increase the number of minority practitioners. However, shifts in population demographics have not been paralleled by changes in the cultural composition of health professions, where there is a serious scarcity of bilingual and bicultural providers (Lynch & Hanson, 1993). The shortage of minority practitioners is unlikely to change markedly in the foreseeable future. Refugees and immigrants who were trained health care professionals in their own countries often arrive in the U.S. and discover that their professional qualifications are not recognized (Rogler, 1994). To resume their medical careers, refugees must undertake professional retraining, but many refugees lack the financial resources to pursue retraining or are impeded by a lack of facility with English. At the same time, the number of minority students entering health-related training programs has not kept pace with the number of minority consumers of services (Atkinson, Spratley, & Simpson, 1994; Lynch & Hanson, 1993; Trevino, Sumaya, Miranda, Martinez, & Saldana, 1994).

In considering the issue of health care provision to minority populations, two underlying contextual issues warrant discussion: (1) the relationship between poverty, minority status, and health risk; and (2) experiences associated with migration, acculturation, and racism.

Relationships among Poverty, Minority Status, and Health

Not all minority children come from impoverished backgrounds, but poverty is a reality for many minority children in this country. In turn, the experience of poverty affects health care needs and resource availability for minority children and their families (Garcia Coll, 1990). In 1991, almost 22 percent of children in the U.S. lived below the poverty threshold (U.S. Bureau of the Census, 1992), a rate double that of most other industrialized nations. Poverty has pervasive effects on the lives of children and on the relationships between children and their parents or caretakers. For many parents, poverty and economic loss diminish their capacity for consistent and involved parenting. Coping with poverty often produces psychological distress, such as depression and anxiety, that affects parenting skills. Thus, poverty and economic loss influence children indirectly through their impact on parental behavior (McLoyd, 1990).

Poverty and deprivation also affect children more directly. Poverty places children at risk for adverse developmental, medical, and behavioral outcomes. Lack of prenatal care, poor prenatal nutrition, and inadequate pediatric health care contribute to increased health risks for poor and minority children (Chan, 1990; Rounds, Weil, & Bishop, 1994). Children living in poverty experience a double jeopardy. First, they are exposed to increased biological risks such as low birth weight, *in utero* infections, lead poisoning, failure to thrive, chronic ear infections, and asthma. Second, they are exposed to higher levels of family stress, inadequate resources, and higher incidence of parental depression (McLoyd, 1990). Finally, these risks have a greater impact on poor children because parents, families, and poor communities lack many of the ameliorating factors that are available to children from higher socioeconomic backgrounds (Kaplan-Sanoff, Parker, & Zuckerman, 1991).

Poverty in the U.S. falls largely along racial and ethnic lines. Minority children bear a disproportionate share of the burden of poverty and economic decline and are at greater risk than White children for emotional and health problems associated with poverty (McLoyd, 1990). For example, low birth weight and prematurity contribute to mortality rates among African-American infants that are almost double those of White infants (Garcia Coll, 1990). Although 22 percent of children in the U.S. lived in poverty in 1991, the percentages were higher for minority children, with 46 percent of African-American children and 40 percent of Hispanic children living in poverty (U.S. Bureau of the Census, 1992). While impoverished White children are more likely to live in episodic poverty, impoverished African-American and Hispanic children are more likely to live in persistent poverty that has a more pervasive impact on their health and adjustment. Most research on the effects of childhood poverty focuses on urban poverty, despite the fact that childhood poverty is also high in rural and suburban areas (Gabarino, 1992; Huston, McLoyd, & Garcia Coll, 1994).

Poverty is associated with poorer health, inadequate housing, limited availability of health care, homelessness, exposure to environmental toxins, and greater risk of living in residential areas where violence is commonplace (Huston et al., 1994). Poor nutrition also places impoverished children in the U.S. at risk for health problems that affect their development. The extreme effects of poor nutrition in developing countries are depicted frequently and dramatically in the media. However, inadequate nutrition among poor children in the U.S. also confers significant health consequences (Huston et al., 1994). In the U.S., iron deficiency anemia affects more than 20 percent of African-American and Hispanic children under the age of two (Pollitt, 1994). Prevalence rates of iron deficiency anemia are higher for minority children than for White children (Garcia Coll, 1990), and are increasing for all ethnic groups except Whites and Asians (Pollitt, 1994). Iron deficiency anemia often appears in concert with high blood levels of lead. Lowered performance on intellectual, developmental, and cognitive tasks is associated with iron deficiency anemia in children. Performance improves when iron stores are replenished (Pollitt, 1994).

Accidental injuries are the leading cause of childhood disability in the U.S. Similar to other health risks, poverty and minority status are associated with greater injury mortality in children. Olson, Becker, Wiggins, Key, and Samet (1990) found that Native American children in New Mexico had higher mortality rates from accidental injury than children from all other ethnic groups. Native Americans in New Mexico, similar to other minorities across the U.S., are more likely to experience poor housing, overcrowding, poor nutrition, lack of education, and limited access to medical care. In addition, poverty affects the ability of parents to maintain safe environments for their children. Across all ethnic groups in New Mexico, motor vehicle accidents, drownings, and fire accounted for most of the accidental injury mortality in children (Olson et al., 1990). Risk for childhood injury from motor vehicle accidents was related to alcohol abuse, poorly maintained vehicles, hazardous rural driving conditions, and lack of child restraints in vehicles—conditions exacerbated by poverty. Drownings were more frequent among impoverished children, probably due to limited access to safe recreational or swimming areas. In addition, children living in poverty are more likely to live in substandard housing that is more susceptible to fire. Finally, successful treatment of accidental injuries often depends on receiving immediate medical care that may not be available to impoverished rural families with limited access to telephones and emergency services.

Children, whether impoverished or not, are dependent on their parents and caregivers to attend to their health care. Impoverished parents frequently have greater life stressors, fewer resources, and more difficulty accessing health care than parents who are more affluent. As a result, impoverished children often suffer delays in obtaining health care, receive less adequate treatment once they enter the health care system, and have a poorer prognosis. Poor children receive less preventive health care and enter the acute care system later, resulting in greater need for high cost, high technology care that places a heavy financial and emotional burden on the family (Guendelman, 1983).

Childhood asthma is a common chronic illness in childhood that illustrates the interaction between minority status, poverty, and children's health (Wissow, Gittelsohn, Szklo, Starfield, & Mussman, 1988; Weitzman, Gortmaker, & Sobol, 1990). Approximately 12 percent of African-American children and 9 percent of White children in the U.S. suffer from asthma. Despite similar prevalence rates, the asthma death rate for African-American children is almost six times that of White children (Wissow et al., 1988). Morbidity and mortality from childhood asthma increased in the past decade, primarily among African-American and impoverished children (Butz et al., 1994) and particularly among inner-city children (Call, Smith, Morris, Chapman, & Platts-Mills, 1992).

Despite numerous studies that corroborate this racial disparity in childhood asthma morbidity and mortality, socioeconomic and environmental conditions are more powerful explanatory factors than race. For example, hospitalizations for asthma were three times greater for African-American children than for White children in Maryland. However, when socioeconomic status was controlled, African-American and White children had identical rates of asthma-related hospitalizations (Wissow et al., 1988). Differences in asthma prevalence between African-American and White children in the Child Health Supplement to the 1981 National Health Interview Survey disappeared when social and environmental variables were controlled (Weitzman, Gortmaker, & Sobol, 1990). The evidence clearly indicates that children living in poverty have higher rates of asthma than children living in more affluent circumstances. In the United States, African-American children have a higher probability of living in poverty than White children (Weitzman, Gortmaker, & Sobol, 1990).

The relationship between poverty and childhood asthma is complex. Poverty is associated with increased prevalence and greater severity of childhood asthma, less preventive health care, and higher rates of hospitalization for asthma-related complications. Poverty is also associated with increased exposure to allergens that precipitate asthma. Mite sensitization is a major risk factor for asthma. In Atlanta, 86 percent of inner-city African-American children were exposed to high levels of mite and cockroach allergens in their homes and a high proportion of African-American children with asthma were sensitized to those allergens (Call et al., 1992). Despite the respiratory problems experienced by these children, their families lacked the resources for control of the offending allergens. Controlling mite and cockroach allergens requires removing carpets and upholstered furniture, commercial spraying, and providing plastic covers for pillows and mattresses. Low-income families with limited access to information about environmental management of asthma, and who live in rental or subsidized housing, may not be able to tear out carpeting or get access to efficient vacuum cleaners, rendering allergen control impossible (Butz et al., 1994; Call et al., 1992).

Poverty is also associated with under-diagnosis of childhood asthma, delays in receiving medical care, and more frequent use of emergency treatment (Butz et al., 1994). Under-diagnosis and delayed care, in turn, are associated with more severe symptoms and more frequent hospitalizations (Wissow et al., 1988). Successful asthma management requires preventive care and regular communication between families and health care providers. However, Butz and colleagues, in a study of asthmatic African-American children in Baltimore, found that use of regular preventive health services was rare, even though 81 percent of the children had symptoms severe enough to require asthma-control medication, and 29 percent had visited an emergency room for asthma-related complications in the preceding six months. Almost one-quarter of families reported they were unaware of a local clinic where care was available and didn't have a telephone to arrange a visit with a health care provider, leading to the use of emergency rather than preventive services for their children.

Health Implications of Racism, Acculturation, and Migration

Minority children are affected by racism, the stresses of acculturation, and migration and pre-migration experiences. These factors have a direct and an indirect impact: direct through the child's personal experience and indirect through the impact on the child's caregivers.

In the U.S., ethnic status is intertwined with the experience of racism. Racial and ethnic minorities cope with prejudice and discrimination, and repeatedly encounter negative stereotypes and limited views of their capabilities, aspirations, and expectations (Julian, McKenry, & McKelvey, 1994). Children and adults are affected differently depending on their experiences with racism and their personal resources. For example, the impact of encountering overt racism may be different for a child who is supported by a nurturant family than for a child whose self-worth is not affirmed within the family. Contrary to popular belief, African-American children from middle class families may be more exposed to overt racism than African-American children from lower socioeconomic status families, since middle-class African-American children have more contact with White children than African-American children who live in segregated neighborhoods (Robinson, 1989).

Historically, ethnic and cultural differences were viewed as pathological deviations from the White, Anglo-American norm (Spencer, 1990). Biological models purporting to explain racial and cultural differences legitimized assumptions about inferiority in groups that differed from White norms and ignored cultural, structural, and environmental explanations. Psychological and intellectual tests for children were based on norms from White, middle-class children and normative standards for child development were Eurocentric. Given that intellectual and cognitive testing often provided a basis for decisions about remedial care, educational programming, and residential placements, the use of White, middle-class normative standards had a profound effect on educational opportunities and aspirations for minority children (Spencer, 1990). Racial and cultural bias in testing has been the subject of passionate debate for many years (Marion, 1980), culminating in attempts to develop "culture-free" or "culture-appropriate" tests and limiting the use of intellectual and cognitive tests for educational and placement decisions. This creates ethical and practical dilemmas for professionals searching for objective standards to use in placement decisions affecting minority children. [While it would be tempting to dismiss biological models of racial inferiority as an historical phenomenon, a recently published book, *The Bell Curve: Intelligence and Class Structure in American Life* (Herrnstein & Murray, 1994) has resurrected vociferous debate about the inherent intellectual inferiority of African-Americans.]

Minority children and their families face a dual adjustment as they learn to live within their own culture and to function within the majority culture (Rounds, Weil, & Bishop, 1994). The ethnic culture imparts knowledge, values, and attitudes that influence coping within the family and the community (Pinderhughes, 1982). At the same time, minority group members are exposed to majority culture through institutions, mass media, advertising, public schooling, and exposure to mainstream fashions, holidays, and cultural heroes (de Anda, 1984). Bicultural socialization involves resolving conflicts between values and behaviors important in the two cultures. The success of bicultural adaptation varies greatly across individuals and cultures. For individuals and groups, bicultural adaptation is more successful when there is a high degree of commonality between cultures, when cognitive and problem-solving approaches are similar, when cultural models for adaptation are available, when individuals have facility in both languages, and when there is similarity in physical appearance between cultural or racial groups (de Anda, 1984).

For example, African-American culture has been influenced by mainstream American culture, African culture, and adaptations to racism, poverty, and oppression (Pinderhughes, 1982). Differences in exposure to these sources of culture produce diversity among African-American families. Some children and families resolve conflicts among these three value systems by identifying exclusively with one cultural system; others by attempting to integrate multiple systems. Because few African-Americans perceive themselves as being wholeheartedly welcomed into mainstream American culture, many African-American families have revived traditional African cultural values such as affiliation or collectivity (Pinderhughes, 1982).

Bicultural adaptation presents opportunities for conflict not only between members of majority and minority cultures, but also between generations within minority families. Parents and older family members of ethnic minority groups may strive to retain their traditional beliefs and values within the home and ethnic community in the face of overwhelming changes produced by their migration into a new culture. In contrast, children and adolescents from ethnic minority groups, by virtue of their greater exposure to mainstream American culture and language through schools and interactions with other young people, may seek to cast aside older ethnic traditions and values in favor of mainstream American behaviors and values. Hispanic adolescents exposed to mainstream American culture have found themselves alienated from older generations and the Hispanic community and criticized for becoming "agringado" (de Anda, 1984). Hispanic and mainstream American cultures differ in their views of appropriate ways for young adults to express maturity and responsibility. In the majority Anglo-American culture, young adults are expected to demonstrate responsibility and maturity by moving away from the family home and establishing an independent life before marriage. In contrast, in Hispanic culture, young adults are expected to demonstrate maturity and responsibility by remaining at home and contributing to the family, notably by providing for greater opportunities for their younger siblings. Leaving the family home to develop an independent life prior to marriage would be considered evidence of disregard for crucial family responsibilities (de Anda, 1984).

Differing values provide opportunities for misunderstanding between members of mainstream American and Hispanic cultures and between older, less acculturated Hispanic family members and more acculturated Hispanic youths. These intergenerational conflicts are often played out in the offices of school psychologists, social workers, and family practitioners. An Anglo-American counselor or health care provider who advises an Hispanic youth to move away from the family home to establish independence might contribute inadvertently to generational conflict and lose credibility with the family.

Immigration into a new country and a new culture introduces simultaneous family stressors, including economic hardship, limited job opportunities, unfamiliarity with the language and culture, education and qualifications which may not be recognized in the new country, and severed ties with family and social networks. As mentioned earlier, family relationships change when children and parents adapt to the new culture at different rates, resulting in intergenerational conflict (Elfert, Anderson, & Lai, 1991; Timberlake & Cook, 1984). Acculturation difficulties often are compounded by pre-migration experiences, particularly for refugees who were forced to flee their native countries with little preparation and few resources (Timberlake & Cook, 1984).

Refugees and immigrants often enter the health care system with health problems that differ from those of Anglo-American patients, and health care practitioners may be unfamiliar with the health problems encountered by patients from differing cultures. Refugees from Central America struggle with health problems ranging from malnutrition, parasitic infections, gastroenteritis, tuberculosis, and severe tooth decay, to post-traumatic stress disorder subsequent to torture and loss of family members (Magar, 1990; Pickwell & Warnock, 1994). Refugee children from Central America are susceptible to infections and enteric pathogens because of malnutrition, underdeveloped immune systems, poor hygiene practices, and close contact with adults and other children in overcrowded living conditions. In addition, refugee children rarely receive adequate immunizations, either in their home country, or after arrival in the U.S. Refugee children from Southeast Asia present with similar physical health problems, including tuberculosis, parasitic disease, hemoglobinopathies, hepatitis B, goiter, anemia, and low stature and weight (Fox, Cowell, & Montgomery, 1994). Studies of migrant and seasonal farm worker women, including Latina, Anglo, African-American, and Haitian, documented high rates of low birthweight, meningitis, seizures, pneumonia, burns, and dehydration among their children. In addition, fewer than half the children had received adequate immunizations against childhood illnesses (Watkins et al., 1994). One of this chapter's authors (JS) housed two exchange students from the Ivory Coast with her family in a small community in the southern U.S. Although malaria is endemic in West Africa, it is less common in the United States. When one of the youths experienced a recurrence of malaria, local health providers were not only uninformed, but believed that the disorder was highly contagious. In addition, medications were unavailable and had to be flown from a city many miles distant. Despite the fact that the youth was well informed about malaria and knew what medication had been used successfully in the past, he was unable to communicate his knowledge to health care workers who were less informed about his malady since it was not customarily seen in their practices.

Many refugee children, like their parents, experienced trauma escaping from their homes and subsequent confinement in crowded refugee camps. The negative effects of violence and trauma on adult survivors are well documented. However, until very recently, little information was available on the effects of violence and trauma on children, particularly refugee children. For refugee children, the effects of pre-migration violence and trauma are compounded by post-migration stressors such as low socioeconomic status, intergenerational conflict, acculturation, racial prejudice, language difficulties, and academic deficits. Practitioners who are not familiar with the child's history may find themselves dealing with a complex health care picture that includes psychosocial and physical stressors before and after migration.

Recent research with adolescent refugees who fled to the U.S. after the Pol Pot regime showed that traumatized Cambodian children exhibited symptoms markedly different from those of traumatized children from other cultural and ethnic groups (Kinzie, Sack, Angell, Manson, & Rath, 1986; Sack, Angell, Kinzie, & Rath, 1986).

More than four years after their arrival in the U.S., half of the Cambodian youths showed symptoms of depression and post-traumatic stress disorder. Many reported nightmares, exaggerated startle reactions, survivor guilt, sleep disturbances, concentration problems, loss of energy and interest, pessimistic outlook, and brooding—classic symptoms of post-traumatic stress disorder. American youths who had been exposed to violence and trauma showed symptoms of social impairment and antisocial, disruptive, or oppositional behavior. In contrast, none of the Cambodian youths exhibited antisocial behavior, truancy, or disruptive behavior in school. Rather, their symptoms were characterized by denial and avoidance, consistent with traditional Cambodian values of passive acceptance. In the classroom, the Cambodian students with post-traumatic stress disorders or depression were characterized by daydreaming, withdrawal, nonparticipation, and reduced academic performance. Anglo-American educators and clinicians, accustomed to the disruptive behavior of American youngsters exposed to trauma, might easily misinterpret or minimize symptoms of post-traumatic stress disorder in Cambodian refugees (Kinzie et al., 1986; Sack et al., 1986).

CROSS-CULTURAL PEDIATRIC CARE

In delivering cross cultural health care to children, the "identified patient," in the narrow sense of the word, is the child. However, it is the family that identifies symptoms, makes a decision to seek help, determines the appropriate source of care, seeks out assistance, interacts with health care providers, and is responsible for carrying out treatment regimens. Cultural considerations impact heavily on all aspects of the family's attempts to obtain health care for the child and on the health care provider's attempts to provide services to the child. Therefore, the needs of the child cannot be considered in isolation from the needs, resources, and constraints affecting the family.

Perspectives held by the family and by health care providers often differ and may give rise to misunderstandings that complicate their collaboration on the child's behalf. Minority children may receive poorer-quality health care for a variety of reasons, including cultural, linguistic, and institutional barriers to obtaining care, communication problems, and cultural insensitivity on the part of health care providers. Parental compliance with treatment recommendations is strongly related to their satisfaction with the provider. Satisfaction, in turn, extends largely from the family's experience of personal warmth and effective communication on the part of the provider. When this chain is disrupted, health care provision for the child is invariably affected.

Many health care providers express frustration in offering health services to families from dissimilar cultural and linguistic backgrounds. Health care professionals often feel that their ability to provide quality care is compromised by (1) linguistic differences; (2) differing cultural beliefs about help-seeking, illness, and appropriate treatment; and (3) parental noncompliance with their recommendations. At the same time, minority families may require more time and greater efforts from the health care provider before either the practitioner or the family can resolve the cultural differences that affect the child's treatment. For example, cultural reticence about communicating openly with authority figures may be misinterpreted, leading the practitioner to conclude that minority families are uncooperative or unconcerned about the welfare of their children. This, in turn, will affect the health care provider's expectations in future encounters with minority children and their families.

The challenges inherent in cross-cultural health care are experienced by the child and the family seeking care, by the individual practitioner providing care, and by health care institutions. Cross-cultural health care practice is affected by sociopolitical issues, by institutional demands and philosophies, and by the actions and beliefs of individual health practitioners, as well as by the children and families themselves. When values and expectations are congruent, all parties find the encounter satisfying. However, when there are differences in the expectations of the patient, provider, or setting, health care delivery is affected. In the next sections, we will examine each of these topics, focus on ways in which each affects cross-cultural care, and discuss possible solutions.

Aspects of Cross-Cultural Health Care That Are Affected by the Sociopolitical System

Health care providers are members of a unique "medical" culture with its own beliefs and values. However, first and foremost, they are members of a larger culture and are influenced by the beliefs and values inherent in the surrounding sociopolitical system. Although many health care providers from the majority Anglo-American culture feel that the values and beliefs within their own culture do not obscure their view of the values and beliefs of other cultures, Anglo-American majority culture is not neutral. One of the most pernicious effects of a majority culture is that it is perceived as essentially neutral by members of that culture, whereas persons from other cultures clearly recognize its inherent biases (Christensen, 1992).

Until very recently, most models of child development confounded socioeconomic background with ethnicity. Minority children and families who differed from majority norms were subject to remedial actions recommended by majority group professionals who had little understanding of the factors underlying ethnic differences (Garcia Coll, 1990; Spencer, 1990). Minority children are exposed to home environments characterized by cultural beliefs and practices different from those in Anglo-American homes. Although ethnic differences in child-rearing practices and beliefs are often viewed as deviations from the norm of Anglo-American child-rearing practices, it is more productive to view ethnic child-rearing practices as instrumental in shaping the competencies required of adults in different cultural groups. Minority group mothers often differ from Anglo-American mothers in their style of teaching and interacting with their children. However, different parenting styles of ethnic mothers assist their children to acquire communication and cognitive skills that are functional in the cultural and environmental contexts in which minority children live (Garcia Coll, 1990).

Harwood (1992) compared concepts of desirable and undesirable childhood attachment among Anglo and Puerto Rican mothers. The Anglo mothers were White, non-Hispanic, born and educated in mainland U.S., and spoke English as their first language. The Puerto Rican mothers were born in Puerto Rico, spoke Spanish as their first language, and had resided in mainland U.S. for a mean of 8 years. All mothers rated vignettes of attachment behavior in toddlers exposed to unfamiliar situations. In rating the behavior of toddlers, Anglo mothers focused on the presence or absence of individual autonomy. In contrast, Puerto Rican mothers focused on the child's ability to maintain proper demeanor in public. Overall, Anglo mothers focused on the development of personal competencies and independence and Puerto Rican mothers focused on the close bond between mother and child. This study illustrates the potential for conflict between parents and health care providers from different ethnic groups, where adults are likely to focus on different aspects of a child's behavior and interpret behavior differently depending on their own cultural backgrounds and contexts. An Anglo mother is apt to view a Puerto Rican toddler as clingy and baby-like, while a Puerto Rican mother is apt to view an Anglo toddler as undisciplined and badly behaved.

Another sociopolitical issue that affects minority patients arises from stereotyping. In this section, we will discuss the overall cultural impact of stereotyping; in a later section of the chapter, we will discuss the impact of stereotyping of minority group members by health care practitioners. Stereotyping can be defined as a conception about a person or group that obscures recognition of individual differences within the group (Lum, 1982). Stereotyping takes two forms: stereotyping across minority groups and stereotyping within minority groups. Stereotyping across minority groups occurs when members of other cultures ascribe particular characteristics to members of one minority group relative to other minority groups. For example, Blacks are commonly stereotyped as loud, disruptive, and prone to violence; Mexicans as shiftless and passionate; Asians as compliant, law-abiding, and passive; and Native Americans as childlike, irresponsible, and dangerous (Lum, 1982). Stereotyping within cultural groups occurs when the diversity within cultural and ethnic groups is not recognized and when all individuals from a particular minority group are assumed to share common characteristics, without recognition of their individuality.

Asians and Pacific Islanders in the U.S. provide a vivid illustration of stereotyping. Asian and Pacific Islanders are often stereotyped as "a model minority," obscuring dramatic differences in cultural origins, immigration history, and length of stay in the U.S. (Gould, 1988). The majority culture's belief in the ready assimilation of Asian and Pacific Islanders has led many individuals to question the appropriateness of offering the same protections and social services to Asians and Pacific Islanders that are offered to other disadvantaged minority groups. The stereotype of the "model assimilated minority" obscures reality for many Asians and Pacific Islanders in the U.S (Gould, 1988).

The tendency to view Asian and Pacific Islanders as essentially similar belies the fact that there are more than twenty Asian and five Pacific Islander groups represented in the 1980 U.S. census. The major groups include Chinese, Filipino, Japanese, Vietnamese, Korean, Asian Indian, Hawaiian, Guamian, and Samoan. Each of these major groups is ethnically, culturally, and linguistically different. In addition, they differ in their circumstances of migration and in their acculturation into U.S. mainstream culture, including economic culture. For example, although Japanese, Chinese, Filipinos, Koreans, and Asian Indians exceeded the national median income in 1980, Hawaiians, Guamians, Samoans, and all other Asian and Pacific Islanders fell below the national median income (Gould, 1988).

In addition to differences between ethnic subgroups, dramatic variation exists among individuals within specific ethnic groups. Although the Japanese had the lowest percentage of families with incomes below the poverty level (4.2 percent), 40.7 percent of Japanese poor families were headed by single females. Among the Chinese, whose median incomes exceeded the national median in 1980, 10.5 percent of families fell below the poverty line. These differences within and across ethnic groups of Asians and Pacific Islanders are obscured when the majority culture stereotypes all Asian and Pacific Islander groups as similar in characteristics and needs.

Stereotyping also occurs within Black and Hispanic racial groups. A black woman and her child entering a physician's office in the U.S. are likely to be assumed to be African-American and acculturated to mainstream America. In fact, they may be recent or long-standing immigrants from Jamaica, Trinidad, Haiti, or other Caribbean countries, members of one of hundreds of tribal groups from dozens of African countries, Canadian descendants of runaway slaves, or immigrants from Britain or other European countries. Similarly, individuals who are considered by virtue of their common language and Spanish surnames to be members of a homogeneous Hispanic group must be recognized as members of a variety of Hispanic subgroups with highly divergent characteristics, countries of origin, customs, degree of acculturation, and immigration histories (Schur, Bernstein, & Berk, 1987). Hispanic groups in the U.S. include refugees from a wide variety of Central and South American countries, Mexicans, Cubans, and Puerto Ricans.

Institutional Barriers to Cross-Cultural Care

Institutional barriers affect access to services and delivery of effective health care for minority children and their families.

Access Barriers

Financial, institutional, and systemic barriers often prevent families from obtaining health care for their children, particularly among low-income, culturally diverse families in rural areas (Cornelius, 1993; Malach & Segel, 1990). Institutional barriers are compounded by linguistic and cultural barriers, often resulting in underutilization of health services for children of minority families (Chan, 1990; Garcia Coll, 1990). Barriers affecting access to medical care for children include the cost of medical care, availability of health care providers, and travel and waiting time, in addition to impediments created by differences in education, income, attitudes toward health care delivery, language, and knowledge

about health care (Cornelius, 1993). In addition, the lack of appropriate outreach and culturally sensitive service models hamper minority families' access to health care (Chan, 1990).

Affordability and availability are major barriers to health care access affecting minority children. Data from the 1987 National Medical Expenditure Survey (Cornelius, 1993) showed that while 45 percent of African-American and 39 percent of Hispanic children in the U.S. lived in poverty, fewer than half of these children were reached by Medicaid, a public insurance program designed primarily for the poor. In 1987, 38 percent of poor White children were without health insurance, compared with 30 percent of poor African-American children and 49 percent of poor Hispanic children (Cornelius, 1993). Eligibility for public insurance programs and reimbursement levels for medical care vary dramatically across geographic areas. Sixty-two percent of African-American children live in the southern U.S. where, in many states, low payment thresholds for Aid for Families with Dependent Children reduce the number of families eligible for Medicaid (Cornelius, 1993).

Limited availability of health care providers creates additional barriers to medical care access for minority children. Between 1978 and 1987, Medicaid participation rates by pediatricians dropped from 85 percent to 77 percent, reducing the availability of pediatric care for poor children (Cornelius, 1993). Residents in impoverished inner city and rural areas have a smaller range of choices for health care providers than residents in more affluent urban areas. Given the scarcity of outreach programs and community facilities for minority families, access to health care for minority children is all too often limited simply because families do not know where to go for health care services (Chan, 1990).

Affordability and availability affect the percentage of minority group children who have access to a "usual source of medical care." In 1987, uninsured children were twice as likely as insured children to have no usual source of care. Twenty-eight per cent of uninsured African-American children had no usual source of care, compared with 25 percent of uninsured Hispanic children and 19 percent of uninsured White children. For children from many minority groups, public health facilities or hospital emergency rooms constitute their usual source of care. In contrast, 90 percent of children with private health insurance had a physician as a usual source of care. In one year, 55 percent of insured children had a routine visit to a health care provider and 87 percent had a dental visit. Among uninsured children, only 18 percent of White children, 11 percent of African-American children, and 11 percent of Hispanic children had a routine visit to a health care provider. Twenty-eight per cent of uninsured White children reported a dental visit, compared to 19 percent of uninsured African-American children and 14 percent of uninsured Hispanic children (Cornelius, 1993). These figures illustrate the disparity in use of medical services among insured and uninsured children from different ethnic groups.

Hispanic immigrants to the U.S. under-utilize health care relative to members of other minority groups and are less likely to have a usual source of health care for their children (Zambrana, Ell, Dorrington, Wachsman, & Hodge, 1994). Compared to Cuban and Mexican immigrants to the U.S., Puerto Ricans are more likely to rely on hospital outpatient departments or emergency rooms as their usual source of care and are least likely to have private health insurance (Schur, Bernstein, & Berk, 1987). The experiences of Hispanic immigrants described below illustrate the unmet health and social needs and the barriers experienced by many minority group members in gaining access to health care.

Zambrana et al. (1994) surveyed Hispanic mothers (Mexican and Central American immigrants) who brought a child to a pediatric emergency room. Many of the mothers delayed seeking health care, despite the perceived seriousness of their children's symptoms. Mothers reported that their children had been sick an average of 9.7 days before the current emergency room visit. Although two-thirds of the mothers reported their child had a usual source of health care, 36 percent relied on a pediatric emergency room, and 43 percent relied on public health facilities as the usual source of care. Fewer than 8 percent identified a private physician as their usual source of pediatric care. Mexican immigrants were 1 1/2 times more likely than Central American immigrants to use the emergency room for routine pediatric care.

The study provided a gloomy picture of pediatric health care for immigrant Mexican and Central American children in Los Angeles, with delays in seeking treatment compounded by reliance on settings, such as emergency rooms and public health facilities, that offer little continuity of care. Hispanic mothers reported structural, financial, cultural, and linguistic barriers to obtaining health services. The mothers identified barriers such as long waits in public clinics, long waits for appointments, lack of health insurance, high costs for medical care, lack of bilingual and bicultural health service providers, and lack of confidence in American-style health care. They also described personal barriers, such as limited English language skills, financial problems, lack of adequate employment, depression or nervousness, and feelings of being overwhelmed and unable to cope with everyday life, that interfered with their ability to obtain health services for their children. A major concern for undocumented immigrants was the fear of being discovered and deported if they sought care for their children from a health facility (Magar, 1990; Pickwell & Warnock, 1994; Zambrana et al., 1994). Other research confirms this picture of limited access to health services for Hispanic immigrants in the U.S. However, these limitations are not restricted to a single minority and are more likely a common denominator affecting many racial and cultural minorities.

California's Proposition 187, which withholds all but emergency health services from undocumented immigrants, promises to add to the misery of immigrant families needing health care services for their children. Fears of deportation and markedly decreased access to medical services will undoubtedly lead to delays in seeking treatment for even life-threatening medical conditions and will reduce access to preventive services such as prenatal care, childhood immunization, and well-baby clinics.

Barriers to Effective Practice

Once a minority family negotiates the access barriers and enters the health care system, other impediments arise to interfere with service provision. All too often, health practitioners are neither bilingual nor bicultural, jeopardizing communication between providers and their patients (Chan, 1990) and increasing the likelihood of diagnostic errors due to miscommunication (Rogler, 1993; Rogler & Cortes, 1993). When there are significant language barriers between practitioners and their patients, interpreters may provide a satisfactory solution. Because of the shortage of trained medical interpreters in most health care settings, interpreters are often lay translators recruited from minority communities or bilingual family members pressed into service as translators. However, even under the best of circumstances, using interpreters to translate between patients and providers can be fraught with difficulties.

Differences in specific cultural background and socioeconomic status between interpreters and patients may lead to problems. Highly educated or acculturated translators may be reluctant to translate accurately if the translator feels that the patient's statements reflect ignorance or superstition. In addition, translators may speak a formal or "textbook" version of the language that is unfamiliar to the families they are attempting to serve (Lynch & Stein, 1987). Many recent immigrants to the U.S. are not literate even in their primary language. Lay translators are apt to know little about medical terminology and may have difficulty translating precise medical terms or instructions, particularly since many

Western medical terms and assumptions about illness do not translate into other languages or cultural belief systems. Family members have difficulty translating information that is considered sensitive or taboo (Clark, 1983). An adolescent son pressed into service as an interpreter may have difficulty translating information about his mother's pregnancy or delivery of a younger sibling, information which may be vital to a pediatrician examining the younger child, but taboo for the older son.

The context within which health care is provided in this country is often foreign and overwhelming to individuals from other cultures. In many health care institutions, the physical setting is formal, bureaucratic, and foreign to many minority group members. Crowded waiting rooms, sterile offices, intimidating equipment, medical charts, forms to be filled out, and a bewildering variety of individuals from receptionists to nurses to physicians to lab technicians await minority families seeking health care for their children.

Another major barrier to effective service delivery is the approach to time that characterizes Western health care institutions (Rogler & Cortes, 1993). Appointments are usually scheduled well in advance, with little attention to the patient's schedule, transportation difficulties, child-care needs, or occupational responsibilities. Few clinics or health care institutions offer evening or weekend treatment hours that would be more convenient for wage-earning families with small children. This may explain the over-reliance on emergency rooms for treatment since they are one of the few health care facilities that are available 24 hours a day, seven days a week. In addition to scheduling appointments at times that are convenient for health care providers but inconvenient for children and their parents, the formal medical system places great emphasis on remembering appointments scheduled long in advance, showing up on time (often only to sit in a crowded waiting room), scheduling repeat diagnostic appointments the relationship of which to the problem at hand may be unclear to the patient, and allotting limited time for appointments. Individuals seeking treatment may find it difficult to understand the long waits typical in many health care facilities, particularly the public institutions that provide services to poor and minority parents. It may appear incongruous to a family to wait several weeks for an appointment and then sit for several hours in the waiting room, taking time from other responsibilities.

For members from minority groups with a "present" rather than a "future" orientation to time, scheduling appointments long in advance of pressing need may be foreign. In addition, for minority ethnic or racial groups who value rapport and require time in which to "tell their story," the standard 20-minute appointment may be unacceptably short. Patients may leave feeling that the health care provider was brusque and preoccupied with time to the detriment of developing a therapeutic relationship with the child and family. In many clinics and public health care facilities, families seldom see the same health care practitioner at subsequent visits. Families must adapt, not only to health care practitioners who are likely to be from different cultural, linguistic, and socioeconomic groups, but also to a different therapist or practitioner at every visit (Rogler & Cortes, 1993). Similarly, members of many minority groups find that the Western treatment model where different "aspects" of the patient are handled by different practitioners is culturally unacceptable.

If the formal medical system appears impersonal and segmented to members of many minority groups, it is of little surprise that many minority patients "drop out" of the formal system and seek treatment from sources that may be more culturally compatible. Approximately half of Hispanics seeking assistance for mental health problems drop out of treatment after the first session, an attrition rate dramatically higher than for individuals with similar problems but from mainstream American culture (Rogler & Cortes, 1993). Health practitioners with little appreciation of the structural, cultural, and linguistic barriers facing Hispanic families seeking health services might be tempted to disparage Hispanic families for their apparent lack of commitment to treatment.

Other barriers interfere with the ability of minority families to follow the health care regimens that are prescribed for their children. Grover, Berkowitz, and Lewis (1994) interviewed English-speaking and Spanish-speaking parents who brought children to the emergency room of a large, urban hospital. Before departure, parents were questioned about their child's diagnosis, medications, care instructions, and follow-up appointments. For both English-speaking and Spanish-speaking parents, recall was poor. Overall, only 38 percent of parents recalled how to administer all medications and only 24 percent of parents recalled the names of prescribed medications.

Such low recall has implications for subsequent compliance with treatment regimens, since the care a child receives at home depends on parental understanding of the diagnosis, treatment, and schedule for follow-up appointments. Written instructions did not enhance recall, perhaps because many parents had difficulty understanding written instructions. Grover, Berkowitz, and Lewis (1994) suggested that at least part of the explanation for poor levels of parental recall may lie in the typical emergency room setting. The nursing staff that typically reinforces medication and care instructions often do so at noisy discharge desks, surrounded by distractions and interruptions, making it difficult for parents to comprehend and retain instructions. These findings suggest that many of the children who routinely receive their health care in public clinics and emergency rooms may not receive adequate treatment after they return home.

Parental dissatisfaction with medical care is also implicated in poor compliance with medical instructions, since compliance is lower when parental expectations about the interaction with the health care provider are not met (Francis, Korsch, & Morris, 1969; Schwartz-Lookinland, McKeever, & Saputo, 1989). Dissatisfaction is related to parental perceptions of a lack of warmth from the practitioner, failure to acknowledge parental concerns and expectations, unclear explanations of the diagnosis and cause of illness, and the practitioner's use of medical jargon (Schwartz-Lookinland, McKeever, & Saputo, 1989). The practitioner's demeanor toward patients and ability to communicate are vitally important to ensure parents' subsequent compliance with treatment instructions for their children.

Poor compliance with medical regimens is costly in terms of continued poor health, discomfort and inconvenience for the child, repeated diagnostic tests, and increased costs to the family and the health care system. Schwartz-Lookinland et al. (1989) evaluated a program to enhance compliance with an antibiotic regimen among Hispanic mothers whose children were diagnosed with otitis media. Hispanic parents prefer short-term therapy and administer medication only while the child is symptomatic, which may result in an incomplete course of antibiotic treatment. All mothers enrolled in the study received careful explanations of otitis media and instructions for administering antibiotics with an oral medication syringe. A Spanish-speaking nurse practitioner provided explanations, instructions, and demonstrated the oral syringe. All mothers demonstrated correct use of the medication syringe during the visit. Mothers in the experimental group also received two handouts, one written in Spanish and a second with pictorial instructions for mothers with limited reading skills. There was no difference in compliance between mothers in the experimental group and the control group. In both groups, 60 percent to 70 percent of the mothers administered at least 80 percent of the prescribed medication.

Schwartz-Lookinland et al. (1989) speculated on the reasons for the high compliance in both conditions, since many of the families were undocumented aliens who had little previous exposure to American medical care. However, at the health clinic where the study was conducted, families were served by a Spanish-speaking nurse practitioner who saw the mother and child on each visit to the clinic, resulting in familiarity and continuity of care. In addition, medical services and medications were provided without cost, reducing temptation for mothers to save medication for use on another occasion or with another child.

In fairness to practitioners, it is also important to focus on institutional barriers that interfere with providers' abilities to provide quality services for minority patients. Rigid schedules, crowded waiting rooms, the lack of time to spend with individual patients and their families, fragmented services, cumbersome referral systems, lack of continuity in care, too few case managers, and a shortage of skilled interpreters all affect the care a practitioner is able to provide to minority patients. Many barriers are related to lack of cultural sensitivity in planning health service institutions. However, many are the result of financial constraints and the need to provide services to large numbers of patients with limited staff and resources. This is particularly true in the public health institutions and hospital emergency rooms that typically serve impoverished and uninsured minority children and their families. Providing adequate cross-cultural health care can be frustrating and difficult for practitioners under the best of circumstances. However, with limited resources, difficulties increase and minority families may be blamed for the practitioners' frustrations. For example, a medical resident (who, interestingly, was a minority group member herself) at a busy public institution described her feelings about providing services to minority patients and their families. "When we're feeling relaxed, benevolent, on top of things, we can naturally find such patients 'interesting,' 'poignant,' 'exotic,' or 'just like us.' But when we happen to get upright, bone-tired, dizzy from hours without sleep, and umpteen patients behind? They may suddenly turn into time-consuming monsters, 'irresponsible,' 'deceptive,' 'childish,' 'unreasonable,' and so on. And in that case, goodbye to our cross-cultural good intentions. Sure, it's a muddle, unpleasant, guilt-making, you name it, but hey, welcome to the r-e-a-l world!" (Marcus & Marcus, 1993, pp. 338–339).

Shortage of Minority Health Care Providers

The shortage of minority health care providers is a serious problem in the U.S. (Atkinson, Spratley, & Simpson, 1994; Trevino et al., 1994). Although the number of minority students entering training programs for health-related professions has increased in the past few years, the increase has not kept pace with the increase in the population of medically underserved minority group members. In 1968, only 4 percent of U.S. medical students were members of minority groups. By 1989, this increased to 15 percent (Trevino et al.). However, fewer than 10 percent of physicians in the U.S. are African-American, Hispanic, or Native American, despite the fact that those groups comprise 22 percent of the population (Atkinson, Spratley, & Simpson, 1994). In 1991, only 2.4 percent of physicians in the U.S. were of Hispanic origin, a minority group which grew at five times the rate of the general population between 1980 and 1990 (Trevino et al.).

A shortage of minority health care providers reduces the availability of health care for members of minority groups and reduces the probability of culturally sensitive and appropriate treatment. Black and Hispanic physicians are more likely to practice in low-income, underserved areas and to serve patients from minority groups (Atkinson, Spratley, & Simpson, 1994; Davidson & Montoya, 1987). About three-quarters of Mexican American physicians trained in Californian medical schools between 1971 and 1977 practiced in Critical Health Manpower Shortage Areas. In contrast, fewer than 10 percent of White, non-Hispanic medical students planned to pursue medical practice in shortage areas (Trevino et al., 1994). This is true for other health professionals as well. Of minority students graduated from California dental schools between 1969 and 1975, 85 percent served patient loads that were more than 50 percent minority and more than one-third had patient loads that were more than 90 percent minority (Trevino et al.). Training larger numbers of minority group medical practitioners, including physicians, speech pathologists, psychologists, and health educators, might yield more effective treatment outcomes and higher treatment compliance among minority patients. Training health care providers from minority groups also has the potential to improve access to culturally sensitive and high-quality health care services for minorities in the U.S.

Practitioner Level Issues Affecting Cross-Cultural Health Care

The previous section described institutional parameters that affect the ability of minority families to obtain health care for their children and that affect the quality of health care provided to minority families. The quality of care, family satisfaction, and provider satisfaction is largely determined by the interaction between the prac-

titioner and the family seeking health services. The practitioner must be willing to take into account the entire psychosocial context of the family and the child (Lum, 1982). In this section, we will focus on practitioner characteristics and behaviors that influence the health care transaction.

Health Care Beliefs

Health care practitioners, by and large, are trained within a biomedical perspective and provide their services from within that framework of beliefs. In delivering cross-cultural care, all too often the practitioner operates from one set of beliefs about health, illness, and treatment and the patient (in this case, the child and his or her caregivers) operates from an incompatible set of beliefs. Although incompatible assumptions can arise when the family and the health provider are members of the same culture, the potential for misunderstanding and miscommunication is more pronounced when the family and provider are from different cultural backgrounds. Differences between medical and lay cultures are compounded by differences between majority and minority cultures.

A useful structure for understanding culturally different conceptions of illness, disease, and treatment is provided by Kleinman and his colleagues (Kleinman, 1978; Kleinman, Eisenberg, & Good, 1978) who distinguish between "illness" and "disease." "Disease denotes a malfunctioning in or maladaptation of biological and/or psychological processes. Illness, on the other hand, signifies the experience of disease (or perceived disease) and society's reaction to disease. Illness is the way the sick person, his family, and his social network perceive, label, explain, evaluate, and respond to disease" (Kleinman, 1978, p. 88). Because health care providers focus on biological malfunctioning and patients and their families focus on the experience of illness, providers and families bring different perspectives, experiences, and expectations to the health care interaction. Health care providers trained in the biomedical model focus on identifying the malfunction, determining its proximal cause, and devising a treatment. In contrast, patients focus on their experience with the disease or condition. The patient's experience of illness may not conform to the health care provider's conception about disease management, particularly if the patient is a member of a minority group that does not subscribe to a Western biomedical model of disease and treatment.

Health care systems operate within three domains: the professional domain that includes nursing, medicine, and other professionals; the popular domain that includes the family and social network; and the folk domain that relies on nonprofessional and traditional healers (Kleinman, 1978). Each domain is a sociocultural system with its own beliefs, values, norms, and explanatory models of illness and health. Patients and health care providers are likely to hold different beliefs about the causes, severity, and course of illness, and about optimal treatment. Failure to recognize conflicting perspectives predisposes the provider and the patient to misunderstanding, with an increased risk of ineffective treatment, particularly when the health care provider and the patient are members of different cultural or racial groups.

For an example, we can look to the experience of Chinese immigrant families with ill or disabled children. These families find themselves caught between familiar Chinese medical traditions and unfamiliar Western biomedical beliefs about disease and treatment. Elfert, Anderson, and Lai (1991) compared Euro-Canadian families and Chinese immigrant families faced with chronic pediatric illness or disability. Not surprisingly, Chinese parents were more dissatisfied with treatment than Euro-Canadian parents. A disabled child's Chinese father described the contrast between Western and Chinese medicine as "their [Chinese] type of cure is almost like digging up the roots, so that once you take up the whole root there won't be any more problems. Western medicine . . . it's like taking out the stem but not the roots" (Elfert, Anderson, & Lai, 1991, p. 117). Chinese families experienced conflict between the goals of Western medicine and traditional Chinese medicine. Western medical practitioners sought to manage what they perceived as a chronic illness; in contrast, traditional Chinese practitioners sought to cure the "root" of the problem, restoring the child to normal.

These two systems of medicine have fundamentally contradictory goals. Given this incompatibility, it is not surprising that Chinese families and Anglo-American providers find themselves at odds with one another. A likely scenario is that families will be dissatisfied with the progress of treatment and feel misunderstood regarding their concerns for their child's future, while providers will be mystified by the family's apparent indifference to management of the child's disability. Another example of misunderstanding between these two cultures is that Chinese immigrant parents may discontinue appointments for diagnostic procedures that health care providers consider essential. However, the parents, who have a different view of medical treatment, do not perceive any relationship between the diagnostic procedures (which do not produce a "cure") and their goal of returning the child to normal (Elfert, Anderson, & Lai, 1991). Their cultural system leads Chinese families to

expect that practitioners will provide direct interventions and immediate symptom relief. When this expectation is not fulfilled, Chinese families may be unwilling to embark on prolonged assessments or diagnostic tests that are, in terms of their goals, ineffectual.

Western medical practitioners who assume that extensive testing prior to treatment is simply good medical practice may find themselves dismayed when ethnic families do not share this assumption. Mainstream health practitioners also are likely to encounter different views from their minority patients about what constitutes "sickness." Practitioners define sickness in terms of laboratory and other tests, which may have little meaning to patients in the absence of culturally defined symptoms of sickness, such as pain (Clark, 1983). When these different assumptions about diagnosis and treatment are not recognized and discussed by the health practitioner and the family, cultural differences may be overlooked in favor of less helpful attributions such as "That doctor doesn't know what he's doing; my child is still sick" on the part of parents and "Minority parents just don't care about their children; they won't even come in for tests" on the part of health care providers.

Stereotyping

An earlier section in this chapter discussed the effects of racism and stereotyping on minority health care consumers. In this section we will discuss some of the issues that arise when providers stereotype children and their families based on race or ethnicity. Health care providers with limited cross-cultural knowledge or experience are apt to be unfamiliar with the great linguistic, ethnic, and cultural diversity that exists within broadly-defined cultural and ethnic groups. One of the authors of this chapter (JS) once studied the traditional and Western medical care systems in Cameroon, West Africa. Within the country, there are 236 distinct ethnic groups, each with medical traditions closely tied to its subculture (St. Lawrence & Azevedo, 1989). Many providers are unfamiliar with the differences between nationalities, much less the tremendous diversity within nationalities. As a result, there is often little recognition of the tremendous cultural diversity that exists among different Hispanic/Latino, Southeast Asian, or Black cultures.

As mentioned earlier, Southeast Asians and Pacific Islanders are all too often viewed as a monolithic group, despite the tremendous racial and ethnic diversity that exists within these broad groups. Within Southeast Asia, each country has several languages, including a national language and languages spoken by ethnic subgroups. The dominant language of a particular individual may be the national language or the language of his or her ethnic subgroup. Redick and Wood (1982) describe a Vietnamese youth newly arrived in the U.S. who was unable to communicate with the interpreter hired by the agency that sponsored his relocation. Unknowingly, the sponsor had engaged a Cambodian interpreter. Redick and Wood stress that not only are there numerous ethnic and linguistic groups represented under the rubric of "Southeast Asian," many of these groups have long histories of conflict with one another. Well-intentioned but uninformed attempts to provide interpreters may result not only in misunderstanding, but also in conflict when linguistic and ethnic diversity are not taken into account.

Culturally competent practice with African-Americans, as well as other minority groups, requires sensitivity to the risk of stereotyping. Health care providers frequently make sweeping generalizations about African-American families without regard to the differences in individual families (Dillon, 1994). Given the cultural heterogeneity in African-American families, there is no "typical African-American family." Middle-class African-American families may be assumed to be impoverished, and responsible and concerned parents may be assumed to be irresponsible and uncaring, based on negative stereotypes of African-American families. Canino and Spurlock (1994) describe African-American parents who were not contacted about problems their child was having in school. When the parents finally learned about the school's attempts to remediate the problems, they discovered that they had not been contacted because of stereotyped assumptions that African-American families do not care about the education of their children.

Communication Skills

A practitioner's ability to develop an effective working relationship with the family is critical to the success of interventions with children, regardless of whether the practitioner and family hail from different cultural or ethnic groups (Kalmanson & Seligman, 1992). A critical requirement in developing an effective working relationship is the practitioner's ability to communicate successfully with family members. Many health care providers focus on the instrumental elements of communication with patients—the provider's ability to elicit information from the family, explain diagnostic procedures and treatment, and instruct family members in caregiving skills. However, equally critical is the ability to listen perceptively and to inspire trust and confidence, thereby enhancing the willingness of parents to comply with treatment procedures for the child (Kalmanson &

Seligman, 1992). Effective communication between the health care provider and the family is central to effective cross-cultural health care.

Communication between mainstream practitioners and ethnic minority patients is complex and difficult. Patients need time to "tell their story," so that practitioners develop an understanding of the context in which the health problem occurs. Context includes beliefs about health and illness, worries, concerns, resources, and the myriad everyday problems that face minority families and their children. Marcus and Marcus (1993), in describing communication between mainstream practitioners and minority patients, argue that "each medical misfortune comes embedded in a dense narrative which contains opposed assumptions, hoarded misinformation, nostalgia for native remedies, and chronic skepticism about our good will and competence" (p. 336). Presenting symptoms frequently mask cultural and psychosocial problems that cannot be addressed unless the practitioner is able to listen effectively, provide continuity of care, and allow time to build rapport. Unfortunately, dealing with the complex social and health needs of minority children and their families takes time. By virtue of their cultural and linguistic differences, minority patients are apt to require additional time and energy, which the provider may not have available.

Parents with ill or disabled children experience concern and anxiety that can be compounded by fears of interacting with health care practitioners. A frequent complaint of minority families is that health care providers use complex medical jargon that is difficult to understand, particularly for individuals with limited facility in English. Minority parents may feel confused or intimidated by medical language or may feel that their childrens' problems are viewed as evidence of parental shortcomings. Health care providers who fail to recognize the intense emotions experienced by parents of sick or disabled children may find that parents appear to distance themselves from providing care for the child, avoid asking questions, or fail to follow through on recommendations (Kalmanson & Seligman, 1992). Providers may feel frustrated with parents, who in turn feel dissatisfied with the practitioner, culminating in a spiral in which both parties feel resentment and the child may not receive the treatment she or he needs.

Providers must take time to provide emotional and concrete support for parents. While some instances of poor cross-cultural communication result from linguistic differences between provider and family, the effects of linguistic differences are compounded by poor communication skills on the part of providers. In particular, failing to attach importance to effective listening, taking insufficient time to develop rapport with families and children, not allowing families and children time to "tell their story," and making limited efforts to understand the unique cultural and socioeconomic situation of the family interfere with forming an effective therapeutic alliance on the child's behalf.

Providers can benefit from familiarity with the differences in patterns of nonverbal communication between different cultures (Clark, 1983). Being unaware of the "messages" contained in different patterns of nonverbal communication across cultures can predispose health care providers and patients to misunderstandings and negative attributions. For example, a well-intentioned White health care provider might go out of his or her way to enhance rapport with an African-American family, only to discover that every attempt has backfired. Unfortunately, the well-intentioned health care provider is likely to resort to methods that would be effective with White families and their children—making direct eye contact, speaking informally, using first names, explaining professional qualifications, and smiling. Unfortunately, those rapport-enhancing behaviors are likely to be misinterpreted by African-American families.

McNeely and Badami (1984) illustrate numerous misunderstandings between members of White majority and African-American minority cultures arising from differences in nonverbal behavior and communication styles. When listening, White Americans gaze directly at the person speaking, whereas African-Americans look away frequently. Within each culture, these patterns of eye contact are attentive and respectful to the listener. However, the well-intentioned health provider making direct eye contact while his African-American patients are speaking is likely to be perceived as hostile or aggressive. Conversely, the practitioner is apt to misinterpret the African-American style of looking away while he is speaking as evidence of disinterest, rudeness, or lack of alertness. Differences in patterns of eye contact between cultures have the potential to create difficulties in establishing trust and rapport between parents and health care providers from different cultural groups.

African-Americans and White Americans also have different methods for establishing credibility and professional status. The White health practitioner is likely to refer to training and degrees to reassure the African-American family about his or her qualifications. However, to the African-American family, formal training and degrees are less important in establishing credibility than personal experiences and presentation. The White professional may feel surprised and dismayed when African-American parents appear more interested in personal information about the provider, such as years of

experience, residence in the community, marital status, and familiarity with ethnic groups than in his or her impressive academic qualifications (McNeely & Badami, 1984). This is also true for Asian families (Fong, 1994).

The White health care provider may routinely use first names to create an atmosphere of equality and comfort. However, African-Americans prefer to be addressed by surnames and titles and prefer a pattern of formality that certifies that the relationship is one of equality and respectful distance. African-American patients may feel that they are being denied respect, particularly if the professional introduces him or herself by title and surname and addresses the patient by first name. For African-Americans, this practice hearkens back to a history of slavery and racism where only Whites were addressed by surnames and titles. Conversely, White care professionals may misinterpret African-American requests to use titles as arrogant, distant, and unfriendly (McNeely & Badami, 1984). This preference for formal address was observed by one of this chapter's authors (GE) in her work with the public health care system in Kenya. In general, Western health care professionals used an informal style of address which created discomfort, not only among Kenyan patients who were uncertain of the qualifications or roles of the *wazungu* (White) doctors, but also among Kenyan health care professionals.

Whites indicate their intended friendliness by smiling at strangers and White health professionals are likely to smile at patients to enhance comfort and rapport. However, African-Americans are likely to interpret "social smiling" as superficial and insincere. Health care providers may find that smiling to create rapport in an early interaction with an African-American child and family may be counterproductive if the family perceives the practitioner to be superficial and insincere, and views the smile as evidence that White people cannot be trusted (McNeely & Badami, 1984). Compared to White Americans, African-Americans are more likely to evidence "ecosystem distrust," a "tendency to distrust institutions, white people, and even other blacks" (McNeely & Badami, 1984, p. 25). Whites may perceive distrust as evidence that African-Americans are paranoid, hypersensitive, or antisocial; whereas, for African-Americans, distrust is perceived as adaptive for survival in an often hostile world.

Another example of the potential for confusion and misunderstanding implicit in different patterns of nonverbal communication across cultures was experienced by the second author of this chapter (JS) during a summer in India. In the U.S., nodding the head up and down communicates agreement, whereas wagging the head from side to side expresses disagreement. In India, the meaning attached to these simple head movements is reversed. The basic, culturally embedded assumptions about the meaning attached to this simple gesture led to several confusing interactions before the reasons behind the repeated misunderstandings became clear. Similarly, different cultures attach different meanings to the physical space between participants in an interaction. In some cultures, close contact and touching are expected, while in others the same proximity and behavior is likely to be misinterpreted as aggression or over-familiarity. When providers are insensitive to the nuances of nonverbal communication, both parties to the interaction may feel uncomfortable, which interferes with good communication.

Patient and Family Characteristics Affecting Cross-Cultural Health Care

Family Structure and Cultural Beliefs

Health care providers must be familiar with differences in family values and beliefs, family structures, and parenting styles across ethnic and racial groups. Mainstream health care practitioners are likely to assume that "ideal" family structures and values are those of mainstream American culture, without recognizing the strengths and diversity in family structures and values common to racial and ethnic minorities.

The importance of recognizing cultural differences in family structures and values can be illustrated by the example of Asian families. Within Asian families, the individual's primary responsibility is to the family; individual identities and desires are secondary to the well-being of the family. The family is hierarchical in roles and duties; the father and other elderly persons in the family are undisputed authority figures, whose responsibility for family decision-making must be respected. Publicly challenging family authority figures is forbidden. Asian families seldom seek help from individuals outside the extended family or community. Seeking help, including Western-style health care, can result in a "loss of face" for the father and for the entire family. Problems, emotions, and conflicts within the family are seldom expressed directly, but are likely to be expressed indirectly, for example, in the form of somatization of physical symptoms. Communication is likely to be indirect and nonverbal rather than direct and verbal.

Health care practitioners providing services to Asian families must be aware of the numerous opportunities for misunderstanding that grow out of the differences between Asian and mainstream American conceptions of appropriate family structures and values. A provider who encourages family members to express emotions or criticism openly is likely to create discomfort and guilt within the family and to lose credibility. Health care providers must view the entire family as the client in any interaction, being careful to include elderly family members and other authority figures in decision making. Mainstream American health care providers are accustomed to dealing directly with the child and his or her mother. In providing services to an Asian family, directing questions or instructions to the mother rather than to the father or other elderly family members is apt to produce family discord and discomfort and result in a loss of credibility for the health care provider. This is particularly true for female health care practitioners, who must defer to the male authority figure in the family and resist the impulse to "empower" female family members at the expense of the existing family structure of authority (Fong, 1994).

Unlike the nuclear family of mother, father, two children, a station wagon, and a dog which is considered the "norm" for mainstream American culture, racial and ethnic minorities show a variety of family structures that are different to practitioners from the White majority culture, but that are adaptive within the context of specific minority cultures. Much has been written about a common "pathological" family structure among African-Americans, in which the family unit is comprised of a single mother, her children, and often the maternal grandmother (Nichols-Casebolt, 1988). Focusing on the ways in which this family unit differs from the White majority "norm" obscures the strengths inherent in this family structure in the African-American community (Pinder-hughes, 1982).

Differences in family structure, roles, and responsibilities often become apparent in interactions between family members and health care providers. A majority group health care provider who schedules a family visit to discuss health care strategies for a minority child might be amazed to discover a waiting room filled with members of the extended family and significant family friends, all of whom have a legitimate cultural stake in the health care decisions made on behalf of the child. Majority group health care providers in hospitals often complain bitterly about the disruptions created by minority group family members, without recognizing that each person "cluttering up the halls and getting in the way" feels a cultural responsibility to provide support and assistance to a hospitalized family member. Support and assistance from family members are particularly critical for minority group members and recent immigrants who may feel overwhelmed by the experience of high technology American hospital care (Guendelman, 1983).

In addition to family structures and roles, parenting styles differ between ethnic and racial groups. Parenting styles of middle-class White families are perceived as the standard against which child-rearing practices of other cultures are compared. However, parenting styles that may be functional for middle-income White families may be inappropriate for families from other cultural groups. Middle-class White parenting emphasizes individual differences, competition and accomplishment, the future rather than the present, emotional detachment, and material well-being (Julian, McKenry, & McKelvey, 1994). In contrast, African-American families have developed parenting styles based on a history of racial prejudice and discrimination. African-American families raise their children to survive in a hostile environment, which requires parenting skills and values different from those of Anglo-American parents. African-American families emphasize respect for authority, a strong work ethic, achievement, balance between the rights of individuals and the needs of the group, a sense of family duty, emotional expressiveness by males and females, and a strong religious orientation. Mexican-American families focus on the dominance and authority of male family members, traditional roles for women, reinforcement of sex role distinctions, strong kinship bonds, centrality of children, and repression of feminine attributes in males (Julian, McKenry, & McKelvey, 1994).

Despite these group characteristics, parents from specific ethnic groups differ markedly among themselves (Julian, 1994). However, ethnic parents emphasize self-control and doing well in school for their children, perhaps reflecting the prejudice and racism experienced by ethnic parents and the need for racial socialization. These values are contrary to stereotypes of minority parents, who are assumed to have little interest in self-control or education for their children.

Cultural Differences in Patterns of Help-Seeking

Patterns of help-seeking differ across cultural groups as a result of differences in their health beliefs (to be discussed in the next section) and differences in their access to health care resources. Differences in perceived health needs and reliance on traditional cultural practices can affect a child's entry into the health care system. This, in turn, affects utilization of health care services and the extent to which prevention and health-promotion activities are adopted (Garcia Coll, 1990).

In examining cultural determinants of entry into the health care system, the concept of "pathways" to health care is useful (Rogler & Cortes, 1993). Health care practitioners often accept the presence of a child and a family seeking treatment without giving much thought to the process by which that child and family arrived in the waiting room or the reasons why other families with children exhibiting similar problems may not seek treatment. Culture-specific pathways determine which child is presented for treatment and the expectations of the family seeking treatment. Help-seeking pathways are "the sequence of contacts with individuals and organizations prompted by the distressed person's efforts, and those of his or her significant others, to seek help as well as the help that is supplied in response to such efforts" (Rogler & Cortes, p. 555). Pathways include formal and informal sources of assistance and differ dramatically across cultures.

A pathway starts with recognition of a problem, a judgment that is profoundly affected by culture. For medical problems involving children, the family is the starting point on the help-seeking pathway. However, the family's culture determines how and when problems are perceived (Clark, 1983). Not only must symptoms be recognized by the family, but they must be viewed as undesirable and help-seeking efforts perceived as likely to be fruitful before the family will enter the help-seeking pathway. For example, first-generation Hispanic immigrants of lower socioeconomic status may perceive undesirable symptoms in their children, but may also subscribe to a belief that individual actions are largely ineffectual in influencing the outcome of events (Rogler & Cortes, 1993). Such beliefs allow for the perception of distress, but inhibit efforts to alleviate the distress. It is well documented that White children use more medical care than non-White children. A typical explanation is that White children have better access to health care services than do non-White children. However, even when socioeconomic status is controlled, non-White mothers have a higher threshold for seeking health services in response to symptoms in their children (Riley et al., 1993).

For many ethnic or cultural minorities, the first step on the help-seeking pathway is not the professional health care system. Rather, the initial steps depend on a culture-specific help-providing system built on a network of personal contacts. This informal system provides information about help-seeking, social support for children and families coping with health problems, and enforces conformity with the community's standards for appropriate help-seeking. When the informal system is extensive and the lay culture markedly different from medical culture, as is often the case in Hispanic and other minority cultures, seeking treatment from the medical sector may be delayed, even when timely treatment-seeking is important (Rogler & Cortes, 1993). Health care providers who are unfamiliar with these informal help-seeking networks may be frustrated and mystified by parents' apparent delays in seeking medical services for their children.

For many cultural groups, the involvement of "outsiders" in family problems is contrary to their community's norms for help-seeking and may bring shame or stigma to the family (Fong, 1994; Rounds, Weil, & Bishop, 1994). In Hispanic communities, initial help-seeking pathways include the extended family, friends, neighbors, and folk healers (Delgado & Humm-Delgado, 1982). Initial attempts at help-seeking are directed to this informal network. Seeking help from the formal medical system occurs only if the informal networks fail to provide relief. In addition, accessing the formal network may occur only if the linguistic and structural barriers within the formal system are not too formidable.

Similarly, for Asian families in the U.S., the family and extended family are the primary sources of support. Enlisting the aid of "outsiders" may bring loss of face and shame to the elders in the family, making the family reluctant to seek outside help (Fong, 1994). Asian families are more likely to accept help from outsiders when providers are perceived to be sensitive to the values and structure of Asian families; sensitive to needs for confidentiality and privacy; willing to provide concrete resources such as money, jobs, housing, health care, and education; and willing to allow the family to assess the trustworthiness and credibility of the practitioner through "personal" questions (Fong, 1994). For mainstream health practitioners, accustomed to their credentials garnering automatic trust and respect from patients and their families, personal questioning may be perceived as a lack of trust or as simple nosiness. However, establishing credibility through responding to personal questioning is vital for developing a working relationship with Asian families.

Mainstream health care providers may also find themselves surprised and frustrated to discover that families seek alternative forms of treatment for their children in addition to accessing the formal medical system (Clark, 1983). Providers who assume that the child's medical problem is "turned over" to a medical practitioner for treatment may find it difficult to accept the roles of folk healers and religious practitioners in providing health care for the child. Family members from ethnic and racial minorities often arrange adjunct forms of care to ensure that family members have access to a full range of possible cures (Clark, 1983). For Westernized medical practitioners unfamiliar with these systems, the inclusion of other sources of medical care may raise questions about the family's commitment to Western-style medical care, trust in the medical practitioner, and willingness to carry through with medical recommendations. Health care providers may be predisposed to view other sources of care as interfering with appropriate medical treatment, rather than as culturally important means of providing treatment and support for the child and the family.

One of the authors of this chapter (GE) experienced this integration of different sources of health care in Kenya, where patients frequently combine traditional and Western medical treatment. Kenyan mothers of young children with diarrhea rely on traditional cures from older mothers, recommendations of herbalists, and treatment by Western-style medical practitioners at primary care clinics. Frequently, mothers combine antibiotics and oral rehydration salts recommended by the local clinic with traditional uji porridge recommended by older women in the village and herbs procured from traditional herbalists.

Marcus and Marcus (1993) describe a recent Guatemalan immigrant to the U.S. who brought her infant son for treatment of low-grade anemia and diarrhea at the same time that she consulted with traditional healers. Medical practitioners reported frustration at her apparent lack of trust in American medicine. "One moment you think a woman like that's in compliance. The next you find she's been running to a folk healer behind our backs, either to hurry things up, or as a fail-safe backup against our own lousy measures, which so far haven't done a thing for her. Only we don't know that because she hasn't been able to say so" (p. 338). This example illustrates not only the reliance on traditional folk medicine by members of many minority groups, but also shows the difficulties immigrant parents may have in communicating with an Anglo-American health care provider.

Alternate sources of medical care frequently result from differing cultural beliefs about the causes and cures of various illnesses and injuries. Members of different cultural and ethnic groups have different beliefs about the causes of illnesses, ranging from beliefs about the immediate causes (such as pathogens or malignancies), the underlying causes (such as exposure to infection, smoking in the home, or high blood cholesterol levels), and ultimate causes (such as genetic susceptibility, stress, environmental hazards, diet). Western medical practitioners tend to focus on immediate and underlying causes for illness and disease, whereas many cultural and ethnic groups focus on ultimate causes. In the area of ultimate causes, folk systems of medicine provide explanations, diagnostic aids, and curative measures that are not available from the mainstream health care system (Clark, 1983). Cultural views of levels of causation may result in a family member bringing a child to a mainstream medical practitioner for treatment of the "immediate cause" while simultaneously consulting a traditional healer who will deal with the "ultimate cause" (Clark, 1983)—much to the frustration of many mainstream health care practitioners.

A comparison between Hispanic and Black children in an outpatient mental health clinic in New York illustrates the operation of help-seeking pathways for minority children (Canino, Gould, Prupis, & Shaffer, 1986). Despite similarities in symptoms and psychosocial stressors for Black and Hispanic children, Hispanic children were less likely to be admitted to the outpatient mental health clinic through a routine referral from schools, parents, or pediatric health programs, and more likely to be admitted following referral from emergency services. Two-thirds of Hispanic children entered the outpatient clinic following emergency referral, compared to about 40 percent of Black children. Canino et al. (1986) suggested that the pattern of emergency admissions reflected a specific health-seeking behavior on the part of Hispanic parents, who might be more likely to view the local hospital emergency room as a stage in the formal help-seeking pathway. A high proportion of Hispanic and Black children in that study had been seen previously by different psychiatrists, indicating that even when minority families gain access to the mental health system, they may experience difficulties obtaining continuity of care (Canino et al., 1986).

Children and adolescents rely on caregivers and representatives of other institutions (e.g., schools, social welfare agencies) to direct them into pathways of health care seeking. In the case of adolescents with psychiatric problems, this reliance on others may lead to racial and cultural bias in patterns of referral. Fabrega, Ulrich, and Mezzich (1993) compared symptom profiles of Black and White adolescents at psychiatric intake. After controlling for socioeconomic status, no differences emerged in levels of stress or social impairment between these two groups of adolescents. However, White adolescents showed greater levels of clinical morbidity at intake and Black adolescents were diagnosed with higher levels of "social aggression" and conduct disorders. Fabrega and colleagues speculated that differences in symptom profiles at intake reflect differences in how the social system

(i.e., schools and welfare agencies) perceives symptoms in adolescents from different racial groups. They argue that the lower symptom levels among Black adolescents suggest that Black adolescents are shunted to psychiatric facilities earlier than White adolescents and that social systems are less tolerant of psychiatric symptoms in Black adolescents. Adults in positions of authority may be less comfortable with behavior problems at home or in the school for Black adolescents and may disproportionately refer them for psychiatric services for conduct disorders. In this sense, adult representatives of institutions serving adolescents may direct Black adolescents toward seeking mental health services sooner than White adolescents.

Among individuals and their families who successfully negotiate entry into the formal help-seeking pathway, structural, cultural, and linguistic elements within the system may produce high levels of attrition (see the earlier discussion of institutional barriers to effective treatment). Treatment attrition may occur when the natural help-seeking pathways channel children and their families into more culturally and linguistically compatible help-providing networks and away from formal help-providing networks. Health practitioners who understand the operation and structure of these natural help-seeking pathways will be able to forge culturally-sensitive alliances with their patients that enable medical care to be accepted as part of the traditional help-seeking pathway (Rogler & Cortes, 1993).

Health Beliefs

This topic was addressed earlier from the perspective of the health care practitioner; in this section we will focus on cultural differences in patients' health beliefs that affect their decisions to seek treatment from the mainstream health care system. For example, Native American cultures view illness in ways that differ markedly from a Western biomedical model (Malach & Segal, 1990). Native Americans may not accept biomedical explanations that contradict cultural beliefs about the interconnectedness of spirit, mind, and body (Rounds, Weil, & Bishop, 1994). In addition, Native Americans often view biomedical assessment and treatment procedures as offensive or culturally inappropriate, reducing their willingness to comply with these measures in the treatment of their children.

Immigrant Chinese families provide another example of a culture with markedly different beliefs about appropriate methods to cure common ailments. Traditional Chinese medical practitioners believe that many diseases are caused by imbalances in fluids or airs. Imbalances may be treating by rubbing the surface of the skin or by using herbal remedies (Timberlake & Cook, 1984). Skin-rubbing, when practiced correctly, brings blood to the surface of the skin and often causes bruising. To Chinese people familiar with these practices, bruises are a sign of successful treatment. To health care providers unfamiliar with these practices, bruises may be misinterpreted as signs of child abuse (Redick & Wood, 1982). Such misinterpretations of common cultural practices have created serious problems for families who found themselves being investigated for child abuse after seeking traditional and culturally familiar treatment for a child.

Health beliefs and cultural values also have a profound impact on a family's adjustment to a child's handicapping condition. Most research on the impact of chronic illness or disability in children has been conducted with majority group families, and there is relatively little information available to guide practitioners who work with families from diverse cultural and ethnic groups. Parents who give birth to a handicapped child are assumed to go through stages of shock, disbelief, grief and mourning, followed by the search for a cause and a cure for the disability. However, this model of family adaptation was generated from research with Anglo-American parents and the responses of parents from other cultures might be quite different (Marion, 1980). For Mexican-American or African-American families with extended family networks, protectiveness and acceptance may be a more typical reaction to the birth of a handicapped child. In contrast, Chinese immigrant families viewed their disabled child more negatively than did Euro-Canadian parents and appraised the illness or disability as having more global effects on the child's present and future life, raising concerns about the child's education, success, social relations, and ability to assume family responsibilities (Elfert, Anderson, & Lai, 1991). These concerns extend from the traditional structure and roles in Chinese families.

In a comparison of the reactions of Black, Hispanic, and White mothers to the birth of a handicapped child, Hispanic mothers were more likely to express a sense of self-sacrifice than mothers from other ethnic groups. For example, Hispanic mothers made comments such as "He's my whole life now" or "I live my whole life for him" (Mary, 1990, p. 3). Hispanic mothers also reported that Hispanic fathers were unlikely to acknowledge or discuss the child's disability, leaving the mother feeling lonely and isolated. Self-sacrifice by Hispanic mothers and denial by Hispanic fathers suggest that Hispanic

mothers may shoulder more of the emotional burden of the child's handicap than mothers from other ethnic groups (Mary, 1990).

Responses to Racism

Providing effective health services for minority children requires trust and collaboration between families and health care providers and self-disclosure on the part of families. Developing collaboration and trust can be profoundly affected by the family's experiences with racism. Families are expected to disclose personal details of family circumstances, child-rearing practices, finances, and previous attempts at help-seeking. Despite the expectations of health care providers, self-disclosure outside an individual's cultural group is unlikely to occur in the absence of trust and rapport between the provider and the family.

The long history of racism on the part of Whites and distrust on the part of African-Americans affects open communication between African-American families and White health care providers. Avoiding self-disclosure to Whites is a long-standing protective mechanism by African-Americans (Rounds, Weil, & Bishop, 1994; Siegel, 1974). White health care providers who do not understand this consequence of racism are likely to make negative attributions for the family's apparent unwillingness to cooperate. For example, it is commonly heard in professional settings that "these people just don't care about their children" (Harry, 1992b, p. 124). In addition, logistical constraints and stressful circumstances associated with poverty and minority status may interfere with the ability of parents to participate in their child's treatment in ways that majority group health professionals deem appropriate. African-American parents may be perceived as disinterested when, in fact, they are overwhelmed by other life stresses and feel mistrustful about interactions with the majority culture health system (Harry, 1992b).

The experiences of minority parents with the special education system illustrate many negative aspects of interactions between White health care professionals and ethnic families. Researchers have documented the low participation rates of ethnic parents in decisions concerning special education placement for their children (Harry, 1992b). Low rates of participation led many majority professionals to assume that ethnic parents do not care what happens to their children in school, a view counter to the actual importance attached to education in many minority families. In fact, low rates of participation are related to distrust of a White-dominated school system which has systematically shunted minority children into special education placements, often against the wishes of their parents; to the overwhelming impact of cumulative stressors on impoverished and minority parents; to difficulties in scheduling appointments and arranging child care and transportation to enable minority parents to attend educational planning meetings; and finally, to low knowledge of parental rights and special education procedures on the part of minority parents (Harry, 1992a; 1992b).

African-American, Hispanic, and other minority parents often disagree with the diagnostic labels applied to their children by White professionals but feel powerless to affect the labeling process (Harry, 1992a, 1992b). Minority parents have a broader definition of "disabled" than is tolerated by schools and professionals. Minority parents may agree that their child's performance is delayed, but do not necessarily perceive the difference as disabling. Because minority families often have limited educational and career expectations for their children, the lack of a high level of academic and educational achievement may not be considered a problem (Harry, 1992b).

Terms such as "retardation" often have unfortunate connotations to parents whose first language is not English. As one Puerto Rican mother explained, "For me, retarded is crazy; in Spanish that's 'retardado.' For me, the word 'handicap' means a person who is incapacitated, like mentally, or missing a leg, or who is blind or deaf, who cannot work and cannot do anything . . . a person who is invalid, useless . . . But for Americans, it is a different thing—for them, 'handicap' is everybody!" (Harry, 1992a). In addition, minority parents with limited formal education and little facility in English may find it impossible to understand how a child who has surpassed his or her parents in formal education and who is fluent in two languages can be considered learning disabled (Harry, 1992a). Unfortunately, White professionals lose credibility with minority group parents by labeling minority children in ways that their parents do not comprehend and by assuming that disagreement on the part of parents represents denial of the reality of the professional's judgments (Harry, 1992a; 1992b). Under these circumstances, it is not surprising that minority parents who feel powerless to deal with the White majority school system register their displeasure by withdrawing from participation with White professionals who appear to hold all the cards.

Professionals often disparage ethnic parents, appearing to believe that poverty and limited formal education are synonymous with limited intelligence and common sense (Harry, 1992b). Professionals may reflect these beliefs by having less contact with ethnic parents than with mainstream parents and by offering fewer services to minority children. Minority parents may be relegated to the role of consent-givers, rubber-stamping decisions made by White professionals on behalf of minority children.

Migration Experience

Providing health services for refugee children and their families demands an understanding of the effects of migration and relocation. Refugees flee familiar environments, often without the opportunity for psychological, financial, or other preparation (Timberlake & Cook, 1984). As a result, refugees commonly experience a loss of identity as well as the emotional pangs of separating from loved ones. Many refugees also experienced the dependency, loss of control, lack of privacy, and dehumanizing effects of refugee camps. Resettlement stresses in their host countries interact with stressful pre-migration experiences. These resettlement stresses can include cultural differences, language and communication problems, inadequate housing and finances, and rejection from within the host culture. Underemployment is a particularly salient problem for many refugee families. Many recent Southeast Asian refugees who had professional careers in their countries of origin were forced into menial labor after their immigration into the U.S., partly because of language impediments and partly because of differences in professional requirements between their country of origin and the U.S. (Rogler, 1994). An example is the loss of status and income faced by a South Vietnamese general who was forced to work as a janitor after immigrating to the U.S. (Lum, 1982).

Central American refugees often enter the U.S. with pressing health and social needs. Although many Central American refugees have family members resident in the U.S., as many as 25 percent of Central American refugees are homeless and up to 60 percent have no permanent address (Magar, 1990). Many homeless and transient refugees include families with infants and young children. In addition, many Central American refugees are undocumented immigrants who are dependent on public services for health care at a time when budget cuts are reducing public health services in many areas of the country. Refugees experience widespread mental and physical health problems. However, since undocumented immigrants do not receive the screening services available to other refugees, conditions such as parasitic infections and tuberculosis flourish. The provisions of California's Proposition 187 promise to reduce even further the already limited medical services available for undocumented immigrants and their families.

SOLUTIONS FACILITATING CULTURALLY COMPETENT CARE PROVISION

Earlier in this chapter, the problems that influence cross-cultural care were described: overriding sociopolitical issues, institutional barriers, and factors related to individual practitioners and to families from different cultures. Just as problems can arise at the social, institutional, and individual level, solutions must address each of those levels. In the next sections, we will describe some potential solutions that can enhance individual practitioners' efforts to provide competent care to patients from diverse cultural and linguistic backgrounds.

Sociopolitical Solutions

Solutions at this level are complex, for they must address the twin problems of poverty and racism and their interaction in the lives of individuals from minority cultures. As we noted earlier in this chapter, poverty creates "double jeopardy" for minority children, exposing them to greater health risks at the same time that it limits resources to ameliorate those risks. Unless the pernicious effects associated with poverty, poor health, limited education, job instability, barriers to health care access, and lowered aspirations can be addressed, minority families will continue to face difficult choices, for example, the choice between food and medication for a sick child. Minority groups share similar aspirations as mainstream American culture, but all too often lack the means to obtain those goals (Julian, McKenry, & McKelvey, 1994).

Changes must occur at a global, as well as national, sociopolitical level. Many would agree that long-standing policies of exploiting Third World countries contributed to their current economic and political disarray, resulting in increased immigration as people flee their countries of origin for safety or economic opportunity. One solution to such mass emigrations is to improve conditions in economically disadvantaged and politically unstable countries. Clearly, a comprehensive discussion of all possible solutions to the global problems of poverty and racism is well beyond the scope of this chapter. However, since these affect the interaction between individual providers and their patients, changes are needed in the larger sociocultural systems that give rise to these problems, as well as at the level of individuals.

Institutional Changes to Enhance Cross-Cultural Service Delivery

Solutions at the institutional level will require willingness to reexamine the institutional barriers that affect access to health services and service delivery. Malach and Segal (1990) offer suggestions to improve health care access for minority groups, including a host of structural changes at the institutional level. One solution is to increase the number of community-based settings that deliver health care. This has several obvious benefits since parents are more likely to learn about services that are located in their local communities and are more likely to use health care services for their children if transportation barriers are removed. Health care institutions can be encouraged to reexamine policies and procedures that were developed for institutional convenience but that pose barriers to access. Extending clinic hours to include evenings and weekends might be unpopular with clinic staff, but could increase access for families with conflicting job and child care responsibilities. Expanded hours could alleviate problems in overcrowded emergency rooms where many minority families seek non-emergency care for their sick children outside regular office hours. When the child's problem requires an interdisciplinary approach, scheduling appointments with different practitioners on the same day would be helpful for families with transportation problems and conflicting child-care and work responsibilities. Reducing waiting times and making child care available in clinics would benefit caretakers of young children, many of whom are daunted by the prospect of hours spent in a crowded waiting room with a sick child and other accompanying children for whom alternative care was not available.

Effective case management systems can offer children and their families a sense of continuity in health care. Ideally, a single case manager would be responsible for the needs of a family, coordinating services and referrals and reducing the risk that a family "falls between the cracks" in a complex network of uncoordinated services. Simplifying eligibility requirements for services and simplifying registration forms and paperwork would also be productive. For example, many Native American families find the bureaucracy and paperwork in Anglo-American health care institutions so burdensome that they leave without obtaining services (Malach & Segal, 1990). It is helpful to remain sensitive to the fact that many members of minority groups have limited education and limited facility in English, rendering complex paperwork virtually impossible. Some health care institutions have increased their bilingual and bicultural staffing to reduce cultural barriers and increased their use of interpreters and translators. These are costly solutions and require funds and commitment on the part of institutions to provide culturally sensitive health care services to minority group members. Another potential solution is to utilize cultural guides, community members who assist health care providers to understand and provide culturally sensitive services (Rounds, Weil, & Bishop, 1994). This approach requires collaboration and cooperation between health care institutions and members of local ethnic communities.

In the next section, we will describe several innovative models for providing accessible and integrated health care services to cultural and ethnic minorities. The first example is the Child Development Project at Boston City Hospital (Kaplan-Sanoff, Parker, & Zuckerman, 1991). This project offers coordinated programs that address medical and social service needs of poor families. The program is based on a "two for one" model of service, meeting the health and educational needs of children while simultaneously supporting the training and social needs of their mothers and other caregivers in the same visit. The assumption is that when treating a child for medical problems, the family is the "patient" and the needs of the child and the needs of the family must be addressed. Rather than dealing with medical problems in isolation, the Child Development Project makes use of the family's presentation of a child in need of treatment to assess and provide comprehensive services to the entire family. Services are directed at undoing some of the "double jeopardy" that we mentioned earlier in this chapter. For example, drug treatment for mothers may be provided in the same session as medical treatment for the child.

The Child Development Project offers a multidisciplinary approach to the family's health care and includes providers from a variety of health care and related disciplines. Case managers coordinate services for the family, including consultation with outside practitioners. Services are provided in settings where families already go for treatment, reducing travel between settings and multiple visits. As much as possible, schedules for appointments are coordinated to reduce travel. While the Boston City Hospital program may be beyond the resources of many health care facilities, it provides a model of integrated services that improve access and outcomes for minority families.

Another innovative approach to providing services to minority families is the community health worker model, similar to the "barefoot doctor" or "village health worker" approaches common to many developing countries. Indigenous helpers from the community are recruited, trained, and supervised to provide culturally appropriate outreach into the community. Lay workers are trained to educate parents about common childhood diseases and appropriate treatment resources and to assist parents in obtaining services for their children. Community health workers serve as a bridge between low-income or minority families and the health care system. In many community programs, lay health workers carry out three important tasks: (1) locating patients; (2) providing emotional and practical support to families, such as child care, transportation and assistance in obtaining medical supplies; and (3) providing health education and referral services (Butz et al., 1994).

For example, lay health workers were recruited from low-income African-American communities in Baltimore and Washington, D.C. and trained to provide community outreach to low-income and minority parents of children with asthma (Butz et al., 1994). Community health workers, who were supervised by an experienced public health nurse, were trained in anatomy and pathophysiology of the respiratory system, recognition of asthma symptoms, medical treatment for asthma, environmental control measures, smoking cessation for parents, basic parenting skills, referral to community resources, and the importance of primary health care. The community workers were successful in visiting families in their homes, developing trust and rapport, and providing basic asthma-management information and referrals. A similar approach has been used to train lay workers in Hispanic communities that had low utilization of health services and high proportions of undocumented workers (Watkins et al., 1994). Community health workers are not substitutes for other medical care providers. However, they provide important services to low-income and minority families by reducing some of the barriers that impede access to care for their children.

Another innovative approach to improving service delivery to minority groups is developing partnerships between health care professionals, community-based agencies, and parents. The University-Affiliated Program (UAP) at Children's Hospital Los Angeles collaborates with community-based agencies to establish statewide projects serving Asian, African-American, and Latino parents of disabled children (Chan, 1990). The Multicultural Training-of-Trainers project recruited and trained minority parents to work with bilingual and bicultural health care providers to organize and conduct training programs for parents of disabled children in ethnic communities. Training coordinators were foreign born and fluent in their native languages; parent trainers were selected on the basis on their ethnic community affiliations, native language proficiency, experience as the parent of a child with a disability, ability to serve as an effective group leader and parent advocate, and commitment to their roles as parent helper, trainer, and liaison. Parent trainers were responsible for recruiting parents of children with disabilities from local communities and organizing and facilitating monthly parent workshops with the training coordinators.

Parent participants benefited from the opportunity to meet and interact with other parents who spoke the same language, had similar cultural backgrounds, and experienced similar needs, problems, and concerns. Parent groups provided emotional support to reduce the sense of isolation and shame frequently felt by parents of disabled children (Chan, 1990). In addition, parents were provided with educational materials written in their native languages and communicated with health care professionals who were bilingual and understood the family's culture. Trainers and group facilitators educated parents about community resources and parental rights to services for their children. The project was designed for sustainability through its connection with existing community organizations and by recruiting parent trainers from within those communities.

The formal medical network can also become involved in innovative community outreach programs by offering services at locations that are already popular and trusted in the community. For example, in an Hispanic area of New York City, an HIV testing center was relocated to a Botanica, a shop specializing in herbal remedies, when it was learned that many individuals in need of testing or counseling already patronized the Botanicas. Similarly, public health nurses in Los Angeles provide screening and referral services to undocumented Central American refugees in homeless shelters, acting as a liaison between the refugees and public health and social services (Magar, 1990).

These innovative programs illustrate ways in which medical service institutions can change to make their services more accessible and culturally appropriate for members of minority groups. Coordinating services to address the myriad needs of minority families, offering services at times and places that are convenient for struggling families, and engaging the minority community in collaboration to provide sensitive and appropriate health care services may increase utilization of health services by impoverished and minority families. These innovative services reflect the recognition that if patients and families have difficulty finding their way to health services, then perhaps health services should find their way to the families. However, this view is contrary to mainstream models of health care in which patients seek out and adapt to medical services offered in medical settings such as physicians' offices and hospitals. Offering innovative services demands a willingness to rethink the traditional relationship between health care providers and patients and a willingness to deal with change in "the way we've always done it."

Changes in institutional research and professional training are also needed. Research into the impact of migration, acculturation patterns, minority family structures, and on differences in parenting styles can improve understanding of the cultural and social environments that affect minority groups. Research is also needed to determine effective ways of providing cross-cultural health care. In writing this chapter, the scarcity of empirical evaluations relevant to effective clinical practice was notable. In the absence of such research, even well-intentioned practitioners are "flying by the seat of their pants."

Even where a body of research on clinical practice with minority group members exists, as it does in social work, the focus and conclusions of research are open to question. McMahon and Allen-Meares (1992) surveyed 117 articles on social work interventions with minority groups published in four major social work journals in the 1980s. These 117 articles represent 6 percent of the 1,965 articles published in those journals during that time. Seventy-eight percent of the articles focused on individual interventions to assist minority clients to adjust to their situation or to sensitize social workers to the particular cultural values and beliefs of minorities and only 22 percent recommended institutional interventions or policy changes. A central assumption of much of this literature was the "ideology of assimilation," the idea that minority group members should integrate into the mainstream of American society (McMahon & Allen-Meares, 1992, p. 536). McMahon and Allen-Meares concluded that the literature on social work practice with minorities in the 1980s was superficial and devalued minority values by expecting minority clients to accept and assimilate the social and family values of majority society. Most of the literature failed to address the social context of minority group members, including poverty, lack of resources, and the effects of racism. McMahon and Allen-Meares argue that the focus of social work research in the 1980s hampered social workers in their attempts to interact effectively with minority clients and to become advocates for larger-scale sociopolitical change.

Institutional accommodations are needed to include cross-cultural training in pre-service training and continuing education for health care providers from all disciplines. Increasingly, health practitioners and educators are acknowledging the need to educate future and current generations of health practitioners in cross-cultural sensitivity and cross-cultural competency. For example, the annual meeting of the Association of Behavioral Sciences and Medical Education in October, 1994 had as its theme "Cultural Diversity in Medicine: Challenges and Opportunities." Practitioners and educators from a broad range of health-related disciplines discussed the need for training curricula that will prepare students for practice among ethnically diverse populations. Despite this recognition of the importance of cross-cultural training, few pre-service or continuing education programs in medicine or health-related disciplines include cross-cultural training in their curricula.

Allison, Crawford, Echemendia, Robinson, and Knepp (1994) surveyed clinical and counseling psychology training programs approved by the American Psychological Association (APA). Despite numerous APA resolutions, task forces, conferences, and specific guidelines for cross-cultural training in doctoral-level programs in psychology, few training programs offer culturally competent training for clinical and counseling psychologists. Recent graduates from doctoral-level training programs reported minimal to moderate exposure to minority faculty members, limited access to courses focused on cultural diversity, and few opportunities for working with clients from diverse cultural groups. Not surprisingly, few recent graduates rated themselves as competent in providing services to clients from diverse cultural and racial groups. On a brighter note, although recent graduates reported limited opportunities for cross-cultural training during graduate school and internship, more than 70 percent reported receiving additional training in cross-cultural competency after receiving their degrees. This suggests that not only do counseling and clinical psychologists in practice perceive a need for additional training in cross-cultural competency but that resources exist for providing at least some continuing education training for psychology practitioners.

Similarly, in 1991 and 1992, deans of all 126 medical schools in the U.S. were surveyed to determine the percentage of schools that offered formal cultural-sensitivity training courses to medical students (Lum & Korenman, 1994). Of the 98 schools that responded to the survey, only 13 percent offered independent courses in cultural awareness. Disappointingly, only one school reported that the course was required for all students. In all other schools, cultural awareness courses were optional and had low student enrollments (between 5 and 10 percent of the students). Approximately 60 percent of the schools reported that cultural-sensitivity information was integrated into other required or optional courses and most schools reported that there was a "low to medium" likelihood that clinical faculty provided cultural-sensitivity information during clinical clerkships. Most schools recognized a fairly high likelihood that their students would interact with minority patients, and most perceived their recent graduates to be only "somewhat prepared" to handle the special demands of practice with minority patients, yet only 34 percent of schools had plans to implement cultural-sensitivity programs within their medical curricula. Seventy-three percent of the schools reported that they had faculty who were prepared, academically or by virtue of experience, to teach cultural-sensitivity training programs. It is difficult to understand this conundrum—medical schools acknowledging a training need, having faculty capable of filling that need, and yet few schools having plans to fill that need.

In some cases, the impetus for change within training curricula has come from students. Students who are faced with the specter of cross-cultural practice for which they feel ill-prepared have recognized the need for training in cross-cultural medical practice. In 1984, after a survey of first-year students at the University of Southern California School of Medicine showed that half the students felt unprepared to handle the cultural barriers between themselves and their patients, a group of students designed and implemented a workshop to increase awareness of lifestyle differences and to improve the ability of students to provide medical care appropriate to the ethnic and sociocultural backgrounds of their patients (Mao, Bullock, Harway, & Khalsa, 1988). Students were overwhelmingly positive toward the program and felt that it sensitized them to the importance of considering sociocultural issues as an integral component of medical practice.

Training in cross-cultural competency will require recognition on the part of faculty and institutions that such training is important in improving the quality of services for minority patients. The need for cross-cultural training must be buttressed by professional regulatory bodies. Without support (or coercion) from regulatory bodies, it is unlikely that cross-cultural training will become widespread. Social work and psychology are examples of health-related professions in which regulatory bodies demand pre-service training in cross-cultural competence. However, as noted earlier, demands by regulatory bodies do not necessarily translate into adequate cross-cultural training opportunities for students. An important aspect of change is recruiting minority students and faculty members into health care training programs (Bernal & Castro, 1994). Without placing special emphasis on recruiting minority students and faculty, including provisions for minority scholarships and grants, programs are unlikely to meet the need to train practitioners who are comfortable and competent in cross-cultural practice (Lum, 1982). In turn, the growing community needs for cross-cultural health care will remain unmet.

Practitioner-Level Solutions for Increasing Cross-Cultural Competence

Changes at the level of individual practitioners will require recognition of the need for professional training in cross-cultural competence. However, given that training in cross-cultural competence in not readily available for practitioners in the field, how can the "average practitioner" enhance his or her cultural competence?

A good place for practitioners to begin is with self-examination, evaluating themselves as ethnic persons of a particular culture (Pinderhughes, 1982). It is important (and often difficult) for practitioners from the mainstream culture to recognize that their culture is not, in fact, a neutral background against which the diversities within other cultures are revealed. Instead, each culture represents a complex set of assumptions, biases, experiences, and perceptions that shape views of other cultural and ethnic groups. Many White professionals who feel that they have no culture per se are unaware of the effect of their own culture on their relationships with members of other cultures (Christensen, 1992). A time-honored adage states that it is difficult for fish to understand water. In the same vein, it is difficult for individuals immersed in a particular culture to understand how it shapes their perceptions of other cultures.

During the process of cultural self-examination, practitioners can begin to understand how their culture influences their perceptions of, feelings about, and behavior toward members of other ethnic, racial, and cultural groups. A particularly salient issue that arises in health care practice is the relationship between power and ethnicity. Majority providers are part of a sociocultural system that systematically oppressed and discriminated against members of other racial and ethnic groups. For health care providers from the mainstream culture, an awareness of how they benefit from that system can be illuminating. For health care providers from other cultures, understanding ethnicity and power must include an awareness of themselves as victims and beneficiaries of the sociopolitical system (Pinderhughes, 1982).

Many majority group members, including health care providers, assume that minority group members come from inferior cultural backgrounds that must be discarded. This attitude profoundly affects minority children, who, through their exposure to majority culture, become conditioned to accept the values of a culture that disparages their parents' culture. Dissonance between foreign-born parents and American-born children is inevitable. Lum (1982) described the example of Juan Morales, the son of Mexican immigrants to the U.S. Juan was raised in a White middle-class community, but his parents spoke only Spanish and his first exposure to English came after he started school. Due to difficulty in acquiring English as a second language, he was repeatedly placed in slow-reader groups and ridiculed by his classmates for his halting English and his Spanish accent. He was torn between the Spanish culture of his family and the Anglo-American culture of his school peers, who belittled his Spanish culture. Until he was befriended by a Mexican-American educator who helped Juan develop an appreciation for his Spanish culture and language, Juan was caught between two worlds, fitting comfortably into neither.

Too often, individuals from the mainstream culture seem to believe that the responsibility for dealing with cultural differences lies only with individuals from minority groups. Expecting members of different ethnic groups to merge into a homogenous cultural mainstream belies the impact of their experiences with migration, negates the effect of racism and poverty, and ignores the richness of a culture composed of many smaller cultures. Many health care providers expect ethnic families to change their culture and lives to fit with the views and values of health care professionals from mainstream America. Christensen (1992) quotes health care providers who feel strongly that minority group members must assimilate into mainstream culture. One professional said, "I feel families need to be encouraged to learn the primary language of the country in which they live, and professionals who make adjustments to enable the family to maintain their inability to communicate keep them dependent on the system." Another professional commented that "some cultures seem very appreciative and others seem to expect that everything will be given to them and fall in the 'poor me' syndrome" (Christensen, p. 55). Health care practitioners who place the burden for change on "them" rather than us may be ignoring the fact that in many areas of the U.S. today, White Anglo-Americans are becoming the "minority group."

In addition to becoming aware of their own attitudes and values about other cultures, practitioners can make other efforts to increase their cross-cultural sensitivity and competence. Practitioners can seek information about minority cultures seen in their clinical practices, become more familiar with culturally sensitive services and organizations in the community, enlist assistance from community groups that can provide cultural guidance, or employ translators to assist families' interactions with the health care system. In addition, practitioners can seek cross-cultural experiences outside working hours and on vacations. Few health care practitioners may view leisure activities as a route to understanding cultural differences. However, attending cultural festivals and events, reading books by authors from diverse cultural backgrounds, attending foreign movies, and even eating at ethnic restaurants can "flesh out" their understanding of diverse ethnic or cultural groups (Rounds, Weil, & Bishop, 1994).

Community and Minority Group Solutions

Many authors suggest that minority communities can aid in developing culturally sensitive health care systems. Malach and Segel (1990) suggest a number of ways that minority communities can become involved in improving minority health services. In addition to developing community-based organizations and facilities to serve minority clients, minority group members can seek to serve on advisory boards for health care institutions and facilities. Community groups can provide cultural guides, individuals who are familiar with the minority language and cultural system, to institutions that serve minority clients. Cultural guides can function as translators, helpers, and intermediaries to assist recent immigrants and other minority group members to gain access to appropriate health care and other services. An example of this kind of minority group involvement in providing culturally sensitive health care for immigrants and minority group members is a Canadian organization called "Mosaic." Mosaic assists new immigrants in acculturating to the Canadian system of health and social services, by helping immigrant families become connected with physicians and health care facilities, by assisting in child care and transportation, and by accompanying new immigrants to health care appointments to interpret and translate. In addition, Mosaic guides, who are themselves immigrants, are familiar with the myriad health and social services available to newcomers to Canada and serve as valuable referral sources for new immigrants.

A TRAINING MODEL FOR CROSS-CULTURAL COMPETENCE

Rounds, Weil, and Bishop (1994) describe five essential elements for culturally competent health care. These elements are useful as a prototype for effective cross-cultural training programs. The first element, *acknowledging and accepting diversity*, includes developing appreciation of the diversity within and across cultural groups as well as accepting cultural differences without judgment. The second element is *conducting a cultural self-assessment* to understand how our own culture imposes a perceptual screen that affects the way we perceive and interact with other cultural and ethnic groups. At an agency or institutional level, cultural self-assessment includes evaluating whether culturally sensitive beliefs are reflected in policies for hiring, staffing, and operating procedures. The third element, *understanding specific differences between and among cultural groups*, emphasizes understanding cultural patterns of interaction, family structures, and beliefs about health and illness that affect health care services. The fourth element is *acquiring knowledge and experience specific to minority cultures* that the health care provider is likely to encounter in his or her practice. The fifth element involves using the information and self-knowledge that was garnered in the previous four steps and *putting it into practice*, developing skills for interacting successfully with patients from diverse cultural groups, and adapting entrenched health care practices to the needs of different groups.

A number of training programs in cross-cultural competence have been developed by government agencies and private organizations to train Americans who live and work in foreign countries. Similar principles and training procedures can be adapted for health care training so practitioners will be prepared to provide services to patients from diverse cultural groups. Brislin and Yoshida (1994) describe an empirically evaluated program based on 40 years of experience in training cross-cultural competence for business people, missionaries, health providers, and consultants who live and work in foreign countries. Their model program, which is compatible with the Rounds, Weil, and Bishop (1994) model described above, incorporates training in self-awareness, general cultural knowledge, specific cultural knowledge, and communication skills that facilitate effective interactions with individuals from other cultures. A large literature on cross-cultural training exists; the challenge is for health care institutions and individual practitioners to harness this literature and translate it into practice.

SUMMARY

Cultural and racial diversity in the U.S. is increasing rapidly, bringing with it the demand for changes in health care provision. Health care practitioners, most of whom are members of the Anglo-American majority culture, increasingly will find themselves providing services for members of other racial and cultural groups whose first language is not English and who may have markedly different beliefs about illness, help-seeking, treatment, and the relationship between health practitioners and health care consumers. Cross-cultural health care places additional demands on health care practitioners and parents to provide effective care for minority children in need of health services.

Provision of health care services for minority children in the U.S. is profoundly influenced by the relationship between minority status, poverty, and racism. Minority children and poor children are exposed to greater health risks than children from White majority culture, but are less likely to have access to timely and appropriate health care, including preventive services. Minority parents, in turn, face cultural and institutional barriers to gaining access to culturally sensitive, accessible, and affordable health care services for their children. Differences in ethnic and cultural backgrounds between parents and providers often result in communication problems that negatively affect the health services received by minority children.

In contrast to the view that the problems inherent in cross-cultural health care services must be solved at the level of the individual family and practitioner, a broader view is that solutions to the problem of providing quality health care services for minority children must include changes at the sociopolitical and institutional levels as well as at the personal level. The process of change demands much from families, practitioners, institutions, and communities as they pursue a better understanding of the broad diversity within cultures, learn to value differences across cultures, and develop a willingness to work together to produce solutions to the shared problem of providing effective health care for minority children.

REFERENCES

Allison, K. W., Crawford, I., Echemendia, R., Robinson, L., & Knepp, D. (1994). Human diversity and professional competence: Training in clinical and counseling psychology revisited. *American Psychologist, 49*, 792–796.

Atkinson, D. D., Spratley, E., & Simpson, C. E. (1994). Increasing the pool of qualified minority medical school applicants: Premedical training at historically Black colleges and universities. *Public Health Reports, 109*, 77–85.

Berlin, E. A., & Fowkes, W. C. (1983). A teaching framework for cross-cultural health care. *The Western Journal of Medicine, 139*, 934–938.

Bernal, M. E., & Castro, F. G. (1994). Are clinical psychologists prepared for service and research with ethnic minorities? *American Psychologist, 49*, 797–805.

Brislin, R., & Yoshida, T. (1994). *Intercultural communication training: An introduction.* Thousand Oaks, CA: Sage Publications.

Butz, A. M., Malveaux, F. J., Eggleston, P., Thompson, L., Schneider, S., Weeks, K., Huss, K., Murigande, C., & Rand, C. S. (1994). Use of community health workers with inner-city children who have asthma. *Clinical Pediatrics, 33*, 135–141.

Call, R. S., Smith, T. F., Morris, E., Chapman, M. D., & Platts-Mills, T. A. E. (1992). Risk factors for asthma in inner city children. *Journal of Pediatrics, 121*, 862–866.

Canino, I. A., Gould, M. S., Prupis, S., & Shaffer, D. (1986). A comparison of symptoms and diagnoses in Hispanic and Black children in an outpatient mental health clinic. *Journal of the American Academy of Child Psychiatry, 25*, 254–259.

Canino, I. A., & Spurlock, J. (1994). *Culturally diverse children and adolescents: Assessment, diagnosis, and treatment.* New York: Guilford Press.

Chan, S. (1990). Early intervention with culturally diverse families of infants and toddlers with disabilities. *Infants and Young Children, 3*, 78–87.

Christensen, C. M. (1992). Multicultural competencies in early intervention: Training professionals for a pluralistic society. *Infants and Young Children, 4*, 49–63.

Clark, M. M. (1983). Cultural context of medical practice. *Western Journal of Medicine, 139*, 806–810.

Cornelius, L. J. (1993). Barriers to medical care for white, Black, and Hispanic American children. *Journal of the National Medical Association, 85*, 281–288.

Davidson, R. C., & Montoya, R. (1987). The distribution of services to the underserved: A comparison of minority and majority medical graduates in California. *Western Journal of Medicine, 146*, 114–117.

Davis, L. E., & Gelsomino, J. (1994). An assessment of practitioner cross-racial treatment experiences. *Social Work, 39*, 116–123.

de Anda, D. (1984). Bicultural socialization: Factors affecting the minority experience. *Social Work, 29*, 101–107.

Delgado, M., & Humm-Delgado, D. (1982). Natural support systems: Source of strength in Hispanic communities. *Social Work, 27*, 83–89.

Dillon, D. (1994). Understanding and assessment of intragroup dynamics in family foster care: African American families. *Child Welfare, 73*, 129–139.

Elfert, H., Anderson, J. M., & Lai, M. (1991). Parents' perceptions of children with chronic illness: A study of immigrant Chinese families. *Journal of Pediatric Nursing, 6*, 114–120.

Fabrega, H., Ulrich, R., & Mezzich, J. E. (1993). Do Caucasian and Black adolescents differ at psychiatric intake? *Journal of the American Academy of Child and Adolescent Psychiatry, 32*, 407–413.

Fong, R. (1994). Family preservation: Making it work for Asians. *Child Welfare, 73*, 331–341.

Fox, P. G., Cowell, J. M., & Montgomery, A. C. (1994). The effects of violence on health and adjustment of southeast Asian refugee children: An integrative review. *Public Health Nursing, 11*, 195–201.

Francis, V., Korsch, B. M., Morris, M. J. (1969). Gaps in doctor-patient communication. Patients' response to medical advice. *New England Journal of Medicine, 10*, 535–540.

Gabarino, J. (1992). The meaning of poverty in the world of children. *American Behavioral Scientist, 35*, 220–237.

Garcia Coll, C. T. (1990). Developmental outcome of minority infants: A process-oriented look into our beginnings. *Child Development, 61*, 270–289.

Gould, K. H. (1988). Asian and Pacific Islanders: Myth and reality. *Social Work, 33*, 142–147.

Grover, G., Berkowitz, C. D., & Lewis, R. J. (1994). Parental recall after a visit to the emergency department. *Clinical Pediatrics, 33*, 194–201.

Guendelman, S. (1983). Developing responsiveness to the health needs of Hispanic children and families. *Social Work in Health Care, 8*, 1–15.

Harry, B. (1992a). Making sense of disability: Low-income, Puerto Rican parents' theories of the problem. *Exceptional Children, 59*, 27–40.

Harry, B. (1992b). Restructuring the participation of African-American parents in special education. *Exceptional Children, 59*, 123–131.

Harwood, R. L. (1992). The influence of culturally derived values on Anglo and Puerto Rican mothers' perceptions of attachment behavior. *Child Development, 63*, 822–839.

Herrnstein, R. J., & Murray, C. (1994). *The bell curve: Intelligence and class structure in American life*. New York: The Free Press.

Huston, A. C., McLoyd, V. C., & Garcia Coll, C. (1994). Children and poverty: Issues in contemporary research. *Child Development, 65*, 275–282.

Julian, T. W., McKenry, P. C., & McKelvey, M. W. (1994). Cultural variations in parenting: Perceptions of Caucasian, African-American, Hispanic, and Asian-American parents. *Family Relations, 43*, 30–37.

Kalmanson, B., & Seligman, S. (1992). Family-provider relationships: The basis of all interventions. *Infants and Young Children, 4*, 46–52.

Kaplan-Sanoff, M., Parker, S., & Zuckerman, B. (1991). Poverty and early childhood development: What do we know, and what should we do? *Infants and Young Children, 4*, 68–76.

Kinzie, J. D., Sack, W. H., Angell, R. H., Manson, S., & Rath, B. (1986). The psychiatric effects of massive trauma on Cambodian children: I. The children. *Journal of the American Academy of Child Psychiatry, 25*, 370–376.

Kleinman, A. (1978). Concepts and a model for the comparison of medical systems as cultural systems. *Social Science and Medicine, 12*, 85–93.

Kleinman, A., Eisenberg, L., & Good, B. (1978). Culture, illness, and care: Clinical lessons from anthropologic and cross-cultural research. *Annals of Internal Medicine, 88*, 251–258.

Lum, C. K., & Korenman, S. G. (1994). Cultural-sensitivity training in U.S. medical schools. *Academic Medicine, 69*, 239–241.

Lum, D. (1982). Toward a framework for social work practice with minorities. *Social Work, 27*, 244–249.

Lynch, E. W., & Hanson, M. J. (1993). Changing demographics: Implications for training in early intervention. *Infants and Young Children, 6*, 50–55.

Lynch, E. W., & Stein, R. C. (1987). Parent participation by ethnicity: A comparison of Hispanic, Black, and Anglo families. *Exceptional Children, 54*, 105–111.

Magar, V. (1990). Health care needs of Central American refugees. *Nursing Outlook, 38*, 239–242.

Malach, R. S., & Segel, N. (1990). Perspectives on health care delivery systems for American Indian families. *Children's Health Care, 19*, 219–228.

Mao, C., Bullock, C. S., Harway, E. C., & Khalsa, S. K. (1988). A workshop on ethnic and cultural awareness for second-year students. *Journal of Medical Education, 63*, 624–628.

Marcus, L., & Marcus, A. R. (1993). Multiculturalism in the real world. *Family Systems Medicine, 11*, 335–341.

Marion, R. L. (1980). Communicating with parents of culturally diverse exceptional children. *Exceptional Children, 46*, 616–623.

Mary, N. L. (1990). Reactions of Black, Hispanic, and white mothers to having a child with handicaps. *Mental Retardation, 28*, 1–5.

McLoyd, V. C. (1990). The impact of economic hardship on Black families and children: Psychological distress, parenting, and socioemotional development. *Child Development, 61*, 311–346.

McMahon, A., & Allen-Meares, P. (1992). Is social work racist? A content analysis of recent literature. *Social Work, 37*, 533–539.

McNeely, R. L., & Badami, M. K. (1984). Interracial communication in school social work. *Social Work, 29*, 22–26.

Nichols-Casebolt, A. M. (1988). Black families headed by single mothers: Growing numbers and increasing poverty. *Social Work, 33*, 306–313.

Olson, L. M., Becker, T. M., Wiggins, C. L., Key, C. R., & Samet, J. M. (1990). Injury mortality in American Indian, Hispanic, and non-Hispanic white children in New Mexico, 1958–1982. *Social Science and Medicine, 30*, 479–486.

Pickwell, S. M., & Warnock, F. (1994). Family nurse practitioner faculty clinical practice with undocumented migrants. *Family and Community Health, 16*, 32–38.

Pinderhughes, E. B. (1982). Family functioning of Afro-Americans. *Social Work, 27*, 91–96.

Pollitt, E. (1994). Poverty and child development: Relevance of research in developing countries to the United States. *Child Development, 65*, 283–295.

Redick, L. T., & Wood, B. (1982). Cross-cultural problems for southeast Asian refugee minors. *Child Welfare, 61*, 365–373.

Reiss, D. (1993). Culture and poverty. *Psychiatry, 56*, 321–323.

Riley, A. W., Finney, J. W., Mellits, E. D., Starfield, B., Kidwell, S., Quaskey, S., Cataldo, M. F., Filipp, L., & Shematek, J. P. (1993). Determinants of children's health care use: An investigation of psychosocial factors. *Medical Care, 31*, 767–783.

Robinson, J. B. (1989). Clinical treatment of Black families: Issues and strategies. *Social Work, 34*, 323–329.

Rogler, L. H. (1993). Culture in psychiatric diagnosis: An issue of scientific accuracy. *Psychiatry, 56*, 324–327.

Rogler, L. H. (1994). International migrations: A framework for directing research. *American Psychologist, 49*, 701–708.

Rogler, L. H., & Cortes, D. H. (1993). Help-seeking pathways: A unifying concept in mental health care. *American Journal of Psychiatry, 150*, 554–561.

Rounds, K. A., Weil, M., & Bishop, K. K. (1994). Practice with culturally diverse families of young children with disabilities. *Families in Society: The Journal of Contemporary Human Services, 38*, 3–14.

Sack, W. H., Angell, R. H., Kinzie, J. D., & Rath, B. (1986). The psychiatric effects of massive trauma on Cambodian children: II. The family, the home, and the school. *Journal of the American Academy of Child Psychiatry, 25*, 377–383.

Schur, C. L., Bernstein, A. B., & Berk, M. L. (1987). The importance of distinguishing Hispanic subpopulations in the use of medical care. *Medical Care, 25*, 627–641.

Schwartz-Lookinland, S., McKeever, L. C., & Saputo, M. (1989). Compliance with antibiotic regimens in Hispanic mothers. *Patient Education and Counseling, 13*, 171–182.

Siegel, J. M. (1974). A brief review of the effects of race in clinical service interactions. *American Journal of Orthopsychiatry, 44*, 555–562.

Spencer, M. B. (1990). Development of minority children: An introduction. *Child Development, 61*, 267–269.

St. Lawrence, J. S., & Azevedo, M. (1989). Health care conditions in Cameroon and Chad. In M. Azevedo (Ed.), *Cameroon and Chad in historical and contemporary perspectives* (pp. 119–137). Lewiston, NY: Mellen Press.

Timberlake, E. M., & Cook, K. O. (1984). Social work and the Vietnamese refugee. *Social Work, 29*, 108–113.

Trevino, F. M., Sumaya, C., Miranda, M., Martinez, L., & Saldana, J. S. (1994). Increasing the representation of Hispanics in the health professions. *Public Health Reports, 108*, 551–558.

U.S. Bureau of the Census. (1992). Poverty in the United States, 1991. *Current Population Reports, Series P-60, No. 181*. Washington, DC: Government Printing Office.

Watkins, E. L., Harlan, C., Eng, E., Gansky, S. A., Gehan, D., & Larson, K. (1994). Assessing the effectiveness of lay health advisors with migrant farmworkers. *Family and Community Health, 16*, 72–87.

Weitzman, M., Gortmaker, S., & Sobel, A. (1990). Racial, social, and environmental risks for childhood asthma. *American Journal of Disabilities in Children, 144*, 1189–1194.

Wissow, L. S., Gittelsohn, A. M., Szklo, M., Starfield, B., & Mussman, M. (1988). Poverty, race, and hospitalization for childhood asthma. *American Journal of Public Health, 78*, 777–782.

Zambrana, R. E., Ell, K., Dorrington, C., Wachsman, L., & Hodge, D. (1994). The relationship between psychosocial status of immigrant Latino mothers and use of emergency pediatric services. *Health and Social Work, 19*, 93–102.

CHAPTER 4

LEGAL ISSUES IN THE PEDIATRIC SETTING

Betty Pfefferbaum

INTRODUCTION

The Child in Context

Important reciprocal interactions occur within families from the moment a child is conceived. These interactions change as children and parents mature. Children and their families also function within a broader social milieu comprised of other individuals and family units organized through a complex structure of customs and laws. Recognizing this, our society distributes authority and responsibilities accordingly among children, their parents, and the state. Legal issues emerge in each of these units and influence interactions among them. Of particular concern are the seeming contradictions between the child's autonomy and the need for protection, and between the family's privacy rights and its social and fiscal responsibilities.

While not necessarily an appropriate marker for ability, age is often used to designate legal milestones. Children are granted rights and responsibilities gradually and must meet certain age requirements before driving, drinking, marrying, voting, and holding public office. Ideally, social policies and laws emanate from some guiding theory of cognitive and emotional development, while civil and criminal legal actions are decided with full attention to individual capacities and differences (Group for the Advancement of Psychiatry, 1989).

Parents have great freedom in managing their families and in making decisions that affect their children. In return, they are responsible for their children's care and support. The state protects parental decisions but intervenes if necessary to guard the safety and well-being of the child (Mnookin & Weisberg, 1995).

The concept of children's rights creates, a tension that derives from concern that children might be granted premature autonomy in areas like consent for medical treatment or, alternatively, be shielded from liability for their criminal acts. The unfortunate politicization of this issue has not elevated the debate; rather, it threatens to undermine the establishment of services for children.

This chapter examines legal issues in the pediatric setting, keeping in mind the complex interactions among children, their families, and the state. Of particular interest are the issues of confidentiality and record keeping, informed consent, malpractice, divorce and custody, discipline and abuse, child witnesses, and special education. Discussion of these issues should acquaint pediatric and mental health professionals with current issues, legal doctrines, and statutory and case law. In many areas, the law is unsettled and may vary from state to state. An understanding of legal reasoning and arguments, as well as legislation and judicial decisions, should enhance the professional's clinical judgment.

CONFIDENTIALITY AND THE MEDICAL RECORD

The Professional Relationship

The doctor-patient relationship can be established in several ways, through express or implied contract or when the professional undertakes to provide care. Express written contracts, previously uncommon, are becoming more important as managed care proliferates. Traditionally, an implied contract formed the basis of the relationship. In legal terms, an implied contract is created when a patient consults a doctor and the doctor accepts the offer by examining the patient. In managed care settings, there may be an express contract between the professional and the institution and another between the patient and the institution, with an implied contract between the patient and the doctor. A professional relationship is also established when a doctor renders treatment (that is, undertakes to care) even absent a contract or expectation of payment. In any case, the professional has a fiduciary obligation, guided by law and ethics, toward the patient.

The Goals of Confidentiality

The mental health professional owes a duty of confidentiality to the patient with respect to information disclosed in the professional relationship. The duty of confidentiality is based on both legal and ethical principles. The goal of these principles is to protect the patient's privacy while promoting open communication. The legal cause of action for breach of confidentiality may be based on an implied covenant of confidentiality, invasion of privacy, the physician's fiduciary duty, and licensing and privilege statutes. In addition, the professional who fails to protect patient confidentiality risks ethics charges and licensure restrictions (Macbeth, Wheeler, Sither, & Onek, 1994).

The goals of confidentiality are no less important when the patient is a minor. This is particularly true for adolescents who, as part of the process of individuation, may desire privacy and confidentiality in their relationships and may seek opportunities to discuss issues without parental knowledge or consent (English, 1990). The duty of confidentiality is complicated in situations involving children and adolescents, however, by differ-

ences among jurisdictions regarding who controls disclosure.

It is important for the professional to address the issue of confidentiality with patients and their parents early in the course of treatment. It is sometimes tempting to share mental health information with pediatric staff. This should be done with caution and with knowledge of, and agreement with, the patient and parents.

Confidentiality is not extended to information indicating the patient's propensity to cause harm to self or others. When disclosure of information is "less vital" but would potentially benefit the family, the therapist may encourage the patient to disclose the information or obtain the patient's permission to disclose it (Schetky & Benedek, 1992, pp. 60–61). Most patients understand the limits of confidentiality, although adolescents may be less candid if they fear the professional is a conduit through which information will pass to adults with whom they experience conflict.

Who Controls Disclosure?

Jurisdictions differ with respect to who controls disclosure of information, particularly when parents are divorced or divorcing or when the patient is an adolescent. The clinician is advised to seek counsel about disclosure in divorce situations. With respect to treatment of adolescents, states have differerent laws governing disclosure, whereby in some states (1) adolescents control disclosure if they have the right to consent to care, (2) disclosure to the parents is denied if the minor objects, (3) professionals may notify parents even in the face of objections by the minor, or (4) parents are allowed access to records without addressing potential conflicts between parents and children (English, 1990). Furthermore, a number of federal and state statutes protect a minor patient's confidentiality for certain specified areas, including HIV status, mental health, and substance abuse. Clinicians are advised to familiarize themselves with state and federal law pertinent to these issues (Macbeth et al., 1994).

Testimonial Privilege

Testimonial privilege is a legal concept sometimes confused with confidentiality. The physician-patient privilege is designed to protect the patient's confidentiality and represents the patient's right to prevent physician disclosure in court (Nurcombe, 1991). The patient may authorize the disclosure of information, thereby waiving the privilege. If the patient's physical or mental condition is at issue, most jurisdictions consider the privilege to have been waived. State statutes and case law should be reviewed because the testimonial privilege does not exist in all jurisdictions; it may not extend to non-physician health care providers (Furrow, Johnson, Jost, & Schwartz, 1991); and it may not apply to family and group therapy (Macbeth et al., 1994).

Duty to Report

Conflict may arise between the duty of confidentiality and the duty to disclose certain information. State statutes may require the reporting of suspected child abuse and certain communicable diseases, and statutes and case law may impose a duty to warn identifiable persons who are objects of a patient's threat (Furrow et al., 1991).

The Medical Record

It is important for professionals to document their involvement with patients. This motivates them to keep a medical record and raises the issue of the patient's or parent's right to information contained in the record. Concern about divulging information in records to patients is based on the belief that patients may not understand the information, may be upset by it, or may use it in harmful ways. Records may contain confidences of third parties, and granting access to records might discourage openness in record-keeping and increase administrative costs. On the other hand, patient access arguably enhances compliance and understanding, improves the professional relationship, and helps assure continuity of care (Furrow et al., 1991).

Medical records are not the property of the patient but belong instead to the provider who created them. There is, however, growing support for a duty to disclose information contained in the record to the patient. Statutes and case law in some states permit patient access to records and some courts have acknowledged that the patient has a property right in the information the record contains (Furrow et al., 1991). This may be problematic in situations involving mental health records because of the potential harm to the patient or others created by disclosure of certain information. Therefore, it is important that the recorder of information use care in choosing what and how to document and in communicating this information to interested parties. Dual record keeping is not advised and concealment is against the law if discovery is legally mandated (Simon, 1992).

INFORMED CONSENT

The doctrine of informed consent emphasizes individual autonomy. It protects patients by involving them in decisions about their care and by encouraging providers to consider patient wishes with respect to treatment. Informed consent is complicated when the patient is a child because it requires the capacity for comprehension and decision-making and because it must also respect parental authority. Mental health professionals may have an important role in providing informed consent, particularly for young children or when there is conflict between child patients and their parents.

Competence

Informed consent requires that the patient be competent to make decisions. To be competent, one must possess "requisite physical, mental, natural or legal qualifications" (Black, Nolan, & Nolan-Haley, 1990). Courts are hesitant to specify standards of competence (Furrow et al., 1991) and legal definitions of competence resist identifying minimum standards for understanding or decision-making.

Competence may be difficult to establish in adults and presents even greater problems in children and adolescents. Theories of cognitive development have been used to develop general guidelines, commonly based on age, with little attention to individual variation. Some suggest that competence of minors to give informed consent be ascertained by comparing the minor's decision with those of legally competent adults or with decisions by hypothetical, reasonable, or rational decision-makers. Few studies exist, however, that compare children and adults on decision-making capability (Gardner, Scherer, & Tester, 1989).

An individual's emotional state, prior history, and experience are among factors that influence comprehension and decision-making necessary for informed consent. Further complicating the issue, competence is not absolute; competence for decision-making in one area may not generalize to other areas (Gardner et al., 1989; Group for the Advancement of Psychiatry, 1989).

Informed Consent of Minors

The general rule is that parental consent must be given for the medical treatment of minors. This is based on respect for parental authority and family privacy and the fact that parents are legally and financially responsible for the care and support of their children (Mnookin & Weisberg,

1995). In addition to obtaining parental consent, it is often advisable to provide age-appropriate information and to obtain formal or informal assent of the child.

In situations involving divorce, consent should be obtained from the parent with legal custody. State legislation addresses specific situations in which parents are absent. States identify who may consent for delinquent, abused, neglected, and foster children, and every state provides for court intervention in situations of neglect by parents who refuse medical intervention for their children (English, 1990). In fact, parents may be charged with criminal offenses if they prevent their children from receiving care.

Exceptions to Parental Consent

A variety of exceptions allow treatment without consent. These include exceptions for emergencies and therapeutic privilege. The exception for emergency treatment logically applies to minors as well as adults. In an emergency involving a minor, however, the clinician is advised to notify parents as soon as possible after intervening and to obtain consent for further treatment. The therapeutic privilege allows treatment if the doctor reasonably believes that disclosure would not be in the patient's best interest and that disclosure would interfere with treatment.

Statutes in most jurisdictions provide that married or emancipated minors may consent to treatment. Emancipated minors are youth who are married, in the military, or living apart from their parents and fiscally independent.

Public policy dictates that minors be allowed to consent to treatment for certain conditions that are often identified by statute. These include contraception and pregnancy, sexually transmitted and other communicable diseases, substance abuse, and emotional problems. Statutes in some states actually forbid the notification of parents when minors seek treatment for substance abuse or venereal disease without their parents' knowledge (Holder, 1987). Clinicians are urged to review their state laws related to these conditions.

The Mature Minor Doctrine

The mature minor doctrine is a common law rule of increasing importance in health care. It allows the clinician to treat consenting adolescents who are mature, able to understand the nature and consequences of treatment, and capable of making decisions. When possible and practical, it is recommended that the clinician also notify the minor's parents.

The clinician relying on the mature minor doctrine should document the basis for using the doctrine with information demonstrating the adolescent's maturity and decision-making capacity. Factors demonstrating maturity include, for example, information that the minor initiated the health care contact, asks appropriate questions, understands pertinent information, and communicates effectively. Decision-making capacity involves understanding and reason, voluntariness, and an appreciation of the implications of the decision (Leikin, 1989; Sigman & O'Connor, 1991). Capacity may vary according to the specific decision involved and is evidenced in the process of obtaining informed consent, the youth's reasoning, and the voluntariness of the decision (Sigman & O'Connor, 1991). The mental health professional is uniquely qualified to assist in assessments of the adolescent's maturity and decision-making capacity.

Clinicians are advised to review the law related to informed consent by minors in their states of practice. Some states have adopted specific legislation regarding consent by minors. In other states, case law protects the clinician. The risk of liability associated with the treatment of mature minors without parental consent is minimal if the minor is an older adolescent who understands the proposed treatment and its risks and benefits and who can give informed consent, if the medical care is necessary for the patient's benefit, and if there is a good reason for not seeking parental consent (English, 1990).

A court's willingness to accept a minor's consent is likely to vary with the severity and risk of the illness and treatment. Courts are apt to allow minors to consent to procedures of relatively low risk, but may be unwilling to allow their consent to high-risk procedures, such as organ donation, or to interventions without therapeutic value (Sigman & O'Connor, 1991). Therefore, the clinician should document the risks and benefits associated with treatment and with failure to treat.

Most statutes and cases related to the mature minor doctrine address situations involving care for physical disorders. Similar rules would presumably apply to mental health intervention but might not protect qualified and licensed health care providers working in community mental health facilities or in facilities without physician coverage, such as drug treatment centers using former addicts as therapists (Holder, 1991).

Abortion

Laws related to abortion are of particular concern and are highly controversial. The current status of parental notification and consent for abortion by minors depends on state law. States may require parental notice or consent for abortion in minors if they also provide a "judicial bypass" or alternate method of consent whereby the minor may seek a timely and anonymous court order to determine her maturity. If determined to be mature, the minor must be allowed to make her own decision. If determined to be immature, the court must decide if the abortion is in the minor's best interest (*Bellotti v. Baird II*, 1979).

The American Medical Association's Council on Ethical and Judicial Affairs (1993) and others (Holder, 1987) have expressed concern for pregnant adolescents in dysfunctional families and for victims of sexual and physical abuse who may fear the repercussions of disclosure to parents. In counseling teens, the professional must be prepared to address their sexual interests and activities and their reproductive options and to assess potential parental support or rejection, all the while respecting the need for privacy (American Medical Association Council on Ethical and Judicial Affairs, 1993).

Information to Be Disclosed

In order to make an informed decision about consent, the patient must have sufficient information. In most jurisdictions, a professional standard, based on customary practice in the community or on a reasonable practitioner, determines what must be disclosed. In some jurisdictions, disclosure must include any information relevant to the individual's decision, independent of medical practice (Macbeth, Wheeler, Sither, & Onek, 1994).

In an increasing number of jurisdictions, the clinician is required to disclose "material" information. As articulated in *Canterbury v. Spence* (1972), "material" information is that which a reasonable individual would need in order to make a decision. A "subjective lay standard" used in some jurisdictions is even stricter, requiring the clinician to divulge all information which the particular patient would want in order to make a decision (Simon, 1992).

It is generally recommended that the following information be disclosed: the diagnosis or nature of the condition that requires treatment; the nature and purpose of the proposed treatment; the probability of success, risks, and benefits of the proposed treatment; alternatives to the proposed treatment and their attendant risks and consequences; and the prognosis with and without the proposed treatment (Furrow et al., 1991; Nurcombe, 1991). Not all risks must be disclosed. The need to disclose a risk depends on its severity and the probability of it occurring, the likelihood of treatment success, and the availability of other less dangerous treatments (Simon, 1992).

Refusing Treatment

Mental health professionals are commonly consulted when children or adolescents are noncompliant with medical treatment. These cases may occur in situations involving religious affiliation or terminal illness. It is essential to determine if treatable or reversible factors such as depression, need for support, or risk-taking are the cause of noncompliance (Hartnett, 1994).

Presumably an adolescent would have the right to refuse "completely elective treatment," but the same is almost certainly not true for necessary or lifesaving treatment (Holder, 1987, p. 3401). The professional is encouraged to review state statutory and case law, particularly in situations where treatment might be lifesaving. Every state has legislation providing for judicial jurisdiction over children in order to supersede parental decisions about medical treatment (Mnookin & Weisberg, 1995). These statutes are typically vague, giving courts substantial discretion.

Commitment

Mental health professionals will be consulted when psychiatric hospitalization or commitment of minors is necessary. In-patient mental health treatment of minors presents unique issues related to parental authority and the autonomy of youth.

The United States Supreme Court addressed the issue of involuntary commitment of minors in *Parham v. J. R. and J. L.* (1979). The *Parham* Court espoused the view that parents act in the best interests of their children and supported parental decision-making in psychiatric hospitalization, requiring only that the admitting physician make an independent evaluation of the child's condition and need for treatment and complete periodic reviews of the need for treatment (*Parham*, 1979). The Court noted that it would allow "informal, traditional medical investigative techniques" (p. 607) in interviewing a child and failed to indicate how formal or frequent postcommitment review must be. The *Parham* Court rationalized the lack of procedural safeguards, noting that such procedures discourage parents from seeking treatment, increase tension within families, and burden health care providers with legal maneuvering when they should be involved in patient care.

States have established mechanisms for emergency, short-term and/or long-term commitment of adults, and provide procedural safeguards, such as judicial hearings and counsel, to protect patients. States vary greatly, however, with respect to involuntary commitment procedures for minors. Some states require no more than those procedures set down in *Parham*; others provide safeguards similar to those granted to adults (Wizner, 1991). Professionals must, therefore, be familiar with laws of the state of practice.

Informed Consent for Psychotherapy

There is a growing trend to obtain informed consent for psychotherapy. Informed consent is useful in psychotherapy for several reasons. It serves a "preventive" function by discouraging potentially harmful psychotherapy through increased participation of patients in choosing the therapeutic method. It encourages professionals as a group to examine the merits of their therapies. It also serves as a theory of legal recovery to compensate patients who are harmed from a defect in the informed consent (Horowitz, 1984).

The elements of negligent informed consent—standard of care, breach, causation, and injury—are difficult to prove in psychotherapy cases. The standard of care may vary greatly. It may be difficult to prove that a therapist's breach caused the injury. An intervention may not be obvious or easily articulated and the potential for misinterpretation and distortion are great. The impact of psychotherapy is often intangible and injury is difficult to substantiate, particularly if the patient was emotionally disturbed at the outset. Harm is often emotional and may be difficult to prove except in extreme situations (Horowitz, 1984).

Legal Causes of Action

The basis of the legal action related to consent is found in tort law under theories of battery and negligence. Battery involves nonconsensual intentional touching. Under the battery theory, the plaintiff's case is relatively easy to establish because it is unnecessary to prove harm or to ascertain the standard of care; the plaintiff need only prove that an unauthorized touching, and thus the injury, occurred. The battery cause of action arises when no consent was given, the clinician exceeds the consent given, or the consent was not informed (Cowan & Bertsch, 1984). Under a battery cause of action, punitive

damages may be awarded even when actual damages are minimal (Furrow et al., 1991).

Negligence involves failure to do what a reasonable and prudent person in similar circumstances would do, or doing something a reasonable and prudent person in similar circumstances would not do. To prove negligence with respect to consent, the patient usually must prove that (1) there was a therapeutic relationship, (2) the clinician had a duty to disclose certain information, (3) there was a failure to provide this information and that failure cannot be excused, (4) the patient would not have consented to treatment had the information been provided, and (5) failure to disclose the information was the proximate cause of the patient's injuries (Rozovsky, 1990).

Some states have enacted specific legislation governing informed consent. This legislation varies with respect to standards for disclosure and non-disclosure, but typically makes failure to obtain informed consent negligence (Cowan & Bertsch, 1984; Rozovsky, 1990; Simon, 1992).

MALPRACTICE

The possibility of malpractice and charges of malpractice threaten all clinicians and influence the way they practice. While mental health professionals were once relatively immune to the threat of legal action, this is no longer the case. In recent years, areas of potential liability, the number of suits, and the size of awards have all increased. It is essential, therefore, that mental health professionals have some understanding of the law related to malpractice.

The Theory of Negligence

A malpractice charge is usually brought as a tort claim of negligence, though it may be based on other legal theories such as contract law (King, 1986). Negligence involves conduct falling below a standard of care that causes injury to the patient. The elements for a cause of action in negligence are (1) a relationship between the clinician and patient giving rise to a duty of care owed by the clinician to the patient, (2) breach of the duty, (3) injury to the patient, and (4) causation. Each of these elements has specific legal meaning.

The clinician owes a duty of care to a patient with whom there is a professional relationship. The nature of the duty is based on the standard of care. Courts base the standard on an "average practitioner" or a "reasonably competent" practitioner (King, 1986, p. 75). The general rule is that the clinician must possess and exercise the knowledge, skill, and care that would be exercised by a reasonable or competent member of the profession in the same or similar circumstances. Specialists are held to higher standards than general practitioners. Historically, standards of care were based on evidence about the prevailing care in the defendant's community; regional and national standards are now common. Professionals generally are not liable for mere errors in judgment if they exercise reasonable care.

Standards of care used to establish malpractice are often vague and unpredictable, and clinical practice requires professional judgment. This introduces a considerable element of subjectivity. Expert testimony is typically required to establish the professional standard and that the defendant's conduct represented a departure from that standard.

Courts differ with respect to how this standard of care is measured, but for the most part, it is determined by the profession. As society becomes more sophisticated about health care issues, however, the allocation of decision-making responsibility may change (King, 1986). This gives rise to the question of whether the profession's standard of care should conclusively establish the legal standard or should simply serve as evidence of due care. The Washington Supreme Court decision in *Helling v. Carey* (1974) heralded a landmark break with precedent when the Court examined the complexity, costs and risks with or without a procedure and held that the medical standard of care must give way to a higher standard if reasonable prudence so requires.

To prove a claim of malpractice, the plaintiff must demonstrate actual harm suffered by the patient and a causal relationship between the defendant's alleged negligence and the harm suffered. Harm may be physical, such as an adverse effect of medication, physical injury, or suicide; or it may be psychological, which is usually more difficult to prove. To establish causation, most courts require the plaintiff to prove that the injury would not have occurred absent the negligent act and that there was a direct and foreseeable link between the conduct and the injury.

Malpractice in Mental Health

Areas of concern with respect to malpractice in mental health cases include the use of medication and adverse drug reactions, such as tardive dyskinesia with antipsychotic medication or tics with stimulants, suicide or threats of violence, failure to obtain informed consent, and unilateral termination of care. Treatment with medication, decisions to hospitalize, concerns about suicide and violence, informed consent, and termination of care

warrant special attention and documentation of the clinician's decisions and rationale for those decisions.

Psychopharmacology

With increasingly precise diagnoses, the development of standards of practice by professional organizations and the proliferation of drugs, there is a growing emphasis on the use of medications. Failure to use medications, or their inappropriate use, creates potential liability. The situation is complicated for drugs that have not been approved for use in children.

There are numerous sources of potential liability associated with the use of medication, including diagnosis; rationale for a drug's use; choice of a particular agent; a history of previous response, side effects, or allergic reactions; the determination of other medical conditions contraindicating the use of medication; informed consent; administration of the drug; concurrent use of other medications; use of drugs in ways or age groups not recommended; monitoring of the drug's effects and side effects; and decisions about when to discontinue the drug (Nurcombe & Partlett, 1994). The physician's rationale and informed consent should always be documented. Documentation of expert consultation and literature review may also be helpful.

Suicide

Suicide, like other malpractice concerns, will result in liability if the professional breached the duty of care stemming from a failure to exercise the skill and care of the average or a reasonably competent practitioner in the same or similar circumstances. Typical issues addressed by courts with respect to suicide involve claims that the professional did not adequately assess the potential for suicide, that appropriate treatment and reasonable precautions were not taken, and that the treatment plan was not appropriately implemented. Courts generally recognize how difficult it is to predict dangerousness and that clinical judgment may vary with respect to the management of any particular patient (Macbeth, Wheeler, Sither, & Onek, 1994). Health care professionals who exercise reasonable care and document their decision-making are not likely to be found liable for errors in judgment.

The duty to protect a patient from suicide arises when there is a foreseeable risk that a patient would endanger him/herself. Liability may result from failure to respond to signs or symptoms indicating the potential for suicide or from failure to respond to new information or developments. This is especially true in the case of hospitalized patients, with liability likely to result from failure to institute adequate precautions, premature discharge of suicidal patients, and inadequate follow-up after discharge. The duty to protect also applies to outpatients, though the difficulty in controlling patients in the outpatient setting is generally recognized. Liability with respect to the suicidal outpatient might result from failure to hospitalize, inappropriate use of medication, abandonment, and failure to warn family members (Macbeth et al., 1994).

The professional must conduct a thorough evaluation of the suicidal patient, often requiring that information be obtained from a variety of sources, including family members and previous records. A risk analysis may be useful. This analysis should include assessment of various factors such as interpersonal relationships, home environment, depressive and psychotic symptoms, impulsiveness, prior history of suicidal ideation and behavior, family history of suicide, drug and alcohol abuse, and the therapeutic alliance (Simon, 1992).

A recent Maryland case, *Eisel v. Board of Education of Montgomery County* (1991), involved the suicide of a teenager whose friends had notified school personnel of the youth's suicidal ideation. Finding a duty to use reasonable means to prevent a suicide, the appellate decision noted that a jury might find that the duty included warning the child's parent. Reasoning that the foreseeability, certainty, and potential severity of harm were very great and that the state's interest in preventing teen suicide placed schools "at the forefront of the prevention effort" (p. 453), the court in *Eisel* concluded that school counselors have a duty to use reasonable means to attempt to prevent a suicide when they have been given notice of a student's suicidal intent. Obviously, the mental health professional must balance this duty against the duty of confidentiality, though confidentiality is typically not extended to indications that a patient may cause harm to self or others.

Violence and the Duty to Warn

Professional liability associated with warning about potentially violent behavior dates to the *Tarasoff v. Regents of the University of California* (1976) case. The duty to warn has subsequently been clarified by both case law and state statutes. *Tarasoff* allowed the victim of a violent patient to recover when the professional knew, or should have known, that the patient was likely to commit violence against the victim and failed to take reasonable steps to prevent the violence (Macbeth et al., 1994). When the intended victim is known, the therapist must warn him/her.

Tarasoff further provided that the therapist could discharge the duty by warning the intended victim or "oth-

ers likely to apprise the victim of the danger," notifying the police, or taking "whatever other steps are reasonably necessary under the circumstances" (p. 340). The court refused to establish "any hard and fast rule" with respect to determining a potential victim's identity (p. 345, footnote 11).

In a later case involving the murder of a child by a juvenile offender with known dangerous and violent propensities, who had threatened to murder a child in the neighborhood, the California Supreme Court refused to impose a duty to warn when the victim's identity was unknown (*Thompson v. County of Alameda*, 1980). Some courts, however, have found professionals liable for violence against unidentifiable victims based on failure to restrain the patient, premature discharge, or failure to institute involuntary commitment (Macbeth et al., 1994). Some courts have also extended liability to situations involving the unintentional harming of another (Macbeth et al., 1994; Simon, 1992). Other courts have refused to impose liability in situations in which the victim is aware of the danger (Macbeth et al., 1994).

In many states, legislation now defines the duty to warn and professional immunity. Confidentiality statutes in some states provide exceptions for disclosure of certain information in particular situations. State provisions should be reviewed and the limits of confidentiality should be addressed with patients and parents.

The assessment of dangerousness may be complicated. The mental health professional must obtain information from a variety of sources: the patient, significant others, and current and past treatment records (Monahan, 1993). The clinician should (1) take a careful history regarding previous violence and the potential for violence, (2) utilize that information in making treatment decisions, (3) obtain mental health or legal consultation when in doubt, (4) institute commitment proceedings when appropriate, (5) assess the credibility of threats and availability of lethal means, (6) warn potential victims, (7) take steps to assure that appropriate follow-up occurs, (8) emphasize the responsibility of the patient and family members, and (9) document assessments, decisions, and discussions (Macbeth et al., 1994).

Abandonment

The clinician, having established a relationship with a patient, may be liable for abandonment if he/she unilaterally and abruptly or prematurely terminates the relationship and the patient suffers harm as a result of the termination (Macbeth et al., 1994; Nurcombe, 1991). Clinicians who simply provide an opinion to a primary care physician are not obligated to provide continuing care unless they have agreed to treat the patient (Nurcombe, 1991). Therapist absences must be discussed with the patient and plans must be made to provide for the patient's care during those absences (Macbeth et al., 1994). Termination should not occur when the patient is in a crisis or if termination will precipitate a crisis.

Except in emergency situations, therapists may terminate the therapeutic relationship if they provide reasonable notice, offer to assist in locating another therapist, and make records available to the new therapist (Simon, 1992). The therapist's efforts, and cautions associated with termination, should be documented. The potential liability associated with abandonment is so great that some authorities recommend that in the event of unilateral termination, the clinician should discuss the reasons for termination with the patient, give the patient names of other providers and sufficient notice to locate another provider, and send the patient a certified letter (return receipt requested) documenting termination (Nurcombe, 1991; Simon, 1992).

DIVORCE AND CUSTODY

Psychological Adjustment of Children to Divorce

While children do not typically present, in the pediatric setting, with complaints directly related to divorce and custody, those issues may underlie or complicate medical conditions. The mental health professional may have an important role in identifying, assessing, and treating divorce and custody issues.

Children suffer immediate and long-term psychological effects associated with their parents' separation and divorce. Psychological adjustment is related to the child's age and developmental stage, expectations of the parents, perception and understanding of the divorce, and mechanisms for coping (Wallerstein, 1989). Studies indicate that children fare better if they have continuing relationships with both parents, if their parents are able to resume parenting after the initial crisis, and if the divorce brings diminution of parental conflict. Abused children improve if separated from the abusive parent. Large numbers of children remain distressed years after their parents' divorce. This is particularly true if the custodial parent remains troubled or experiences diminished parenting capability, or if conflict between the parents does not dissipate (Wallerstein, 1989).

Custody Decisions and Legal Standards

Custody may be granted to one or both parents. Parents may share legal (parent who makes important decisions) and/or physical (parent with whom the child resides) custody. Studies addressing the effects of joint custody are not conclusive: joint custody may work well for parents who choose it and are committed to it, but there is no evidence that it is better for children; and it may even be deleterious if chosen for the wrong reasons (such as to decrease financial settlements or child support payments) or if judicially imposed (Nurcombe & Partlett, 1994).

At common law, children were the property of their fathers and fathers were given preference in the event of divorce. During the nineteenth century, a preference favoring maternal custody, at least for young children, was established with the "tender years" doctrine. Most courts now use some variation of the "best interests of the child" standard, though they may be influenced by other factors.

The "best interests" standard typically takes into consideration a variety factors, including the wishes of the parents and child, the ability of the parties to parent effectively, the relationships within the family, the child's adjustment, any mental and physical conditions of those involved, and the willingness and ability of the parents to encourage close and continuing relations with the other parent. When the "best interests" standard fails to dictate a clear choice between parents, some states give preference to the primary caretaker, who is defined with respect to rather specific functions in relation to the child (Nurcombe & Partlett, 1994).

Race, Religion, and Morality in Custody Decisions

Few divorce and custody cases reach the level of the United States Supreme Court, but the Court has decided that race is not a permissible consideration in custody decisions (*Palmore v. Sidoti*, 1984). While courts may consider religious preferences and issues in determining custody, the First Amendment requires constraint in this area. Moral issues which used to be emphasized in custody suits are now generally irrelevant unless they directly affect the child.

Custody Evaluations

Mental health professionals participate in the judicial determination of custody by providing custody evaluations. They may become involved at the request of either or both parents or the court. Experts are advised to ascertain what questions the parties or judge want answered, and whether they can be answered, and should provide objective and impartial evaluations to be used by both parties and the court rather than by one party alone (Schetky & Benedek, 1992). Clinicians should not perform custody evaluations for individuals they treat and should not treat those evaluated for custody (Nurcombe & Partlett, 1994). Parents should be advised that they must waive the privilege of confidentiality because of the nature of the evaluation (Schetky & Benedek, 1992).

The custody evaluation is intended to assess (1) relative strengths of parents with respect to parenting, (2) quality of the parent-child relationships, (3) and the best interests of the child. This involves assessment of the parents, the child, and the parent-child relationships, keeping in mind that parents may be unduly critical of their partners and defensive about their own behavior (Schetky & Benedek, 1992).

Custody evaluations are not formal psychiatric evaluations of the parents (Schetky & Benedek, 1992). If a parent suffers from a psychiatric illness, the expert should emphasize the individual's parenting abilities and any limitations on those abilities rather than make a diagnosis (Herman, 1990).

The child should be seen in sessions alone and with each parent. Sessions with the child and parent together provide an opportunity to observe their interactions. When interviewing the child, it is unwise to directly ask about his or her preference for custody as this burdens a child at a sensitive time. When a child volunteers a preference, it should be noted and considered; the clinician should recognize, however, that the child may have been directly or indirectly pressured to make the choice or statement. Sessions with other persons important to the child may be helpful if both parents agree (Schetky & Benedek, 1992).

Special Issues

One area of increasing concern involves custody actions in which a biological mother consents to adoption without the biological father's knowledge and consent. In *Michael H. v. Gerald D.* (1989), the United States Supreme Court expressed its strong support for the primacy of families when it held that the biological mother's husband's rights to fatherhood were superior to the biological father's rights in a situation involving a child conceived during an adulterous affair. More recently, however, the courts have shown greater deference to the rights of biological parents in situations involving children

given up for adoption in infancy. In two highly publicized cases, *Baby Jessica* (*Deboer v. Deboer*, 1993) and *Baby Richard* (*O'Connel v. Kirchner*, 1995), the United States Supreme Court refused to respond in situations in which children, adopted during infancy without the knowledge and consent of the biological father, had been returned to their biological parents.

Modern technology has complicated the law with respect to custody in cases involving, for example, artificial insemination and surrogate contracts. Parental rights and responsibilities in these situations are determined by state case law and statute. Typically, a contract or agreement stipulates that a sperm donor gives up, and is relinquished from, the rights and responsibilities of fatherhood. If married, the woman's husband becomes the legal father, particularly if he is party to the contract. Suits involving surrogate mothers are complicated by the woman's unique role during the pregnancy and birth of the child. The *Baby M* case (*In the Matter of Baby M.*, 1988) raised as many questions as it answered and state law addressing these issues varies greatly. Mental health professionals involved in cases involving these newer technologies are advised to participate only with legal counsel.

DISCIPLINE AND ABUSE

Parental Discipline

As part of the concept of family privacy, our society and law allow parents considerable latitude in the discipline of their children. Punishment is viewed as a means of correcting, educating, and controlling children. External intervention may occur under conditions of suspected abuse. Proceedings against a parent may occur in juvenile, civil, or criminal proceedings. State case law and statutes typically look at the following factors to determine if discipline has been excessive: characteristics of the child such as age, sex, physical and mental condition, and ability to understand and appreciate the intent of the punishment; the nature of the offense; and characteristics of the punishment, such as the purpose for its use, the means used, its reasonableness, and the degree of force involved. Punishment that is excessive, cruel, malicious, degrading, or protracted is suspect (Mnookin & Weisberg, 1995).

Corporal Punishment in Schools

State case law and statute or local school district and school regulations determine whether corporal punishment may be administered in schools. Courts have long justified corporal punishment in schools based on the need to maintain order and control in the classroom. The use of corporal punishment in schools has withstood challenges based on the rights of parents to make decisions about the punishment of their children, on Eighth Amendment cruel and unusual punishment grounds, and on procedural due process grounds (*Baker v. Owen*, 1975; *Ingraham v. Wright*, 1977).

The United States Supreme Court has provided for minimal procedural due process in corporal punishment in schools. Under usual circumstances (1) a student has the right to notice which may include as little as the previous ineffective use of other methods to gain control and being informed beforehand that specific behavior could result in the use of corporal punishment; (2) a teacher or principal using corporal punishment must do so in the presence of a second school official who must be informed, in the student's presence, of the reason for the punishment before its use; (3) the student need not be afforded a formal opportunity to present his or her side to the second official; and (4) one using corporal punishment must, upon request, provide to the child's parent a written explanation of the reasons for the punishment and the name of the second official present (*Baker v. Owen*, 1975).

Abuse and Neglect

Mental health professionals may be asked to evaluate and treat children and families in which there are concerns about abuse and neglect. In 1992, over 2.9 million children were reported for maltreatment, representing an increase of 50 percent over rates in 1985 (McCurdy & Daro, 1994). The incidence of abuse and neglect in adolescents is as high or higher than that of younger children. Maltreatment of adolescents is less likely to be reported and adolescents are less likely to be perceived as innocent victims. Maltreatment in adolescents is associated with increased risk of premature sexual activity, unplanned pregnancy, emotional disorders, substance abuse, and incarceration. It is recommended that all adolescents be routinely asked about a history of emotional, physical, and sexual abuse and that special attention be paid to those with a history of psychiatric conditions, substance abuse, and irresponsible sexual behavior (American Medical Association Council on Scientific Affairs, 1993).

Reporting Abuse

All states require that suspected child abuse be reported and provide civil and/or criminal sanctions against those who fail to report. State law determines the entity to which the report must be made, typically the state children's protective services or health and human services agency, the police, or the prosecutor. Despite the fact that most states provide immunity to those making good faith reports, professionals are sometimes reluctant to report because they do not believe abuse occurred, they recognize how difficult it is to substantiate, they do not want to alienate families, they do not want to become entangled in the legal system, and they dislike the punitive nature of the system.

State statutes define what constitutes abuse or neglect and when reports must be made. For example, some jurisdictions require reporting of any indication of possible abuse; some require reporting when the professional has reason to believe or suspect that abuse occurred; and some require reporting only if the one making the report has had professional contact with the alleged victim (Macbeth et al., 1994). The practitioner is advised to familiarize him or herself with the laws of the state of practice.

Evaluating Sexual Abuse

The American Academy of Child and Adolescent Psychiatry (1988) has published guidelines for the clinical evaluation of children and adolescents for whom sexual abuse is suspected. The evaluation of sexual abuse is designed to determine if abuse has occurred, if the child needs protection, or if the child needs treatment for medical or emotional problems. Evaluations should be performed by child and adolescent psychiatrists or psychologists with experience in the area. The professional conducting the evaluation should not also treat the child. Multiple interviews should be avoided and the number of people involved should be as few as possible. The interview should take place in a relaxed, nonthreatening environment. The history should be obtained from the parent or caretaker and should include, among other things, an assessment of the child's credibility and alliances with the parents. Psychological testing of the child and parents may be helpful. Drawings are helpful. A physical examination should be performed preferably by a pediatrician or family physician the child knows (American Academy of Child and Adolescent Psychiatry, 1989).

State law determines the admissibility of evidence involving anatomical dolls and videotaped interviews. The use of dolls is sometimes helpful for eliciting the child's terminology and for children who cannot verbalize or draw the events being discussed. Videotaping can help preserve the child's initial statements, decrease the likelihood of duplication, and persuade a defendant to plead guilty (American Academy of Child and Adolescent Psychiatry, 1988).

Professionals rely on a variety of sources to substantiate allegations of abuse, including the history of the symptoms, the child's verbal report and presentation, the phenomenological experience of abuse, and corroborating evidence. Various indicators of credibility have been identified, including consistency of descriptions, detail, and evidence of the child's perspective in the descriptions; verbal descriptions that demonstrate a progression of activities involving elements of secrecy, bribery, and coercion; delayed disclosure and possible retractions; affect congruence; evidence of the ability to differentiate fact from fantasy; reenactment of sexual themes in activities such as play or drawing; symptoms of stress and/or inappropriate sexual behavior; medical indicators; and corroborating evidence (Heiman, 1992).

It is sometimes impossible to determine if abuse occurred because the child may be too young to provide a history, the abuse may have happened too long ago, there may be contamination by too many interviews, or the child may have been unduly influenced by one parent and no longer know what to believe (American Academy of Child and Adolescent Psychiatry, 1988). Furthermore, there is increasing concern about false accusations. False accusations have been reported in cases involving family conflict and dissolution (Schuman, 1986; Yates, 1987). Kaplan (1990) identified "several adult illusions about childhood" to explain why children are commonly believed to tell the truth: they are considered unable to describe things they have not witnessed, they are thought to have little to gain by not telling the truth, and they are thought to have perception similar to adults (pp. 661–662). He further identified specific reasons children might not tell the truth: misperception, confabulation, fantasy, lying, and of course, psychiatric conditions such as psychosis and hysteria. Goodwin and colleagues (1978) attribute false accusations of incest to "opportunistic lies rather than the symptoms of a specific hysterical or delusional state" (p. 270).

A guardian *ad litem* may be appointed to represent the best interests of the child if custody is an issue. The clinician does not have the responsibility of deciding disposition, but the evaluation may help the protective service agency in making that decision. The decision will be based in part on whether or not the family believes and can protect the child, the child's wishes, and the willingness of the perpetrator to take responsibility for his or her behavior and seek professional attention

(American Academy of Child and Adolescent Psychiatry, 1988).

False Memories

The issue of recovered memories of sexual abuse has created significant controversy. Some states have passed legislation allowing for the tolling of the statute of limitations until the time of discovery of the injury, allowing suits to be brought by adult women against alleged perpetrators of sexual abuse during their childhood. The theory of recovered memories is highly controversial, however, and more recent suits against therapists have created much debate and concern (Loftus & Rosenwald, 1993). Perhaps the most publicized case was *Ramona v. Ramona* (1994), in which a patient's father sued the therapist for implanting false memories of child sexual abuse. The decision is the first in which a court has found a duty by the therapist to a third party (Loftus & Rosenwald, 1993).

CHILDREN AS WITNESSES

Children are now routinely called to testify in legal proceedings about their experiences. The typical situation involves victims of abuse. Mental health professionals may be consulted to assess or treat children following abuse, to prepare them for testifying, or to assist them following legal proceedings. The consultant should have an understanding of what is likely to occur during investigation and adjudication of a case.

Abuse cases involve either civil or criminal proceedings or both. Child protection proceedings are designed to protect children while criminal proceedings focus on the guilt or innocence of alleged perpetrators. A child victim has no status as a party and, therefore, no guaranteed constitutional rights in criminal cases, where the presumption of innocence is in the defendant's favor. The burden of proof in civil cases is typically a "preponderance of evidence," while in criminal cases it is "beyond a reasonable doubt." Child protection cases are presumably less traumatic for witnesses because the court may be closed, hearsay evidence is less restricted, and the proceedings are not adversarial. Nonetheless, these experiences are likely to be stressful.

The National Institute of Justice reviewed three major research studies examining the emotional effects of testifying on child victims of abuse. The studies demonstrate that these children suffer stress and anxiety prior to their involvement in the court process, most of them improve over time regardless of their court experiences, and maternal support is associated with improvement (Whitcomb, Goodman, Runyan, & Hoak, 1994). Court experiences force confrontation with the trauma; they conceivably provide a sense of empowerment; and they may bring closure to an unfortunate set of events. Little is known, however, about specific aspects of the court experience itself, the effects of preparation, or changes in court procedures.

In the last decade, the United States Supreme Court has decided a number of cases involving child witnesses and has clarified its position with respect to several significant issues concerning children's testimony. These decisions provide useful information for clinicians working with children involved in court situations.

Memory and Suggestibility

A key issue regarding child witnesses is related to their ability to remember trauma and the quality of their memories. Child witnesses of parental homicide have been shown to have vivid memories, at least for certain elements of the event (Pynoos & Eth, 1984). Likewise, victims of abuse may recall events of the abuse long after it has ended and may recall them with such intense affect that the individual appears to re-experience aspects of abuse (Gelinas, 1983).

Suggestibility is an important related issue, especially when the witness is a child. Data on the comparative suggestibility of children and adults are far from conclusive and the debate about the suggestibility of children remains highly controversial. Some authorities suggest that a child's memory may be altered by post event information brought about through questioning and the interview process (Loftus & Davies, 1984). Because of concerns about suggestibility, leading questions are not usually allowed in eliciting testimony from witnesses. Exceptions are sometimes made for child witnesses, however, because of the need to provide support during difficult testimony.

Competence

All persons who appear as witnesses must be competent to testify. Competence has traditionally been associated with age, and in the court setting, standards are imposed on children that far surpass those imposed on adults. The assumption that competence occurs at a specific age oversimplifies a complex issue because, in reality, competence is a highly individual phenomenon. Under the Federal Rules of Evidence and many analogous state competence provisions, all persons are now presumed to be competent as witnesses. A trial judge may make individualized determinations of competence for young children or other problematic witnesses (Weinstein & Berger, 1987) by examining the witness in chambers to assess factors such as his or her understanding of the concept of truth, appreciation of the obligation to speak truthfully in the court setting and the gravity of the oath, capacity to form and retain accurate impressions of the incident on trial, and ability to communicate and respond to questions about the incident (*United States v. Lightly*, 1982).

Court Closure

Criminal defendants and the public both have constitutionally protected rights to public trials, but these rights are not absolute. Even though the defendant's right to an open court is explicitly guaranteed by the Sixth Amendment, the right must be balanced against a variety of factors, such as the necessity to protect witnesses (*Waller v. Georgia*, 1984). In 1982, in *Globe Newspapers v. Superior Court* (1982), the United States Supreme Court struck a Massachusetts statute that required court closure in cases involving child sexual abuse victims. The Court held that, absent a compelling state interest and means narrowly tailored to achieve those interests, the public's constitutional right to an open trial may not be abridged. The Court would, however, allow a case-by-case assessment of individual children and closure if necessary to protect a child witness (*Globe Newspaper v. Superior Court*, 1982).

Confrontation

The Confrontation Clause of the Sixth Amendment of the Constitution provides the defendant the right "to be confronted with the witnesses against him" (United States Constitution, Amendment VI), a right that has created great concern when children testify. The Confrontation Clause provides for cross examination and allows the jury the opportunity to observe the witnesses and assess their credibility.

The United States Supreme Court has examined the right to face-to-face confrontation in the context of child sexual abuse cases twice in recent years. In *Coy v. Iowa* (1988), the Court held that face-to-face confrontation is protected by the Constitution and refused to decide whether there could be any exceptions to the Confrontation Clause.

In *Maryland v. Craig* (1990), the Court explored the possibility of exceptions to the face-to-face confrontation noting that the right is not absolute. A state's interest in the child victim's physical and psychological well-being may, in some cases, outweigh a defendant's right to a face-to-face encounter with the child. Before the right to confrontation can be abridged, however, the state must demonstrate necessity on an individual case-by-case basis. The emotional distress to an individual child must be more than "de minimis"; it must be so severe that the child cannot reasonably communicate (*Maryland v. Craig*, 1990, p. 3169). A state's interest in protecting the child from courtroom trauma in general, however, is not sufficiently compelling to abrogate a defendant's constitutional right to confront a witness. The state must show that the trauma is caused by the presence of the defendant, but the showing of necessity does not require the trial court to actually observe the child witness in the defendant's presence or to explore less restricted alternatives. In *Craig*, expert testimony was used to establish a child's need for protection. The child, therefore, need not necessarily attempt to testify in the defendant's presence, and the judge's decision may be based on recommendations from experts or other data.

Hearsay

Hearsay is a statement that was made, or assertive conduct that occurred, out of court that is offered at trial to prove the truth of the facts asserted (Federal Rule of Evidence). Hearsay is particularly important in the prosecution of child sexual abuse cases that are difficult to prove because there are often no witnesses to the abuse. The child victim is frequently the only one available to testify to the actual occurrences. The child victim may not be an ideal witness, however, because of age, immaturity, or emotional distress.

In general, hearsay statements are not permitted as testimony because they were not made under oath and are not subject to cross-examination and because they deprive the jury of the opportunity to observe the demeanor of the declarant. Hearsay information may be critical in proving a case, however, and may be admitted into evidence under exceptions to the hearsay rule.

Many states have enacted hearsay exceptions allowing hearsay statements about the abuse made by the victim to others outside of court. One hearsay exception allows statements made while undergoing medical diagnosis or treatment; another hearsay exception allows for "excited utterances" involving spontaneous statements made while excited. In some states, a residual, or "catch-all," exception to the hearsay rule allows evidence of out-of-court statements that satisfies specified criteria ensuring reliability.

Several recent United States Supreme Court cases have examined whether the reliability guarantees specified in traditional hearsay exceptions are sufficient to protect the criminal defendant's right to confrontation. In *Idaho v. Wright* (1990), the Supreme Court examined the testimony of a pediatrician in a child sexual abuse case and noted that hearsay statements are admissible if they represent traditional hearsay exceptions, such as statements made for purposes of medical diagnosis or treatment or excited utterances, or if they possess "indicia of reliability." The Court identified a number of factors that indicate trustworthiness: spontaneity, consistency, the child's mental state, lack of a motive to fabricate, and content or terminology of a statement that is unexpected of a young child.

Of significance to clinical practice, the Court refused to mandate that particular guidelines be used in professional interviews. Instead, the Court stated that the critical inquiry is whether the child was likely to be telling the truth when the statement was made. The relevant circumstances for consideration of reliability are those surrounding the making of the statement "and that render the declarant particularly worthy of belief" (*Idaho v. Wright*, 1990, p. 819). Evidence that corroborates the statement, such as physical evidence of abuse, is not to be considered in determining whether the statement is reliable.

In *White v. Illinois* (1992), the Court addressed the issue of whether the Confrontation Clause requires that the state either produce the declarant at trial or show that the declarant is unavailable before admitting hearsay testimony. The Court observed that some hearsay statements that represent traditional hearsay exceptions, such as statements made in the course of medical diagnosis or treatment or excited utterances, might be more trustworthy than in-court statements. The Court explained that statements that are admissible under the traditional hearsay exceptions are so trustworthy that cross-examination can be expected to add little to their reliability. The Confrontation Clause does not bar such testimony, even absent a finding of the declarant's unavailability.

SPECIAL EDUCATION

Historical and Legal Perspective

Children with disabilities commonly present in the pediatric setting. Mental health professionals are frequently consulted to assist in evaluating the special education needs of these children. It is important, therefore, to understand the historical and legal basis of special education in this country. Educational philosophy and policy related to children with disabilities has changed significantly over the last century. In the late 1800s, children with disabilities were segregated, largely for the benefit of teachers and other children. As concern emerged about the children with disabilities themselves and the education they received, segregation was justified as a mechanism for protecting them. By the mid-1900s, paralleling concerns about racial segregation, the deleterious effects of segregation were recognized and mainstreaming was endorsed (Rothstein, 1990).

Congress began providing for the special education needs of children with disabilities at the federal level in the 1960s, with the Elementary and Secondary Education Act (Public Law No. 89-10) and amendments to it. This legislation was enacted to encourage states to develop resources and train personnel for educating individuals with disabilities (*Board of Education of the Hendrick Hudson Central School District v. Rowley*, 1982). While not itself a funding statute, Section 504 of the Rehabilitation Act of 1973 mandated that schools receiving federal funds not discriminate against individuals with disabilities. Section 504 case law further requires accommodation to avoid discrimination (Rothstein, 1990).

Basing their decisions on the equal protection and due process provisions of the Fourteenth Amendment, two District Court cases, *Pennsylvania Association for Retarded Children v. Pennsylvania* (1971) and *Mills v. Board of Education of District of Columbia* (1972), provided the model for the due process requirements now associated with special education (Rothstein, 1990). The Education for All Handicapped Children Act of 1975 (Public Law No. 94-142) established federal guidelines for education of children with disabilities and provided financial subsidies for state and local educational programs that follow the federal guidelines (Rothstein, 1990).

The Education for All Handicapped Children Act

The Education for All Handicapped Children Act (EAHCA) is based on the constitutional provisions of equal protection and due process (Rothstein, 1990). It is guided by the principles that all children with disabilities are entitled to an education; such education must be provided in the least restrictive appropriate environment; such education must be individualized and appropriate

to the child's needs; and such education must be free (Rothstein, 1990). These principles are protected by procedural safeguards (Rothstein, 1990).

In 1986, the Education of the Handicapped Act Amendments of 1986 (Public Law No. 99-457) modified the federal legislation by establishing policy for early intervention programs and by extending the rights and protection of the Act to three year olds. The Amendments increased financial support for preschool services and provided incentives for states to develop early intervention programs for infants and toddlers and their parents. States were required to organize interagency coordinating councils to develop and oversee early childhood plans for children with disabilities from infancy to age five, operate registries of children with special needs, and offer and publicize prescreening activities for children with suspected developmental problems (Purvis, 1991).

The EAHCA mainstreaming mandate requires that children with disabilities be educated in the "least restrictive environment" (Public Law No. 94-142, Section 300.550). The education must be individualized and guided by an Individualized Educational Program (IEP), which is a written statement addressing the individual child, developed in a meeting between educational representatives, the parent(s) and, if appropriate, the child (Public Law 94-142, Section 300.344). The IEP includes a statement of the child's current performance, annual goals, and short-term objectives; an assessment of the child's capacity to participate in regular educational activities; specification of educational services to be provided as well as the necessary transition services; projected implementation dates and duration; and criteria and procedures for annual (or more frequent) evaluation (Public Law No. 94-142, Section 300.346).

The term "handicapped children" is defined by the statute to include children with mental retardation, specific learning disabilities, hearing impairment, speech or language impairment, visual impairment, serious emotional disturbance, orthopedic impairment, and other health impairment, who because of these disabilities, "need special education and related services" (Public Law No. 94-142, Section 300.5). Terms within this definition, however, are "undefined and extremely broad," making it important to review the regulations and interpretations in the state of practice (Nurcombe & Partlett, 1994, p. 77).

Under the federal legislation, the term "specific learning disability" refers to a disorder of the "basic psychological processes involved in understanding or in using language, spoken or written, which may manifest itself in an imperfect ability to listen, think, speak, read, write, spell, or to do mathematical calculations" (Public Law No. 94-142, Section 300.5). Specific learning disabilities do not include learning problems "which are primarily the result of visual, hearing, or motor handicaps, of mental retardation, of emotional disturbance or of environmental, cultural, or economic disadvantage" (Public Law No. 94-142, Section 300.5(b)(9)). Most states specify criteria for qualification for learning disability services which should be reviewed by the clinician (Purvis, 1991).

The conditions included under the category of "serious emotional disturbance" are heterogeneous and subjective. The category commonly includes children with attention and behavior problems. Children with schizophrenia are covered but children who are socially maladjusted are not covered unless they have an accompanying psychological condition (Rothstein, 1990). To qualify, a child must exhibit one or more of the following for "a long time period and to a marked degree which adversely affects educational performance": (1) an inability to learn unexplained by intellectual, sensory, or health factors; (2) an inability to establish or maintain satisfactory interpersonal relationships with peers and teachers; (3) inappropriate behaviors or feelings under normal circumstances; (4) a general pervasive mood of unhappiness or depression; or (5) a tendency to develop physical symptoms or fears associated with personal or school problems (Rothstein, 1990).

The meaning of terms such as "free appropriate public education" (Public Law No. 94-142, Section 300.4) and "related services" (Public Law No. 94-142, Section 300.13) used in the legislation have been clarified by judicial interpretation. "Free appropriate education," as interpreted by the United States Supreme Court in *Board of Education of the Hendrick Hudson Central School District v. Rowley* (1982), is intended "to open the door of public education to handicapped children on appropriate terms" (*Rowley*, 1982, p. 192). According to the *Rowley* Court, the EAHCA mandates "access to specialized instruction and related services which are individually designed to provide educational benefit" to children with disabilities (p. 201). *Rowley* limited the "free and appropriate education" language; the Court refused to find "congressional intent to achieve strict equality of opportunity or services" (p. 198) or to require "the furnishing of every special service necessary to maximize each handicapped child's potential" (p. 199). For children educated in regular classes of the public school system, a child's individual plan "should be reasonably calculated to enable" the child to pass from one grade to the next (p. 204). The Court supported local control when it ruled that reviewing courts may not "substitute their own notions of sound educational pol-

icy for those of the school authorities which they review" (p. 206).

The EAHCA defines "related services" to include transportation and "such developmental, corrective, and other supportive services as are required to assist a handicapped child to benefit from special education" (Public Law No. 94-142, Section 300.13). Such services include speech pathology and audiology, psychological services, physical and occupational therapy, recreation, social services, counseling, and medical services unless the medical services are for diagnostic and evaluation purposes. The United States Supreme Court addressed the meaning of "related services" in *Irving Independent School District v. Tatro* (1984) when it found that clean intermittent catheterization (CIC) for a child with spina bifida qualified as "related services" because without it during the school day, the child would be unable to attend school and, therefore, unable to benefit from special education. The Court described CIC as a "supportive service" rather than a "medical service" serving only diagnostic or evaluation purposes (p. 890), noting that CIC made possible "meaningful access to education" as envisioned by Congress when it enacted the legislation (p. 891). The Court explained that the exclusion for medical services may have stemmed from a desire to spare schools the burden of providing unduly expensive and complicated services but found that CIC in this case was not intended solely for purposes of diagnosis and evaluation. The Court clarified that "only those services necessary to aid a handicapped child to benefit from special education must be provided, regardless of how easily a school nurse or lay person could furnish them" (p. 894). Furthermore, "school nursing services must be provided only if they can be performed by a nurse or other qualified person, not if they must be performed by a physician" (p. 894).

Procedural Safeguards of the Education for All Handicapped Children Act

The procedural safeguards of the Education for All Handicapped Children Act (EAHCA) are substantial and include the right to an independent evaluation, notice, parental access to records, an impartial hearing with representation, and review through the state educational agency and ultimately the courts (Public Law No. 94-142, Section 502-512).

The EAHCA contains a "stay-put" provision which, in the absence of an agreement by the parties, requires that the child with a disability remain in the current placement until completion of review proceedings. In *Honig v. Doe* (1988), the United States Supreme Court addressed the "stay-put" provision in light of a "dangerousness" exception. *Honig* involved the indefinite expulsion of two emotionally disturbed youth for violent and disruptive behavior related to their disabilities. The Supreme Court rejected the "dangerousness" exception to the "stay-put" concept and noted alternative mechanisms available to schools to deal with disruptive youth.

State Statutory Schemes

States must meet the Education for All Handicapped Children Act (EAHCA) requirements in order to receive federal funding for special education. All states currently comply. Some states provide even more detailed programming than that required by the federal legislation by extending the age requirements, categories for service entitlement, and procedural safeguards (Rothstein, 1990).

Mental health professionals are consulted for various purposes related to special education. They may serve as school consultants to evaluate and treat children who qualify for services, assist in developing Individualized Educational Programs (IEPs), or serve as expert witnesses at later administrative or judicial hearings. Such involvement requires familiarity with the federal legislation. It is also imperative that state and local statutes and regulations be followed.

SUMMARY

The relevance of law to the lives of children and families increases as our society becomes more complex. The health care system, where law and policy are now prominent, is one area in which that relevance becomes evident. Mental health care is perhaps even more replete with legal and policy issues. It is crucial, therefore, that mental health care providers understand the principles upon which the law related to children and families is based, be familiar with trends in the development of that law, and arm themselves with sufficient knowledge to make reasoned decisions and interventions.

Mental health providers are taught to make clinical judgments. Legal, ethical, and social issues and positions form the basis of many of those judgments and yet remain largely obscure. Once revealed, that foundation increases clinical acumen and guides decision-making. The law related to children and families is based largely on state case law and statute, making it wise for the provider to familiarize himself or herself with appropriate practice in his or her state of practice. There are commonalities in approach among some or all jurisdictions, at least with respect to many issues. If a position or practice is at variance with established law, it is imperative that the provider carefully consider appropriate options and document his or her position and choice.

REFERENCES

American Academy of Child and Adolescent Psychiatry Council on Rights and Legal Matters. (1988). Perspective: Guidelines for the clinical evaluation of child and adolescent sexual abuse. *American Academy of Child and Adolescent Psychiatry, 27*, 655–657.

American Medical Association Council on Ethical and Judicial Affairs. (1993). Mandatory parental consent to abortion. *Journal of the American Medical Association, 269*, 82–86.

American Medical Association Council on Scientific Affairs.(1993). Adolescents as victims of family violence. *Journal of the American Medical Association, 270*, 82–86.

Baby Jessica, 501 N.W.2d. 193 (Mi 1993).

Baker v. Owen, 395 F.Supp. 294 (M.D.N.C.), *aff'd without opinion*, 423 U.S. 907 (1975).

Bellotti v. Baird II, 443 U.S. 622 (1979).

Black, H. C., Nolan, J. R., & Nolan-Haley, J. M. (1990). *Black's Law Dictionary*. St. Paul: West Publishing Co.

Board of Education of the Hendrick Hudson Central School District v. Rowley (Rowley), 458 U.S. 176 (1982).

Canterbury v. Spence, 464 F.2d 772 (D.C. Cir. 1972).

Cowan, D. H., & Bertsch, E. (1984). Innovative therapy the responsibility of hospitals. *Journal of Legal Medicine, 5*, 219–251.

Coy v. Iowa, 487 U.S. 1012 (1988).

Deboer v. Deboer, 114 S.Ct. 11 (1993).

Eisel v. Board of Education of Montgomery County, 597 A.2d 447 (Md. 1991).

English, A. (1990). Treating adolescents: Legal and ethical considerations. *Adolescent Medicine, 74*, 1097–1112.

Federal Rule of Evidence, Rule 802.

Furrow, B. R., Johnson, S. H., Jost, T. S., & Schwartz, R. L. (1991). *Health law: Cases, materials and problems*. St. Paul: West Publishing Co.

Gardner, W., Scherer, D., & Tester, M. (1989). Asserting scientific authority: Cognitive development and adolescent legal rights. *American Psychologist, 44*, 895–902.

Gelinas, D. J. (1983). The persisting negative effects of incest. *Psychiatry, 46*, 312–332.

Globe Newspapers v. Superior Court, 457 U.S. 596 (1982).

Goodwin, J., et al. (1978). Incest hoax: False accusations, false denials. *American Academy Psychiatry Law, 6*, 269–270.

Group for the Advancement of Psychiatry (1989). *How old is enough? The ages of rights and responsibilities.* New York: Brunner/Mazel.

Hartnett, T. (1994). Mature enough to decide. *Medical Ethics Advisor, 10*, 97–101.

Heiman, M. L. (1992). Annotation: Putting the puzzle together: Validating allegations of child sexual abuse. *Journal of Child Psychology and Psychiatry, 33*, 311–329.

Helling v. Carey, 519 P.2d 981 (Wash. 1974).

Herman, S. P. (1990). Special issues in child custody evaluations. *Journal of the American Academy of Child and Adolescent Psychiatry, 29*, 969–974.

Holder, A. R. (1987). Minors' rights to consent to medical care. *Journal of the American Medical Association, 257*, 3400–3402.

Holder, A. R. (1991). Legal issues in professional liability. In M. Lewis (Ed.), *Child and adolescent psychiatry: A comprehensive textbook* (pp. 1139–1145). Baltimore: Williams & Wilkins.

Honig v. Doe, 484 U.S. 305 (1988).

Horowitz, S. (1984). The doctrine of informed consent applied to psychotherapy. *Georgia Law Journal, 72*, 1637–1664.

Idaho v. Wright, 497 U.S. 805 (1990).

Ingraham v. Wright, 430 U.S. 651 (1977).

In the Matter of Baby M., 537 A.2d 1227 (1988).

Irving Independent School District v. Tatro, 468 U.S. 883 (1984).

Kaplan, J. M. (1990). Children don't always tell the truth. *Journal of Forensic Sciences, 35*, 661–662.

King, J. H. (1986). *The law of medical practice: In a nutshell.* St. Paul: West Publishing Co.

Leiken, S. (1989). A proposal concerning decisions to forgo life-sustaining treatment for young people. *Journal of Pediatrics, 115*, 17–22.

Loftus, E. F., & Davies, G. M. (1984). Distortions in the memory of children. *Journal of Social Issues, 40*, 51–67.

Loftus, E. F., & Rosenwald, L. A. (1993). Buried memories shattered lives. *American Bar Association Journal*, Nov., 70–73.

Macbeth, J. E., Wheeler, A. M., Sither, J. W., & Onek, J. N. (1994). *Legal and risk management issues in the practice of psychiatry.* Washington, D.C.: Psychiatrists' Purchasing Group, Inc.

Maryland v. Craig, 110 S. Ct. 3157 (1990).

McCurdy, K., & Daro, D. (1994). Child maltreatment. A national survey of reports and fatalities. *Journal of Interpersonal Violence, 9*, 75–94.

Michael H. v. Gerald D., 491 U.S. 110 (1989).

Mills v. Board of Education of the District of Columbia, 348 F. Supp. 866 (D.D.C. 1972).

Mnookin, R. H., & Weisberg, D. K. (1995). *Child, family and state: Problems and materials on children and the law.* Boston: Little, Brown.

Monahan, J. (1993). Limiting therapist exposure to *Tarasoff* liability: Guidelines for risk containment. *American Psychologist, 48*, 242–250.

Nurcombe, B. (1991). Malpractice. In M. Lewis (Ed.), *Child and adolescent psychiatry: A comprehensive textbook* (pp. 1127–1139). Baltimore: Williams & Wilkins.

Nurcombe, B., & Partlett, D. F. (1994). *Child mental health and the law.* New York: The Free Press.

O'Connel v. Kirchner, 115 S.Ct. 891 (1995).

Palmore v. Sidoti, 466 U.S. 429 (1984).

Parham v. J. R. and J. L., 442 U.S. 584 (1979).

Pennsylvania Association for Retarded Children v. Pennsylvania, 334 F. Supp. 1257 (E.D.Pa. 1971).

Public Law No. 89-10, Elementary and Secondary Education Act.

Public Law No. 94-142, Education for all Handicapped Children Act of 1975.

Public Law No. 99-457, Education of the Handicapped Act Amendments of 1986.

Purvis, P. (1991). The public laws for education of the disabled: The pediatrician's role. *Developmental and Behavioral Pediatrics, 12*, 327–339.

Pynoos, R. S., & Eth, S. (1984). The child as witness to homicide. *Journal of Social Issues, 40*, 87–108.

Ramona v. Ramona, (Napa County Superior Court, No. 618981, 1994).

Rothstein, L. F. (1990). *Special education law.* New York: Longman.

Rozovsky, F. A. (1990). *Consent to treatment: A practical guide.* Boston: Little, Brown.

Schetky, D. H., & Benedek, E. P. (1992). *Clinical handbook of child psychiatry and the law.* Baltimore: Williams & Wilkins.

Schuman, D. C. (1986). False accusations of physical and sexual abuse. *Bulletin of American Academy of Psychiatry & Law, 14*, 5.

Sigman, G. S., & O'Connor, C. (1991). Exploration for physicians of the mature minor doctrine. *Journal of Pediatrics, 119*, 520–525.

Simon, R. I. (1992). *Clinical psychiatry and the law.* Washington, D.C.: American Psychiatric Press.

Tarasoff v. Regents of the University of California, 551 P.2d 334 (Cal. 1976).

Thompson v. County of Alameda, 614 P.2d 728 (Cal. 1980).

United States v. Lightly, 677 F.2d 1027 (4th Cir. 1982).

United States Constitution, Amendment VI.

Waller v. Georgia, 467 U.S. 39 (1984).

Wallerstein, J. S. (1989). Separation, divorce, and remarriage. In M. D. Levine, W. B. Carey, A. C. Crocker, & R. T. Gross (Eds.), *Developmental-behavioral pediatrics* (pp. 241–255). Philadelphia: W. B. Saunders Company.

Wallerstein, J. S. & Corbin, S. B. (1991). The child and the vicissitudes of divorce. In M. Lewis (Ed.), *Child and adolescent psychiatry: A comprehensive textbook* (pp. 1108–1118). Baltimore: Williams & Wilkins.

Weinstein, J. B., & Berger, M. A. (1987). *Weinstein's Evidence Manual*, para. 10.01(02), at 10-5 to 10-6.

Whitcomb, D., Goodman, G. S., Runyan, D. K., & Hoak, S. (1994). The emotional effects of testifying on sexually abused children. National Institute of Justice.

White v. Illinois, 112 S. Ct. 736 (1992).

Wizner, S. (1991). Legal considerations in the psychiatric hospitalization of children and adolescents. In M. Lewis (Ed.), *Child and adolescent psychiatry: A comprehensive textbook* (pp. 1118–1123). Baltimore: Williams & Wilkins.

Yates, A. (1987). Should young children testify in cases of sexual abuse? *American Journal of Psychiatry, 144,* 476.

CHAPTER 5

PSYCHIATRIC EMERGENCIES IN THE PEDIATRIC SETTING

Eileen P. Ryan

INTRODUCTION

There are few genuinely life-threatening emergencies in pediatric psychology and psychiatry. This chapter will focus on the two most likely to be encountered by the pediatric clinician—the suicidal patient and the "agitated" patient. Such emergencies are often intimidating to non-psychiatric physicians and practitioners. Since the majority of pediatric patients in need of emergency psychiatric intervention are adolescents, much of the following discussion will concern the thirteen-and-above age group, although alterations in approach necessary for younger children will be addressed where applicable. The goal of this chapter is to facilitate the education of clinicians in pediatric medical settings regarding the management of children and adolescents in crisis.

Emergencies in pediatric psychiatry are frequently defined by the child's caretakers. The equilibrium in a family may shift; suddenly a situation which was previously manageable or tolerable becomes overwhelming, and a psychiatric "emergency" is born. Nurses and physicians in non-psychiatric medical settings frequently encounter the same phenomenon. Patients with symptoms that have been present for several days may suddenly appear in the emergency department or contact the physician on call in the early morning hours. Similar challenges face the evaluating clinician whether the chief complaint is depression or abdominal pain.

Children and adolescents in crisis must be considered as both individuals and members of a family. Therefore,

it is crucial that parents or other caretakers be involved in the evaluation. This must be accomplished in such a way as to acknowledge the child's or adolescent's individuality and convey respect for privacy. The clinician should meet with the child alone for at least part of the interview, without other adults present. The parents' pivotal role in the child's life must also be respected. The family's involvement and participation is crucial if the clinician expects any treatment plan to be successful, whether the recommendation is for hospitalization or outpatient services. When parents are dissatisfied with their child's psychiatric care, be it evaluation or treatment, inevitably a major complaint is that they were not sufficiently involved by the clinicians and/or there was insufficient communication. Parents, even those who are extremely troubled themselves or are considered "difficult," can be tremendous allies of the pediatric team if encouraged and allowed to be. On the other hand, if ignored or provoked, they likely will respond negatively and either directly or indirectly thwart the clinician's efforts.

Agitation can be contagious, and physicians, including psychiatrists, are not immune. Frequently, psychiatric emergencies evoke strong emotions in adults entrusted with the child's care as well as understandable urges to assuage the patient's discomfort immediately. The pediatric clinician must approach these emergent situations in the same manner as any other medical emergency. The first priority in any psychiatric emergency must be stabilization and ensuring the patient's safety and the safety of others. Evaluation of the chief complaint should actually be in progress during stabilization. The nuances of psychiatric diagnosis and categorization need not be a priority for the emergency room clinician. It is far more important to determine that a child or adolescent is suicidal and in need of hospitalization than to decide whether the patient has a major depressive episode versus an adjustment disorder with disturbance of mood. Likewise, recognition that an agitated psychotic adolescent is also delirious and in need of further medical assessment is more critical than the immediate differentiation of schizophrenia from a psychotic bipolar presentation.

SUICIDE

Suicide is the second most common cause of death in American adolescents, accounting for about 12 percent of the mortality among young people between the ages of 15 and 24 years (Centers for Disease Control, 1985). There has been a dramatic three-fold increase in the rate of completed suicide among 15- to 19-year-olds over the past forty years, with the rate of completed suicide among younger children remaining relatively stable. The upsurge of suicide in the 15- to 19-year-old population has resulted in increased research examining risk factors for both completed suicide and suicidal behavior, particularly in the adolescent population. In 1991, however, 266 children between the ages of 5 and 14 committed suicide in the United States (National Center for Health Statistics, 1993), and it is likely that suicidal ideation and suicidal behavior (but not completed suicide) is as common in children as in adolescents.

The prevalence of suicidal ideation in community samples of pre-adolescents has been found to be between 8.9 percent and 17.9 percent at any given time (Pfeffer, Newcorn, Kaplan, Mizruchi, & Plutchik, 1988). As many as 4 percent of high school students have made a suicide attempt within the past twelve months, and 8 percent have made an attempt at some time in their lives (Smith & Crawford, 1986). An even higher prevalence of suicidality has been found in children and adolescents undergoing treatment for psychiatric disorder. Psychological autopsies of adolescent suicide completers have consistently found that 90 percent to 98 percent of suicide victims suffered from one or more psychiatric illnesses (Brent et al., 1988; Ryland & Kruesi, 1992; Shaffi, Steltz-Lenarsky, Derrick, Beckner, & Wittinghill, 1988; Shaffer, 1974).

Suicidal behavior is more difficult to quantify than completed suicide, given the lack of a national registry;

however, a study of an academically select public high school in New York City revealed that of the 9 percent of students who had actually made a suicide attempt, 64 percent had made at least two attempts and fewer than half of the attempters came to the attention of mental health professionals (Harkavy Friedman, Asnis, Boeck, & DiFiore, 1987). A much lower percentage of suicide attempts in the general population receive medical attention: only 12 percent by some estimates (Smith & Crawford, 1986). Pediatricians, family practitioners, and other clinicians working with children and adolescents need to become adept at identifying and referring suicidal and potentially suicidal youth.

An understanding of risk factors for suicidal behavior and completed suicide is crucial for clinicians working with the pediatric population. There is considerable overlap between those who attempt and those who complete suicide, but the victims and attempters are two distinct groups, and so risk factors and characteristics for each group will be discussed separately. In this chapter, the terms "suicidal behavior" and "suicide attempt" are used interchangeably and refer to any *behavior* or *action* associated with suicidal thoughts. The terms "suicidal thoughts" and "suicidal ideation" reflect any *thinking* about suicide.

Clinical Features

Age

Adolescents by far are more at risk for completed suicide than are younger children. Most studies indicate that completed suicide in children under the age of 10 is rare, and that the increase in the suicide rate has not occurred in the 10- to 14-year age range, but rather in the 15- to 19-year-old range (Shaffer & Fisher, 1981). There are several possible reasons why younger children do not complete suicide with the frequency of adolescents despite the similar prevalence of suicidal thoughts and impulses. Cognitive immaturity that limits the child's ability to plan and execute a genuinely lethal attempt may be protective (Shaffer & Fisher, 1981). Greater involvement of family and teachers in the lives of younger children than in the lives of adolescents may also be a factor, as well as the decreased prevalence of affective illness in children.

In children, suicidal behavior may more often reflect chronic family problems, including early separation from parents, inadequate mothering or nurturing, and/or emotional, physical, or sexual abuse. Suicidal children often see themselves as expendable and are frequently depressed and lonely.

Gender

As with adults, the completed suicide rate for males is much higher than for females (Brent, 1989a). Boys tend to choose more violent and lethal means to commit suicide (i.e., firearms and hanging). Girls attempt suicide more frequently than boys in a ratio of 4:1 (Hoberman & Garfinkel, 1988), which may be related to the greater prevalence of affective disorders in females, the tendency of girls and women to use less violent and irreversible means of suicide (e.g., overdoses and wrist cutting), their greater willingness to seek help, and perhaps a higher degree of impulsivity in boys.

Race and Ethnicity

White adolescent boys complete suicide at a rate 3 to 5 times higher than blacks, yet Native Americans, Asians, and Hispanics have an even higher suicide rate than whites (Sulik & Garfinkel, 1992), which may be related to forced cultural assimilation. The rate of completed suicide in young black adolescents has increased substantially and is comparable to that of whites in the urban Northeast and Midwest United States (Dillihay, 1989; Shaffer & Fisher, 1981).

Method

The most frequent method used in completed suicide in both male and female adolescents is firearms. The availability of firearms has been noted to be higher in the homes of completers than attempters (Brent et al., 1988), indicating that the availability of a lethal, irreversible means to a suicidal adolescent increases the risk that he or she will complete suicide. Reduced accessibility of the firearms (hiding, storage in a locked gun cabinet, etc.) is not effective in eliminating the risk (Brent et al., 1988). Suicidal adolescents are still able to find and use firearms, contrary to the beliefs of many parents. The suicide rate by firearms has increased faster than the rate of suicide by other methods. Girls are also becoming more likely to use firearms than in the past.

The combination of alcohol and firearms is particularly deadly. Suicide victims who used firearms were five times more likely to have been drinking than victims utilizing other methods (Brent, Perper, & Allman, 1987b). One study found that the percentage of all 15- to 19-year-old suicide victims with detectable blood alcohol levels during a 24-year study period rose nearly four-fold, from 12.9 percent in 1968 through 1972 to 46 percent in 1978 through 1983 (Brent et al., 1987b).

The most common method used in suicide attempts is overdose, which accounts for 71 percent (Brent et al., 1988). Girls attempt to overdose more frequently than boys, but the rate of lethal overdoses has been found comparable for both sexes (O'Brien, 1974). Adolescents who attempt suicide by planned, irreversible, violent means (firearms, hanging, jumping) seem to resemble actual suicide completers with respect to psychiatric diagnosis and family history and are more likely to complete suicide in the future (Brent et al., 1988).

Precipitants

Similar precipitants exist for both completed and attempted suicide. It is a serious error to assume that children and adolescents who engage in suicidal behavior in response to a disciplinary crisis (including legal charges or consequences such as detention) or an interpersonal crisis (e.g., break-up with a girlfriend or boyfriend) are not at genuine risk. Accumulation of life stressors and exposure to suicide and suicidal behavior have also been noted to be precipitants to completed suicide on psychological autopsy. Sexual and physical abuse and family discord can also be significantly involved in suicidal behavior (Brent, 1989a).

Risk Factors

Psychiatric Risk Factors

The vast majority of children and adolescents who complete suicide suffer from at least one major psychiatric disorder, although less than one-third have had any mental health contact in their lives (Brent et al., 1988). The most significant psychiatric risk factors associated with completed adolescent suicide are major depression, mixed bipolar disorder, substance abuse, and conduct disorder (Brent et al., 1988; Brent et al., 1993b). Substance abuse appears to be a more significant risk factor when combined with affective illness than when alone (Brent et al., 1993b). Comorbidty with other psychiatric disorders such as conduct disorder or attention deficit/hyperactivity disorder appears to confer greater risk in general.

Even suicide victims without apparent individual psychiatric pathology are more likely to demonstrate psychiatric risk factors compared to community controls, including a greater likelihood of previous suicide attempts, family history of affective illness, lower rates of psychiatric treatment, cumulative life stressors over the past twelve months prior to the suicide, and a greater prevalence of an available loaded gun in the home (Brent, Perper, Baugher, & Allman, 1993d). Suicidal ideation thus needs to be taken seriously and thoroughly evaluated even if clear psychopathology is not evident. Prevention of suicide in this group is probably best achieved by restricting firearm availability, particularly loaded firearms (Brent et al., 1993d).

Suicidal behavior is a significant risk factor for completed suicide. Adolescent suicide completers were much more likely than controls to have made previous suicide attempts (Shaffer, Garland, Gould, Fisher, & Trautman, 1988; Shaffi et al., 1988). Adolescents who have attempted multiple times are three times more likely to complete suicide than those who have made only a single attempt (Kotila & Lonnqvist, 1989).

An increasing body of evidence points to the presence of personality disorders in suicide victims, particularly cluster B (impulsive-dramatic) and cluster C (avoidant-dependent) disorders (Brent et al., 1994). Anxiety disorder, both alone and comorbid with affective disorder, has been reported as a risk factor for completed suicide and suicidal behavior in adults (Weissman, Klerman, Markowitz, Quellette, & Phil, 1989; Allgulander & Lavori, 1991), but studies of adolescents have produced mixed results (Brent et al., 1993b; Marttunen, Aro, Henriksson, & Lonnqvist, 1994; Shaffii, Carrigen, Whittinghill, & Derrick, 1985; Shaffer, 1974) perhaps owing to the high rate of comorbid anxiety disorder in this population, obscuring the impact of anxiety disorder alone as a risk factor for suicide.

Family History and Environment

A high prevalence of suicide has been reported in the families of adult psychiatric patients who later went on to complete suicide (Roy, 1983). A study of suicidal prepubertal children (Pfeffer, Normandin, & Kakuna, 1994) reported an association with suicidal behavior in their families, although no first-degree relative had committed suicide. There was an association between suicidality in prepubertal children and a first-degree relative with antisocial personality disorder, assaultive behavior, and substance abuse. Fifty percent of the mothers of child psychiatric in-patients who had attempted suicide had made a suicide attempt themselves. Although some studies have not found an association between suicidal behavior in children and adolescents and a family history of affective disorder (Pfeffer et al., 1994; Puig-Antich et al., 1989), other studies have reported a strong positive association (Brent et al., 1988; Shaffer, 1974; Shafii et al., 1985).

Suicide victims are noted to have suffered more maltreatment and parental loss or separation than normal controls (Shafii et al., 1985). Loss of a parent, especially before the age of 12, has been noted among suicide attempters (Pfeffer, 1986). Similarly, Brent and colleagues (1993a) reported a higher prevalence of loss of a relative to death in 13- to 18-year-old suicide attempters versus non-attempters. The home environments of suicide attempters as a group have been reported to be less supportive, with more hostile, less empathic family members than those of non-suicidal psychiatric or community controls (Brent, 1986). As a group, suicide attempters have been sexually and/or physically abused more than psychiatric or community controls. In young children, the association between suicidal behavior and abuse may be particularly strong (Brent, 1986). Runaways have often experienced abuse and are also at high risk for suicidal behavior (Deykin, Alpert, & McNamara, 1985; Rotheram, 1987).

Exposure to Suicide

Over the past decade, a growing body of data supports the concern that exposure to suicide confers an increased risk for suicide and suicidal behavior. Imitation is the most common explanation given for outbreaks of suicide and suicidal behavior far in excess of the expected frequency in several schools and communities, statistical evidence of clustering of suicides (Gould, Wallenstein, & Kleinman, 1990), and the reported increased rate of suicide following news stories or fictional docudramas about suicide (Gould & Shaffer, 1986). More recent research (Brent et al., 1993c) indicates that exposure to the suicide of a friend or acquaintance confers increased risk of new-onset major depression, post-traumatic stress disorder (PTSD), and suicidal ideation, but not an increase in suicide attempts. They question whether suicide contagion may be mediated by depression triggered by the loss of a friend to suicide rather than imitation. The responses of exposed adolescents in the study indicated that the friends of suicide completers were reluctant to inflict the sort of emotional pain they were experiencing on friends and family. On the other hand, television dramas and even news reports often portray adolescent suicide victims as highly sympathetic, romanticized figures. Brent and colleagues (1993c) suggest that adolescents exposed only to sanitized media portrayals may identify with these portraits of misunderstood, tortured martyrs without grasping the actual aftermath of suicide, especially the toll inflicted on friends and loved ones.

Medical Illness

Epilepsy is the only medical illness that has been linked conclusively to completed suicide and suicidal behavior (Brent, Crumrine, Varma, Allan, & Allman, 1987a; Brent, 1986; Brent, 1989a). The increased risk may be related to use of phenobarbital. Epileptic children and adolescents, ages 6 to 16 years, treated with phenobarbital versus carbamazepine were studied and compared (Brent et al., 1987a). Those treated with phenobarbital had a much higher prevalence of major depressive disorder (40 percent versus 4 percent) and suicidal ideation (47 percent versus 4 percent) compared with patients treated with carbamazepine.

There is some indication that HIV positive status and AIDS may be linked with suicidal risk in adults (Marzuk et al., 1988). This has been inadequately studied in children and adolescents. Suicidal behavior, including completed suicide, may be increased in gay adolescents. In one study (Rotheram-Borus, Hunter, & Rosario, 1994), 39 percent of adolescent gay and bisexual males presenting at a New York City social service agency had made a suicide attempt, and of those more than half had tried to kill themselves more than once. Also, up to 80 percent of individuals who discover that they are HIV positive have suicidal ideation (Krener & Miller, 1989). Reports indicate that the suicide rate of middle-aged men with AIDS is 21 to 36 times the rate of men without AIDS (Marzuk et al., 1988; Kizer, Green, Perkins, Doebbert, & Hughes, 1988).

Table 5.1. Identification of Youth At-Risk for Suicide

Age:	Adolescents more likely to complete
Gender:	Males more likely to complete suicide; females more likely to attempt

Psychiatric Risk Factors:
  Major depression
  Bipolar disorder, especially mixed type
  Substance abuse
  Conduct problems/ADHD
  Psychosis
  Comorbid affective disorder (ADHD, conduct disorder, substance abuse)

Family Risk Factors:
  History of abuse or neglect
  Family history of suicide
  Family history of psychiatric disorder

Environmental Risk Factors:
  Availability of firearms
  Interpersonal loss (especially in psychiatrically vulnerable individuals)
  Exposure to suicide (especially in psychiatrically vulnerable individuals)
  Social isolation/poor social adjustment
  Interpersonal conflict
  Legal problems/disciplinary crises
  School failure
  Lack of acculturation (?)

Previous suicide attempts or suicidal threats

Medical Risk Factors:
  Epilepsy, especially with phenobarbital use
  HIV positive status

Assessment of Suicidality

Overview

An appreciation of what constitutes suicidal risk (Table 5.1) is absolutely imperative if the clinician is to competently assess suicidality. Ignorance of risk factors compromises the evaluation as well as the interpretation of information obtained from the child or adolescent and the family. When clinicians called on to assess suicidality are unskilled at eliciting pertinent, valid information or in interpreting the significance of the data gleaned from the interview, one of two possibilities is likely. The first is an overly rigid, albeit safe, approach in which any child or adolescent who admits to any suicidal thoughts is considered in imminent danger and immediately hospitalized for "evaluation and treatment." The second approach, perhaps the one with greater potential for disaster, involves discounting the child's suicidal risk, a practice that is often based on prejudices or myths

regarding what constitutes "real" suicidality. For example, it is all too common for suicidal behavior in conduct-disordered adolescents, especially those with a history of legal charges, to be dismissed as "manipulative." The clinician's awareness of the increased risk that conduct disorder and disciplinary crises confer for completed suicide should prompt a thorough clinical evaluation of the adolescent's suicidality. A history of multiple unsuccessful suicide attempts might lead the unsophisticated clinician to automatically assume that the child or adolescent isn't "serious" and is "looking for attention," again a hasty, uninformed conclusion with possible deadly consequences. Clinicians who consistently err on the side of underestimating or dismissing certain youths' potential for suicide are frequently insulated from the consequences of their incompetence by the low incidence of completed suicide in this population, allowing such clinicians to continue along blithely believing that they are skilled rather than just lucky.

False positives, the over-prediction of suicidal risk is both inevitable, given the low base rate for suicide in the general population, and desirable since the consequences of an error in clinical judgment (false negative predictions) can have disastrous consequences. However, the over-inclusive approach, while protecting the clinician from the emotional and possibly legal consequences of a child's suicidal behavior, may rob the child or adolescent and their family of their liberty while mandated evaluation and treatment occur. Another risk of insensitive and/or inappropriately mandated "treatment" is alienation of the patient and/or family from future psychiatric intervention. Many clinicians, including many mental health professionals, believe that the costs of mandated treatment, including involuntary hospitalization, are small compared with the risk of completed suicide, but such judgments need to be made on a case-by-case basis, and there is no substitute for common sense and informed clinical reasoning.

Because the predictors of suicidal risk are inexact, researchers are working on detection of a biological marker which might more accurately predict a predisposition toward suicidal behavior. Preliminary findings indicate that patients with major depressive disorder may have a dysfunctional serotonin neurotransmitter system, and that low levels of serotonin in the central nervous system may be associated with an increased risk for the most lethal suicidal acts (Mann & Arango, 1992). The activity level of serotonin may regulate both mood and the threshold for impulse and suicidal behavior. At the present time, however, there is no substitute for solid clinical skill.

The Clinical Interview

If suicidal ideation is elicited from a child or adolescent, specialty consultation is advisable; however, familiarity with assessment is crucial not only with respect to determining the level of urgency of consultation, but also to enable the pediatric clinician and staff to manage the child and family in the meantime, whether it be for minutes or 24 hours or more.

Frequently the clinician will be faced with a situation in which suicidality is suspected, but the child or adolescent has not directly presented with suicidal behavior or suicidal complaints. Although the clinician must ask about suicidal ideas and behavior directly, the questioning must be done sensitively. Interviews can be quite constrained in an emergency setting or when the clinician is pressed for time. General "goals" include:

Safety. The safety of the child must be ensured. The child should not leave the office or emergency room

until the evaluation has been completed by the clinician if there is any concern about active suicidality. The child also should not be left alone, especially if there is equipment that the child can use for self-harm. Delirious or actively suicidal patients on a pediatric ward may require a 24-hour sitter. The sitter must clearly appreciate the risks and should be someone who can be trusted not to leave the patient unattended even for a few minutes. If immediate hospitalization is not necessary and the child is able to agree to a "no-suicide contract," caretakers must be willing and able to provide the appropriate level of supervision recommended by the clinician, even if that requires constant supervision. They must also be able to respond appropriately to changes in clinical status. If the clinician does not believe that family members are reliable, that is an additional reason to hospitalize a child.

Establishing rapport. The clinician must establish rapport with the child or adolescent and the family. The child should be interviewed alone at some point. This is absolutely crucial, even in the prepubertal child, as frequently children and adolescents will not reveal suicidal thoughts with a parent or other adult present. The parents should also be interviewed without the child present because they may have concerns and information which can be helpful to the clinician and which they are unwilling to discuss in front of the child. Contact the child's therapist if the child has one.

From the moment of introduction, the typical child or adolescent is evaluating whether the clinician can be trusted. For the first 5 to 10 minutes, depending how much time is available, the patient should be encouraged to discuss the problem, difficulties which precipitated an evaluation, or the concerns presented by the adults. Premature structuring of the interview should be avoided. Interrupting the child to ask more specific questions can be inhibiting, and the clinician may miss important clues which may provide a smooth and gentle segue into sensitive areas. For example, consider the 15-year-old boy presenting for a school physical who complains only of fatigue. Asking the adolescent to describe the fatigue and explain how it has interfered with his life may open the door for eliciting depressive symptoms (Table 5.2), which in turn can be used as a stepping stone into an exploration of suicidality. It is the clinician's responsibility to establish an atmosphere of trust where the child or adolescent feels safe to reveal sensitive, sometimes painful and embarrassing information. Obviously, this takes some time. For the pediatrician, family physician, or pediatric clinician who already knows the patient and family, and perhaps has a history of several years of

Table 5.2. Signs and Symptoms of Depression

Depressed mood

Irritability or anger

Depressed, unhappy, or sullen facial expression

Slowness of body movements

Slowed speech, increased number or length of pauses during speech, decreased amount of speech, low volume of speech

Agitation or an increase in purposeless movement

Sleep disturbance (increased sleep or decreased sleep with delayed falling asleep, sleep continuity disturbance, and/or early morning awakening)

Fatigue or lack of energy

Decreased enjoyment of previously pleasurable activities

Appetite increase or decrease with weight changes

Tearfulness

Aches and pains/somatic complaints

Social withdrawal

Concentration difficulties

Decreased school performance

Feelings of guilt, worthlessness, helplessness and/or hopelessness

---

mutual trust, this task may be significantly easier. Regardless of how well, or for how long, the clinician has known the patient, however, the clinician is well advised to "ease" into the area of suicidality. This is not an encouragement to be indirect or "skittish" about discussing suicide, but rather a reminder that suicidal ideation and behavior are sensitive and often disturbing topics for most people to discuss. The suicidal adolescent who is fearful of the reactions of others is more likely to admit to suicidal thoughts with an empathic, sensitive, patient clinician.

Setting priorities. Determine the most crucial question(s) or problem(s) in need of evaluation. For example:

- Is this child or adolescent psychotic, suicidal, and/or depressed?
- Can the child or adolescent return home with parents? If hospitalization is recommended and refused, is commitment against the child's will indicated? What about against the family's will?
- Is there an organic component to the presentation? Delirious patients are often agitated and may experi-

ence psychotic symptoms. Delirious individuals may also be at extremely high risk for dangerous, self-harmful behavior even if genuine suicidal intent is not present. The fluctuating nature of delirious patients' confusion, disorientation, and perceptual abnormalities makes underestimation of risk possible.

- Although determining the specifics of diagnosis may not be of crucial importance in an emergency situation, the clinician should query as to the presence of symptomatology of disorders that confer additional risk (e.g., mania or hypomania indicating possible bipolar disorder, conduct disorder symptomatology, depression, substance abuse). To the non-psychiatric clinician, this may appear to be a formidable task, but can often be accomplished quickly and efficiently with the use of probe questions (Shea, 1988). Examples of probe questions for depression (Table 5.2) include, "Do you ever feel like you're more sad or unhappy than other kids your age?" or "Do you think you're more mad a lot more of the time than your friends?" Probe questions for psychosis may include "Do you ever experience things that other people don't, like seeing things or hearing things?" or "Do your thoughts ever get so intense that they almost seem like voices?" Specifically ask the adolescent how much they drink alcohol and what drugs they use. This may be more successful than querying "Do you drink?" in that the positive assumption on the part of the clinician may increase the patient's willingness to convey information about activities which are frequently criticized by adults. Conduct disorder symptomatology can be elicited by specific questions regarding shoplifting, lying, legal charges, vandalism, fire setting, and fighting. Parents are frequently better historians than children or adolescents when it comes to observable behaviors. Children and adolescents are frequently better historians when it comes to describing their own internal experiences. It is quite common and understandable that a concerned, involved, empathic parent might not be aware of a child's suicidal thoughts or urges. A probe question for anxiety might be "Do you think you're more nervous or worried than other kids your age?" Probe questions are utilized to assess if more thorough questioning about an area or disorder is needed. For example, an affirmative answer, or even some hesitation, to a probe question about depression or psychosis should alert the clinician that additional questions should be asked before the presence or absence of a disorder can be put to rest.

Direct Assessment of Suicidal Risk

The question of whether or not a child or adolescent is suicidal must be asked directly, but can be approached in three steps (Shea, 1988): (1) the clinician must set the stage (as described earlier), (2) the clinician must ask directly about suicidal thinking, and (3) the clinician must carefully explore the extent of suicidal ideation, including plans and behavior. There is a spectrum of suicidal ideation, from nonspecific thoughts or passive death wishes (e.g., "I wish I was dead") to more specific suicidal thoughts (e.g., "I'll kill myself"), to suicidal ideation with a concrete plan, to actual suicidal behavior. When questioning about suicidality, the examiner should move from general and nonthreatening questions to more specific queries, especially if the answers to the more general questions were positive or equivocal (Table 5.3). As a general rule the clinician should not accept the first negative answer. If the child or adolescent answers "no" to queries regarding passive death wishes or suicidal thoughts, the clinician should follow up with a question referring to "even fleeting" thoughts, or with a younger child follow up with questions regarding thoughts they may have had about parents or others "being better off" without them.

Clinician:	Given how depressed you've been feeling lately, have you ever felt like life isn't worth living?
Adolescent:	Not really.
Clinician:	What thoughts have you had?
Adolescent:	Well, just that everyone would probably be better off without me. My parents wouldn't have to go through the shame of having a son who got kicked out of school. My girlfriend would realize how

Table 5.3. Eliciting Suicidal Ideation

1. Has there ever been a time when you felt that life was not worth living?

2. Have you ever thought that your family or others might be better off without you?

3. Have you ever wished you were dead?

4. What thoughts have you had?

5. What ways or plans have you thought of to hurt or kill yourself?

6. How close have you come to harming or killing yourself?

7. Have you ever harmed/hurt yourself on purpose or tried to kill yourself?

much I really care about her, and I wouldn't have to put up with any of this crap anymore.

Clinician:	If the pain really gets to be too much, what would you do to end it?
Adolescent:	A gun—quick, painless, no chance for screw up.
Clinician:	Are you able to get hold of a gun if things come to that?
Adolescent:	My father has guns, but they're locked up. It would be hard to get at them.
Clinician:	How close have you actually come to killing yourself?
Adolescent:	About a week ago I was pretty drunk. I thought about smashing the gun cabinet open with a baseball bat.

In the above dialogue, the clinician smoothly leads the adolescent from an admission of passive death wishes to concrete plans to kill himself. Although more extensive questioning is necessary, even in this brief passage there is enough information to place this adolescent at high risk—access to a firearm, alcohol abuse, suicidal intent with a clear plan and irreversible means, depression, hints of an interpersonal crisis, and school problems. Clearly, this is an adolescent who requires swift psychiatric intervention and probable hospitalization. Whether or not to hospitalize the adolescent and whether (if he is unwilling to be hospitalized voluntarily) he should be committed involuntarily are complicated decisions which require more extensive interviewing with both the adolescent alone and with the family.

The evaluation of imminent risk is a crucial part of the suicide assessment. The long-term and immediate treatment goals will become more apparent as specific information is obtained.

- Does the adolescent belong to one or more "high risk" groups discussed earlier (Table 5.1)?
- Does the adolescent have a specific suicide plan or plans in mind?
- What is the actual potential lethality of the child's or adolescent's plan(s)? Obviously plans which involve potentially lethal and irreversible methods (firearms, hanging) confer greater risk for completed suicide. However, the clinician must explore the specifics of the plan in the context of that particular child's or adolescent's situation. For example, if the child is contemplating an overdose, what would he or she take and how much? What medication is available in the home, and what is the accessibility? Information that a parent or sibling is taking potentially toxic

medication such as tricyclic antidepressants should raise serious safety concerns.

- What is the patient's perception of the lethality of the plan? This may need to be asked directly, as children and even some adolescents may be ignorant of the actual risks of overdosing on some medications. For example, many children and adolescents (and even adults) perceive acetaminophen as a relatively "safe" drug for overdose, and know nothing of the risk of liver toxicity. The child or adolescent's cognitive level and capacity should also be taken into account. A mentally retarded adolescent may actually believe that attempts to strangle herself with her hands or immerse her head under water in a sink could be successful, and present with high suicidal intent.
- Has the child or adolescent taken any steps toward suicide? All other factors being equal, an adolescent who stands on a bridge looking over as he thinks about jumping is at greater risk for imminent danger (all other factors being equal) than the boy who thinks about jumping off a particular bridge but never goes anywhere near it, who in turn is more potentially dangerous than the adolescent who thinks about suicide but has no specific plan.
- How capable is the family of offering support and supervision? It is one thing to minimize the child's suicidal behavior prior to an explanation by the clinician of the child's status and suicidal risk, but after the clinician's concern has been made clear to the family, do they still minimize or deny the threat?
- Does the child or adolescent have access to firearms? This is a crucial question to ask of every child and family when there is any question of suicidal ideation or even passive death wishes. As previously noted, the risk of completed suicide is much greater for suicidal adolescents who have a firearm, particularly a loaded firearm, in the home.

If the child has already made a suicide attempt, similar areas require careful exploration:

- How exactly did the child or adolescent attempt suicide? It is not enough to know that the child overdosed. It is not even enough to know that the child overdosed on aspirin. The clinician must get the specifics of which medication(s) and how many pills were taken. If the child or family do not know, specifically query as to whether it was more than 10, more than 20, etc., or whether it was more than a handful, the whole bottle, etc.
- What were the circumstances of the suicide attempt? Was it planned and executed thoughtfully so as to

avoid detection? Was it impulsive? Did the child or adolescent engage in any behavior in anticipation of death (e.g., giving away possessions)? Nonimpulsive suicide attempters and those who premeditated and planned their attempts seem to be significantly more depressed and hopeless than impulsive attempters (Brown, Overholser, Spirito, & Fritz, 1991).
- Did the child or adolescent communicate before the suicidal behavior? Was the suicide attempt carried out in isolation, and if so, was that purposeful on the part of the adolescent, or was there someone present or nearby, possibly indicating greater ambivalence or the desire to communicate rather than a genuine desire to die?
- Was the attempt timed in order to make intervention unlikely (e.g., after a parent left for work in the morning, leaving the adolescent—who claimed to be ill and unable to attend school—alone until evening)?
- Were precautions taken against discovery (e.g., door locked)? After the attempt, did the child or adolescent have second thoughts and try to contact someone, and if so, what was the time interval between the attempt and the revelation? If the child did not have second thoughts and tell someone, what feelings were generated by discovery (e.g., relief, anger, gratitude, disappointment)?
- What was the purpose of the act according to the child or adolescent? Was there truly a wish to die; escape an intolerable situation and/or feeling state; communicate anger, love, or despair; or influence others in some way?
- A suicide note may communicate more serious intent and a greater degree of planning, but the lack of a suicide note does not indicate lower risk. Most completed child and adolescent suicides appear to be the result of highly impulsive acts carried out by those with access to a lethal means (Hoberman & Garfinkel, 1988), and it follows that significantly suicidal children and adolescents may not have the forethought to consider leaving a note.

Confidentiality

Clinicians are frequently more preoccupied with confidentiality than are children and adolescents. It is misguided and dangerous to keep parents in the dark about their child's suicidal ideation or behavior. Blanket assurances of confidentiality are seldom, if ever, helpful in eliciting information that would not have been revealed otherwise. However, for the child or adolescent who has been given false assurances, the sense of betrayal experienced when suicidality must be revealed to caretakers can be enormous. It is best to steer clear of promises that cannot and should not be kept. Remember that the clinician's ability to convey respect, trust, and empathy is much more likely to encourage the sharing of sensitive and painful information than any generic promises of secrecy.

Management

When the clinician has elicited and evaluated positive suicidal ideation or a history of suicidal behavior, it is crucial to remain nonjudgmental. Suicide remains a highly stigmatizing behavior both for the victim and the family. The clinician who is able to convey empathy and concern is more likely to obtain valid information from all parties, as well as influence the course of events that follow. For example, if the clinician considers immediate hospitalization to be necessary, voluntary hospitalization with both a willing adolescent and family who understand its necessity and purpose is preferable to being faced with the prospect of involuntary commitment.

The "no-suicide contract" (Table 5.4) has become a popular and sometimes useful tool in both the out-patient and in-patient settings. The clinician should obtain a no-suicide promise or agreement in which the child or adolescent promises not to engage in self-harmful or suicidal behavior and to tell a parent or caretaking adult if suicidal urges return or intensify. Although it is important to document the fact that a no-suicide agreement has been obtained in the medical record, a no-suicide agreement's primary purpose is the benefit provided to the patient, not any kind of medicolegal "protection." Frequently when children and adolescents become suicidal, they are in a heightened affective state which may seriously compromise their ability to "think through" a problem. Suicidal thoughts and/or behaviors may have become a way of coping with problems and the over-

whelming, intolerable feelings generated. A clear, specific plan for dealing with suicidal thoughts and/or the thoughts and feelings that develop prior to experiencing suicidal impulses can serve as an anchor—something to "hold on to" if the patient begins to drift toward suicidality. The child's or adolescent's ability to anticipate future situations which might precipitate suicidal urges and to plan ahead for how to cope with them is a crucial piece of negotiating a no-suicide agreement (Rotheram, 1987). An inability to do so should signal to the examiner that the child or adolescent may be in imminent danger of suicide (Rotheram, 1987) and prompt emergency mental health consultation.

As mentioned earlier, it is crucial to inform the family regarding the extent of the child's suicidality. This will not be a problem if no false assurances regarding confidentiality have been provided to the child or adolescent. Typically, children and adolescents are relieved to have their parents informed about the extent of their suffering.

Knowledge and experience in the evaluation and treatment of pediatric psychopathology is a must for the clinician who undertakes to manage these patients, since a large proportion will probably suffer from a psychiatric disorder which requires specialized treatment. In addition to specialized training, a high level of comfort (but not complacency) in dealing with suicidal individuals is necessary, as well as the time and availability that management of such a patient will require. Clinicians must be aware that these patients and their families can strain the clinician's emotional and physical resources. The safest course of action is to obtain specialty consultation. Ideally, the clinician should arrange the consultation appointment for within 48 hours of the initial evaluation or sooner if clinically indicated. A definite appointment time increases the likelihood of compliance. Again, it is important to highlight that if the clinician has any concerns or questions about the child's imminent risk of dangerousness and specialty consultation is not immediately available, hospitalization is indicated.

One of the most important interventions that a clinician can make for suicidal children and adolescents is the *strong recommendation to the family that all firearms be removed from the home*. A family's reluctance to do so should be considered quite worrisome and may indicate the family's inability and/or unwillingness to provide unqualified support for their child, as well as some denial of the significance and seriousness of their child's suicidal behavior.

If a specialty consultation is obtained, it is quite appropriate and advantageous for the pediatrician or family physician to be involved in the decision, along with

---

Table 5.4. No-Suicide Agreement

1. Child or adolescent promises not to harm self.

2. Child or adolescent will inform parent(s), therapist, clinician, or other responsible, supportive adult if suicidal thoughts/urges are experienced.

3. Child or adolescent will inform "alternate adult" if "primary" adult (step #2) is unavailable or cannot be contacted.

4. Child or adolescent will go to an emergency room if no one is available to help or child remains suicidal.

5. Parents and/or other caretakers (preferably those who may be serving as supports in steps #2 and #3) are contacted and aware of situation.

the child or adolescent and family, about what the next step should be. A conference call may be arranged, or the consultant may wish to call immediately after interviewing the patient and family individually, and before meeting with them again as a group to convey impressions and recommendations.

No child or adolescent who makes a suicide attempt should be discharged home directly from the emergency department or pediatrician's or family physician's office, even if their medical condition is stable. A brief 24- to 48-hour hospitalization on the pediatric unit during which psychiatric consultation can be obtained may be all that is necessary for the majority of children and adolescents. Out-patient interventions can also be arranged during this time and should begin within a day or two of discharge from the hospital, when the patient or family is at their most receptive and accepting of the need for help. Referral to a child and adolescent psychiatrist for ongoing treatment instead of to other mental health professionals is recommended if the child or adolescent (1) is or may be psychotic, (2) has or may have a serious mood disorder, (3) requires detoxification, (4) has a co-existing medical condition which may be contributing to the psychiatric symptomatology, or (5) may require psychopharmacologic intervention (Brent, 1989a).

Hospitalization clearly communicates to the child and family that the suicide attempt and the suffering that provoked it is being taken seriously. Many suicide attempters have chaotic family situations and caretakers who are unable and/or unwilling to offer genuine empathy and practical support. Typically, the emergency department setting is not conducive to performing the detailed evaluation necessary to determining continued suicidal risk, which requires a thorough assessment of the suicide attempt as well as the patient's mental status, an assessment for the presence of psychopathology, and a family assessment. Indications for psychiatric hospitalization (Brent, 1989a) are presented in Table 5.5. Children and adolescents with serious psychiatric disorders and/or those who present with risk factors which place them in imminent danger of continued suicidal behavior are candidates for psychiatric hospitalization.

AGITATION

Agitation is, simply put, an increase in the frequency of purposeless, non-goal-directed motor behavior. It is usually the expression of an intense mood state and can reflect anger, depression, anxiety, or euphoria (Taylor, 1986). It may also reflect frustration and fear, as in the confused and disoriented patient. Agitation may be noted as pacing, hand wringing, picking at clothes or bed sheets, randomly touching things, frequently shifting body movements, leg shaking, and so on. Agitation is an imprecise term which may convey little more than that the child or adolescent is "not acting right" or is disruptive and noncompliant. Careful differential diagnosis is crucial. Treatment failure as well as significant morbidity and even death can result if the etiologic diagnosis goes unrecognized. Agitation may progress to overt aggression or even dangerous violence in the older adolescent, especially if ignored or inappropriately treated in its early phases.

When it comes to assessment, clinicians must be flexible and practical, yet able to resist inappropriate compromise. Emergencies frequently strain the boundary between necessary efficiency and dangerous expediency. The first step in approaching the agitated child or adolescent must be clarification of exactly what the term "agitation" means in that particular patient. Is the six-foot-tall male adolescent who has waited in the emergency department for several hours genuinely agitated or "only" angry, loud, and noncompliant? Clearly the approach to this boy differs from the approach to the delirious postoperative patient. It is sometimes very difficult to differentiate delirium, dementia, psychosis, depression, mania, anxiety, and disruptive behavior disorders from one another. Sometimes two or more conditions coexist, further complicating the clinical picture.

Table 5.5. Indications for Psychiatric Hospitalization

Inability to make or maintain a no-suicide contract/agreement

Active suicidal ideation with plan and intent

Suicide attempt with genuine intent to die and/or high potential lethality

Previous suicide attempts

Psychiatric disorder
    Psychosis
    Bipolar (manic-depressive) illness
    Severe depression
    Substance abuse
    Severe aggression

Sexual, physical, or emotional abuse

Severe parental psychiatric illness

Family unable or unwilling to protect and monitor patient

Previous noncompliance with, or failure of, outpatient treatment

Adapted by permission from Brent, D.A. (1989). Suicide and suicidal behavior in children and adolescents. *Pediatrics in Review, 10*, 269–275.

A physical examination is crucial in the assessment of the agitated child or adolescent, as well as a history that is as complete as is reasonable and possible to obtain. It can be quite difficult to elicit a cohesive history from an agitated patient, and therefore other historians become especially important. The setting of the examination may affect the quality of the interview and information obtained. Agitated patients are often distractable. The clinician should attempt to eliminate distracting stimuli such as interruptions or noise as much as possible and talk with the child or adolescent in a quiet setting. It may be advisable to allow parents or relatives to remain with the patient, especially with young children. Even if there are concerns that the parent may be contributing to a child's or adolescent's agitation, careful reconsideration of this conclusion is prudent, especially where young children are concerned. Fear and pain (mental as well as physical) may exacerbate agitation. The comforting presence of a parent may slightly disinhibit a frightened child, but there is little to be gained and much to lose by depriving a fearful, agitated child of parental support.

It is wise to keep in mind that staff are sometimes more troubled by a parent's watchful, questioning, sometimes critical presence than is the child. In a study assessing emergency nurses' levels of knowledge and comfort with the specific medical needs and conditions of pediatric patients, nurses reported psychiatric emergencies as one of the areas of greatest discomfort and least knowledge (Fredrickson, Bauer, Arellano, & Davidson, 1994). Curiously, most nurses queried seemed to believe quite strongly that parents should not be allowed to stay with the child in the emergency department for painful procedures such as reducing fractures, lumbar punctures, and even sutures. Some comments indicated a sense that if the child was extremely distressed, then the parent must somehow be responsible.

Differential Diagnosis

The mind/body enigma rears its ugly head persistently in the evaluation of the agitated patient. It is convenient and useful to think in terms of "organic" versus "nonorganic" causes of agitation, while realizing that such reductionistic thinking has major limitations and pitfalls. *The Diagnostic and Statistical Manual of Mental Disorders* (DSM-IV) (4th edition) (American Psychiatric Association, 1994) is the official psychiatric classification system in the United States. Its authors address the dilemma posed by dichotomous thinking in the introduction, where it is stated that even the term

"mental disorder" implies a distinction between "mental" and "physical" disorders that is "reductionistic" and "dualistic." With these reservations and caveats duly noted, it nevertheless appears to be true that a practical, informed dualism is often useful in clinical settings.

It is critical to remember that psychiatric emergencies are medical emergencies. Patients should not be treated differently just because the presentation happens to appear to be "psychiatric." An aura of almost palpable crisis is no reason to abandon the basics. The clinician will need a solid differential diagnosis, just as with a patient presenting with respiratory distress. A history of the current problem, past medical and psychiatric history, history of drug or alcohol use, a history of what medications the patient is taking, and physical examination including vital signs are at the very least necessary when presented with an agitated child or adolescent. Illicit substance abuse should always be considered in the differential diagnosis of agitation, especially in adolescence, and the adolescent needs to be interviewed about this privately, but false assurances of confidentiality should not be provided. Further laboratory and other diagnostic testing and consultation should be ordered based on information obtained from the history and physical exam. As noted previously in this chapter, in an emergency setting or situation, it is seldom necessary or advisable to deliberate about diagnostic nuances. A major task for any evaluating clinician presented with an agitated child or adolescent is to seriously consider and, if at all possible, determine whether the agitation is "organic" or "nonorganic" in etiology. A brief differential diagnosis of agitation in the pediatric patient is presented in Table 5.6. The clinician is reminded that there are a myriad of medical conditions and disorders, including intoxication and withdrawal syndromes, which can produce emotional, cognitive, and behavioral symptomatology in both the adult and pediatric populations.

Delirium

Children and adults over the age of 60 are said to be at increased risk for delirium (Mikkelson, 1994), but persuasive data regarding an increased risk for children are lacking. Delirium appears to be common in sick children and may herald a rapidly deteriorating physical condition (Prugh, Wagonfeld, Metcalf, & Jordan, 1980). Children may be more likely than adults to experience delirium and hallucinations in response to fever and infection (Prugh et al., 1980). Unfortunately, there is little formal research on delirium in children; however, even in the adult population where it may be the most

Table 5.6. Differential Diagnosis of Agitation in the Child or Adolescent

I. Delirium
   A. Secondary to a general medical condition
   B. Secondary to substance intoxication
   C. Secondary to substance withdrawal

II. Dementia

III. Psychotic disorders
   A. Schizophrenia, schizoaffective disorder
   B. Affective disorders
      1. Agitated depression
      2. Mania
      3. "Mixed" bipolar presentation
   C. Secondary to a general medical condition
   D. Substance induced

IV. Affective disorders (without psychosis)
   A. Agitated depression
   B. Mania
   C. "Mixed" bipolar presentation
   D. Secondary to a general medical condition
   E. Substance induced

V. Anxiety
   A. Situational/Post-traumatic
   B. Anxiety disorder
   C. Secondary to a general medical condition
   D. Substance induced

VI. Disruptive behavior disorder
   A. Conduct disorder with or without ADHD
   B. Oppositional defiant disorder with or without ADHD

common psychiatric syndrome found in a general medical hospital (Wise, 1987), delirium remains an under-researched phenomenon.

Terms such as "acute confusional state," "ICU psychosis," "encephalopathy," and "delirium" are often used interchangeably. Some would reserve the term delirium for syndromes which include confusion, agitation, autonomic instability, and hallucinations (Adams & Victor, 1981). In this chapter the term delirium will be defined more broadly, as by Wise (1987), as "a transient, essentially reversible dysfunction in cerebral metabolism that has an acute or subacute onset and is manifest clinically by a wide array of neuropsychiatric abnormalities" (p. 91). As noted in DSM-IV (American Psychiatric Association, 1994), delirium refers to a disturbance of consciousness (i.e., reduced clarity of awareness of the environment) associated with reduced ability to focus, sustain, or shift attention, as well as changes in cognition (such as memory deficits or disorientation).

The hyperactivity, distractibility, and other behavioral disturbances of delirium in children are often easily dismissed as "normal" reactions to the stress of hospital-ization and serious illness, or mistakenly attributed to "acting out" (Prugh et al., 1980). Especially in very young children, the agitation, confusion, and hallucinations of delirium are less obvious and threatening than in older patients (Adler, 1992). The phenomenology of delirium in children has not been well studied, and there is much that we do not know. How frequently is agitation (versus hypoactivity or a mixed state) encountered in delirious children? How prevalent are paranoid delusions, frequently encountered in delirious adults (Lipowski, 1967)? Postcardiotomy adult patients have a reported incidence of delirium of 13 to 67 percent (Dubin, Field, & Gastfriend, 1979), whereas children appear to have a negligible incidence (Kornfeld, Zimberg, & Malm, 1965). Although it seems that the clinical picture of delirium in children and adolescents appears to be similar to that in adults, it is frequently missed in children, especially in its milder forms and early stages (Prugh et al., 1980). Subclinical delirium is particularly difficult to diagnose.

The presence of pre-existing brain damage, burns, and drug or alcohol abuse/withdrawal confer additional risk, lowering the threshold for the development of delirium. Sleep deprivation and sensory deprivation or overload may also facilitate the development of a delirium. The child in the intensive care unit (ICU) certainly does not lack for stimulation; however, it is stimulation which is often confusing and relentless. Sleep-wake cycles are often disrupted in the hospital setting and almost always disrupted in the ICU, contributing to the risk. Studies of adult transplant patients indicate that up to 50 percent have experienced delirium postoperatively (House, Trzepacz, & Thompson, 1991; Trzepacz, Brenner, & Van Thiel, 1989). Delirium and adjustment disorders are the most common psychiatric disorders seen in adults subsequent to liver transplantation (Trzepacz, Maue, Coffman, & Van Thiel, 1986).

Clinical features of delirium

   Prodrome Onset is usually rapid over hours or days. Prodromal signs and symptoms (restlessness, anxiety, irritability, and sleep disturbance) are often missed.

   Fluctuating Course Signs and symptoms wax and wane throughout the day and night. The child who seems fine on morning rounds may be agitated and disoriented an hour or two later. Confusion and agitation tend to be more marked at night.

   Disorientation Orientation to time is the most sensitive indicator and is typically affected before orientation to place or person. The severity of the delirium will determine the extent of disorientation.

Memory Impairment   Memory impairment is most severe for new information.

Attentional Deficit   The delirious child or adolescent is very easily distracted and must work hard at sustaining attention. If someone walks into the room, the patient will typically focus on that person and forget the question the examiner asked. Attentional difficulty may manifest itself as an inability to focus on the interview, perseveration, and/or requests that the clinician "repeat the question."

Sleep-Wake Disturbances   Patients may frequently sleep or "catnap" during the day and be awake at night when staffing is sparse and without the orienting presence of family and daytime routine. Sleep deprivation may then exacerbate disorientation and confusion. Nightmares and/or vivid dreams are also common, possibly related to side effects of medications.

Disorganized Thinking   Disorganization is often reflected in speech which may be fragmented, or if delirium is severe, rambling and incoherent. Reasoning is illogical and faulty and may be difficult to evaluate in the younger child or in the child with developmental disabilities. Parents and other caretakers can be invaluable resources in assisting the clinician in comparing current status with baseline.

Disturbances of Arousal and Psychomotor Abnormalities   Fluctuations in the patient's level of consciousness typically coincide with psychomotor abnormalities. The patient may be in a *hypoactive state* (apathetic, somnolent, quietly confused). Frequently hypoactive delirium is ignored unless the child or adolescent is uncooperative, and the delirium may be mistakenly diagnosed as depression and inappropriately treated. The delirious patient may be in a *hyperactive state* (agitation, hypervigilance). The delirium may also be missed, particularly in younger children and in children with a known history of ADHD, where a hyperactive delirium may be dismissed as disruptive behavior or simple oppositionality. The patient may be in a *mixed state* in which he or she alternates between hyperactive and hypoactive delirium.

Altered Perceptions   Misperceptions are noted in most patients and may take the form of illusions, or misperceptions of real external stimuli (e.g., an intravenous [IV] line or Foley catheter mistaken for a snake). Strangers may be misperceived as family members, and this phenomenon may serve the oddly adaptive function of converting the strange and threatening into the familiar and comforting. Hallucinations and/or delusions may be noted. Delusions are typically poorly formed and not systematized. Visual hallucinations seem to occur more frequently, at least in adult delirium, than do auditory hallucinations, and tactile hallucinations are the least frequent (Wise, 1987). New-onset hallucinations, especially of a visual nature, should immediately trigger the clinician to consider delirium in the differential diagnosis, as should hallucinatory phenomenon in a different sensory modality than "usual" in a child or adolescent known to have a history of hallucinations. For example, the presence of visual hallucinations in an adolescent who has experienced auditory hallucinations of a derogatory nature (but never before visual hallucinations) during several episodes of a psychotic depression should always raise suspicion that an organic process is now involved.

Dysgraphia/Constructional Apraxia/Dysnomia   In adults, dysgraphia has been shown to be one of the most sensitive indicators of delirium (Chedru & Geshwind, 1972; Wise, 1987). Asking the older child or adolescent to write a sentence may reveal clumsiness, perseveration, the inability to orient and align letters properly, and spelling impairments (Wise, 1987). Of course, this exercise becomes even more useful to the clinician if there is a parent available to assist the clinician in assessing motor, spatial, and linguistic impairments from baseline. An inability to name familiar objects may reveal dysnomia. For the child or adolescent who is able to tell time, draw a large circle on a blank sheet of paper and ask the patient to draw the face of a clock and show the hands to be at 10 minutes before 2 o'clock. Prugh et al. (1980) found that significant constriction in Bender-Gestalt Item #7 was a distinguishing feature between hospitalized delirious and nondelirious children.

Emotional Ability   Fear, anxiety, and apprehension are very common and may fluctuate in response to the level of confusion and disorientation. Sadness and apathy may also be seen, particularly with hypoarousal.

Abnormal Movements   Motor abnormalities such as tremor (usually absent at rest and apparent on movement), asterixis, myoclonus, and symmetric reflex and muscle tone changes may often occur depending on the underlying cause and severity of the delirium.

Autonomic Activation   Autonomic activation may accompany delirium, but not uniformly. Signs of tachycardia, hypertension, and fever may be noted. Autonomic activation is particularly common in toxic-metabolic and withdrawal states.

Differential diagnosis of delirium. If the clinician always considers delirium in the differential diagnosis when evaluating the agitated child or adolescent, including when the patient has a known psychiatric disorder, half the battle is won. The differential diagnosis of delirium is exhaustive and not within the scope of this discussion, but it is essentially the same as that of any organic mental disorder. Briefly, consideration must be given to *infections* (i.e., cerebral and systemic); *metabolic derangements* (i.e., hypoglycemia, electrolyte imbalance, uremia, hypoxia, dehydration, hypoperfusion, diabetic ketoacidosis, hepatic failure, and inborn errors of metabolism); *toxins* (i.e., alcohol, virtually any drug with potential CNS effects, heavy metals such as lead, manganese, and mercury, pesticides and hydrocarbons); *CNS disorders* (i.e., seizures including postictal states, neoplasms, trauma, bleeding, increased intracranial pressure, and cerebral vascular insufficiency); *trauma* (i.e., head trauma, heat stroke, burns, post-op states; *withdrawal states; endocrine abnormalities* (i.e., hyper- and hypothyroidism, hyperparathyroidism, and adrenal insufficiency); *deficiencies* (i.e., B_{12}, folate, niacin, thiamin, hypovitaminosis, and hypervitamosis); and *serious systemic disease* (including congestive heart failure, renal and hepatic failure) (Campo, 1993; Slaby, 1994). Very rarely, patients with psychiatric disorders such as schizophrenia and mania may present with delirium without any underlying "organic cause." However, because of this phenomenon's rarity, it should be considered only after a complete medical, including neurological and psychiatric, workup has been performed. Dementia, as in HIV infection in children and adolescents, may also present with delirium.

Laboratory and other testing. The electroencephalogram (EEG) can be a sensitive indicator of even subclinical delirium in children (Prugh et al., 1980). The typical abnormality found is slowing of the EEG background activity, but in hyperactive states there may be superimposed fast activity, and/or EEG slowing may be completely absent. However, EEG interpretation in children is difficult owing to the great variability of the normal range (Prugh et al., 1980), and therefore comparison with a child's premorbid EEG may be most helpful if available (Campo, 1993). It is important to keep in mind

that a diffusely slow tracing can help make the diagnosis of delirium, but a normal or fast record does not rule it out (Popkin, 1986). Sometimes an EEG cannot be obtained on an emergency basis; hence the importance of history and physical examination, including mental status. A study of adult "psychiatric patients" presenting to an emergency department revealed that there was failure to document mental status in 56 percent of the patients, and that the most frequent deficiency in the medical evaluation was in the neurological examination. Four percent of the patients required acute medical treatment within 24 hours of psychiatric admission, and it was determined that the emergency department history and physical examination should have identified an acute condition in 83 percent. The chart was documented "medically clear" in 80 percent of patients in whom a medical disorder should have been identified. Interestingly, patients less than 55 years of age had a four times greater chance of a missed medical diagnosis, probably reflecting an increased level of suspicion for organic etiologies in geriatric patients (Tintinalli, Peacock, & Wright, 1994). In addition to whatever laboratory testing the clinician determines to be necessary, a toxic screen for drugs is indicated even in very young children.

Dementia

Dementia is defined as a disorder of decline in multiple cognitive functions from the child's or adolescent's previous intellectual level (McHugh & Folstein, 1988). There is impairment of both short- and long-term memory, impairment in abstract thinking, impaired judgment, other disturbances of higher cortical function, and/or personality change (American Psychiatric Association, 1994). These symptoms do not occur only in the presence of reduced ability to maintain or shift attention as in delirium. Dementia does not have the fluctuating course observed in delirium. Delirium and dementia can co-exist, further complicating the clinical presentation. The disturbance must be severe enough to interfere with school performance, social activities, or relationships with others.

Pediatric clinicians may be unfamiliar with evaluating a condition which is found primarily in the elderly; however, some neuropsychiatric disorders such as AIDS dementia complex (ADC) are associated with dementia. ADC, a subcortical dementia, may occur at any point in the course of the illness and is more likely to occur as the illness progresses (Price et al., 1988). Early symptoms include impaired attention and concentration, memory loss, slowed information processing, mild frontal lobe dysfunction, and difficulty with performance of complex sequential mental activities (Krener & Miller, 1989). The MRI or CT frequently is normal but may show cortical atrophy and ventricular dilation; the MRI may reveal discrete areas of increased signal in the white matter (Krener & Miller, 1989). Neuropsychological testing is indicated and will reveal more profound and specific deficits than found on routine cognitive screening as part of the mental status examination. Dementia in children, including ADC, may be accompanied by a variety of behavioral changes including apathy, social withdrawal, and change in personality. In a minority of patients, anxiety, hyperactivity, and inappropriate behavior may occur (Price et al., 1988). Treating anxiety and/or agitation with a benzodiazepine could result in a delirious response, as the presence of dementia increases the risk of developing delirium.

Other disorders in which dementia may be seen are Huntington's disease, a variety of inherited enzyme defects such as Gaucher's and Niemann-Pick disease, metachromatic leukodystrophy, and mucopolysaccharidoses, toxic lead exposure, adrenoleukodystrophy, ceroid lipofuscinosis, mitochondrial encephalomyopathies, and Wilson's disease (Campo, 1993).

Psychosis

Psychosis is not a diagnosis; it is a syndrome with an extensive differential diagnosis, including organic and nonorganic disorders. Psychosis can be defined as a break down of the perceptual, cognitive, or rationalizing functions of the mind to the extent that the person experiences reality very differently from others within the same culture (Shea, 1988). Delirious patients may be psychotic; that is, they may experience psychotic symptoms as part of their delirium. Individuals experiencing an acute exacerbation of a major psychotic mental disorder (i.e., schizophrenia, schizoaffective disorder, psychotic mania, and psychotic depression) are not by definition delirious. However, a major mental disorder does not confer immunity against the development of delirium. This simple and seemingly obvious fact is frequently forgotten by clinicians. History obtained from both the child or adolescent, if possible, and from parents or caretakers is often of crucial importance in determining whether the child or adolescent is experiencing an acute exacerbation of a chronic illness or something new with a clinical presentation superimposed on, and perhaps influenced by, the underlying chronic mental disorder. The development of delirium in a patient with a pre-existing psychiatric disorder should always result in a careful evaluation for the presence of a physical disease or other factors that have produced the delirium. For example, delirium may signal the development of neuroleptic malignant syndrome in a schizophrenic patient on chronic neuroleptic therapy.

Shea describes "soft" and "hard" signs of psychosis (Shea, 1988). Hard signs of psychosis include delusions, hallucinations, gross disorientation, bizarre mannerisms and body language, and moderate or severe formal thought disorder. Typically, soft signs were present before hard psychotic symptoms and signs crystallized. Soft signs may persist and can be an important clue to the clinician that a psychotic process may be present. Soft signs include:

- Unusually intense affect (e.g., the adolescent may become enraged when recalling a mild snub earlier in the day); angry affect and agitation
- Glimpses of inappropriate affect (e.g., sudden giggling for no reason)
- Guardedness or suspiciousness
- Vagueness
- Evidence of a very mild thought disorder (circumstantiality and tangentiality)
- Preoccupation with an incident from the distant past
- Expectation of familiarity from the interviewer
- Inappropriate eye contact (staring, refusing to make eye contact, or fleeting, furtive eye contact)
- Long latency before responding (frequently indicating an additional effort to make the answer as "normal" as possible, versus thought blocking in which the patient may stop in midstream)

Children and adolescents with primary psychotic disorders not secondary to delirium or some other organic cause frequently present as psychiatric emergencies. The psychotic symptomatology of a major depression, bipolar disorder, and schizophrenia typically develop over weeks or months. Unfortunately, the insidious unfolding of the psychotic process is usually ignored, denied, or misconstrued by others. The clinician involved with a psychotic child or adolescent should be aware that psychosis is usually an extremely painful state. Typically the realization that one's reality is different from that of friends and family is a terrifying and isolating experience. Adolescents especially may suffer frightening auditory hallucinations and delusional ideation without telling anyone as long as they possess sufficient contact with reality to hide the more blatant signs of psychosis. Given the fact that psychotic process tends to develop slowly, it is relatively easy for parents or teachers, or even peers, to rationalize or misconstrue incipient, evolving psychosis. For example, the psychotically depressed adolescent who begins to spend more and more time in her room may be misperceived as just irritable and going through a "teenage phase." Declining school performance may be chalked up to "moodiness" over a breakup with a boyfriend. A new-found interest in religion may initially be welcomed by parents, who may then find themselves feeling increasingly distanced and uncomfortable with the teenager's intense preoccupation with sin.

The psychotic child or adolescent is often brought unwillingly for evaluation and treatment after some major incident occurs (e.g., bizarre behavior which can no longer be rationalized, assaultive behavior, or suicidal behavior). A history of the child's or adolescent's last several weeks or months viewed retrospectively will usually reveal that psychotic symptomatology has been present for some time. In fact, sudden onset of psychosis (over hours or days) in a child or adolescent with or without a psychiatric history should raise suspicions of an organic process, as should visual, tactile, olfactory, or gustatory hallucinations.

Most acute psychotic presentations with agitation as a prominent feature occur in adolescents who are developing or have developed schizophrenia, schizoaffective disorder, bipolar disorder, or a severe depression with psychotic features. Brief psychotic reactions to highly stressful situations are possible, as well as psychotic symptomatology as the result of illicit substance abuse, hence the recommendation that all children and adolescents presenting with an altered mental status have a urine toxicology screen. Amphetamine psychosis and delusional states from cocaine and other sympathomimetic agents may be indistinguishable from a nonorganic psychiatric disorder such as schizophrenia on the basis of clinical features alone, and symptoms of psychosis are not uncommon in chronic amphetamine abusers. In a predisposed individual, a hallucinating panic state may occur after a single dose of amphetamine (Slaby, 1994). Other non-psychiatric medical disorders can be responsible for the development of psychosis, and the possibility of undiagnosed physical disease should be considered in every patient who presents with acute psychosis.

Affective Disorders

Depression and mania have been reported in children and adolescents for many years. However, in the past many clinicians doubted their existence, believing that children, for theoretical reasons such as immaturity and unformed personality structures, could not experience extremes of mood (Weller & Weller, 1991). Mania is typically observed in bipolar disorder, but can also be precipitated by organic derangements. Hypomania (an abnormality of mood falling somewhere between euthymia and frank mania) is easily missed and typically is recalled only after the child or adolescent has suffered a major episode of depression or full-blown mania. Children and adolescents may present in a mixed bipolar state, with a mixture of both manic and depressive symptomatology.

Bipolar disorder can be very difficult to diagnose in the pediatric age group, even for experienced mental health professionals. Typically, the diagnosis is not made until the child or adolescent has undergone an extensive evaluation, often during a psychiatric hospitalization. Depressive symptomatology is listed in Table 5.2. Manic symptoms include inflated self-esteem or grandiosity, decreased need for sleep, increased talkativeness or pressure to keep talking, racing thoughts or flight of ideas, distractibility, increased activity or psychomotor agitation, and excessive involvement in pleasurable activities that have high potential for painful consequences (Weller & Weller, 1991). Three or more of those features accompanied by elevated, expansive, or irritable mood is necessary to make a diagnosis of mania (Weller & Weller, 1991). Pediatric bipolar patients may present with conduct problems, marked irritability, and explosiveness, which may seem out of character to the patient and family members.

Anxiety

Anxiety is a universally familiar feeling state, unlike psychosis and mania. Although anxiety is a common human experience, it is also present in many psychiatric disorders and can have an organic etiology. The clinician will note that the presentation of the anxious child or adolescent is very different from that of the agitated psychotic or delirious patient. Even older preschool children are able to identify emotions such as scared, mad, sad, happy, and nervous, and can distinguish between being "just a little bit scared" and "very scared." Obviously, subtle qualitative emotional differences are beyond the very young child's repertoire. Children usually will be able to articulate for the examiner how they feel and what makes or made them scared, nervous, or anxious, if such a specific stressor exists. Physical signs and symptoms are common in severe anxiety and include palpitations, tachycardia, flushing, pallor, hyperventilation, shortness of breath, increased perspiration, paresthesia, tremulousness, muscle tension or cramps, diarrhea, nausea, abdominal pain, headache, chest pain, easy startle, insomnia, nightmares, dizziness, fainting, and urinary hesitancy. The child will usually be able to articulate feelings of fright, tension, upset, or nervousness. In panic anxiety, the child may feel overwhelmingly frightened, and experience a sense of dread or impending doom.

Disruptive Behavior Disorders

Practically every psychiatric disorder noted in children and adolescents, ranging from mental retardation to schizophrenia, can manifest itself as a disorder of conduct (Lewis, 1991). Because conduct disorder has a poor prognosis and there is no treatment which has been demonstrated to be clearly efficacious, it is a diagnosis that a clinician should not make lightly, especially after a single evaluation in an emergency setting. Nevertheless, the pediatric clinician may be presented with an angry, violent, or potentially violent adolescent with a long history of resorting to aggression or intimidation when feeling threatened or thwarted. Even if it is learned that a particular child or adolescent has a history of delinquent behaviors, the evaluation in a crisis setting should proceed in essentially the same way as that for the previously mentioned disorders. An organic etiology for the child's "agitation," which might be more aptly described as "fury," should be considered as vigilantly as in any other patient. Trauma of one sort or another to the central nervous system (CNS) is extremely common among especially aggressive juvenile delinquents and adult aggressive offenders (Lewis, 1991). Conduct disorder or oppositional defiant disorder may be comorbid with ADHD. The impulsivity, low frustration tolerance, and social skills deficits characteristic of ADHD may further lower the child's or adolescent's threshold to become aggressive when feeling threatened, frightened, or angry.

Mental Status Examination

The mental status examination, analogous to the physical examination in emergency medicine, is a direct objective examination of the patient's behavior as well as the clinician's inferences from what the patient says and does. Expertise in performing a detailed mental status examination develops only with extensive experience and training, but in its briefer version, the mental status examination is an essential diagnostic tool for all physicians and clinicians in the position of evaluating patients in medical and non-medical settings. The mental status examination of children and adolescents requires tailoring to age, as well as developmental and cognitive level, with respect to how questions to the patient are framed as well as how responses are interpreted. For example, to the question, "What brought you to the hospital?," the response of "a car" in an adult or older adolescent is considered pathologically concrete, but is developmentally appropriate for a 6-year-old.

Although physicians spend many years mastering the art and science of physical diagnosis, relatively little attention is paid during medical education and training to the mental status examination. This is quite unfortunate since the inability to distinguish between the delirious adolescent and the anxious adolescent can have consequences just as deadly as those that might stem from the physician's inability to distinguish cardiac pain from GI distress.

A detailed discussion of the mental status exam is beyond the scope of this chapter; however, a brief review of the mental status exam is presented as it may pertain to the agitated child or adolescent. The pediatric clinician need only proceed in the evaluation of agitation as he or she would proceed when confronted with any nonspecific medical sign or symptom—in an organized and systematic manner.

General Appearance and Behavior

During the clinician's observation of the child, the specifics of the child's agitation are noted. A child who is restless and unable to sit still will stimulate thoughts about ADHD, mania or hypomania, anxiety, psychosis, or an organic disorder. Is the hyperactivity purposeful or nonpurposeful? Equally important is noting the child's or adolescent's level of consciousness. Is the child drowsy or lethargic (suggesting delirium and raising suspicion of organic etiology, including intoxication)? Does the child or adolescent seem confused out of proportion to the situation? Does the child appear to be in pain or complain of pain (often associated with anxiety)? Is the child or adolescent able to attend to the clinician's questions as appropriate to age and developmental level? If attention is poor and the patient seems distractable, does this distractibility wax or wane during the examination? Contrast and compare what is observed during the evaluation with information from parents or caretakers. What do they think about the child's presentation, including level of distractability and attention span? Is this usual or clearly a change for a child?

The child's attitude toward the clinician may also be useful. Children, especially younger children, usually react to clinicians cautiously at first, but may also appear extremely guarded and suspicious, irritable, indifferent, tearful, tense, or overly friendly and familiar. Momentary lapses of attention (staring, blinking, shuddering) may indicate seizure activity. Specifically look for automatisms, noted in partial complex seizures. Frequently children will be agitated and confused when postictal rather than only somnolent. Mannerisms may also provide a clue. Tics may indicate an anxiety disorder or Tourette's disorder. Are tremors noted? If the child is noted to be clumsy, poorly coordinated, and awkward, parents should be asked if this is a chronic condition.

Speech and Stream of Thought/Thought Process

Speech reflects the patient's thought processes. Normal speech and thought process should be spontaneous, goal directed, clear, logical and coherent given the child's age and developmental level. Thought process is often easier to infer from speech in school-age children and adolescents than in the very young child.

Thought process has three major clinical dimensions: actual thought content, speed of thinking, and ease of flow (Lewis, 1991). A disturbance in any of these dimensions may be severe enough to constitute a thought disorder. Lewis (1991) classified the causes of a thought disorder in a child or adolescent as follows:

- Psychological (e.g., acute massive psychological stress reaction)
- Genetic (e.g., inborn errors of metabolism)
- Traumatic (e.g., postconcussion syndrome)
- Infectious (e.g., viral encephalitis and brain abscesses)
- Toxic (e.g., amphetamines, corticosteroids, hallucinogens)
- Deficiencies (e.g., pellagra)
- Endocrine (e.g., thyrotoxicosis)
- Multiple (e.g., pervasive developmental disorder, schizophrenia)

When the clinician detects evidence of a thought disorder, elements of the history as well as additional information obtained in the mental status examination will assist in narrowing the differential.

Vague speech may be observed in numerous disorders. While this finding is not very specific, it should alert the examiner to the possibility or probability of a thought disorder. In an adolescent, the examiner must question the patient's motive. Perhaps this is an adolescent who is harboring a psychotic thought process but is still enough in touch with reality to be concerned about the perceptions of others. Such adolescents usually demonstrate a paucity of speech. They are usually guarded and quite afraid to reveal what they are thinking, lest others perceive them as "crazy." Psychotic adolescents are usually terrified, and all too easily can misperceive innocuous comments and situations, becoming more terrified and overwhelmed. Such agitation can easily escalate into violence. The clinician who is aware of this potential and able to sensitively convey concern and empathy, as well as the hope of providing help, is in a much better position to avert an escalation.

In mania, the clinician may note loud, circumstantial, tangential, pressured, overly productive speech which is extremely difficult to interrupt. The patient may be giddy and silly one moment and then become tearful and talk of suicide the next. Mixed bipolar states are not uncommon in children and adolescents with bipolar disorder. The patient looks distressed and may pace or engage in much purposeless and/or repetitive movement. The agitated psychotically depressed patient may present with speech which is pressured or hesitant, retarded, and under-productive, or may be mute.

Disordered, irrelevant, incoherent, rambling speech is often observed in delirium and specific organic states, including intoxication.

In children and adolescents the presence of a language disorder, either receptive (compromising the patient's ability to understand what is said) and/or expressive (compromising the patient's ability to communicate affect and cognitions) can also compromise the clinician's ability to obtain information from the child or adolescent. A number of investigators have shown that children with psychiatric disorders frequently also suffer from speech and language disorders (Gualtieri, Koriath, VanBourgondien, & Saleeby, 1983; Baker & Cantwell, 1987). In almost all cases, the communication disorder has its onset prior to the psychiatric disorder (Baker & Cantwell, 1987). Frequently, communication disorders in psychiatrically impaired children go undetected (Cohen, Davine, Horodezky, Lipsett, & Isaacson, 1993).

Affect and Mood

Affect is the feeling state of the patient as observed by the clinician. Mood is a symptom, reported by the child or adolescent, regarding the current feeling state.

In schizophrenia, affect may be inappropriate to the situation. In depression, mood is depressed and affect is often consistent. In mania it is elevated. However, symptoms of mania and depression can often co-exist in mixed bipolar states. The clinical picture of mania and depression in older adolescents is frequently similar to that seen in adults. However, teenagers, and especially younger manic children (under the age of 9), often present with irritability and emotional lability rather than the euphoria and grandiosity typically noted in adult mania (Carlson, 1983). Hyperactivity, pressured speech, and distractibility are seen at all ages and are frequently misdiagnosed as ADHD. Dysphoria, hypomania, and agitation may be interwoven in the early cycles of prepubertal bipolar disorder.

Individuals with anxiety as their primary problem will be able to describe their anxiety and the situations that prompt it. In emergency settings agitation may be observed in an anxious child who is being forced to confront a highly anxiety-provoking stimulus, for example, the child with a severe separation anxiety disorder or school phobia who is being forced to go to school. The child may become overwhelmed, hyperventilate, experience perioral numbness and tingling, or may faint, resulting in an emergency department visit or trip to the physician's office in a highly anxious state.

Affective lability may be seen in organic mental syndromes, with marked mood shifts, inappropriate outbursts, or rage reactions out of proportion to the provoking stimulus.

Thought Content

As noted earlier in this chapter, all children and adolescents must be screened for suicidal ideation. Delirious patients are at considerable risk for self-harm and even suicide given their propensity for misperceiving environmental stimuli and for impulsivity. Agitated, psychotic, or suicidal delirious patients should have a "24-hour sitter" with them at all times who is aware of the risks and can be trusted to not leave the patient unattended even for a few minutes. Homicidal ideation may be present and should be queried about, but is far less frequent.

Delusions may be present in psychiatric disorders of both nonorganic and organic etiology. The delusional ideation of the delirious patient is usually poorly formed and of a paranoid nature, often precipitated by perceptual abnormalities, also so common in delirium. For example, a delirious child may hear X-ray technicians in the hall discussing taking another patient downstairs and become convinced that the technicians are kidnappers. Delusional ideation that comes on rapidly should immediately arouse suspicion about an organic process. "Functional" nonorganic psychotic process typically has an insidious onset.

Shea (1988) describes the "life cycle" of a delusion, which begins with a delusional mood. Here the patient, more typically an adolescent than a younger child, begins to sense or feel that things are somehow different or not quite right. Colors may seem more intense and whispering may seem louder. The patient may become preoccupied with the meaning of other's gestures or facial expressions. Delusional mood typically evolves slowly into delusional perception. At this point, the patient may have ideas of reference and believe that previously innocuous stimuli have special significance. They may believe that peers are talking about them and secretly signaling to one another. By the time the delusional ideation has evolved into a concrete delusion, the adolescent "knows" that there is definitely a conspiracy, and is clear about who is involved and why. In other words, an elaborate fixed belief system has evolved from those initial inklings that "something" was different. Family input will often support a history of gradual escalation of paranoia. In retrospect, the family may be able to recall that the patient began acting differently and tried to involve family members in their belief system and behaviors.

Delusions may be paranoid, somatic ("My intestines are rotting away"), nihilistic ("The world is coming to an end"), grandiose ("I've been sent by God to save to humanity"), despairing ("I'm an awful person and deserve to die"), or persecutory ("The mafia is after me"). Delusional patients are often quite agitated, especially as they become aware that others do not believe them or are skeptical. Clinicians who directly confront a delusional belief system may find themselves quickly incorporated into it as one of the "enemy." It is generally not appropriate to directly confront the delusional belief system early on, especially in an agitated patient. Instead, the clinician can empathize with how distressed, angry, or fearful the patient is over these occurrences, and provide support, but need not agree with or reinforce the delusion. Be aware that ideas of reference may be normal up to a point in children and adolescents. The adolescent who believes that peers became silent when he walked into a room recently because they had been talking about him is not necessarily suffering a thought disorder. Most adolescents struggle with self-consciousness and extreme reactivity to the opinions of others, particularly peers.

However, more intricate ideas of reference should raise concerns, especially if they are held onto with complete conviction. Few studies have objectively studied the experience of delusions in children, and those that are available report conflicting results. It is possible that the presence of delusions in childhood and early adolescence are relatively infrequent and may rise after age 17, when schizophrenia in young persons becomes more prevalent (Bettes & Walker, 1987). Delusions can also be a consequence of non-psychiatric medical disorders, including metabolic disorders, deficiency states, and drug intoxication (Cummings, 1985).

Perception

Perceptual distortions can be present in the agitated child and adolescent and may exacerbate the level of agitation. Illusions are false sensory perceptions of actual external stimuli, such as misinterpreting a curtain blowing in the breeze as a man climbing in the window at night. They can be seen in extremes of hunger, thirst, or fatigue, and also in delirium, intoxication (especially with hallucinogens), and epilepsy, as well as any acute psychiatric condition (Nurcombe, 1991). Unless the clinician makes specific queries regarding the circumstances of the experience and considers other explanations, the illusion is likely to be mistaken for a hallucination.

Hallucinations are false sensory perceptions not associated with real external stimuli. Hallucinations which occur as an individual falls asleep (hypnagogic) or awakens (hypnopompic) are encountered in normal individuals and are not seen as distinctly pathological. Hallucinations appear to be rare in children under age 6 or 7, even in organic states (Caplan & Tanguay, 1991). Hallucinations in children and adolescents resemble hallucinations in adults, including hallucinations commanding harm to self or others. Mumbling voices and other auditory hallucinations have been reported in children, as well as visual hallucinations of frightening figures and shapes and scenes (Burke, DelBeccaro, McCauley, & Clark, 1985). Hallucinations in children and adolescents are encountered in delirium and can be associated with numerous medical conditions already noted. Hallucinations should automatically bring to mind a differential diagnosis which includes organic etiologies, especially in the case of visual, olfactory, tactile, somatic, or gustatory hallucinations. Although hallucinations in childhood are usually pathological, there is some controversy in the literature on this point (Lewis, 1991). Young children experiencing severe stress may hallucinate briefly. Acute brief reactions after the death of a parent may also be associated with hallucinations, usually involving the dead parent. External conflicts rarely, if ever, precipitate hallucinations in adolescents and adults (Lewis, 1991).

In psychotic depression, the hallucinatory content is consistent with depression—negative, hopeless, critical (e.g., a voice saying the child is bad and should commit suicide). In manic psychosis, signs and symptoms of mania are also present and content is consistent with mania.

Although not a reliable diagnostic differentiation, hallucinations in schizophrenia are often more fragmented, incoherent, and bizarre. Bodily complaints and paranoid delusions are also common. Disorganized and illogical thinking, as well as inappropriate affect are also often present.

Other perceptual distortions include depersonalization (feelings of unreality and strangeness about one's self) and derealization (a sense of unreality about one's surroundings). These phenomenon can occur in a variety of situations, including psychosis of any etiology, non-psychotic mental disorders such as panic disorder, or in individuals experiencing extreme stress or suffering from post-traumatic stress.

Cognitive Functioning

This is perhaps the most important part of the mental status examination when faced with an agitated child or adolescent and when evaluating the possibility of organic involvement. Tact is required as adolescents can be especially sensitive to and fearful of cognitive impairment. However the clinician should not apologize for testing memory, orientation, or other relevant cognitive parameters. Although not studied or validated for use in the adolescent population, the Mini Mental State Examination (Folstein, Folstein, & McHugh, 1975) is an excellent clinical screening method of assessing cognitive impairment and documenting cognitive change in adults, including the geriatric population (Figure 5.1). A score of 20 or less is found essentially only in patients with dementia, delirium, schizophrenia, or a severe affective disorder (Folstein, Folstein, & McHugh, 1975). This screening tool is probably most helpful in the hands of a pediatric clinician who has previously seen the patient and has some grasp of the patient's baseline functioning. It can be used to follow a patient's progress serially over time.

(Add points for each correct response)

Orientation		Score Points
1. What is the	Year?	1
	Season?	1
	Date?	1
	Day?	1
	Month?	1
2. Where are we	State?	1
	County?	1
	Town or City?	1
	Hospital?	1
	Floor?	1

Registration

3. Name three objects, taking one second to say each. Then ask the patient all three after you have said them. Give one point for each correct answer. Repeat the answers until patient learns all three.   3

Attention and Calculation

4. Serial sevens. Give one point for each correct answer. Stop after five answers. Alternate: Spell WORLD backwards.   5

Recall

5. Ask for names of three objects learned in Q. 3. Give one point for each correct answer.   3

Language

6. Point to a pencil and a watch. Have the patient name them as you point.   2

7. Have the patient repeat "No ifs, ands or buts."   1

8. Have the patient follow a three-stage command: Take a paper in your right hand. Fold the paper in half. Put the paper on the floor.   3

9. Have the patient read and obey the following: CLOSE YOUR EYES (Write it in large letters.)   1

10. Have the patient write a sentence of his or her choice. (The sentence should contain a subject and an object and should make sense. Ignore spelling errors when scoring.)   1

11. Enlarge the design printed below to 1.5 cm per side and have the patient copy it. (Give one point if all sides and angles are preserved and if the intersecting sides form a quadrangle.)   1

Years of education = _____ _____ = Total 30

From Folstein, M.F., Folstein, S.E., & McHugh, P.R. (1975). "Mini-mental state": A practical method for grading the cognitive state of patients for the clinician. *Journal of the Psychiatric Resident, 12*, 189–198. Reprinted with permission.

Figure 5.1. Mini-mental state examination

Judgment. The history may provide information regarding whether the patient is demonstrating good or poor judgment. Parents or caretakers should be asked if the child's level of judgment has deteriorated recently, and specific examples should be sought. Asking how a child or adolescent behaves in troublesome situations has traditionally been used to evaluate judgment (e.g., What would a child or adolescent do if smoke was seen in a crowded theater?).

Orientation. In delirium, orientation to time is the first to be impaired, followed by place and lastly by orientation to person, which becomes impaired only in extreme cases.

Attention, concentration, and memory. Attention and concentration are usually tested by subtracting 7s from a hundred, but most younger children and many adolescents are unable to comply with this request in the best of circumstances. Ask the child or adolescent to spell "world" and then spell it backward. Or give the child or adolescent a series of numbers to remember and then repeat immediately and in a few minutes. The patient who reveals extreme deficits in attention and concentration is unable to filter relevant from irrelevant material and is therefore extremely distractible. In a child or adolescent, it is important to distinguish between attentional deficits and lack of cooperation.

Deficits in memory include:

- Immediate—child or adolescent cannot register what has just been said
- Short-term—unable to retain information for five minutes
- Recent—unable to recall events in the past weeks or month
- Long-term (remote)—unable to remember significant events that took place months ago

At age 8, the child should be able to count 5 digits forward or 3 digits backward; a 10-year-old can count 6 digits forward and 4 digits backward (Lewis, 1991). Minor problems may indicate anxiety, but very poor performance may indicate brain damage, mental retardation, or delirium.

Calculation and counting. Again, without someone to provide information on the patient's baseline functioning in this area, even poor performance is likely to contribute little to differential diagnosis. For example, a 10-year-old unable to do simple addition clearly has a problem, and a developmental learning disability in arithmetic is only one possibility. If a parent is able to inform the clinician that the child was an excellent math student in a regular 5th grade class, the case for an organic etiology becomes stronger.

Management Issues

Appropriate treatment of the agitated child or adolescent depends on the etiology of the agitation. Fortunately, there is usually less pressure to prematurely sedate an agitated child or adolescent than an agitated adult. Prematurely medicating agitation is analogous to providing analgesia for another relatively nonspecific entity—abdominal pain. Analgesia, prior to a thorough examination of abdominal pain, may obscure important signs and symptoms. Although pharmacologic intervention may play an important role in the management of the agitated pediatric patient, it is only one potential strategy, and each clinical situation must be evaluated and treated individually. In general, intervention should follow careful assessment, but common sense and flexibility are also important in emergency situations. For example, it is frequently very difficult, and at times impossible, to perform a decent physical examination on someone who is highly agitated or violent, and the clinician should not compromise safety in attempting to do so. Hopefully, verbal maneuvers will be able to calm the patient sufficiently, but if not, physical and/or chemical restraint may be necessary.

Signs such as hyperreflexia, nystagmus, pupillary changes, vital sign abnormalities, and slurred speech may offer clues to an organic etiology during the physical examination.

Particularly with the agitated, potentially violent patient, the clinician need not, and should not, face this crisis alone. The pediatric clinician should be willing to call on staff as well as specialty consultation. If the crisis occurs in the clinician's office, the resources of local emergency services, including the police, may be necessary, particularly if the family also becomes "agitated" for whatever reason. With any patient who presents with a psychiatric crisis, it is useful to have an established, comfortable relationship with a psychiatric consultant who can be reached by phone in order to describe the problem and ask advice. If the patient is sent to the emergency department (ED), it is important to speak directly with the ED physician.

One of the major differences between pediatric and adult crisis intervention is the dependence of children and even adolescents on the family for basic needs to an extent that most adults are not. Therefore, it is especially important that the family be included in crisis intervention, stabilization, and treatment. Parents should be looked upon as allies, people who care deeply for the child and who can be rallied into offering support for the child and adolescent no matter what the disposition.

Verbal Strategies

Verbal strategies are important regardless of the cause of the patient's agitation. Some useful points to remember are:

- Try to get as much information as possible from parents or caregivers; it is amazing how distorted some information can become in translation, even with the most competent intermediaries. Unfortunately, some professionals continue to adhere to archaic and unproductive notions about parental responsibility for a child's emotional distress. This criticism can be easily conveyed to parents, increasing their sense of helplessness and powerlessness, and reinforcing their own feelings of guilt and shame.

- Approach the child or adolescent in a calm manner and introduce yourself. Speak softly and concretely. Try not to use long sentences with multiple clauses. The agitated patient does best with short, specific questions and directives.

- Listen to the patient. Avoid interrupting if at all possible during the first few minutes. Valuable information regarding the child's mental status can often be obtained without asking a single question.

- Facilitate the child's talking. If the patient is reluctant to give more than yes-or-no answers to questions, try a more open-ended approach ("Tell me more about that," or "What are you worried about right now?"). Open-ended questions are more difficult to answer with a "yes" or "no" or a one-word response. Empathic maneuvers ("Uh-huh," head nodding, etc.) and statements ("This must be hard for you," "You've been through a lot.") should be utilized and can be quite helpful in establishing an atmosphere of trust (Shea, 1988). Especially in the early stages of the psychotic process, adolescents are often very much aware of how different their reality has become relative to others' reality. The clinician's ability to convey that others have experienced similar problems and the clinician is comfortable talking about them can be a powerful tool in eliciting trust and compliance.

- Avoid direct, intense eye contact, especially with an agitated adolescent who may be potentially violent and dangerous. Paranoid individuals who are psychotic and/or delusional frequently interpret prolonged eye contact as a challenge. A paranoid male adolescent may interpret prolonged eye contact from a male clinician as a dare or provocation to physical confrontation or as conveying a homosexual interest. Likewise, the "staring" of a young female clinician may be misinterpreted as a "come on." Any of these perceptions are almost guaranteed to exacerbate the patient's anxiety and agitation with possible escalation into violence. Avoid getting too physically close very early on in the evaluation. This may also be perceived as frightening or threatening and result in the child's striking out. Be aware that children and adolescents as a rule tolerate long silences and pregnant pauses poorly. The psychotic adolescent may become increasingly paranoid or agitated regarding the significance of the examiner's silence.

- Talk to the patient softly in a nonjudgmental manner. Avoid critical or provocative remarks or even statements which could be easily interpreted as critical (e.g., "Why in the world did you do that?").
- Do not make promises that you cannot or should not keep. Sometimes clinicians feel pressured into false reassurances of confidentiality, especially in emergency situations where time is such a crucial element.

Delirious patients are typically extremely distractible, which contributes to their level of agitation. The clinician should attempt to limit distracting, overly stimulating noise and interruptions as much as possible. Orienting devices such as a clock can be helpful as well as the presence of a familiar comforting adult who can provide necessary reassurance, orientation, and reality testing. If possible, it is best to have one nurse or staff person tend to the patient rather than several. Moderate or even dim lighting may be optimal but should be assessed on an individual basis. Bright lighting can be discomforting to the delirious individual, but darkness or even dim lighting can also be disorienting to children prone to misperceive benign stimuli such as curtains, furniture, etc., in a frightening and threatening manner.

Safety Issues

It is an unfortunate fact that the potential for dangerousness to both self and others in children and adolescents is often minimized or denied. Those who perceive childhood as a time of "innocence" may have difficulty reconciling this view with the reality posed by abused, assaultive, suicidal, and severely mentally ill youth. The pediatric clinician will encounter many agitated youngsters, most of whom are not dangerous. Some, however, may present a threat to themselves or others. Until the clinician has evaluated the patient, it is safest to assume that there is some significant risk.

Aggressive adolescents are especially problematic because of their larger size, especially if they become violent where people are unprepared to intervene. The clinician's top priority must be safety for the patient and safety for others. If the clinician does not feel safe with the patient, fear (especially fear which is denied) will compromise the evaluation and may result in misdiagnosis and/or physical injury or death. A good rule of thumb is that if the clinician feels afraid, there is probably something worth fearing. The presence of hospital security officers should be requested when a severely agitated and potentially violent patient is encountered in an emergency department or pediatric ward. Sometimes the presence of others who will clearly be able to take control of the situation if the patient is unable to stay in control is quite comforting and may assist the patient in calming down or at least in maintaining some control. An understated show of force that avoids provocation is often quite effective in helping the patient maintain control. Frequently patients, adults as well as children and adolescents, are terrified of "losing it"—the loss of control and potential for harming loved ones engenders a sense of overwhelming and terrifying helplessness. At times, pharmacologic intervention is both necessary and helpful.

Pharmacotherapy

It is quite curious and alarming that although the use of psychotropic medication in the emergency treatment of agitation in children and adolescents is common, both clinicians and researchers have virtually ignored this area as a potential target for study. There are no established guidelines for the use of medication in the highly agitated and/or delirious pediatric patient. Pediatric and psychiatric texts tend to offer minimal and rather vague recommendations and guidance which are of little help to the clinician faced with an emergency of this nature. This discussion will attempt to offer the reader some specific and concrete guidance with respect to choosing a pharmacologic agent when faced with a dangerously agitated child or adolescent. Although pertinent references are cited whenever possible (often from the adult literature), the reader is again reminded that there is a paucity of research in this area generally, and especially in the pediatric population. Many of the recommendations are based on the author's personal experience with adults, adolescents, and children in the emergency department of an urban psychiatric hospital and on an inpatient adolescent unit.

Although an effort has been made to provide accurate indications and dosage schedules in this chapter, it is possible they may change as new information becomes available. The reader is cautioned to review the package information data of the manufacturers of the medications mentioned. It is also assumed that prior to using any of the medications discussed in this chapter for the indications listed, the clinician will be familiar with the myriad of potential contraindications, potential drug interactions, side effects, and adverse reactions, a thorough discussion of which is beyond the scope of this chapter.

Common reasons for pharmacotherapy on an emergency basis include:

- Severe, sustained agitation
- Aggression
- Self-injurious behavior which is serious or sustained

Unfortunately, there is no "ideal" medication for the highly agitated child or adolescent. The ideal agent for chemical restraint should (Elliott, 1992):

- Take effect rapidly, preferably within seconds.
- Be convenient to administer and be available as a small pill or chewable tablet and in clear liquid for oral use, as well as be available as a low-volume injectable form.
- Primarily calm and organize the patient with a relatively small amount of sedation. It should be useful for patients with a wide variety of symptoms and disorders.
- Produce no side effects or atypical/idiosyncratic responses. There should be a wide therapeutic window.
- Be compatible with the many other medications, including anticonvulsants, that children and adolescents with medical and psychiatric disorders are likely to be taking.
- Be able to be readministered whenever needed. Therefore, the duration of action should be short, preferably no more than a few hours.

Obviously, no available drug can fulfill all these requirements. Frequently, the clinician is caught in a bind. The child or adolescent may be far too agitated and out of control to provide necessary history or cooperate with the physical exam. No amount of talking, with either the clinician or family members, seems to be helping; in fact, at times the patient appears to become more agitated. The decision may come down to choosing the lesser of two evils. On the one hand, not medicating the patient risks an inadequate physical and psychiatric exam, as well as continued exacerbation of the agitation. On the other hand, the clinician may choose a drug which exacerbates a delirium or overly sedates the pa-

tient, obscuring a possible organic cause for the symptomatology. The clinician must be able to sort through the complexity of such situations with the assistance of history obtained from caretakers and/or others accompanying the patient and information obtained through observation and whatever physical examination is possible. When used appropriately, pharmacologic intervention with an agitated child or adolescent can provide relief of overwhelming, sometimes unbearable psychic pain, perhaps aborting an assaultive incident. Inappropriately utilized, pharmacologic interventions can further undermine a child's or adolescent's limited sense of control, intensifying a sense of powerlessness, or be perceived as punishment for "bad" behavior.

Medication is only one piece of a larger effort to comfort the agitated pediatric patient, especially in the pediatric setting, where it may serve as a temporary means of more thoroughly assessing the etiology of the patient's agitation and preventing physical harm.

Antihistamines. Antihistamines are commonly used in the emergency treatment of "functional" agitation especially in younger children on psychiatric in-patient units. However, there are no controlled studies showing antihistamines to be effective in agitation. Antihistamines have relatively short half-lives (1 to 4 hours in adults), seldom disinhibit patients or produce paradoxical excitement, and have few serious side effects. They can be overly sedating, especially in younger children, and are not especially useful in severely agitated states or in psychosis.

Diphenhydramine has been noted by some clinicians to be an effective anxiolytic in children up to about age 10, in whom it reduces anxiety before producing sedation or lethargy (Green, 1995). However, antihistamines were found to be no more effective than placebo when administered to "disruptive" hospitalized children in a controlled study (Vitiello et al., 1991). It is likely that children who "calm down" after receiving an antihistamine are responding primarily to a placebo effect and perhaps slightly to the sedative effect of the antihistamine. Older children tend to experience sedation, rather than a more specific anxiolytic effect (Fish, 1960). The use of diphenhydramine as a "PRN" for agitation in children or adolescents is not an FDA-approved indication.

Fish (1960) found a dose range of 2 to 10 mg/kg/d with an average of daily dose of 4 mg/kg to be most effective. Practically, most clinicians in an acute situation with an agitated school-aged child use a single dose of 25 to 50 mg. Duration until maximal activity is approximately one hour, and the effects last about 4 to 6 hours.

Contraindications include known hypersensitivity, narrow-angle glaucoma, gastrointestinal or urinary obstruction, and mental status changes which could be secondary to anticholinergic toxicity. Diphenhydramine may exacerbate delirium.

Antipsychotics. Antipsychotics or neuroleptics are frequently used for agitation, especially in in-patient settings. Whereas antipsychotic agents may be helpful for agitation accompanying a psychotic disorder and in delirium (specifically the high-potency neuroleptic, haloperidol), it is debatable as to whether they are most appropriate in other situations. Neuroleptics have many drawbacks as agents in the treatment of agitation, not the least of which is akathesia. Akathesia is the subjective complaint of motor restlessness, which ranges from a sensation of inner tension, often localized in the muscles, to an inability to keep still or lie quietly, resulting in the need to pace or keep moving constantly. Akathesia can be extremely uncomfortable to the point of being intolerable. It is easily misperceived as an increase in psychotic agitation, which can lead to a resultant increase in the neuroleptic dosage. Questioning children or adolescents directly and specifically about the physical (akathesia) versus emotional sensations they are experiencing if being treated with neuroleptics is often productive. Antiparkinsonian agents may provide some relief but often are only minimally effective. Neuroleptic malignant syndrome, which is life threatening, has been reported in the literature after only one dose of a neuroleptic.

Chlorpromazine, thioridazine, and haloperidol have FDA approval for use with children and adolescents in severe behavioral disorders and nonpsychotic anxiety (see Table 5.7). Some clinicians prefer to use a sedating agent such as chlorpromazine, which has the advantage of low potential for causing dystonic reactions and severe akathisia. Disadvantages include a side-effect profile (high potential for hypotension and anticholinergic effects) which is not conducive to aggressive dosing and can worsen an organic process. Intramuscular administration of chlorpromazine can produce severe hypotension, is quite painful, and is not recommended.

The butyrophenone droperidol is a potent, highly sedating drug used as a premedication for general anesthesia and in the control of agitated psychosis resulting from ketamine anesthesia. It is frequently used in general psychiatric practice in Europe, and although not FDA-approved for this use in adults or children, it is being used in this country safely and effectively in the management of markedly agitated and potentially dangerous (combative or severely self-injurious) adults and adolescents (Resnick & Burton, 1984). Droperidol is not available for administration by mouth. Although both intramuscular (IM) and intravenous (IV) use have been de-

Table 5.7. Antipsychotic Drugs in Agitation

DRUG	SEDATIVE EFFECTS	ANTICHOLINERGIC EFFECTS	EXTRAPYRAMIDAL EFFECTS	DOSAGE
Phenothiazines				
Chlorpromazine (Thorazine)	High	High	Low	25–50 mg po[1]
Thioridazine (Mellaril)	High	High	Low	25–50 mg po[2]
Butyrophenones				
Haloperidol (Haldol)	Low	Low	High	1–5 mg po, IM, IV[3]
Droperidol (Inapsin)	Very High	Low	Medium	2.5–5 mg IM[4]

For severe agitation

[1]Chlorpromazine:
      6–12 yrs ORAL 0.25 mg/kg q 4–6 hrs as needed
             RECTAL 1 mg/kg q 6–8 hrs
      Adolescents: 25 mg po and repeat in 1 hr if necessary.
[2]Thioridazine:
      ages 2–12 yrs: Usual dosage ranges 0.5 mg/kg/d to a maximum of 3 mg/kg/d.
      Usual PRN 25 mg po or less depending on size.
      Adolescents: Maximum of 800 mg/d maintenance treatment to minimize pigmentary retinopathy. 25–50 mg po in severe agitation
[3]Haloperidol:
      ages 3–12 yrs 0.5–1.0 mg PRN agitation IM or po
      Adolescents: 1–5 mg PRN IM or po q 4–6 hrs
[4]Droperidol:
      Over 12 yrs 2.5–5.0 mg PRN IM q 4–6 hrs
      May repeat first dose in 30 minutes
      <12 yrs (preanesthetic dose) 1.0–1.5 mg per 20–25 pounds IM

scribed (Neff, Denney, & Blachly, 1972; van Leeuwen et al., 1977), this author has had experience with only the intramuscular administration of droperidol to control marked psychotic and nonpsychotic agitation in adults and adolescents.

The most striking effect of droperidol is marked sedation, usually within five minutes with peak effects at 30 minutes. If ineffective, the dose may be repeated in 20 to 30 minutes up to a total dose of 10 mg, although there are reports of much higher doses being given to adults—greater than 50 mg IV and IM (Szuba et al., 1992). Half-life is also relatively short at 2 to 4 hours in adults. Droperidol has also been used effectively in the treatment of "bad drug trips" secondary to hallucinogens and amphetamines in adults (Neff et al., 1972). Hypotension and extrapyramidal symptoms (EPS) can occur. Very serious adverse reactions such as laryngospasm and neuroleptic malignant syndrome have also been reported, but are quite rare. EPS are very infrequently reported with droperidol, especially with the low doses usually employed (5 to 10 mg) in agitation; however, two reports in the anesthesiology literature (Melnick, 1988; Schreibman, 1990) noted extrapyramidal reactions (which responded to diphenhydramine) occurring several hours after low-dose droperidol administration. One cannot help but wonder whether akathisia and other extrapyramidal reactions short of acute dystonia have been overlooked or misperceived as continued "agitation" in highly out of control patients.

There are very few clinical situations warranting IM control of agitation in a young child. There are almost always more appropriate interventions, and the smaller size of the young child diminishes the threat of dangerousness. The usual first dose of droperidol employed by this author in dangerously out of control adolescents and adults is 2.5 to 5 mg IM. As the pre-anesthetic dose in children under 12 years of age, a dose of 1.0–1.5 mg per 20 to 25 lbs is recommended (Physicians' Desk Reference, 1996).

Benzodiazepines. Benzodiazepines, particularly the short-acting benzodiazepine, lorazepam, appear to be used commonly for agitation in adults and adolescents. There are no studies to support benzodiazepine use for agitation in children or adolescents. Benzodiazepines have not been utilized commonly in children, especially prepubertal children, secondary to concerns about disinhibition. Despite the oft-noted concern linking benzodiazepines with behavioral disinhibition, there is only one study in the psychiatric literature linking the two (Kraft, Ardalli, Duffy, Hart, & Pearce, 1965), which found a 10 percent incidence of "paradoxical" reactions in 13 out of 130 children treated for a heterogenous mix of psychiatric disorders with chlordiazepoxide. Most of the children who experienced the behavioral disinhibition had neurologic impairment. The anesthesia literature, however, does report frequencies of behavioral disinhibition as high as 23 percent (Rosenberg, Holttum, & Gershon, 1994) with presurgical sedation. In prepubertal children, the behavioral features of disinhibition include over-excitement, hyperactivity, irritability, increased aggression, or even rage outbursts (Coffey, 1990). Sedation and cognitive impairment are also drawbacks to the benzodiazepines. However, well-designed studies of these drugs in the pediatric population are clearly indicated. Studies in the adult literature have indicated that benzodiazepines can be useful in the treatment of severe agitation in both psychotic and nonpsychotic patients, including critically ill delirious adults in combination with haloperidol (Adams, Fernandez, & Andersson, 1986; Dubin, 1988; Modell, Lenox, & Weiner, 1985). Lorazepam may significantly decrease the likelihood of akathisia and dystonia when combined with haloperidol in adults.

Lorazepam is probably the most commonly used benzodiazepine for agitation in adults and adolescents and is available for administration by mouth, IM, or IV. Short-term emergency treatment of aggression in children and adolescents is not an FDA-approved use, and 12 years is the minimum age approved for any use (Green, 1995).

Usual dosage is 1 to 2 mg of lorazepam po, IM, or IV, but 0.5 mg can also be given and the dose titrated. The onset of action in adults for lorazepam is 30 minutes to 3 hours by mouth, 15 to 30 minutes IM, and 1 to 5 minutes IV. Half-life is about 12 hours. If agitation is unrelieved and the situation is acute, the dosage may be repeated in 60 minutes.

Manic adult patients have been successfully managed with lorazepam (po, IM, or IV)—2 to 4 mg every two hours or PRN, and ultimately stabilized on 10 mg or less of lorazepam (two patients required 20–30 mg for several days). The most noticeable side effect was ataxia when the dose exceeded 10 mg per day (Moddell et al., 1985).

The clinician should exercise caution in the use of benzodiazepines when there is a history of alcohol and/or substance abuse. To further complicate matters, benzodiazepines can exacerbate a delirium and psychosis, even though they have been advocated in the treatment of delirium, most frequently in combination with haloperidol in adults. Hallucinations and perceptual abnormalities have also been known to occur.

Haloperidol-Lorazepam combination in psychotic agitation. A combination of haloperidol and lorazepam has been used successfully in controlling psychotic agitation in young adults. The addition of lorazepam may hasten sedation and effect a decrease in agitation while enabling a lower dosage of neuroleptic to be used. The antipsychotic effect of neuroleptics typically does not become apparent for 1 to 3 weeks. The more sedating antipsychotics (e.g., chlorpromazine) are usually limited by hypotension (especially with IM administration) before sedation and/or a significant reduction in agitation is achieved. The higher potency neuroleptics are safer in high doses; however, they are also associated with potentially painful dystonia and akathesia.

In adults, lorazepam 1 to 4 mg can be administered IM combined with haloperidol 5 mg, and if necessary repeated in sixty minutes. This dosage is usually sufficient to quell severe agitation. After the emergency has subsided, lower maintenance levels of lorazepam (up to a maximum of 10 mg per day in adults in three divided doses) can be given with or without haloperidol. Higher doses of lorazepam and haloperidol have been utilized safely and efficaciously in the management of severely agitated psychotic adult and older adolescent patients. Successful treatment was defined as significant reduction in a standardized agitation score within 210 minutes. Thirty-one of 33 patients (aged 17 to 52) were treated successfully within 210 minutes. One patient who failed to respond within that time required 40 mg of haloperidol and 24 mg of lorazepam to respond. Another patient required 65 mg of haloperidol and 8 mg of lorazepam (Garza-Treviño, Hollister, Overall, & Alexander, 1989). The haloperidol-lorazepam combination is also not FDA-approved for the treatment of agitation in children, adolescents, or adults.

Pharmacologic treatment of delirium. When delirious patients become severely agitated and/or grossly psychotic, it may be necessary to treat the delirium pharmacologically (Tesar, Murray, & Cassem, 1985; Adams, 1988; Fernandez, Holmes, Adams, & Kavanaugh, 1988). Delirium may progress to the point where efforts to orient the patient and the best supportive care possible are inadequate. There are several reasons to intervene aggressively to medicate an agitated delirious child or adolescent:

- The confusion and disorientation of delirium is a painful, highly upsetting state.
- Delirious patients are often combative and self-injurious, seriously compromising evaluation and treatment.
- Delirious and agitated patients frequently interfere with equipment, often attempting to disconnect or rip

out intravenous lines, catheters, chest tubes, central and arterial indwelling lines, pacing wires, etc.
- Physical restraint only adds to the patient's profound confusion and fear, usually stimulating further agitation and fueling paranoia.
- The autonomic instability associated with severe agitation (e.g., hyperventilation and tachycardia) may further compromise a tenuous medical situation.

The clinical condition of the patient should guide the decision to treat agitation with medication. The patient who is only mildly agitated and confused, who does not appear to be at physical risk, and who is not seriously disrupting treatment, may not require medication. Close monitoring of the patient's clinical course may be indicated based on the realization that delirium can unexpectedly flare up just as it appears to be fizzling out. If, on the other hand, the patient is paranoid, combative, pulling out lines, and generally compromising treatment, medication may be the most humane way to treat the severe agitation. Physical restraint in this situation, while sometimes necessary for brief periods, will certainly do nothing to calm the patient and will probably increase the level of agitation. Physical restraint with mechanical devices should only be used in the most extreme circumstances and at no time should the child or adolescent be left alone while restrained.

There are no studies of pharmacologic treatment of delirium in children. Despite the absence of double-blind trials in either the pediatric or adult literature, haloperidol has been advocated for the pharmacologic treatment of severe delirium, sometimes in combination with lorazepam. Haloperidol has negligible anticholinergic and hypotensive properties and can be administered parenterally. Although not FDA-approved for use in either adults or children, intravenous haloperidol has been used effectively and safely, often in high dosages (Tesar & Stern, 1986).

Haloperidol can be used orally, IM, or IV in equivalent doses. Interestingly, extrapyramidal side-effects seem to be less common even at high doses when administered intravenously, relative to the oral and intramuscular routes (Sanders, Minnema, & Murray, 1989). This may relate in part to frequent co-administration of a benzodiazepine, typically lorazepam, possibly resulting in the establishment of some γ-aminobutyric acid (GABA)–dopaminergic equilibrium (Murray, 1991).

Adams (1988) described a protocol developed over eight years at two major cancer centers in the United States and Canada in which over 2,000 seriously medically ill adult patients with delirium were treated by intravenous administration of a combination of haloperidol and lorazepam. All of the patients had cancer and were suffering from multiorgan failure. Hourly doses of both haloperidol and lorazepam, up to as much as 10 mg each for as long as fifteen days, have been used safely and effectively in the most critically medically ill patients with delirium. Adams (1988) points out that most textbooks and handbooks recommend "paltry and unrealistic" dosing schedules for neuroleptics in the critical care setting. He refreshingly and unequivocally states that the agitated, delirious, sometimes violent patient needs to be put to sleep in order to aggressively investigate the causes of the delirium and prevent a further downward spiral.

The interested reader is referred to Adams's (1988) article for additional specifics, but briefly he suggests the following approach. Treatment begins with 5 mg of haloperidol followed immediately by 0.5 mg of lorazepam (both injected intravenously in less than a minute). If there is little or no response within twenty minutes, the dose of haloperidol is doubled (10 mg) and 2 to 10 mg of lorazepam is given half-hourly until the patient is sedated (unresponsive to verbal stimuli but responsive to vigorous flexor-extensor movements of the arms). The haloperidol dose is kept constant at 10 mg, and the lorazepam dosage is adjusted to the level of sedation required. When the patient is sedated, haloperidol administration is halved and the time between doses doubled; lorazepam is discontinued. The patient's emergence from sedation is a crucial determinant of how to proceed. If the patient is agitated, both haloperidol and lorazepam should be reinstituted at the previously effective doses and given every 1 to 3 hours to maintain the sedation for the next 10 to 12 hours. When the patient again emerges from sedation, the same evaluation and procedure takes place. Hydromorphone can be added if pain is a complicating feature. Many patients may require bed time dosing after the acute episode has passed (5 to 10 mg IV of haloperidol, and lorazepam 0.5 to 4 mg IV) for up to a week, especially if the patient is in an ICU where sleep disturbance and the day/night routines are more problematic and disorienting. For the mildly agitated delirious patient, the nighttime intravenous dosing of haloperidol and lorazepam may suffice.

Adams makes a point several times of recommending the previously described doses and schedules "regardless of age and sex"; however, there is no specific mention made in the article about pediatric patients. Given what we do know about the pharmacokinetics of neuroleptics and benzodiazepines, some adjustments may be necessary. There is enormous variation in haloperidol plasma levels among same-age children receiving the same milligram-per-kilogram dose, with younger patients on average having lower levels at a given dose

(Teicher & Gold, 1990). There is only very limited data on the pharmacokinetics of benzodiazepines in children, and even less in adolescents, indicating an increased ability to metabolize and eliminate diazepam in children (Kanto, Sellman, Haataja, & Hurme, 1978) owing to faster hepatic biotransformation and renal clearance. Developmental pharmacokinetic principles would suggest that children have faster metabolism and clearance than adults and that by late adolescence adult pharmacokinetic patterns are present (Coffey, 1990).

Clinicians will need to assess each patient individually with respect to dosing, but a sensible rule of thumb might be that for young children start out with 0.5 mg of haloperidol for mild agitation, up to 2 mg for moderate agitation, and 2 to 5 mg if agitation is severe. In larger, older adolescents, 2 mg for mild agitation, 5 mg for moderate agitation, and 5 to 10 mg for severe agitation may be required, although the likelihood of painful dystonic reactions increases with increased dosing of haloperidol, with addition of a benzodiazepine perhaps having a dampening effect. Clinicians should remain alert to the possibility of respiratory depression, as well as other potential side effects or adverse reactions.

During the induction phase, the child should be either in the ICU or have "constant bedside attention" (Adams, 1988) by a physician experienced in the diagnosis and treatment of delirium supported by a knowledgeable, experienced nursing staff. PRN orders are generally not useful or appropriate in the treatment of delirium, anymore than "as needed" orders are in the treatment of severe pain or alcohol withdrawal. Unfortunately, there appears to be considerable resistance especially in the clinical community to definitively abandon or even discourage these outmoded practices.

Midazolam is frequently used in emergency settings but is limited by its penchant for causing severe hypotension. Droperidol is limited by this feature also and is not recommended in the treatment of delirium. In 1988 the Food and Drug Administration issued a report cautioning that midazolam has been associated with respiratory depression and arrest, especially when used for conscious sedation (Dubin, 1988).

SUMMARY

The dramatic rise in adolescent suicide compels pediatric clinicians to develop the knowledge base and assessment skills necessary to identify and, if necessary, initially stabilize youth presenting in crisis. The emergency evaluation and management of the agitated child or adolescent calls on all of the clinician's diagnostic acumen and skill, as there are few other situations in medicine that require more diversified expertise. The agitated adolescent whom the clinician has never met may be suffering from a rapidly progressing metabolic or neurologic disturbance, or be psychotic and paranoid and at risk of exploding into violence. The value of a careful, yet efficient, evaluation, including the gathering of relevant history from the patient and caretakers, physical examination, including mental status examination, and pertinent laboratory and other testing, cannot be over-emphasized.

Psychiatric emergencies are frequently encountered by pediatric clinicians practicing in both the in-patient and out-patient settings. Even where child psychiatric consultation is readily available, the pediatric clinician and staff must often assume the responsibility of initial evaluation and stabilization. It is hoped that the information presented will be of use to pediatric health care providers and mental health professionals.

REFERENCES

Adams, F. (1988). Emergency intravenous sedation of the delirious, medically ill patient. *Journal of Clinical Psychiatry, 49 (suppl. 12),* 22–27.

Adams, F., Fernandez, F., & Andersson, B. S. (1986). Emergency pharmacotherapy of delirium in the critically ill cancer patient. *Psychosomatics, 27 (suppl.),* 33–37.

Adams, R. D., & Victor, M. (1981). *Principles of neurology.* New York: McGraw-Hill.

Adler, R. (1992). Burns are different: The child psychiatrist on the pediatrics burn ward. *Journal of Burn Care and Rehabilitation, 13,* 28–32.

Allgulander, C., & Lavori, P. W. (1991). Excess mortality among 3,302 patients with "pure" anxiety neurosis. *Archives of General Psychiatry, 48,* 599–602.

American Psychiatric Association. (1994). *Diagnostic and statistical manual of psychiatric disorders,* 4th edition (DSM-IV). Washington, DC: Author.

Ayd, F. (1984). IV haloperidol-lorazepam therapy for delirium. *International Drug Therapy Newsletter, 19,* 1–3.

Baker, B. A., & Cantwell, D. P. (1987). Comparison of well, emotionally disordered, and behaviorally disordered children with linguistic problems. *Journal of the American Academy of Child and Adolescent Psychiatry, 26,* 193–196.

Bettes, B. A., & Walker, E. (1987). Positive and negative symptoms in psychotic and other psychiatrically disturbed children. *Journal of Child Psychology and Psychiatry, 28,* 555–568.

Brent, D. A. (1986). Over-representation of epileptics in a consecutive series of suicide attempters seen at a children's hospital, 1978–1983. *Journal of the American Academy of Child Psychiatry, 25,* 242–246.

Brent, D. A. (1989a). Suicide and suicidal behavior in adolescents. *Pediatrics in Review, 10,* 269–275.

Brent, D. A., Crumrine, P. K., Varma, R. R., Allan, M., & Allman, C. (1987a). Phenobarbital treatment and major depressive disorder in children with epilepsy. *Pediatrics, 89,* 909–917.

Brent, D. A., Johnson, B. A., Perper, J., Connolly, J., Bridge, J., Bartle, S., & Rather, C. (1994). Personality disorder, personality traits, impulsive violence, and completed suicide in adolescents. *Journal of the American Academy of Child and Adolescent Psychiatry, 33,* 1080–1086.

Brent, D. A., Kolko, D. J., Wartella, M. E., Boylan, M. B., Moritz, G., Baugher, M., & Zelenak, J. P. (1993a). Adolescent psychiatric inpatients' risk of suicide attempt at 6-month follow-up. *Journal of the American Academy of Child and Adolescent Psychiatry, 32,* 95–105.

Brent, D. A., Perper, J. A., & Allman, C. J. (1987b). Alcohol, firearms, and suicide among youth. *Journal of the American Medical Association, 257,* 3369–3372.

Brent, D. A., Perper, J. A., Goldstein, C. E., Kolko, D. J., Allan, M. J., Allman, C. J., & Zelenak, J. P. (1988). Risk factors for adolescent suicide. *Archives of General Psychiatry, 45,* 581–588.

Brent, D. A., Perper, J. A., Moritz, G., Allman, C., Friend, A., Roth, C., Schweers, J., Balach, L., Baugher, M. (1993b). Psychiatric risk factors for adolescent suicide: A case control study. *Journal of the American Academy of Child and Adolescent Psychiatry, 32,* 521–529.

Brent, D. A., Perper, J. A., Moritz, G., Allman, C., Schweers, J., Roth, C., Balach, L., Canobbio, R., & Liotus, L. (1993c). Psychiatric sequelae to the loss of an adolescent peer to suicide. *Journal of the American Academy of Child and Adolescent Psychiatry, 32,* 509–517.

Brent, D. A., Perper, J. A., Moritz, G., Baugher, M., & Allman, C. (1993d). Suicide in adolescents with no apparent psychopathology. *Journal of the American Academy of Child and Adolescent Psychiatry, 32,* 494–500.

Brown, L. K., Overholser, J., Spirito, A., & Fritz, G. K. (1991). The correlates of planning in adolescent suicide attempts. *Journal of the American Academy of Child and Adolescent Psychiatry, 30,* 95–99.

Burke, P., DelBeccaro, M., McCauley, E., & Clark, C. (1985). Hallucinations in children. *Journal of the American Academy of Child and Adolescent Psychiatry, 24*, 71–75.

Campo, J. V. (1993). Medical issues in the care of child and adolescent inpatients. In A. S. Bellack & M. Hersen (Eds.), *Handbook of behavior therapy in the psychiatric setting*, (pp. 373–405). New York: Plenum Press.

Caplan, R., & Tanguay, P. E. (1991). Development of psychotic thinking in children. In M. Lewis (Ed.), *Child and adolescent psychiatry: A comprehensive textbook*, (pp. 310–317). Baltimore: Williams & Wilkins.

Carlson, G. A. (1983). Bipolar affective disorders in childhood and adolescence. In D. P. Cantwell & G. A. Carlson (Eds.), *Affective disorders in childhood and adolescence*, (pp. 61–84). New York: S.P. Medical and Scientific Books.

Centers for Disease Control. (1985). *Suicide surveillance 1970–1980*. Atlanta: U.S. Department of Health and Human Services, Public Health Service, Violent Epidemiology Branch, Center for Health Promotion and Education.

Chedru, F., & Geshwind, N. (1972). Writing disturbances in acute confusional states. *Neuropsychologia, 10*, 343–353.

Coffey, B. J. (1990). Anxiolytics for children and adolescents: Traditional and new drugs. *Journal of Child and Adolescent Psychopharmacology, 1*, 57–83.

Cohen, N. J., Davine, M., Horodezky, N., Lipsett, L., & Isaacson, L. (1993). Unsuspected language impairment in psychiatrically disturbed children: Prevalence and language and behavioral characteristics. *Journal of the American Academy of Child and Adolescent Psychiatry, 32*, 595–603.

Cummings, J. L. (1985). Organic delusions: Phenomenology, anatomical correlations, and review. *British Journal of Psychiatry, 146*, 184–197.

Deykin, E. Y., Alpert, J. J., & McNamara, J. J. (1985). A pilot study of the effect of exposure to child abuse or neglect on adolescent suicidal behavior. *American Journal of Psychiatry, 142*, 1299–1311.

Dillihay, T. C. (1989). Suicide in black children. *Psychiatric Forum, 15*, 24–27.

Dubin, W. R. (1988). Rapid Tranquilization: Antipsychotics or benzodiazepines? *Journal of Clinical Psychiatry, 12(suppl.)*, 5–11.

Dubin, W. R., Field, N. J., & Gastfriend, D. R. (1979). Postcardiotomy delirium: A critical review. *Journal of Thoracic Cardiovascular Surgery, 77*, 586–594.

Elliot, G. R. (1992). *The use of prns and chemical restraints in children and adolescents*. Paper presented at the 39th Annual Meeting of the American Academy of Child and Adolescent Psychiatry, October 20–25, 1992, Washington, D.C.

Fernandez, F., Holmes, W. F., Adams, F., & Kavanaugh, J. J. (1988). Treatment of severe refractory agitation with a haloperidol drip. *Journal of Clinical Psychiatry, 49*, 239–241.

Fish, B. (1960). Drug therapy in child psychiatry: Pharmacological aspects. *Comprehensive Psychiatry, 1*, 212–227.

Folstein, M. F., Folstein, S., & McHugh, P. R. (1975). "Mini-mental state": A practical method for grading the cognitive state of patients for the clinician. *Journal of the Psychiatric Resident, 12*, 189–198.

Fredrickson, J. M., Bauer, W., Arellano, D., & Davidson, M. (1994). Emergency nurses' perceived knowledge and comfort levels regarding pediatric patients. *Journal of Emergency Nursing, 20*, 13–17.

Garza-Treviño, E. S., Hollister, L. E., Overall, J. E., & Alexander, W. F. (1989). Efficacy of combination of intramuscular antipsychotics and sedative hypnotics for control of psychotic agitation. *American Journal of Psychiatry, 146*, 1598–1601.

Gould, M. S., & Shaffer, D. (1986). The impact of suicide in television movies. *New England Journal of Medicine, 315*, 690–693.

Gould, M. S., Wallenstein, S., & Kleinman, M. (1990). Time-space clustering of teenage suicide. *American Journal of Epidemiology, 131*, 71–78.

Green, W. H. (1995). *Child and adolescent clinical psychopharmacology*. Baltimore: Williams & Wilkins.

Gualtieri, C. T., Koriath, U., VanBourgondien, M., & Saleeby, N. (1983). Language disorders in children referred for psychiatric services. *Journal of the American Academy of Child and Adolescent Psychiatry, 22*, 165–171.

Harkavy Friedman, J. M., Asnis, G., Boeck, M., & DiFiore, J. (1987). Prevalence of specific suicidal behaviors in a high school sample. American *Journal of Psychiatry, 144*, 1203–1206.

Hoberman, H. M., & Garfinkel, B. D. (1988). Completed suicide in children and adolescents. *Journal of the American Academy of Child and Adolescent Psychiatry, 27*, 689–695.

House, R. M., Trzepacz, P. T., & Thompson, T. L. (1991). Psychiatric consultation to organ transplant services. In A. Tasman, S. M. Goldfinger, & C. A. Kaufman (Eds.), *Review of psychiatry, (vol. 9)* (pp. 515–536). Washington, D.C.: American Psychiatric Press.

Kanto, J., Sellman, K., Haataja, M., & Hurme, P. (1978).

Plasma and urine concentrations of diazepam and its metabolites in children, adults, and in diazepam intoxicated patients. *International Journal of Clinical Pharmacology, 16,* 258–264.

Kizer, K. W., Green, M., Perkins, C. I., Doebbert, G., & Hughes, M. J. (1988). AIDS and suicide in California. *Journal of the American Medical Association, 260,* 1881.

Kornfeld, D. S., Zimberg, S., & Malm, J. R. (1965). Psychiatric complications of open heart surgery. *New England Journal of Medicine, 273,* 287–292.

Kotila, L., & Lonnqvist, J. (1989). Suicide and violent death among adolescent suicide attempters. *Acta Psychiatrica Scandanavica, 79,* 453–459.

Kraft, I. A., Ardall, C., Duffy, J. H., Hart, J. T., & Pearce, P. (1965). A clinical study of chlordiazepoxide used in psychiatric disorders of children. *International Journal of Neuropsychiatry, 1,* 433–437.

Krener, P., & Miller, F. B. (1989). Psychiatric response to HIV spectrum disease in children and adolescents. *Journal of the American Academy of Child and Adolescent Psychiatry, 28,* 596–605.

Lewis, D. O. (1991). Conduct disorders. In M. B. Lewis (Ed.), *Child and adolescent psychiatry: A comprehensive textbook* (pp. 561–573). Baltimore: Williams & Wilkins.

Lewis, M. B. (1991). Psychiatric assessment of infants, children, and adolescents. In M. B. Lewis (Ed.), *Child and adolescent psychiatry: A comprehensive textbook* (pp. 447–463). Baltimore: Williams & Wilkins.

Mann, J. J., & Arango, V. (1992). Integration of neurobiology and psychopathology in a unified model of suicidal behavior. *Journal of Clinical Psychopharmacology, 12,* 25–75.

Marttunen, M. J., Aro, H. M., Hennksson, M. M., & Lonngqvist, J. K. (1994). Antisocial behavior in adolescent suicide. *Acta Psychiatrica Scandanavica, 89,* 167–173.

Marzuk, P. M., Tierney, H., Tardiff, K., Gross, E. M., Morgan, E. B., Hsu, M. A., & Mann, J. J. (1988). Increased risk of suicide in persons with AIDS. *Journal of the American Medical Association, 259,* 1333–1342.

McHugh, P. R., & Folstein, M. F. (1988). Organic mental disorders. In J. O. Cavenar (Ed.), *Psychiatry (vol. 1)* (pp. 1–21). Philadelphia: J. B. Lippincott.

Melnick, B. M. (1988). Extrapyramidal reactions to low-dose droperidol. *Anesthesiology, 69,* 424–426.

Mikkelson, E. J. (1994). Organic mental disorders. In J. O. Cavenar (Ed.), *Psychiatry (vol. 2)* (pp. 1–11). Philadelphia: J. B. Lippincott.

Modell, J. G., Lenox, R. H., & Weiner, S. (1985). Inpatient

clinical trial of lorazepam for the management of manic agitation. *Journal of Clinical Psychopharmacology, 5,* 109–113.

Murray, G. B. (1991). Confusion, delirium, and dementia. In N. H. Cassem, *Handbook of general hospital psychiatry* (pp. 89–120). St. Louis: Mosby Year Book.

National Center for Health Statistics (1993). Advance report of final mortality statistics, 1991. *Monthly Vital Statistics Report,* 42. Hyattsville, MD: U.S. Public Health Service.

Neff, K. E., Denney, D., & Blachly, P. H. (1972). Control of severe agitation with droperidol. *Diseases of the Nervous System, 33,* 594–597.

Nurcombe, B. (1991). The development of attention, perception, and memory. In M. B. Lewis (Ed.), *Child and adolescent psychiatry: A comprehensive textbook* (pp. 161–168). Baltimore: Williams & Wilkins.

O'Brien, J. P. (1974). Increase in suicide attempts by drug ingestion. The Boston experience 1964–1974. *Archives of General Psychiatry, 34,* 1165–1169.

Pfeffer, C. R. (1986). *The suicidal child.* New York: Guilford Press.

Pfeffer, C. R., Newcorn, J., Kaplan, G., Mizruchi, M. S., & Plutchik, R. (1988). Suicidal behavior in adolescent psychiatric inpatients. *Journal of the American Academy of Child and Adolescent Psychiatry, 27,* 357–361.

Pfeffer, C. R., Normandin, L., & Kakuna, T. (1994). Suicidal children grow up: Suicide behavior and psychiatric disorders among relatives. *Journal of the American Academy of Child and Adolescent Psychiatry, 33,* 1087–1097.

Physician's Desk Reference. (1996). 50th ed. Montvale, NJ.

Popkin, M. J. (1986). Organic brain syndromes presenting with global cognitive impairment: Delirium and dementia. In G. Winokur & P. Clayton (Eds.), *The medical basis of psychiatry* (pp. 3–19). Philadelphia: W. B. Saunders.

Price, R. W., Brew, B., Siditis, J., Rosenblum, M., Scheck, A. C., & Cleary, P. (1988). The brain in AIDS: Central nervous systems HIV-1 infection and AIDS dementia complex. *Science, 239,* 586–592.

Prugh, D., Wagonfeld, S., Metcalf, D., & Jordan, K. (1980). A clinical study of delirium in children and adolescents. *Psychosomatic Medicine, 42,* 177–195.

Puig-Antich, J., Goetz, D., Davies, M., Kaplan, T., Davies, S., Ostrow, L., Asnis, L., Twomey, J., Iyengar, S., & Ryan, N. D. (1989). A controlled family history study of prepubertal major depressive disorder. *Archives of General Psychiatry, 46,* 406–408.

Resnick, M., & Burton, B. T. (1984). Droperidol vs.

haloperidol in the initial management of acutely agitated patients. *Journal of Clinical Psychiatry, 45,* 298–299.

Rosenberg, D. R., Holttum, J., & Gershon, S. (1994). *Textbook of pharmacotherapy for child and adolescent psychiatric disorders.* New York: Brunner/Mazel.

Rotheram, M. J. (1987). Evaluation of imminent danger for suicide among youth. *American Journal of Orthopsychiatry, 57,* 102–110.

Rotheram-Borus, M. J., Hunter, J., & Rosario, M. (1994). Suicidal behavior and gay-related stress among gay and bisexual male adolescents. *Journal of Adolescent Research, 9,* 498–508.

Roy, A. (1983). Family history of suicide. *Archives of General Psychiatry, 39,* 971–974.

Ryland, D. H., & Kruesi, M. J. (1992). Suicide among adolescents. *International Review of Psychiatry, 4,* 185–195.

Sanders, K., Minnema, A. M., & Murray, G. B. (1989). Low incidence of extra-pyramidal symptoms in the treatment of delirium with intravenous haloperidol and lorazepam in intensive care unit patients. *Journal of Intensive Care Medicine, 4,* 201–204.

Schreibman, D. L. (1990). Treatment of a delayed reaction to droperidol with diphenhydramine. *Anesthesia and Analgesia, 71,* 105.

Shaffer, D. (1974). Suicide in childhood and early adolescence. *Journal of Child Psychology and Psychiatry, 15,* 275–291.

Shaffer, D., & Fisher, P. (1981). The epidemiology of suicide in children and young adolescents. *Journal of the American Academy of Child and Adolescent Psychiatry, 20,* 545–565.

Shaffer, D., Garland, A., Gould, M., Fisher, P., & Trautman, P. (1988). Preventing teenage suicide: A critical review. *Journal of the American Academy of Child and Adolescent Psychiatry, 27,* 675–687.

Shafii, M., Carrigen, S., Whittinghill, J. R., & Derrick, A. (1985). Psychological autopsy of completed suicide in children and adolescents. *American Journal of Psychiatry, 142,* 1061–1064.

Shaffi, M., Steltz-Lenarsky, J., Derrick, A. M., Beckner, C., & Whittinghill, J. R. (1988). Comorbidity of mental disorders in the postmortem diagnosis of completed suicide in children and adolescents. *Journal of Affective Disorders, 15,* 227–233.

Shea, S. C. (1988). *Psychiatric interviewing: The art of understanding.* Philadelphia: W. B. Saunders.

Slaby, A. E. (1994). *Handbook of psychiatric emergencies.* Norwalk: Appleton & Lange.

Smith, K., & Crawford, S. (1986). Suicidal behavior among "normal" high school students. *Suicide and Life Threatening Behavior, 16,* 313–325.

Sulik, L. R., & Garfinkel, B. D. (1992). Adolescent suicidal behavior: Understanding the breadth of the problem. In D. P. Cantwell (Ed.), *Child and Adolescent Psychiatric Clinics of North America, 1,* 197–228.

Szuba, M. P., Bergman, K. S., Baxter, L. R., Guze, B. H., Reynolds, C. A., & Pelletier, L. R. (1992). Safety and efficacy of high-dose droperidol in agitated patients. *Journal of Clinical Psychopharmacology, 12,* 144–145.

Taylor, M. A. (1986). Motor behavior. In G. Winokur & P. Clayton (Eds.), *The medical basis of psychiatry* (pp. 433–441). Philadelphia: W. B. Saunders.

Teicher, M. H., & Glod, C. A. (1990). Neuroleptic drugs: Indications and guidelines for their rational use in children and adolescents. *Journal of Child and Adolescent Psychopharmacology, 1,* 33–56.

Tesar, G. E., Murray, G. B., & Cassem, N. H. (1985). Use of high-dose intravenous haloperidol in the treatment of agitated cardiac patients. *Journal of Clinical Psychopharmacology, 5,* 344–347.

Tesar, G. E., & Stern, T. A. (1986). Evaluation and treatment of agitation in the intensive care unit. *Journal of Intensive Care Medicine, 1,* 137–148.

Tintinalli, J. E., Peacock, F. W., & Wright, M. A. (1994). Emergency medicine evaluation of psychiatric patients. *Annals of Emergency Medicine, 23,* 859–862.

Trzepacz, P. T., Brenner, R., Van Thiel, D. H. (1989). A psychiatric study of 247 liver transplantation candidates. *Psychosomatics, 30,* 147–153.

Trzepacz, P. T., Maue, F. R., Coffman, G., & Van Thiel, D. H. (1986–87). Neuropsychiatric assessment of liver transplantation candidates: Delirium and other psychiatric disorders. *International Journal of Psychiatry and Medicine, 16,* 101–111.

van Leeuwen, A. M. H., Molders, J., Sterkmans, P., Mielants, P., Martens, C., Toussaint, C., Hovent, A. M., Desseilles, M. F., Koch, H., Devroye, A., & Parent, M. (1977). Droperidol in acutely agitated patients. *Journal of Nervous and Mental Disease, 164,* 280–283.

Vitiello, B., Hill, J. L., Elia, J., Cunningham, E., McLeer, S. V., & Behar, D. (1991). Prn. medications in child psychiatry patients: A pilot placebo-controlled study. *Journal of Clinical Psychiatry, 52,* 499–501.

Weissman, M., Klerman, G., Markowitz, J., Quellette, R., & Phil, M. (1989). Suicidal ideation and suicide attempts in panic disorder and attacks. *New England Journal of Medicine, 321,* 1209–1213.

Weller, E. B., & Weller, R. A. (1991). Mood disorders. In M. B. Lewis (Ed.), *Child and adolescent psychiatry: A comprehensive textbook* (pp. 646–664). Baltimore: Williams & Wilkins.

Wise, M. G. (1987). Delirium. In R. E. Hales & S. C. Yudofsky (Eds.), *The American Psychiatric Press textbook of neuropsychiatry* (pp. 89–105). American Psychiatric Press: Washington, D.C.

CHAPTER 6

FACTITIOUS DISORDER BY PROXY

Judith A. Libow
Herbert A. Schreier

DESCRIPTION OF
THE PROBLEM

British pediatrician Roy Meadow (1977) is credited with having first applied the unusual name Munchausen by Proxy Syndrome to the disorder of factitious illness by proxy. He described two very puzzling cases of children whose persistent medical problems led to a very important discovery. Meadow's first case of factitious disorder by proxy involved a six-year-old girl who repeatedly presented with unexplained "urinary tract infections" resulting in extensive, fruitless workups: twelve hospital admissions, six exams under anaesthesia, five cystoscopies, eight courses of antibiotics, 16 specialist consultations, and over 150 laboratory cultures. Eventually, Dr. Meadow decided to test for parental fabrication by collecting specimens under controlled conditions. He found that all 45 urine specimens collected under carefully controlled conditions showed no unusual organisms—yet the 12 specimens collected by the mother were all contaminated! This medical puzzle would likely have gone on for a much longer time had Dr. Meadow not been willing to consider the then radical possibility that a parent could deliberately fabricate a medical illness. The second case reported by Dr. Meadow in his seminal article described the case of a child being overloaded with sodium; unfortunately, the child died while the medical staff was planning a strategy for intervening.

The name "Munchausen by Proxy Syndrome" (MBPS) derives from an 18th-century nobleman, Baron Hieronymus Karl Friedrich Freiherr Von Munchausen, who was a mercenary soldier and teller of tall tales that were later popularized in a bestselling pamphlet written by Rudolph E. Raspe, an embezzler who fled to England and published the stories. Asher (1951) used the name "Munchausen Syndrome" to describe the medical attention-seeking behavior of a group of adult patients who have also been described as "hospital hobos" and "hospital addicts" (Spiro, 1968; Stern, 1980), in their relentless efforts to obtain surgery, medication, and patient status. The "by Proxy" label was later adapted by Meadow (1977) to describe the use of a child as the identified medical patient, by a parent or caretaker. Factitious disorder by proxy has also been described with the use of adult patients (Sigal, Carmel, Altmark, & Silfen, 1988), pediatric patients abused by a nurse (Egginton, 1990), and even a fetus (Goodlin, 1985) as proxy victim. The overwhelming majority of these parents are mothers, with a statistical preponderance as high as 98 percent (Rosenberg, 1987).

Factitious disorder by proxy (American Psychiatric Association, 1994), more commonly known as Munchausen by Proxy Syndrome, is a disorder in which a caretaker systematically fabricates illness in a child or intentionally makes a child ill in order to gain and maintain contact with doctors and/or hospitals (see Schreier & Libow, 1993a). This is a conscious, planned behavior, often compulsively repeated. As in Meadow's (1977) case of the child with "urinary tract infections," it often results in long, expensive and unnecessary medical treatment of the child. The parent is not psychotic or in a dissociative state. Our definition of factitious disorder by proxy, or MBPS, excludes behavior whose primary goal is some direct secondary gain such as winning a custody battle or obtaining disability payments. The very nature of MBPS is that the infant or child is seriously endangered through involvement in a complex relationship between mother and physician which has no simple and obvious motivation. Instead, there is the paradox of the seemingly ideal, caring mother who is later revealed to be threatening the health of her child through often shocking and bizarre fabrications.

There are five main forms of parental fabrication used to convince physicians that youngsters are sick. They fall under the following general categories:

- *Poisoning*   In these often very damaging, and sometimes fatal cases, caregivers have overdosed their children on a broad range of substances, from prescribed medications to household cleaning products. The range of poisonous substances potentially in use is so broad that it is often difficult or impossible for the physician to determine the substance or devise the appropriate screen for toxins. The literature reports use of ipecac, lasix, table salt, fertility drugs, laxatives, steroids, barbiturates, anticonvulsants, antidepressants, and even ethyl alcohol, among others.
- *Suffocation*   These cases of active induction generally present as cases of apnea, respiratory arrest, near SIDS, or other forms of life-threatening illness. Infants or young toddlers have been suffocated via manual pressure, nose-pinching, carotid sinus pressure, use of pillows or plastic bags. Some number of these cases result in the probably unintended death of the child victims. It is suspected that some percentage of SIDS deaths may actually represent cases of MBPS that were never identified (Emery, 1993), as there have been reports of a significant percentage of prior "SIDS deaths" in siblings of children who are known victims of MBPS (Meadow, 1990).
- *Tampering*   In these cases, laboratory specimens, intravenous lines or other medical lines (e.g., indwelling catheters) are deliberately contaminated by the parent. A broad range of substances have been introduced into a child's body or specimens, including fecal matter, menstrual products, saliva, blood, contaminated water, gasoline, "crushed insects," and urine. In an unusual twist on this technique, there have been cases of tampering via *withdrawal* rather

than addition of bodily fluids, as in cases of mothers withdrawing a significant percentage of a child's blood volume via catheters.
- *Adulteration*   These are cases in which a child's body is altered in some way so as to convince the physician that the child is ill. These are generally less sophisticated, more easily identified forms of fabrication, and have included such activities as scratching a child's skin and administering caustic substances to cause rashes, and simulating jaundice via painting with Mercurochrome.
- *Withholding Medication*   In these cases, the caregiver withholds or tampers with the dosages of prescribed medication for a bona fide medical problem, resulting in unexpected exacerbation of illness or an unexplainable series of upturns and downturns in the child's health status. Asthma and seizure medications and insulin are often abused in this manner, in spite of the parent's insistence that she is strictly adhering to the prescribed regimen.
- *Symptom Exaggeration*   In these cases, parents do not actively induce illness through direct tampering or administration of lifethreatening interventions. Instead, they obtain treatment for their child through a careful presentation of symptoms in order to convince the physician to prescribe medication, administer diagnostic procedures, or repeatedly examine and treat the child for nonexistent or exaggerated illness. Parents are often quite successful in obtaining treatment for a myriad of fabricated conditions including allergies, diarrhea, seizures, behavioral and psychiatric problems, apnea episodes and other problems that are often treated without direct observation of each occurrence by the physician. Symptom exaggeration can result in morbidity as serious as that resulting from parental poisoning or suffocation. As in the case of asthma treated with unnecessary steroids, the child can suffer serious morbidity and in at least two cases known to the authors, even death.

INCIDENCE AND PREVALENCE

There are no extant population-based studies of the incidence of factitious disorder by proxy. It is inherent in the very nature of the disorder that detection and confirmation are difficult. There is no central registry of cases, most are not reported, and significant numbers are probably missed entirely. Our clinical experience, however, suggests that MBPS is far from the rare occurrence suggested in the lay media and, at times, in the professional literature.

In a survey of two pediatric subspecialty groups most commonly involved in the presentations chosen by MBPS perpetrators (Pediatric Gastroenterology and Pediatric Neurology), Schreier and Libow (1993b) found that there were 465 cases of MBPS (considered "confirmed" or "seriously suspected") seen by 316 doctors in both specialties. Close to two hundred papers, mostly in the form of case reports, have appeared in the pediatric and child abuse literature and far fewer in the psychological literature. Furthermore, studies by illness category indicate a potentially large number of cases. Warner and Hathaway (1984) suggested that 16 of 301 allergy clinic attendees may have represented factitious illness by proxy cases. Also, of 1,648 children being seen in Belgium with asthma problems, 1 percent were believed by that group to be likely cases of factitious disorder by proxy that were being seriously over-investigated and treated or undertreated sufficiently to cause serious morbidity (Godding & Kruth, 1991). Emery (1993) found that more than 10 percent of children afflicted with sudden infant death syndrome did not die of natural causes and that a small but not insignificant number of these may have represented Munchausen by Proxy Syndrome.

There are also additional factors in the clinical presentation that make it likely that many cases of MBPS will go undetected. First, there often is a reluctance by pediatricians and nurses to believe the diagnosis even when incontrovertible evidence is presented (see Case Illustration). Second, the length of the time from first presentation to diagnosis of MBPS suggests the difficulties in suspecting that abuse is taking place. In one study, for example, over one-third of cases took more than six months to diagnose, and in 19 percent it was more than a year before the factitious illness was recognized (Schreier & Libow, 1993b). Rosenberg's (1987) meta-analysis of several papers indicated that the mean length of time to diagnosis was close to 15 months from the onset of symptoms. Third, when cases are uncovered, there is sometimes a history of another sibling who died of mysterious causes which went completely undetected, likely through the same mechanism as the index child. There are at least two reports of more than seven children dying before the mother was confronted (DiMaio & Bernstein, 1974; Egginton, 1990). In one series by Meadow (1990) involving very serious abuse (suffocation), there were 27 affected children who had 18 siblings who had died of suspicious causes earlier in life.

Anecdotally, the authors know of no pediatric hospital that has not seen at least one or two cases of Munchausen by Proxy, and many hospitals have had considerable experience with multiple factitious illness cases. Having said this, it should be noted that this form of abuse is far less common than the physical and sexual abuse of children in general.

ASSESSMENT APPROACHES

The possibility of factitious disorder by proxy is not suspected simply because a physician is faced with an unexplainable medical problem, and the diagnosis cannot be made simply through the clinical interview of a parent. The determination of MBPS must be based on several essential elements that are observed and documented by medical staff. When taken together, these elements lead to the only possible conclusion: that the parent is creating or exaggerating the medical problem to keep the child "sick." The essential elements can be described as

- *The Medical "Puzzle"*   There is a medical problem that does not respond as expected to repeated treatment, follows an unusual course, is physiologically impossible, or otherwise makes little sense to the treating physician. The unexplainable illness may coexist with known and bona fide illnesses.
- *The "Devoted" Caregiver*   There is a caregiver who appears to be unusually invested in the child's illness or treatment, and may appear to thrive in the medical environment. Her affect in response to her child's medical crises and her enthusiasm for continued, invasive procedures may begin to arouse concern.
- *The Evidence*   There is evidence that connects this caregiver with the child's symptoms, either directly or indirectly. For example: (a) separation of caregiver and child results in significant improvement in the child's condition, (b) the reported symptoms are not observed by anyone but the caregiver, (c) there is direct discovery of toxins in the child or medical paraphernalia in the caregiver's control, and (d) the caregiver is caught administering substances to the child or otherwise actively inducing illness.

Before these elements are confirmed, medical personnel must first suspect a factitious disorder by proxy in order to make the observations and document the data that will establish the diagnosis.

The Medical Puzzle

Suspicions usually begin with a physician or subspecialist who becomes frustrated with the repeated treatment of a child whose symptoms appear to be resistant to diagnosis or treatment. Often laboratory tests or specialized examinations yield puzzling information that does not make sense to the physician. At the same time, the physician may begin to notice that the parent appears to be unusually calm or even apparently cheerful about the child's persistent medical problems, and may seem quite comfortable living for periods of time in the hospital at her child's side. The family history may be filled with unusual medical problems, including odd sibling illnesses, extensive maternal illnesses and tragedies, and perhaps an unexplained death of another child in the family. If physicians admit children to the hospital for tests or observations, they may find that the child's reported medical problems are not observed by medical staff, appear much less severe than described by parents, or are only observed when the mother is visiting or has spent time alone with the patient. Unfortunately, it often takes quite some time for the physician to begin to suspect that something is amiss.

The "Devoted" Caregiver

Mothers with MBPS generally present as devoted, caring parents, often reluctant to leave the bedsides of their sick children. They are often very knowledgeable about medical matters, and are quite willing and able to give detailed presentations of their child's long and puzzling health history. Their interactions with physicians may involve adulatory support or angry, hostile attacks on the doctor's failure to resolve the child's medical problem. Many are emotionally needy and seem to derive obvious pleasure from their interactions with fellow parents in the hospital and through their association with medical staff. In fact, a significant minority of mothers with this disorder are either nurses, nurse's aides, or in some way associated with the medical field (Rosenberg, 1987).

Although empirical research on factitious disorder by proxy is relatively sparse, clinical observations suggest that mothers with the disorder can come from any ethnic or socioeconomic group. Often they will describe long and surprisingly pathological medical histories for themselves and other family members. They may report a happy childhood, but detailed history frequently uncovers the loss of a parent in childhood or a feeling of being less valued than her siblings. They do not present as thought-disordered, and are often very convincing even to mental health professionals. Psychosis in these parents is quite rare. When confronted about factitious behavior, it is very common for these mothers to indignantly deny any accusations of fabrication, and to rally support from family members, neighbors, and even health care staff who are impressed with their devotion to their child.

Husbands of mothers with MBPS are most often described as absent and uninvolved in the lives of their wives and children. Some are divorced from the mother, but even those still married are often overinvolved in work or other activities to such an extent that they play a marginal role in their children's lives. It is not uncommon for husbands to never visit their child during hospitalizations, or to pay enormous medical bills without questioning the discrepancy between the illnesses described and their own observations. Some fathers actively collude in the fabrications of illness.

The child victims of MBPS can be of any age, gender, or birth order. Sometimes a single child is selected for the abuse, and sometimes siblings are abused serially or simultaneously. Little is known at this time about the important factors in the selection of the target child, and it is quite possible that factors other than the characteristics of the child are primary in the mother's selection of a victim.

Very young victims of MBPS abuse do not typically show obvious problems in attachment with their caregiver. The degree of the child's collusion or cooperation with the medical charade appears to be related to his/her age at the time the abuse first began (Schreier & Libow, 1993a), in that somewhat older children have sometimes been coached by parents to produce the factitious symptoms in question.

The Evidence: Steps toward Verifying Suspicions of MBPS

If the physician suspects that the child may be suffering from a caretaker-induced factitious illness, the steps taken to verify this fact are critically important to a correct diagnosis, an appropriate response from protective services systems, and effective resolution of the problem by the legal system.

One of the first important steps for any physician to take—once suspicions of MBPS have been aroused—is to call an interdisciplinary meeting of fellow specialists and other involved health providers, in order to pool data and observations, and develop an effective strategy for information-gathering and intervention. Inconsistencies in observations of the patient, in details of treatment, and in past medical histories given by the parent with MBPS to different providers may emerge at this meeting and help clarify that a problem exists. Pediatric psychologists and psychiatrists have an important role in helping to plan a strategy for further establishing the diagnosis, and developing a plan for protecting the child and parent. If it is decided that there is probable factitious illness involved, nursing staff and child protective services should also be involved in the early stages as well. However, it is critical that hospital staff, including nurses, not only be informed of the plan but also carefully educated about factitious disorder by proxy so that the plan is not compromised by well-meaning staff who cannot believe that such a devoted mother would endanger her child.

If suspicion seems justified, medical records need to be thoroughly reviewed, and checked for verification of all incidents of the suspicious "illness" and important details such as who observed them and the circumstances under which they occurred. For example, a report of repeated medical problems (such as a history of multiple apnea alarms each night) needs to be carefully questioned as to whether anyone else in the home besides the mother actually observes the problem and sees it happening when the mother is not present. At the same time, all suspicions and actual observations of false reporting by the parent, or harmful behavior toward the child, should be carefully documented in the medical chart.

There is a tendency for many medical "facts" reported by a parent to become unquestioningly repeated in medical records, despite a lack of verification from the beginning. Medical records should be requested from other physicians and institutions because they often reveal test results that contradict the caregiver's reports. Even the parent's own suspicious or unbelievable medical history should be verified, if possible, because the discovery of overt lies and exaggerations in the parent's own history will be useful evidence for establishing a pattern of deception.

The creativity and remarkable range of possible fabrications and manipulations by a mother with MBPS sometimes makes it impossible for the physician to directly search for a specific substance or method of illness-induction. However, if poisoning is suspected, the medical staff should consider toxicology screens for as broad a range of substances as is possible. At the same time, the hospitalized child should be carefully monitored by careful nursing observation when the suspected parent is present. All food, drink, and medicines should be administered only by the nursing staff.

In cases of suspected suffocation or life-threatening tampering, the most effective way to protect the child is to monitor the parent actively with video surveillance, in an effort to witness the parent in the act of endangering the child. This allows immediate emergency protective intervention and almost guarantees successful legal action for long-term protection of the child. Video surveil-

lance techniques have been used with great effectiveness in England by Samuels, McClaughlin, Jacobson, Poets and Southall (1992) and is becoming more widely accepted in the United States. Despite legitimate concerns that have been raised about issues of privacy and the parent's legal rights (Zitelli, Seltman, & Shannon, 1987), as well as potential hospital liability for infringement of these rights, there is increasing awareness of the value, necessity, and legality of surveillance in certain life-threatening cases (Frost, Glaze, & Rosen, 1988). This technique is gaining in popularity as increasing protections are being incorporated, including continuous monitoring of the video record, often without sound to enhance family privacy. Video surveillance is likely to become the standard of care in the future for evaluation of the most severe and life-threatening forms of MBPS.

The authors have seen tragic outcomes when factitious illness by proxy is suggested in the differential diagnosis of a puzzling case, but no steps are taken to verify the suspicions. It should be noted that physicians and hospitals leave themselves open to legal action by a spouse of a perpetrator of MBPS if they do not act to investigate the possibility of factitious illness thoroughly.

The Role of the Pediatric Psychologist/Psychiatrist in MBPS

Mental health professionals typically have little special expertise in detecting lying on the part of the parent with MBPS, and a clinical interview alone cannot confirm the diagnosis in the absence of a well-documented medical record. Mothers with MBPS are generally very believable and effective at convincing physicians as well as mental health professionals of their devotion to and concern for their child. However, mental health professionals can play an important role as consultants to the interdisciplinary team conducting the medical investigation of a suspected case, and they can obtain significant family history and clinical observations from an intensive psychosocial interview of the mother and appropriate follow-up with spouse and extended family. Particular areas to cover in the interview with a suspected parent are the mother's work history or occupational aspirations (which often focus on health care), her relationships with physicians and staff in other hospitals, discrepancies between medical knowledge and general knowledge, and a history of loss or sense of deprivation in her family of origin.

Psychological testing of the suspected parent can also be helpful in identifying some of the underlying dynamics, and in developing a profile of the parent for later use in evaluating the parent's progress following a course of psychotherapy. While there is no single or simple profile of the parent with MBPS, preliminary data (Schreier & Libow, 1993a) suggest that these mothers generally have a relatively normal MMPI profile (no T-scores exceeding 70) with a high (F-K) Index and relative elevations in the Character scales, with generally low scores on Social Introversion subscales. Projective test data support the finding of a rigid, denying defensive style with underlying resentment, rebelliousness, passive-aggressiveness, and emotional immaturity.

Pediatric psychologists and psychiatrists are also likely to be called upon to provide psychotherapy for mothers with MBPS, as this type of pathology requires a treating clinician familiar with the disorder as well as the pediatric setting. While the prognosis for these patients is often believed to be rather poor, given intense maternal denial and entrenched character disorders, it is hoped that more case studies and empirical treatment data will provide increasingly useful guidelines for effective therapeutic work.

INTERVENTION STRATEGIES

Once a careful assessment of a medical puzzle provides compelling evidence of factitious disorder by proxy, there are many complex and difficult decisions to be made to ensure the most successful outcome for the child and family. Important steps that remain to be taken include notification of the family, planning for the child(ren)'s protection, legal intervention, long-term case management, psychological treatment, and if feasible, reunification planning.

Notification of the Family

It is always a complex decision to plan the most effective timing and strategy for informing the parent and family of the suspected factitious disorder by proxy. This is generally the first time that the facts of the case as they are understood by the medical staff are revealed and presented in detail to the family. Since the recognition that an illness is being fabricated is generally a process of gradual confirmation via the slow accumulation of confirmatory evidence, medical staff often wonder how much evidence is necessary before the family should be apprised of staff concerns, and how early one should involve law enforcement and child protection authorities. Both the disturbing risk of falsely accusing a

"devoted parent" and concerns about possibly serious ramifications of prematurely revealing one's "hand" in the absence of an "airtight case" often lead to long and unfortunate delays in the notification process.

However, it is important to remember that even in cases where there is entirely convincing evidence of MBPS abuse, such as a mother recorded on videotape smothering her infant, it is common for the parent to angrily and vociferously deny the accusation. Thus, the decision to confront a parent should not be based on acquiring adequate evidence to bring forth a parental confession, but rather it should be based on having adequate evidence to obtain child protective services support and intervention. The notification or informing of the family should be planned collaboratively with the police and protective services so that the child (if necessary) can be taken into protective custody immediately upon informing the parents. If this is not done, there is a serious risk that the family will flee to another medical facility to begin the process anew, or may rapidly up the ante in an even more life-threatening assault on the child to "prove" that he/she is really sick. Preparation of nursing and ward staff to understand the disorder so they are not deceived by the mother's imposture is essential.

Mental health professionals should be actively involved in the notification process so that appropriate support can be offered (both to physician and family), and the parent being confronted can be assessed for possible suicidal response to news of being revealed as an abuser and having her child removed from her custody. We have anecdotal evidence to suggest that including the police in the notification meeting with the family may increase the chance of obtaining a confession by the parent with MBPS.

We recommend that the suspected parent's partner as well as extended family be included in the notification process, so that they are kept actively involved in how and why the institution is taking the various steps to protect the child patient. In informing the family, the reasons for suspicion, the observations made, and the support for the diagnosis of factitious illness should all be simply and directly explained to the family in a nonjudgmental manner. It is helpful to inform the parent that her child will be protected, and will likely be returned eventually to her custody if she is willing to actively engage in treatment to understand and resolve her disorder. It is often the case that the primary pediatricians or family physicians are intensely involved in the parent's imposture, and highly invested in months if not years of medical "treatment" of the child. They should only be alerted in advance, and/or included in the process of notifying the parent, if there is little risk that they will warn the parent or otherwise sabotage the structured plan of the medical staff before all the necessary steps are taken.

Child Protection

Immediate removal of the child is generally the best approach to avoid flight of the family, protect the health of the child, and further establish the validity of the MBPS diagnosis. In most cases, the placement of the child in a foster home allows for rather rapid weaning of the child from unnecessary medications and treatments. Moreover, separation of parent and child allows the clearest differentiation of bona fide medical problems, which are witnessed and persist in the absence of the parent, from those exaggerated or actively induced symptoms which improve dramatically or are found not to exist.

While it is difficult to justify from the psychological standpoint of the child's needs for a secure and familiar family placement, it is very important to make sure the child is placed in a foster setting which is entirely independent of the suspected parent. Even if a father or a grandparent promises to protect the child in his/her own home or the child's own residence, any access of the abusing parent to the target child is likely to provide an unnecessary risk of continuance of the abuse. Few health professionals, let alone family members, can imagine the extreme degree to which these caregivers may go to prove and maintain the appearance of the child's illness, even under careful supervision. And mothers with MBPS are generally skilled enough at insisting on their innocence and creating doubts in others to such a degree that close family members generally require many months or years before they believe the reality of the mother's abuse and accept the fact that the child is truly endangered by that parent. (Family acceptance of MBPS can be further confused by the fact that older children who have been involved in illness fabrication for several years may exhibit some of the same factitious symptoms even after placement out of the home, particularly during or after visits by the perpetrating parent.)

Furthermore, family members generally have never heard of factitious disorder by proxy, and may seriously doubt its validity, given their loyalty to their family member. Consider the fact that even the family physician often requires weeks or months of soul-searching and consultation with peers before finally accepting the sometimes rather obvious conclusion that a mother is deliberately harming her child!

Legal Intervention

While many health care providers find involvement in the legal arena a distasteful chore that they prefer to avoid, collaboration with police investigators and district attorneys is critical to effective protection and treatment of the family. Just as physicians and other health care providers struggle with accepting the validity of MBPS, so too do social workers, lawyers, and judges who are essential to the active protection of the child. The health care provider and mental health consultant have a critical role to play in helping to initially explain and substantiate the diagnosis of MBPS so that immediate protective intervention and psychological evaluation will be mandated by the court.

In most cases, clearcut proof of parental tampering or suffocation, as in video surveillance tapes, will not be available. Thus, the disorder will most likely have to be proven indirectly, in that the child's condition can be explained in no other way than through the parent's deceptions, and is found to improve dramatically by separation from the suspected parent.

Pediatricians, and pediatric psychologists and psychiatrists, may be called upon as expert witnesses to explain factitious disorder by proxy and give expert opinions on specific cases before the court. Unfortunately, mental health professionals unfamiliar with MBPS are often appointed by the court to evaluate mothers diagnosed with the disorder and are sometimes deceived by the parent, reporting back an inability to find any major psychopathology. This is why informal as well as organized opportunities to provide education to the mental health community about MBPS is as important as the training necessary for physicians and other health care providers on the front lines.

Case Management

Once the child is in foster care or placement with relatives who are physically and emotionally distant from the suspected parent, treatment and visitation become primary issues. The authors recommend that all family members older than 3 years of age should be provided individual therapy, with distinctly separate issues to be addressed by the abuser, the spouse, the victim, and the siblings. It is very important that therapists have consent to communicate among themselves, as this will allow the best assessment of progress, of troubling or positive developments within the family, and of the readiness for any eventual family work. A consultant or therapist familiar with MBPS and the treatment pitfalls should be made available to the team of therapists.

If the individual therapy of the parent and her spouse progresses, couples and/or family therapy at a much later stage of treatment, including the children, will be important in eventually reunifying the family. As in cases of familial incest, eventual family therapy is a goal, in order to allow the abuser to directly and fully accept responsibility for the factitious illness behavior, the disruption of family life, and the serious blow to trust and security within the family unit.

Visitation arrangements between parent and child should be decided on an individual basis, with many factors taken into consideration, including age of the child, the child's comfort with ongoing contact, and any risk of continued abuse. While the majority of children abused by mothers with MBPS remain very attached to their parent and eager for continued contact, the authors are aware of some cases in which the child has been extremely angry at the abusing parent, or has actually experienced what appears to be a conditioned illness reaction (in several cases, nausea and vomiting) in response to contact with the parent.

The target child as well as siblings should be placed under the medical supervision of a single physician who is familiar with the particular patient, as well as with factitious disorder by proxy. If the child's longtime primary physician understands and accepts the diagnosis, he/she would be an ideal caregiver for continuity and good management. The fact that many children abused by MBPS actually have bona fide medical disorders and illnesses, in addition to the factitious illness, can further complicate the medical picture and confuse the practitioner. As some pediatricians are reluctant to assess any symptom as factitious in origin once their patient is diagnosed with an actual problem, the physician must be able to treat the child with both real and fabricated illness, and recognize the difference.

Once the target child is in protective custody, with a plan for psychotherapeutic treatment and medical management in place, the child's siblings deserve careful assessment as well. Many parents with MBPS are known to abuse several children in a family simultaneously, or turn to younger children once an older child is removed from their control. A thorough protective services evaluation should include collection of all family medical records, as well as a comprehensive physical and psychological examination of siblings. Certainly, the removal of the target child from the family for protection and the exposure of their parent as an abuser is likely to be traumatic for both the siblings and other family members most directly involved. Siblings are often as des-

perately protective of their mother as the target child, and will also need help in breaking through their denial, collusion, or ignorance of the problem in order to cope with the unfolding tragedy in their household.

Psychotherapy

In general, the prognosis for psychotherapy with patients with factitious disorder by proxy has not been considered a very positive one, as these patients are notoriously resistant, in denial, or primarily motivated to win back their child from the protective services system by cooperating only as much as is absolutely necessary. More recently, therapists have begun to anecdotally report some success in psychotherapeutic treatment. Day (1994) has reported successful treatment outcomes through the careful building of trust in the therapist, a nonjudgmental, problem-solving approach providing practical support and encouraging client dependency, and an eventual working-through of the trauma, with the goal of "identity reformation." Until very recently, another difficulty faced by psychotherapists working with these patients was the absence of any systematic theory of the dynamics of the disorder to guide the development of useful strategies for treatment.

Schreier (1992) and Schreier and Libow (1993a) have presented a model of MBPS as a form of female perversion, referring not to the patient's sexual practices but to her mode of mental functioning. We used the definition of a "perversion" as a strategy intended to correct and revenge a childhood mortification, while keeping the purpose of the perverse acts out of consciousness. This compulsive behavior creates intense anxiety if it is not reenacted repeatedly. In this sense, we proposed MBPS as a form of perversion in which the parent, through the creation or exaggeration of illness in the child, can maintain an intense but ambivalent (needy and hostile) relationship with the physician, who represents a powerful figure who arouses strong fears of rejection and abandonment. Many mothers with MBPS have a history of loss or abandonment by their fathers, and a sense of being unseen and unrecognized in their families of origin. At the same time, many find themselves in unsatisfying marital relationships with distant, uninvolved partners who only validate feelings of invisibility and neglect.

On an interpersonal level, we have also described the relationship between the mother with factitious illness by proxy and the physician as an "imposture" of the devoted mother role. By creating and elaborating upon the role of the martyred mother of a sick child, the mother with MBPS strives to compensate for her own lack of a separate and functional identity. She substitutes instead the socially approved role of "self-sacrificing mother," which earns her both admiration and pity. At the same time, by successfully fooling and controlling the powerful medical staff, the impostor can experience both some nurturance from physicians because of their attention, as well as contempt for their helplessness and failure. Revelation of her childhood wounds and current unmet needs, acknowledgment of the imposture, and acceptance of the need for new modes of interpersonal relating will be a long, slow process. For psychotherapy to be effective, the roots of these dynamics need to be explored with the patient, and a more authentic identity and sense of relationship with others slowly nurtured.

The question arises as to whether a patient so comfortable with lying can form a therapeutic alliance. In some cases, all that can be hoped for is the establishment of a supportive relationship, or a substitute career which provides a certain amount of the needed succor for these patients.

Reunification

Given the long and arduous process of psychotherapy, it is unfortunate that court dates and deadlines for reunification tend to proceed on their own accelerated schedules. The court will generally base its decisions about reunification of mother and child on the recommendations of treating therapists and the assigned caseworker. There is good reason for caution and care in taking this major step, as there have been many indications that reunification can lead to continued abuse or harmful outcomes. Illustrative is a recent study by Bools, Neale, and Meadow (1993), in which it was found that years after their initial involvement with child protective services, children in these families experienced ongoing problems with emotional and behavioral problems, school attendance, concentration, and a substantial number of continued medical fabrications by their parents. And early findings on adult outcomes for children victimized throughout childhood by MBPS (Libow, 1995) suggest that post-traumatic stress symptoms, relationship problems, avoidance of medical care, and low self-esteem may persist for decades after such experiences.

Meadow (1985) indicates that a child is placed more at risk, if reunified with the parent, by many factors, including severe abuse, age younger than 5 years of age, unexplained sibling deaths, mother's lack of understanding of her behavior, and maternal substance abuse. We also suggest some additional criteria in the decision to reunify the child and parent (Schreier & Libow,

1993a). The child should not have a major, bona fide medical problem that would seriously complicate assessment of long-term progress when returned to the mother. The mother with MBPS should have achieved some insight and better relationship and parenting skills from her therapeutic experience, as well as alternative coping strategies. The extended family of the child should accept the parent's diagnosis and demonstrate commitment to the child's future protection. The mother with MBPS should not have a serious thought disorder, organicity, or psychosis, nor be engaged in adult factitious illness behavior. And most important, if the child is returned to the care of this parent, there should be long-term and careful supervision of the child's health and safety. While seemingly obvious, the last requirement is often one of the most difficult to ensure, as the legal system is often guided by a reunification timeline that does not allow for long-term supervision once a limited time period has elapsed. These are issues that our legal and protective services systems will need to address if they are to adequately serve the needs of these children.

CASE ILLUSTRATION

(The following case illustration is adapted from Schreier, H. A., and Libow, J. A., Munchausen by proxy syndrome: A modern pediatric challenge, *The Journal of Pediatrics*, 1994, *125*, S111-114 and reproduced with permission from Mosby-YearBook, Inc.)

Clinical Presentation

"A male infant was born prematurely and was hospitalized for 1 month because of respiratory problems. After he was released from the hospital, he had difficulty feeding and was said by the mother to spit up, vomit and choke, which caused inadequate weight gain. He also had frequent ear infections, respiratory illnesses, and a urinary tract infection and was hospitalized several times.

"The evaluation of the patient in an inpatient setting showed that he had slight gastroesophageal reflux and questionable malabsorption. He gained very little weight during his stay in the hospital. Metoclopramide was prescribed for the feeding problems after gastroesophageal reflux was diagnosed, and he was then released from the hospital. The mother subsequently reported that the medication had no effect on his vomiting, and he did not gain weight despite a high-caloric formula. The infant was readmitted to the hospital, and nasogastric feeding was begun. He showed a small weight gain in the hospital, and vomiting was minimal. Evaluations of gastric, duodenal and esophageal biopsies were normal. After the infant was released from the hospital, the mother continued to report vomiting, which was not controlled with cimetidine. Another esophageal biopsy was performed, the results of which revealed moderate reflux esophagitis. A fundoplication and gastrostomy were performed to treat reflux esophagitis and to provide direct gastrostomy feedings. He gained 1.22 kg during the next 3 months as he remained an inpatient after his recovery from surgery.

"However, after he was released from the hospital, the infant was reported by the mother to have frequent gagging, retching, bloating, weight loss, and irritability. In addition drip feedings were, by history, not tolerated. He was hospitalized again and a variety of medicines and regimens were tried. Independent consultation at a neurologic institute ruled out previously entertained causes for the child's condition. Doctors then considered a diagnosis of chronic intestinal pseudo-obstruction, and total parenteral nutrition was initiated with use of a central venous catheter (Broviac). The child gained weight during his stay in the hospital, but gram-negative bacterial sepsis developed 4 days after he was released. This episode of sepsis was the first of seven that he experienced during the next 4-1/2 months.

"The infected catheter was removed, but the mother reported that the infant continued to have feeding problems, which led to the insertion of another central venous catheter. One week later septic shock developed, and he was admitted to a pediatric intensive care unit. Evaluation of blood cultures revealed the presence of *Klebsiella*, *Enterobacter cloacae*, and *Citrobacter* organisms. Days after completing a successful course of antibiotics, the child experienced another episode of sepsis, this time, however, with a different *Enterobacter* species."

Assessment Findings

"When the infant recovered from the latest episode of sepsis, treatment with cisapride was initiated because of its potential value in managing chronic intestinal pseudo-obstruction. However the trial with cisapride did not improve the symptoms as reported by the mother. Despite the absence of mucosal inflammation or bowel dilation, the physicians assumed that the bacteremias were caused by translocation of organisms through the bowel wall. Numerous diagnostic tests were performed; however, the diagnosis of chronic intestinal pseudo-obstruction could not be confirmed, and no other gastrointestinal

abnormalities were found. Low levels of immunoglobulin IgG4 were detected, but the consulting immunologist did not believe that it was a contributing factor to the child's problems. The infant was released from the hospital again, and subsequently, he returned three times during the following month with gram-negative sepsis.

"The hospital physicians suspected that this might be a case of MBPS, and they sought counsel from experts in this field at a medical center in another state. The infant was placed in an intensive care unit under close observation. Antroduodenal motility studies, which were unavailable in the local hospital, were performed and showed normal motility. Observations for symptoms of chronic intestinal pseudo-obstruction revealed none; the results of a lactose tolerance tests were also normal. The central venous catheter and the gastrostomy tube were removed and the infant began oral feedings."

Treatment Selection and Course

"The mother was confronted with the belief of the doctors that she was causing her child's illnesses. Although the infant initially lost weight during the oral feedings (400 gm) during 3 weeks' time, he gained weight steadily after strictly supervised visits were begun. In the next 6 months, his weight increased by 1.82 kg, placing him in the 50th percentile for weight for his age for the first time. The mother became increasingly anxious rather than relieved. During this time he had three retching episodes, each occurring after a visit with his mother. He continued to have otitis media and upper respiratory illnesses, but no episodes of sepsis, hospitalizations, or feeding problems.

"Experts in gastroenterology and infectious disease were called as witnesses in a custody court hearing. The infectious disease expert attributed the frequency of sepsis due to unusual organisms as a result of outside tampering. Another expert testified that only 10 percent of Broviac-related infections were caused by gram-negative bacteria. In the case of this infant, the number of infections with gram-negative bacteria was much greater than usual, especially because they were always caused by a different organism than the one that had just been treated, and almost invariably, the infection started after the child was sent home with the mother.

"Two consulting gastroenterologists noted that the evidence supporting the absence of a motility disorder was compelling. Absence of this disorder was further supported by the fact that the child was able to be fed orally less than 1 week after the discontinuation of total parenteral nutrition. These same physicians, along with the consulting child psychiatrist, commented that the mother maintained "unbelievable calm" during the multiple near-death experiences of her child, a reaction she also evidenced when being confronted with the belief that she has MBPS—a belief that, at that time, she neither confirmed nor denied.

"In contrast, two different gastroenterologists hired by the parents thought that there was evidence for postprandial hypomotility. This is a condition, as stated by one gastroenterologist, commonly found in cases of chronic intestinal pseudo-obstruction. One noted gastroenterologist for the defense thought that the patient's "remission" of his chronic intestinal pseudo-obstruction, which coincided with the closely supervised removal of the central venous catheter at the tertiary care center, could have been a coincidence and was not related to the mother's removal as caregiver. Another gastroenterologist for the defense believed that the episodes of sepsis were caused by bowel seeding, but offered no explanation as to why the patient did not experience episodes of sepsis before the implantation of a central venous catheter. One of the gastroenterologists for the defense focused on various procedural aspects of the motility studies that were done at the tertiary center. It was his belief that an incorrect formula was administered and that sedation was used for these tests."

Termination and Follow-Up

"The court then brought in another experienced gastroenterologist who reviewed the results of the motility studies. This expert testified that the patient had normal fasting and interdigestive motor activity, with no evidence of antroduodenal hypoactivity. Parenthetically, this expert stated that he knew of no studies of antroduodenal motility in normal children. He also noted that children with antroduodenal motility appear to improve after treatment with cisapride, whereas the patient did not. This expert indicated that the history of other infections (such as otitis) was normal for a child of his age. He further noted that patients with chronic intestinal pseudo-obstruction have an increased frequency of sepsis. However, this court-appointed expert believed that in this case the episodes of sepsis were catheter-related and probably caused exogenously.

"In total, nine doctors testified at the trial. Five nurses who testified described the mother as a caring, loving parent, and several refused to believe the diagnosis of MBPS. The court, however, was persuaded that the diagnosis of MBPS was correct but returned the child to the family where he remains under close supervision.

"This case represents a typical example of the length to which a mother will go to continue the intense and seemingly bizarre relationship with her baby and the medical establishment. The intensity of her denial and the 'circuslike' involvement of attorneys and the media are not uncommon. This leads to enormous expenditure of time and money by numerous professionals and governmental agencies. Because chronic intestinal pseudo-obstruction is a relatively new diagnosis and there is a lack of consensus among gastroenterologists as to what constitutes normal gastrointestinal motility, it is a 'set-up' for the elaboration of a MBPS process. It is only when we understand the individual dynamics of the mother and the ways in which doctors are susceptible to the interpersonal abnormality of these women who 'impersonate' good mothers, that we will be able to improve our often greatly delayed diagnosis of MBPS." (Schreier & Libow, 1994)

This case illustrates many of the difficulties experienced by those involved in MBPS cases. There were literally months of unnecessary medical treatment, with the medical providers unsure of what had happened, even at the end of the long process. The legal system kept turning to more and more experts, and the child's improvement was explained by contentious professionals and family members to support their point of view, even though the most parsimonious explanation was MBPS. There are lawyers and psychiatrists now making a reputation by defending parents in such cases. Hospitals have even been accused of a phenomenon called "institutional Munchausen," in which it is alleged that the staff plant false evidence to implicate a parent when they are convinced of the parent's guilt, but unable to prove it. This disorder is so puzzling and can generate such disbelief and confusion that it is often difficult to sort out the fact and the fiction, even in retrospect.

SUMMARY

Mental health consultants in the pediatric setting will find that cases of factitious disorder by proxy, at the intersection of pediatrics and psychiatry, challenge all of their clinical skills. Factitious illness by proxy is a costly problem in the pediatric setting, in terms of children's morbidity and mortality, abuse of health care resources, stress on physicians, and financial costs. There are challenges at every step of the way, from initial recognition of this dynamic in a child's persistent medical problems, through the gathering of supportive evidence, coordination of an appropriate medical response, intervention by protective service and police authorities, and therapeutic and reunification issues. Continued study of the dynamics of these mothers and effective therapeutic approaches to their treatment will hopefully shed light on ways that physicians and mental health consultants can best respond to the enormous challenges posed by the parent engaged in illness fabrication.

REFERENCES

American Psychiatric Association. (1994). *Diagnostic and statistical manual of mental disorders, DSM-IV* (4th ed.). Washington, D.C.: American Psychiatric Association.

Asher, R. (1951). Munchausen's syndrome. *Lancet, i*, 339–341.

Bools, C., Neale, B., & Meadow, R. (1993). Munchausen by Proxy: A study of psychopathology. *Child Abuse and Neglect, 18*, 773–788.

Day, D. O. (1994, August). *Treatment of Munchausen Syndrome by Proxy*. Paper presented at the Annual Convention of the American Psychological Association, Los Angeles.

DiMaio, V. J. M., & Bernstein, C. G. (1974). A case of infanticide. *Journal of Forensic Science, 19*, 745–754.

Egginton, J. (1990). *From cradle to grave: the short lives and strange deaths of Marybeth Tinning's nine children*. New York: Jove Books.

Emery, J. L. (1993). Child abuse, sudden infant death syndrome, and unexpected infant death. *American Journal of Diseases of Children, 147*, 1097–1100.

Frost, J. D., Glaze, D. G., & Rosen, C. L. (1988). Munchausen's Syndrome by Proxy and video surveillance. *American Journal of Diseases of Children, 142*, 917–918.

Godding, V., & Kruth, M. (1991). Compliance with treatment in asthma and Munchausen Syndrome by Proxy. *Archives of Disease in Childhood, 66*, 956–960.

Goodlin, R. C. (1985). Pregnant females with Munchausen Syndrome. *American Journal of Obstetrics and Gynecology, 153*, 207–210.

Libow, J. A. (1995). Munchausen by Proxy victims in adulthood: A first look. *Child Abuse and Neglect*, In press.

Meadow, R. (1977). Munchausen by Proxy Syndrome: The hinterland of child abuse. *Lancet, ii*, 343–345.

Meadow, R. (1985). Management of Munchausen Syndrome by Proxy. *Archives of Disease in Childhood, 60*, 385–393.

Meadow, R. (1990). Suffocation, recurrent apnea and sudden infant death. *Journal of Pediatrics, 117*, 351–357.

Rosenberg, D. (1987). Web of deceit: A literature review of Munchausen Syndrome by Proxy. *Child Abuse and Neglect, 11*, 547–563.

Samuels, M. P., McClaughlin, W., Jacobson, R. R., Poets, C. F., & Southall, D. P. (1992). Fourteen cases of imposed upper airway obstruction. *Archives of Disease in Childhood, 67*, 162–170.

Schreier, H. A. (1992). The perversion of mothering: Munchausen Syndrome by Proxy. *Bulletin of the Menninger Clinic, 56*, 421–437.

Schreier, H. A., & Libow, J. A. (1993a). *Hurting for love: Munchausen by Proxy Syndrome*. New York: Guilford Press.

Schreier, H. A., & Libow, J. A. (1993b). Munchausen by Proxy Syndrome: Diagnosis and prevalence. *American Journal of Orthopsychiatry, 63*, 318–321.

Schreier, H. A., & Libow, J. A. (1994). Munchausen by Proxy Syndrome: A modern pediatric challenge. *Journal of Pediatrics, 125*, S110–S115.

Sigal, M., Carmel, I., Altmark, D., & Silfen, P. (1988). Munchausen Syndrome by Proxy: A psychodynamic analysis. *Medicine and Law, 7*, 49–56.

Spiro, H. R. (1968). Chronic factitious illness. *Archives of General Psychiatry, 18*, 569–579.

Stern, T. A. (1980). Munchausen's Syndrome revisited. *Psychosomatics, 21*, 329–336.

Warner, J. O., & Hathaway, M. J. (1984). Allergic form of Meadow's Syndrome (Munchausen by Proxy). *Archives of Disease in Childhood, 59*, 151–156.

Zitelli, B. J., Seltman, M. F., & Shannon, R. M. (1987). Munchausen Syndrome by Proxy and its professional participants. *American Journal of Diseases of Children, 141*, 1099–1102.

CHAPTER 7

SOMATIZATION

John V. Campo
Judith Garber

DESCRIPTION OF THE PROBLEM

Definitions

The term *somatization* has generated much confusion and has been used in a number of different ways. First, it has been used as a descriptive term, with somatization being said to occur when physical symptoms are experienced, but medical evaluation reveals no discernible physical pathology or pathophysiologic mechanism, or when physical pathology is present, the physical complaints or associated impairment are beyond what would be expected from the medical findings alone (Kellner, 1991). A related descriptive definition by Lipowski (1988) emphasizes the importance of the suffering individual attributing the experienced physical symptoms to physical disease and seeking medical help. The term has also been employed to refer to a hypothetical mechanism of symptom production or psychological process. A third use of the term has been as the distinguishing label of a categorical psychiatric disorder characterized by multiple unexplained physical symptoms, somatization disorder (American Psychiatric Association, 1994). In many respects, the resulting imprecision in the use of the term across settings parallels the use of similar terms with a long history in psychiatry such as *hysteria* and *conversion*. Unless otherwise specified, the term *somatization* will be used in the descriptive sense throughout this chapter.

Somatization in the Western Medical Tradition

Somatization appears to be rooted in the Western medical tradition (Fabrega, 1990). The prevailing Western biomedical model of disease emphasizes physical disease as the cause of *illness*, the subjective suffering and related behaviors of patients. Physical *disease* is understood in terms of a definable pathology or pathophysiologic process, and is considered to have a natural history and course; it is understood as being reducible to biophysical or biochemical terms (Weiner & Fawzy, 1990). This model has been tremendously important in the evolution of Western medicine, though physicians have found themselves in a quandary when presented with the quite common occurrence of patients who appear to truly suffer from physical symptoms, yet show no evidence of physical disease. A psychological model of illness developed alongside the biomedical model primarily because of such patients, and has been codified in the development of disciplines focused on one model or the other, with traditional medicine taking a primarily biomedical focus, and the mental health disciplines being relegated primarily to the realm of the psychological or the mind (Weiner & Fawzy, 1990).

In contrast to traditional Chinese or Indian medicine, where physical symptoms themselves were the focus of medical practice, the suffering of patients in modern medical settings engenders a search for physical disease, which in many respects becomes a process of verifying or legitimizing the somatic complaints (Fabrega, 1990). There is a tacit assumption that illness associated with evidence of disease is somehow "legitimate" and considered to be beyond the patient's control, whereas illness in the absence of documented disease may be viewed as self-caused and under voluntary control, implying a sort of sociomoral failure of the patient or family, and thus becoming a source of stigma. This is consistent with Weiner's (1993) theory of perceived responsibility and social motivation, which maintains that individuals are generally not held responsible for matters perceived as outside of their control such as "sickness," but are held accountable for symptoms or difficulties that are perceived by others to be controllable. It is thus no surprise that a great many patients and families are insistent on an intensive search for evidence of physical disease when physical suffering is present, not only because of fear of disease per se, but also because of some concern related to the stigma associated with "illegitimate" or medically unexplained physical symptoms.

In our society the physician is regarded as the final arbiter of who is granted the social sanction of the sick role, which traditionally allows the sick individual to be exempted from certain duties and responsibilities, and potentially to be granted certain privileges (Parsons, 1964). For example, there is evidence that parents are more likely to excuse child misbehavior when children exhibit signs of physical illness, especially when the illness is associated with a concrete medical diagnosis (Walker, Garber, & Van Slyke, 1995). Some individuals may exaggerate the presence of physical symptoms under conditions in which their performance is being evaluated, with somatic complaints and physical symptoms sometimes serving a "self-handicapping" function, essentially allowing the individual to minimize personal responsibility for any potential failure and perhaps serving to help maintain self-esteem (Organista & Miranda, 1991; Smith, Snyder, & Perkins, 1983). Pilowsky (1969) has conceptualized "abnormal illness behavior," referring to situations in which a physician determines that a given patient's medical assessment does not explain the symptoms presented, and thus does not legitimize the patient's or family's expectations regarding being granted sick role status.

It is essential to remember that children and adolescents who suffer from medically unexplained physical symptoms often feel profoundly misunderstood by both physicians and mental health professionals. After a visit to the physician, who may embark on a thorough search for evidence of physical disease, they may be told that "nothing is wrong," despite the fact that the child's distress appears to be quite real. As a result, they may feel dismissed, and yet still feel convinced that a serious physical disease has been "missed," which may provoke what has been commonly referred to as "doctor shopping." Mental health professionals may generate similar confusion as a result of efforts to persuade a given patient and family that the child's complaints are the result of a disembodied psychiatric disorder, rather than accepting the description of suffering that was originally presented. Interestingly, patients and families may incorporate the expectations of professionals depending on the setting in which they present, perhaps being more likely to describe their suffering in physical terms in the medical setting and in psychological terms in the mental health setting (Bridges & Goldberg, 1985).

Implications

Review of the literature documents that medically unexplained physical symptoms are common in children and adolescents, though there is a lack of systematic research (Campo & Fritsch, 1994). This area is of great relevance to society for a number of reasons. First, despite the absence of physical disease, the physical suffering of somatizing children and adolescents appears to be quite real. Somatization in childhood and adolescence is associated with significant functional impairment, most notably school problems and frequent school absences (Aro, Paronen, & Aro, 1987; Faull & Nicol, 1986; Hodges, Kline, Barbero, & Woodruff, 1985; Robinson, Alverez, & Dodge, 1990). The persistence of somatic complaints may place children at risk for potentially unnecessary medical investigations and treatments that can result in needless physical suffering or even iatrogenic, or physician caused, disease (Stickler & Murphy, 1979). Unnecessary testing procedures also can have developmental consequences, and can maintain somatization by enhancing the conviction that a particular child is "sickly" (Goodyer & Taylor, 1985; Grattan-Smith, Fairley, & Procopis, 1988).

The importance of physician behavior is emphasized by findings that uncertainty of diagnosis (Walker & Greene, 1991), inadequate medical advice (Bergman & Stamm, 1967), and even excessive physician reassurance (Warwick & Salkovskis, 1985) may be related to the development or maintenance of somatization. There are suggestions that pediatric somatization is associated with increased health care utilization (Belmaker, Espinoza, & Pogrund, 1985; Lewis & Lewis, 1989; Livingston, 1993; Starfield et al., 1984). As such, pediatric somatization is of potentially great cost to society in terms of both human and economic resources.

Adult somatization disorder has been associated with markedly increased health care utilization, increased costs, and decreased productivity (Smith, Monson, & Ray, 1986). Many somatizing adult patients report that they have suffered from similar symptoms since early in life (Kellner, 1986; Pilowsky, Bassett, Begg, & Thomas, 1982), and the majority of Briquet's patients with poly-symptomatic "hysteria" began with their physical suffer-ings prior to age 20 (Mai & Merskey, 1980), suggesting that adult somatization has its roots in childhood. A study of adults hospitalized because of persistent prob-lems with somatization suggests that a history of somatic complaints dating to childhood is associated with poor response to treatment (Shorter, Abbey, Gillies, Singh, & Lipowski, 1992).

Finally, somatization may be one of the more com-mon ways for emotional and behavioral difficulties to present in the primary care setting (Garralda & Bailey, 1987). Given the prevailing biomedical approach in modern medicine, the presence of physical symptoms may actually distract medical providers, or encourage them to pursue investigations within their own area of medical expertise, where they may feel most comfortable and confident. As a result, psychiatric disorders may be more likely to go unrecognized in affected children (Riley & Wissow, 1994).

Nosology

The problems presented by somatization in the clin-ical setting have been operationalized in the *Diagnostic and Statistical Manual of Mental Disorders, fourth edi-tion (DSM-IV)* in the category of *somatoform disorders* (American Psychiatric Association, 1994). Neverthe-less, other diagnostic categories within the DSM-IV, such as panic disorder, generalized anxiety disorder, sep-aration anxiety disorder, and mood disorders may also include various somatic symptoms within the diagnostic criteria that do not appear to have an organic cause apart from the psychiatric disorder itself. The category of so-matoform disorders is defined by the presence of phys-ical symptoms that suggest a physical disorder, but for which explanatory pathophysiologic findings are absent; the reported symptoms should not appear to be inten-tionally produced, and the patient is viewed as not ex-periencing any sense of control over the production of the physical symptoms.

Somatoform disorders are distinguished from facti-tious disorders and malingering. *Factitious disorder* is the diagnosis applied when physical symptoms are feigned or are self-inflicted, with the presumed psycho-logical gain associated with the sick role appearing to be the internal incentive of the patient. *Factitious disorder by proxy* refers to situations in which a parent or care-taker produces, feigns, or simulates disease in a child, with the incentive appearing to be an internal one for the caretaker. *Malingering* refers to the deliberate produc-tion or simulation of physical symptoms in pursuit of an external incentive, such as financial gain, avoidance of particular responsibilities, or avoidance of punishment (American Psychiatric Association, 1994).

There are seven subcategories within the broad cat-egory of somatoform disorder (American Psychiatric Association, 1994). *Somatization disorder* is the somato-form disorder that has generated the most research and at-tention in the adult psychiatric literature. The diagnosis refers to a chronic disorder characterized by recurrent and multiple somatic complaints for which medical attention has been sought, but for which the physical complaints are apparently not due to any physical disorder (American Psychiatric Association, 1994). The criteria have been modified over the years, and are the product of extensive work on the syndrome of "hysteria" or Briquet's Syn-drome by psychiatric researchers in the midwestern United States (see Cloninger, 1994). Prior to the DSM-IV, diagnosis of the disorder was determined by a symptom count from an extensive list of somatic symptoms. For example, in the *Diagnostic and Statistical Manual of Mental Disorders, third edition, revised (DSM-III-R)*, the diagnosis of somatization disorder required 13 symptoms from a list of 35 somatic symptoms grouped into the fol-lowing subcategories: pseudoneurologic (12 symptoms), gastrointestinal (6 symptoms), pain (5 symptoms), car-diopulmonary (4 symptoms), sexual (4 symptoms), and reproductive symptoms (4 symptoms) (American Psy-chiatric Association, 1987). In order for a symptom to be judged significant, it needed to result in functional im-pairment and medical help seeking or self-medication, and could not occur exclusively during a panic attack.

The modified DSM-IV (American Psychiatric Asso-ciation, 1994) criteria de-emphasize the extensive symp-tom counts previously required, with the diagnosis now requiring the following: pain in least four different bod-ily sites or during specific functions such as sexual in-tercourse, menstruation, or urination; a history of two gastrointestinal symptoms other than pain (e.g., nausea, diarrhea, bloating, vomiting other than during pregnancy, or intolerance of several different foods); a history of at least one sexual or reproductive symptom other than pain, such as sexual indifference, erectile or ejaculatory dysfunction, irregular menses, excessive menstrual bleed-ing, or vomiting throughout pregnancy; and a history of at least one symptom or deficit suggesting a neurological disorder not limited to pain, such as sensory impairment, aphonia, impaired coordination or balance, localized weakness or paralysis, difficulty swallowing, difficulty breathing, urinary retention, pseudoseizures, or dissociative symptoms such as amnesia or loss of consciousness. There is currently no consensus as to whether the diagnosis of somatization disorder identifies a unique and specific population, or whether it identifies the far end of a spectrum along a continuum of patients with multiple somatic symptoms.

The diagnosis of somatization disorder as defined in DSM-III and DSM-III-R appears to be rare in the pediatric age group, particularly in prepubertal children (Offord et al., 1987; Walker et al., 1991). Although it is true that children meeting criteria for the diagnosis have been identified (Kriechman, 1987; Livingston & Martin-Cannici, 1985), many investigators have argued that the previously employed diagnostic criteria were inappropriate for children, given the fact that many of the required symptoms were sexual and reproductive symptoms (Garber et al., 1991; Livingston & Martin-Cannici, 1985; Walker et al., 1991).

The diagnosis of *undifferentiated somatoform disorder* is applied when one or more somatic complaints or symptoms are present for at least six months and the disturbance is not accounted for by another mental disorder. The diagnosis is applied to patients with multiple somatic complaints or chronic fatigue who do not meet criteria for somatization disorder. Because this diagnosis requires fewer symptoms and is less rigidly defined than that of somatization disorder per se, it may be more applicable to use in children.

Conversion disorder is diagnosed when one or more symptoms or deficits affecting voluntary motor or sensory function that suggest a neurological or other general medical condition are present, and psychological factors are judged to be associated with the symptom because the initiation or exacerbation of the symptom or deficit are preceded by conflicts or other stresses. The DSM-IV returns to the more traditional definition of conversion disorder referring to pseudoneurologic symptoms, or symptoms that suggest neurological disease. Prior editions of the DSM had allowed for a broader interpretation of when the diagnosis of conversion disorder might be applied, with the emphasis being on conversion as a mechanism of symptom production.

Pain disorder is diagnosed when psychological factors are judged to play an important role in the onset, severity, exacerbation, and maintenance of pain, and may be of either acute or chronic duration; the pain may be present in one or more anatomical sites, and is of sufficient severity to cause significant distress or functional impairment. There are three subtypes: *pain disorder associated with psychological factors*, where psychological factors are judged to play the major role in the genesis or maintenance of the pain; *pain disorder associated with both psychological factors and a general medical condition*, where both psychological factors and a general medical condition are judged to be important in the development or maintenance of pain; and *pain disorder associated with a general medical condition*, which is not considered a mental disorder, is coded on Axis III, and where psychological factors are judged to play no more than a minimal role.

Hypochondrias is diagnosed when an individual fears or believes that a serious physical disease is present, and these fears or beliefs persist despite the reassurance of a physician for a duration of at least six months. A preoccupation with an imagined physical defect in a person who appears normal or who appears to have an obsessive concern regarding a slight physical anomaly may justify the diagnosis of *body dysmorphic disorder*. Finally, the diagnosis of *somatoform disorder, not otherwise specified* is employed in situations where symptoms consistent with somatoform disorder are present, but criteria for any one of the more specific somatoform disorder diagnoses are not met.

There appears to be much inconsistency in the diagnosis of somatoform disorders, though this has not been well studied. Virtually all of the available studies in children and adolescents focus on physical symptoms themselves, rather than systematically employed psychiatric diagnoses (Campo & Fritsch, 1994). The fact that physical symptoms may figure prominently in other DSM-IV categories such as mood disorders and anxiety disorders adds further confusion, as the manual provides little in the way of guidance as to when a somatoform disorder should not be diagnosed. In the absence of diagnosable anxiety or depression, there may be less confusion in applying a somatoform diagnosis, though here too there is the potential for diagnostic uncertainty. For example, a patient with functional gastrointestinal symptoms may be diagnosed with irritable bowel syndrome by one physician, with the psychiatric diagnosis of psychological factors affecting medical condition being applied if the symptoms appear to be related to psychological factors; the same patient might be diagnosed with a somatoform disorder by another physician, who may not consider irritable bowel syndrome a certified physical disease. Furthermore, the diagnosis of a somatoform disorder requires that the symptoms not be intentionally produced or feigned as in factitious disorder or malingering, thereby making such a determination exceedingly difficult in the clinical setting.

INCIDENCE
AND PREVALENCE

A Common Problem

Review of the literature suggests that medically un-explained physical symptoms are quite common in children and adolescents, especially recurrent complaints of pain (Campo & Fritsch, 1994; Garralda, 1996). Most of the available studies are not comprehensive in nature, focusing on some physical symptoms but not others, and most often failing to address whether the reported symptoms are associated with functional impairment or medical help seeking. Furthermore, independent medical assessments designed to determine whether the reported physical symptoms are the result of physical disease are lacking in the more comprehensive studies (Campo & Fritsch, 1994). For example, a community sample of 540 children and adolescents in grades 3 to12 was evaluated by Garber, Walker and Zeman (1991). Nearly half of the sample reported at least one physical symptom during the preceding two weeks, with the most commonly reported symptoms including headaches, low energy, sore muscles, and abdominal discomfort. Factor analysis identified four symptom clusters: cardiovascular, gastrointestinal, pain/weakness, and pseudoneurological. Approximately 1 percent of the sample endorsed at least 13 somatic symptoms, with 15 percent endorsing four symptoms or more. These symptoms were derived from a list of 36 somatic symptoms operationalized for use in children in the form of a self-report instrument known as the Children's Somatization Inventory (Walker & Greene, 1989, 1991; Walker, Garber, & Greene, 1991). Though the vast majority of the symptoms reported are unlikely to have been caused by physical disease, one limitation was the lack of an independent medical assessment of reported symptoms.

All manner of medically unexplained physical symptoms have been reported in the pediatric literature. Headaches are the most commonly reported of painful somatic symptoms across a number of different studies, with 10 to 30 percent of children and adolescents reporting frequent headaches, or headaches on an at least weekly basis (Aro, Paronen, & Aro, 1987; Belmaker, Espinoza, & Pogrand, 1985; Larson, 1991; Oster, 1972; Rutter, Tizard, & Whitmore, 1970). Recurrent abdominal pain is also an extremely common symptom, and has been reported in 10 to 25 percent of school-aged children and adolescents (Apley, 1975; Apley & Naish, 1958; Belmaker et al., 1985; Garber et al., 1991; Oster, 1972). Limb pains and so-called "growing pains" have been

described in 5 to 20 percent of children and adolescents (Apley, 1958; Belmaker et al., 1985; Garber et al., 1991; Larson, 1991; Oster, 1972), and chest pain on a frequent or at least weekly basis has been described in 7 to 15 percent (Belmaker et al., 1985; Garber et al., 1991). Fatigue is also commonly reported (Garber et al., 1991), particularly among adolescents, with 15 percent complaining of daily fatigue, and between one-third to one-half of all adolescents acknowledging fatigue on an at least weekly basis (Belmaker et al., 1985; Larson, 1991). The complaint of dizziness is also reported by 15 percent of subjects in available samples (Garber et al., 1991; Larson, 1991), and gastrointestinal symptoms other than abdominal pain such as nausea and vomiting are also commonly reported symptoms in children and adolescents (Apley, 1975; Garber et al., 1991; Larson, 1991).

Interestingly, symptoms suggestive of a neurological illness in the absence of evident neurological disease, or so-called pseudoneurologic symptoms, are quite rare in community samples of children and adolescents in Western societies (Garber et al., 1991; Rutter et al., 1970; Stefansson, Messina, & Meyerowitz, 1976). Nevertheless, conversion or pseudoneurological symptoms have received a great deal of attention in the literature, with pseudoseizures or non-epileptic seizures, unexplained falls, and faints being the most commonly reported symptoms, followed by gait abnormalities and sensory abnormalities (Goodyer, 1981; Goodyer & Mitchell, 1989; Grattan-Smith, Fairley, & Procopis, 1988; Lehmkuhl, Blanz, Lehmkuhl, & Braun-Scharm, 1989; Leslie, 1988; Maloney, 1980; Spierings et al., 1990; Steinhausen, Aster, Pfeiffer, & Gobel, 1989; Volkmar, Poll, & Lewis, 1984). Cultural factors may be relevant in the presentation of pseudoneurologic symptoms, as studies from Turkey (Turgay, 1980) and India (Srinath, Bharat, Girimaji, & Seshadri, 1993) report that conversion symptoms are a common presentation of psychiatric disorder in those populations.

Polysymptomatic presentations in pediatric somatization are quite common, and the symptoms reported often appear to cluster (Garber et al., 1991). Workers in the Ontario Child Health Study reported on a polysymptomatic somatization syndrome that was identified in 4.5 percent of the boys and 10.7 percent of the girls in the 12- to 16-year-old age group (Offord et al., 1987). Interestingly, the prevalence of polysymptomatic somatization in children younger than 12 was so low that an accurate determination of prevalence could not be made. This reinforces the clinical observation that polysymptomatic presentations are more likely to be encountered with increasing age, with multiple and frequent somatic complaints being reported in 10 to 15 percent of adolescents (Belmaker et al., 1985; Garrick, Ostrov, & Offer, 1988). Although patients often present for medical evaluation with one particular symptom, the prevalence of polysymptomatic somatization is emphasized by the finding that one-third of pediatric patients with recurrent pain suffer from additional somatic symptoms (Apley, 1958; Oster, 1972).

Additional empirical support for a "somatic complaints syndrome" in children and adolescents that is replicable across age and sex groupings is provided by a study employing principal components analysis on parent ratings of over 8,000 children and adolescents aged 6 to 16 years who were referred for mental health services (Achenbach, Conners, Quay, Verhulst, & Howell, 1989). As previously discussed, however, it is important to recognize that full-blown somatization disorder as described in previous issues of the DSM is unusual in children and adolescents, particularly given the number and type of symptoms necessary to make the diagnosis (Campo & Fritsch, 1994). Although hypochondriasis has generated much interest in the adult literature, there are no available studies addressing the prevalence of hypochondriacal concerns in the pediatric population (Campo & Fritsch, 1994; Shapiro & Rosenfeld, 1987).

Age Effects

The prevalence of somatization in general and of specific kinds of somatic complaints may vary with age. It has been suggested that recurrent abdominal pain is the most common medically unexplained physical symptom in early childhood, with headache and limb pain perhaps becoming more prominent with increasing age (Apley, 1975). Oster (1972) has reported that recurrent abdominal pain peaks in prevalence at age 9, with headache peaking at age 12. Pseudoneurological symptoms appear to become more common with increasing age throughout adolescence (Stefansson et al., 1976). Indeed, pseudoneurologic symptoms are considered quite rare before the age of 6, with many workers suggesting that clinicians should be reluctant to make the diagnosis of conversion disorder in a child younger than 6 without painstaking consideration of the presence of physical disease (Grattan-Smith et al., 1988; Lehmkuhl, Blanz, Lehmkuhl, & Braun-Scharm, 1989; Leslie, 1988; Volkmar, Poll, & Lewis, 1984). Polysymptomatic presentations appear to be more common in adolescents (Achenbach et al., 1989; Offord et al., 1987). Unfortunately, although age appears to be an important consideration in pediatric somatization, there are few

comprehensive, systematic longitudinal studies that provide convincing guidance.

Gender

In general, the prevalence of somatization in boys and girls appears to be equal in early childhood, with female symptom reporting becoming predominant during adolescence (Garber et al., 1991; Oster, 1972; Rauste-von Wright & von Wright, 1981; Walker & Greene, 1991). Although the onset of puberty and menarche in girls has been associated with increased somatic symptom reporting (Aro & Taipale, 1987; Belmaker, 1984), the differences between males and females observed during adolescence may also be explained by a decline in symptom reporting by adolescent males (Garber et al., 1991; Oster, 1972). Females are more consistent than males in their reporting of physical symptoms over time (Rauste-von Wright & von Wright, 1981; Walker & Greene, 1991). Girls also appear to be more likely to seek care for their physical complaints than are boys (Lewis & Lewis, 1989). Parents may be more likely to encourage illness behavior in girls than in boys, and mothers appear more likely to encourage illness behavior in their children than fathers (Walker & Zeman, 1992).

Pseudoneurologic or conversion symptoms may represent a special circumstance in that such symptoms appear to be more prevalent in girls, regardless of age (Goodyer & Mitchell, 1989; Looff, 1970). Available studies suggest that pseudoneurologic symptoms are twice as common in females at early ages, with the female to male ratio increasing in adolescence (Lehmkuhl et al., 1989; Leslie, 1988; Thomson & Sills, 1988; Turgay, 1980; Volkmar et al., 1984). It is unclear whether the preponderance of females experiencing conversion symptoms might be suggestive of an etiologic role for sexual maltreatment in a sub-group of this population, but the finding might encourage such speculations, given the association of pseudoneurologic symptoms with sexual maltreatment in a number of reports (Freud, 1962; Goodwin, Simms, & Bergman, 1979; Gross, 1979; LaBarbera & Dozier, 1980).

Sociocultural Factors

The potential impact of social factors, cultural factors, race, and ethnicity on the development of somatization in the pediatric population has been inadequately studied. Although low socioeconomic status and low levels of parental education have been associated with pediatric somatization (Aro et al., 1987; Steinhausen et al., 1989), other studies have failed to show such an association (Stevenson et al., 1988; Walker & Greene, 1991). As mentioned previously, pseudoneurologic symptoms may be more common in non-Western cultures (Srinath et al., 1993; Turgay, 1980).

ASSESSMENT APPROACHES

Medical Issues

High-quality assessment provides the sturdy foundation necessary for later treatment. It is essential for the thoughtful clinician to remember that medically unexplained symptoms may simply be unexplained, and may not be representative of one of the clinical conditions encompassed by the term somatization. It is often fear of undiagnosed physical disease that motivates clinicians, patients, and family members to pursue dangerous and often unnecessary medical tests and procedures. The clinician must be alert to the possibility of previously undiagnosed physical disease in virtually every patient presenting with presumably unexplained physical symptoms, but must also remain aware of the risks associated with excessive medical investigations in such patients. There may be no absolute end to the process of "ruling out" physical disease in many somatizing pediatric patients, emphasizing that clinicians may need to tolerate some degree of uncertainty, particularly early on in the assessment and treatment process (Campo, 1995).

Nevertheless, there are reports of children being diagnosed with conversion symptoms who were later found to be suffering from a physical disease (Caplan, 1970; Rivinus, Jamison, & Graham, 1975). In one study, more than 40 percent of patients diagnosed with conversion symptoms were ultimately found to have a physical disease that explained the original symptoms (Caplan, 1970). More recent samples of patients with conversion symptoms suggest that the risk of missing physical disease in somatizing children is far less, occurring in less than 10 percent of patients with unexplained physical symptoms (Maisami & Freeman, 1987; Spierings, Poels, Sijben, Gabreels, & Renier, 1990; Volkmar et al., 1984). Similarly, children with recurrent abdominal pain are identified as suffering from a physical disease in less than 10 percent of cases (Apley, 1975; Walker et al., 1994). It may be that more accurate diagnostic techniques and procedures, particularly the availability of sophisticated imaging techniques, may reduce the current risk of faulty diagnosis in presumed somatizing patients, though systematic studies of the risk of misdiagnosis are yet to be accomplished. While past reports seem to exaggerate the current risk of misdiagnosis, this should not make the modern clinician complacent.

In addition to being a potential direct cause of the physical symptoms presented by patients with presumed somatization, physical disease may be related to somatization in other ways. Suffering from a chronic medical illness in childhood may increase susceptibility to somatization (Livingston, 1993). The adult literature supports the notion that physical disease may actually serve as a risk factor for the development of somatization, with diseases affecting the central nervous system generating the greatest risk (Kellner, 1986). It is well known that patients with confirmed epilepsy commonly suffer from non-epileptic seizures or pseudoseizures (Fenton, 1986; Williams, Spiegel, & Mostofsky, 1978). Experiencing some of the benefits associated with the sick role may predispose to later somatization (Wooley, Blackwell, & Winget, 1978).

Acute illnesses or accidents in childhood and adolescence also have been associated with pediatric somatization, with a number of reports documenting the merging of a documented physical illness into what might best be considered representative of somatization (Carek & Santos, 1984; Dubowitz & Hersov, 1976; Leslie, 1988; Spierings et al., 1990). Such circumstances were recognized earlier in the century, with Creak (1938) referring to the "hysterical prolongation" of a symptom.

Pediatric somatization has also been associated with the presence of physical illness or disability in a parent or close family member (Belmaker, 1984; Bergman & Stamm, 1967; Poikolainen, Kanerva, & Lonnquist, 1995; Walker et al., 1991; Walker et al., 1994; Zuckerman, Stevenson, & Bailey, 1987). Somatizing children and adolescents may be more likely to have family members who suffer from migraine or other headaches (Apley, 1975; Mikail & von Baeyer, 1990; Robinson et al., 1990). Somatizing adults have been reported to be more likely to have experienced physical illness or hospitalization early in life (Pilowsky et al., 1982). It may be that early exposure to the psychosocial benefits associated with the sick role, either experienced directly or on the basis of the modeling of others, may serve to encourage the development of somatization (Wooley et al., 1978).

The importance of close collaboration with the referring primary care provider or any related medical specialist cannot be overemphasized. Indeed, an assessment that focuses in a non-integrated way on either medical issues or psychological and psychiatric issues will be suboptimal, given the complex interaction between mind and body. It must also be remembered that there may be no absolute end to the process of ruling out physical disease in the pediatric patient with presumably unexplained physical symptoms (Campo, 1995). Though much has been written about the risk of undiagnosed physical disease in such patients, it may be that inappropriate medical investigations, treatments, or procedures pose a far greater risk. Inappropriate tests and procedures may result in physical harm to the patient, and may also strengthen the patient's and family's convictions that a physical disease must be the likely cause of the symptoms under investigation, which can maintain somatization (Goodyer & Taylor, 1985; Grattan-Smith et al., 1988).

The clinician should communicate with any referring medical professionals and attempt to determine whether the patient has had an appropriate medical evaluation and physical examination. Previous medical records should be reviewed carefully. Records hand carried by the patient or parents, however, might best be viewed with some degree of suspicion initially. Hand-carried records might be chosen selectively, or in rare instances might contain alterations, as has been reported to occur in some cases of factitious disorder by proxy. Though there is no general rule as to when medical assessment should be considered complete, it appears reasonable to pursue medical assessment sufficient to result in a reasonable consensus among the collaborating professionals that physical disease is in all likelihood not responsible for the symptoms presented. Given the common intense worries and fears of disease among patients and their families, it is extremely difficult for the clinician to be effective in treatment until the clinician's own worries and concerns have been sufficiently alleviated. Ideally, medical assessment and psychiatric/psychological assessments may proceed concurrently, avoiding the prevailing tendency to pursue psychiatric/psychological assessment only when physical disease has been "ruled out." A concurrent approach may actually help reduce stigma by giving so-called mental disorders a place in the medical differential diagnosis.

Psychological and Psychiatric Assessment

Just as the diagnosis of physical disease requires positive findings, the determination that a given patient's symptoms may be representative of somatization should be based on positive findings rather than simply the exclusion of physical disease (Dubowitz & Hersov, 1976; Friedman, 1973; Goodyer & Taylor, 1985; Maisami & Freeman, 1987). Unfortunately, although there may be many "clues" to the presence of somatization (see Table 7.1), it is most often neither possible nor desirable to demonstrate that a given somatic symptom is "purely" psychological in nature (Campo, 1995). For example, while indifference to the symptom or "la belle indifference" has been described in some patients with conversion disorder (Leslie, 1988; Maisami & Freeman, 1987; Volkmar et al., 1984), this is a quite subjective finding of unclear significance (Dubowitz & Hersov, 1976; Goodyer, 1981; Spierings et al., 1990). It is essential to realize that virtually all of the "clues" to somatization listed in Table 7.1 may also be found in patients with physical disease (e.g., Walker et al., 1993). Nevertheless, a constellation of the "clues" listed may provide greater confidence in the diagnostic process, and be useful to the clinician in exercising clinical judgment (Friedman, 1973).

Somatization may represent one of the most common ways for psychiatric disorder to present within the primary care medical setting, and the population of children with problems representative of somatization is quite heterogeneous. Review of available studies suggests that somatization is frequently associated with evidence of psychopathology in the patient and in family members (Campo & Fritsch, 1994). This common association reinforces the importance of considering psychological/psychiatric issues early in the assessment, and ideally, concurrently with any medical assessment. Patients with physical symptoms often generate inordinate anxiety among mental health professionals, and this

Table 7.1. Clues to the Presence of Somatization

- Contiguity of the symptom with psychosocial stressors
- Intense or ongoing stressors in the life of the child
- Presence of a diagnosable psychiatric disorder
- Association of the symptom with some interpersonal, social or intrapsychic gain for the child
- Appearance of the symptom as a communicative act or as having symbolic meaning
- Existence of a model for the symptom in the family or social milieu
- Violation of known anatomic or physiologic patterns by the symptom
- Responsiveness of the symptom to suggestion, psychological treatment or placebo

(Friedman, 1973; Goodyer & Taylor, 1985)

once again reinforces the importance of multidisciplinary collaboration.

Reports of somatic symptoms on the Children's Somatization Inventory appear to correlate with self-report measures of anxiety, depression, and perceived competence in school-aged children (Garber et al., 1991). Trait anxiety, depression, and alcohol/drug use were associated positively with reports of somatic symptoms by adolescents in a Finnish study (Poikolainen et al., 1995). Studies employing questionnaires also have shown anxiety to be quite common in patients with recurrent abdominal pain as compared to normal controls (Hodges, Kline, Barbero, & Woodruff, 1985; Walker et al., 1993). Children and adolescents with medically unexplained physical symptoms also have been reported to suffer from an excess of depression (Garber et al., 1990; Hodges, Kline, Barbero, & Flanery, 1985; Kashani, Lababidi, & Jones, 1982; Kowal & Pritchard, 1990; Larson, 1991). Children 6 years of age or younger with physical symptoms thought representative of somatization have been noted to have an excess of disruptive behavioral difficulties and hyperactivity (Faull & Nicol, 1986; Stevenson et al., 1988; Zuckerman et al., 1987).

Children with recurrent abdominal pain (RAP) have been the best-studied group, and semistructured psychiatric interviews used in available studies have documented the frequent occurrence of psychiatric symptoms and disorders in patients with recurrent abdominal pain, particularly anxiety disorders (Garber, Zeman, & Walker, 1990; Walker et al., 1993; Wasserman, Whitington, & Rivera, 1988). Walker et al., (1993) found that children with RAP evidenced levels of emotional distress and somatic complaints that were indistinguishable from those of children with documented peptic disease, but higher than those of healthy children and lower than those of children with previously identified psychiatric disorders.

Further support for an association between somatization and psychopathology is provided by studies investigating the presence of somatic symptoms in children who had previously been diagnosed with psychiatric disorder. Children who have been diagnosed with anxiety disorders often suffer from a variety of somatization symptoms (Beidel, Christ, & Long, 1991; Last, 1991; Livingston, Taylor, & Crawford, 1988). Children who suffer from an anxiety disorder with prominent somatic symptoms appear to be more likely to experience school refusal (Last, 1991). Studies also have documented prominent somatic complaints in children and adolescents who have been diagnosed with depression (Carlson & Kashani, 1988; Ryan, Puig-Antich, Ambrosini,

Nelson, & Krawiec, 1987), and somatic symptoms may increase with the severity of depression, regardless of coexisting anxiety (McCauley, Carlson, & Calderon, 1991). Children who have been psychiatrically hospitalized with a variety of diagnoses appear to show high rates of somatic symptoms, particularly headaches and abdominal discomfort (Livingston et al., 1988).

There is no substitute for a careful interview of the child, with additional information being provided by interview of the parents and communication with referral sources, primary health care providers, and the school. There are a number of potential screening tools available to assess children and adolescents for the presence of psychopathology. The Stony Brook Children's Symptom Inventory (Gadow & Sprafkin, 1994) is somewhat unique in that it is a parent reported symptom checklist based on the DSM-IV. Symptoms of particular disorders are grouped together, making the instrument quite useful clinically, as this allows the clinician to quickly identify particular areas of concern simply by scanning the document. An adolescent version of the instrument is also available (Gadow & Sprafkin, 1995).

Psychiatric disorder appears to be more common in the families of somatizing children and adolescents when they are compared to families of children and adolescents without medically unexplained symptoms or physical disorders (Garber et al., 1990; Hodges, Kline, Barbero, & Flanery, 1985; Hodges, Kline, Barbero, & Woodruff, 1985; Lehmkuhl et al., 1989; Routh & Ernst, 1984; Walker & Greene, 1989; Zuckerman et al., 1987). Parents of children with recurrent abdominal pain appear to suffer more anxiety and/or depressive symptoms than the parents of normal controls (Garber et al., 1990; Hodges, Kline, Barbero, & Flanery, 1985; Hodges, Kline, Barbero, & Woodruff, 1985; Walker & Greene, 1989; Zuckerman et al., 1987). Parents of children with recurrent abdominal pain also have been reported to show an increased tendency to suffer from somatization disorder, as well as being more likely to suffer from alcoholism and antisocial behavior (Routh & Ernst, 1984).

The importance of family assessment is reinforced by evidence that somatization is often familial, with somatizing children often sharing a variety of symptoms with other family members (Apley, 1975; Garber et al., 1990; Kriechman, 1987; Mechanic, 1964; Mikail & von Baeyer, 1990; Oster, 1972; Robinson et al., 1990; Routh & Ernst, 1984; Walker et al., 1991; Walker & Greene, 1989). Children with RAP are more likely to come from families where there is a higher incidence of physical illness and greater perceived parental encouragement of illness behaviors than well children or psychiatric controls (Walker et al., 1993). The children of parents with somatization disorder appear to be at greater risk to suffer from medically unexplained physical symptoms and psychiatric disorder than children in control families (Livingston, 1993). In adults, Briquet's Syndrome, a polysymptomatic disorder related to somatization disorder, appears to cluster in the family members of affected patients and in the families of patients with anti-social personality disorder (Cloninger, Reich, & Guze, 1975). It remains unclear as to whether the clustering of somatization within families represents a genetic vulnerability or is the result of environmental factors, although some studies suggest that both environmental and genetic factors may be operative (Bohman, Cloninger, von Knorring, & Sigvardsson, 1984; Cloninger, Sigvardsson, von Knorring, & Boham, 1984). It may be that somatization and psychiatric disorder are linked by a shared vulnerability to certain personality traits that may predispose to somatization and psychiatric disorder (see Campo & Fritsch, 1994).

The parents of somatizing children have been noted in a number of studies to show a tendency toward "overprotection" and fears related to separation (Bergman & Stamm, 1967; Grattan-Smith et al., 1988; Lehmkuhl et al., 1989; Robinson et al., 1990). Such parental fears and behavior may serve to promote a sense of vulnerability in the child that may ultimately result in somatization and/or hypochondriasis (Spierings et al., 1990). Indeed, the health beliefs and practices within a given family appear to be relevant, and a number of writers have emphasized the importance of a family model for the patient's physical symptoms (Grattan-Smith et al., 1988; Leslie, 1988; Maloney, 1980, Mechanic, 1964; Mikail & von Baeyer, 1990; Mullins & Olson, 1990; Spierings et al., 1990; Volkmar et al., 1984; Wood et al., 1989; Wood, 1993).

The attention and interest shown toward a child's physical symptoms by a parent may readily influence the child's response to those symptoms (Lehmkuhl et al., 1989; Mechanic, 1964). This is not especially surprising from a behavioral perspective, and the whole notion of "secondary gain" of a particular symptom refers essentially to the social and familial reinforcement of that symptom (Wooley et al., 1978). The physical symptoms of the child may at times be understood as serving to maintain proximity to important attachment figures (Wooley et al., 1978), or as consequences of the anxiety produced when an important attachment relationship is perceived as being threatened.

Somatization has been viewed by family systems theorists as serving a special "function" within the family system, perhaps allowing the family to avoid conflict, often parental conflict, and allowing the family to preserve its day-to-day functioning (Mullins & Olson, 1990). Indeed, marital conflict is frequently reported within the families of somatizing children and adolescents (Aro et al., 1987; Aro, Hanninen, & Paronen, 1989; Leslie, 1988; Maloney, 1980; Mechanic, 1964; Rauste-von Wright & von Wright, 1981; Zuckerman et al., 1987). Difficulties in family communication have been reported (Faull & Nicol, 1986; Looff, 1970; Maloney, 1980; Wasserman et al., 1988), and the families of somatizing children have been described as being low in support, cohesion, and adaptability (Faull & Nicol, 1986; Walker & Greene, 1987; Walker, McLaughlin, & Greene, 1988). Patients with somatization are nevertheless a heterogeneous group, and it may be inappropriate to generalize. For example, Walker et al. (1993) found that families of RAP patients reported better family relationships than a psychiatric comparison group, and appeared indistinguishable from control families of children without RAP. Somatizing children often perceive themselves as having a poor relationship with one or both parents (Aro et al., 1987, 1989; Rauste von Wright & von Wright, 1981). The physical symptoms experienced by the patient have been viewed by some as serving to communicate physically what cannot be spoken, with the symptoms serving as a form of "body language" or a "plea for help" (Goodyer & Taylor, 1985; Lask & Fosson, 1989; Maisami & Freeman, 1987). Wood (1993) has proposed a biobehavioral family model of pediatric illness that attempts to integrate biological, psychological, and social processes.

The clinician should be careful to consider the presence of current or past psychosocial stressors, as review of available studies suggests that there may be an association between negative life events and somatization in childhood and adolescence (see Campo & Fritsch, 1994). The relationship between negative life events may be complex, with particular types of children—such as those who are low in social competence—being especially vulnerable to somatization in response to life events (Walker et al., 1994). A recent study of adolescents found a positive association between somatic symptom reporting and the presence of a serious illness in the family, parental discord, break-up of a romantic relationship, and school failure (Poikolaonen et al., 1995). Pediatric somatization has been associated with the loss or death of a family member or relative (Aro, 1987; Aro et al., 1989; Greene, Walker, Hickson, & Thompson, 1985; Hodges, Kline, Barbero, & Flanery, 1984; Livingston, 1993; Maloney, 1980; Scaloubaca, Slade, & Creed, 1988). Maloney (1980) reports that the somatizing child's symptoms may at times mirror physical symptoms that were suffered by a lost relative or attachment figure. Most importantly, the clinician should be alert to the possibility of maltreatment in the somatizing child, as there have been a number of reports that associate the development of somatization with prior maltreatment, particularly sexual abuse (Klevan & DeJong, 1990; Livingston et al., 1988; Rimza, Berg, & Locke, 1988).

INTERVENTION STRATEGIES

General Principles

The approach to treatment to be discussed relies upon information provided by clinical case reports and descriptive studies, as well as cumulative clinical experience. Controlled trials of treatment are lacking, with the exception being a few studies that employed self-monitoring techniques and cognitive behavioral methods in the successful treatment of children with recurrent abdominal pain (Finney, Lemanek, Cataldo, Katz, & Fuqua, 1989; Sanders et al., 1989; Sanders, Shepherd, Cleghorn, & Woolford, 1994). Most available treatment reports have focused on single cases or have described multimodal interventions.

Once again, it is important to emphasize that the assessment process lays the foundation for successful intervention. During the assessment, the clinician needs to express a willingness to avoid prejudging the etiology of the patient's symptoms, and to communicate a desire to truly understand the problem, as well as a sense of empathy for the suffering of the patient and the family. It is essential that the reality of the somatizing patient's suffering be acknowledged. The clinician should avoid challenging the subjective reality of the physical symptom, and should not rush to reframe it in purely psychological terms. Acknowledging the symptoms of patients who have come to believe that their suffering may somehow be "illegitimate" or indicative of personal weakness or lack of will is important in helping to frame the problem as one that is understood, and as such, one that can be solved or managed.

The patient's difficulties should be addressed like those presented by any other illness, and the diagnosis stated in a positive manner (Campo, 1995). Formal treatment should only begin following an interactive discussion with patient and family in which the clinician's impression is communicated in a clear and frank manner. The clinician should be careful to avoid communicating any sense of reticence or embarrassment regarding the diagnosis of somatoform disorder or any other re-lated psychiatric disorder, as this may reinforce the very stigma that can interfere with treatment efforts.

Although many children and adolescents who present with medically unexplained symptoms can be confidently diagnosed with a somatoform disorder once evaluation is complete, there are instances in which diagnostic uncertainty persists. A successful treatment response may provide supportive evidence that the patient's difficulties have a significant psychological component and may reflect somatization. Furthermore, a positive treatment response could allow the patient to avoid potentially dangerous and costly medical or surgical evaluations and treatments. It is important in such circumstances for the treating professional to speak openly and frankly with the patient and family members in order to ensure informed consent. Unfortunately, diagnostic uncertainty and the anxieties of treating professionals are often responsible for many treatment failures, with treatment being interrupted repeatedly by a resurgence of patient, family, or clinician anxiety in relation to the physical symptoms. This reinforces the importance of multidisciplinary collaboration, as work with a collaborating professional can help assuage the anxieties of mental health professionals who treat difficult somatizing patients.

Initially, reassurance that the patient's problem will not result in death or physical handicap may be helpful in and of itself, and has been advocated in the treatment of somatizing adults (Kellner, 1991) and children (Goodyer & Mitchell, 1989; Grattan Smith et al., 1988; Maisami & Freeman, 1987; Schulman, 1988; Thomson & Sills, 1988). Excessive reassurance, however, may actually serve to maintain somatization in some patients with obsessional features and hypochondriacal fears, and should be minimized over the long term (Warwick & Salkovskis, 1985). Nevertheless, it is exceedingly difficult to reframe the patient's and family's expectations of treatment without first providing some degree of reassurance that serious physical disease is not likely to be present. Ideally, this may reduce their cumulative anxiety by communicating that the problem presented is common, well understood, and treatable.

Most patients and families think about treatment in terms of a traditional medical model, with the assumption being that the professional will assume responsibility for the patient's "cure." It is essential that the clinician communicate with the patient and family that successful treatment will require a collaborative venture in which the patient, the family, and the professionals will share responsibility for the outcome. It is also important to delineate as clearly as possible what the nature of those individual responsibilities will be. The patient and family should be encouraged to establish realistic goals for treatment, and a promise of cure should be avoided (Kellner, 1991).

While reassuring the patient and family regarding the physical threat posed by the illness, clinicians should be clear regarding the very real functional impairment and interference with daily life that the patient's suffering has engendered. It is also wise for the clinician to communicate that the diagnosis of a somatoform disorder may in fact be "good news," given the physical diseases that might have been possibilities within the differential diagnosis.

Many patients and families have had the experience of being treated by prior clinicians with exaggerated deference, most likely as a result of the clinician's fear that the patient or family may become angry with the suggestion that the patient's complaints were representative of somatization. Many physicians have been tempted to employ placebo in the treatment, or to "play along" with the idea that the patient's problems were indeed caused by physical disease. Such behavior is risky in that patients and families treated in such a manner may become convinced by the physician's behavior that a serious physical disease is truly present, which might later serve to intensify and/or maintain somatization and any associated disability. The use of placebo might increase the likelihood of children viewing themselves as sickly and more vulnerable to physical disease than their age mates.

Traditionally, the treatment of somatizing children has been conceptualized as a two-step process, with the first step involving removal of the symptom, followed by more traditional psychological interventions (Shapiro & Rosenfeld, 1987). Methods employed in symptom removal have included suggestion (Proctor, 1958; Rock, 1971), encouragement (Gold, 1965), or the use of chemical abreaction with medications such as amobarbital (Laybourne & Churchill, 1972). At present, clinical experience argues that withholding other interventions until symptom removal is accomplished is often unproductive, though most workers in the field would agree that helping the patient and family view the presenting symptom or symptoms as being less threatening is ultimately beneficial, decreasing anxiety in the system and allowing other treatment interventions to be introduced (Kellner, 1986; Kotsopolous & Snow, 1986; Lehmkuhl et al., 1989; Maisami & Freeman, 1987; Schulman, 1988).

A *rehabilitative approach* to somatizing children and adolescents is favored, with the patient being encouraged to return to usual activities, and an effort being made to discourage behaviors associated with the sick role (Dubowitz & Hersov, 1976; Leslie, 1988; Maisami & Freeman, 1987; Schulman, 1988). The rehabilitative approach serves an important function in that it allows a shift of responsibility to the patient for a successful return to healthy functioning, which undermines the notion that the patient can only return to school or other important areas of functioning when the symptoms presented have been "cured" by the treating clinician. The patient's role is reframed from one in which the patient is a passive recipient of care to one in which the patient is an active collaborator with the professional and with the family. This approach acknowledges the power of the symptom, as well as the power of sick role expectations, yet makes overcoming the symptom an accomplishment that the patient can be proud of, and that the family can praise and communicate their sense of admiration for the patient's efforts. Several authors have recommended the use of physical therapy in the treatment of certain patients with pseudoneurologic symptoms (Dubowitz & Hersov, 1976; Leslie, 1988; Maisami & Freeman, 1987; Thomson & Sills, 1988), which allows a gradual return of the patient to prior functioning, and which may allow the patient to give up the symptom "with honor" (Bolton & Cohen, 1986).

Psychotherapy

The successful treatment of somatization in children and adolescents is based on sound behavioral principles. The cooperation and collaboration of parents and often family members are essential to successful behavioral treatment. The mainstay of any treatment effort is finding a way to reward the patient for healthy and adaptive behavior. The use of *positive reinforcement* in such an effort has been emphasized by a number of workers in the field (Delameter, Rosenbloom, Conners, & Hertweck, 1983; Dubowitz & Hersov, 1976; Klonoff & Moore, 1986; Lehmkuhl et al., 1989; Maisami & Freeman, 1987; Mansdorf, 1981; Mizes, 1985; Sank & Biglan, 1974).

Coincident with finding a way to positively reinforce adaptive behavior, the rewards associated with the sick role should be minimized. The practice of "minimizing secondary gain" can best be conceptualized as representative of *extinction* or *withdrawal of reinforcement* of the symptom (Delameter et al., 1983). The actual process involved in "minimizing secondary gain" may present many practical problems, as parents may have difficulty with this process, often as a result of some combination of their own fears and concerns that the child may be treated "unfairly," and the influence of family systems issues which may help preserve old patterns of behavior. It should also be mentioned that *time-out* has been utilized in the treatment of somatization, with a case report in the literature of a 10-year-old girl with RAP who was successfully treated by a time-out procedure that resulted in a reduction of pain complaints over the course of treatment (Miller & Kratochwill, 1979). Clinical experience argues that *punishment* per se is not advisable in the vast majority of cases of somatization in childhood, though firmness and a willingness to place expectations upon the child that family members or other professionals might find somewhat "unfair" may be necessary to return the patient to normal functioning. A related approach to those mentioned above consists of lifting restrictions that have been imposed by the illness, such as allowing discharge from the hospital only with functional improvement, or restricting outside activities with peers until functional improvement is achieved; such an approach is representative of *negative reinforcement* (Leslie, 1988). Any successful treatment program will incorporate elements of some of the above-mentioned approaches in all likelihood. Maintaining a longitudinal view and an understanding of the functional disability associated with somatization might help the clinician disabuse family members or other professionals of the common "misplaced sense of kindness" that can perpetuate or maintain childhood somatization.

Cognitive behavioral methods have been utilized. A controlled trial of psychotherapy that employed a cognitive behavioral approach in the treatment of children with recurrent abdominal pain has been reported (Sanders et al., 1989). The authors employed a multimodal treatment method that included differential reinforcement of healthy behavior, cognitive coping skills training, and self-monitoring techniques in school-age children with recurrent abdominal pain. Though the sample size was small, the positive results of the study are encouraging, with the treated group of patients faring significantly better than controls. In an extension of this research, a cognitive-behavioral family intervention was compared to standard pediatric care for 7- to 14-year-old children with RAP, and resulted in higher levels of parental satisfaction with treatment, greater improvements in functionality, higher rates of complete elimination of the pain, and lower levels of relapse at 6- and 12-month follow-up than standard pediatric care (Sanders et al., 1994).

In another small controlled trial of treatment of children with RAP in a primary care setting, multimodal treatment that included self-monitoring of the symptoms, limiting parental reinforcement of illness behavior, relaxation training, administration of a dietary fiber supplement, and strong encouragement of participation in routine activities such as school was successful in reducing complaints of pain, school absenteeism, and health care utilization as compared to an untreated control group (Finney et al., 1989). Interestingly, the reduction in medical care utilization was not accounted for by an effect on RAP-related visits alone, suggesting some reduction in visits for other illnesses and complaints. Though it is unclear which component or copmponents of the multimodal interventions described were effective, such trials are important in that they are more likely to approximate clinical practice and demonstrate that a salutary effect of treatment is possible.

Other authors have discussed the use of self-management techniques such as training in coping and relaxation (Linton, 1986; Masek, Russo, & Varni, 1984), hypnosis (Caldwell & Stewart, 1981; Elkins & Carter, 1986; Williams & Singh, 1976), and the use of biofeedback (Klonoff & Moore, 1986; Mizes, 1985).

Psychodynamic and interpersonal approaches also should be considered, and it is useful for any treatment to be "psychodynamically informed." Just as there may be external gains associated with a particular symptom, there may be internal or intrapsychic gains as well. This has been referred to by psychodynamic writers as the "primary gain" of the symptom, which may allow the patient to avoid potentially troublesome or painful affects, thoughts, or memories (Simon, 1991). Individual expressive psychotherapy is widely employed, although there are no controlled studies of its efficacy. Helping patients to express and identify emotions of which they may have been unaware, and exploring the subjective meaning of the symptom may be helpful. Expressive techniques such as verbal expression and keeping a journal may be especially helpful when somatization follows a traumatic event (Pennebaker & Susman, 1988).

There are no reports regarding the use of group psychotherapy in the treatment of somatizing children and adolescents. A group setting might offer benefits for at least some young patients suffering with somatization, and should be studied further.

The use of family therapy in the treatment of children and adolescents with somatization has generated a great deal of interest and enthusiasm, and appears to make good clinical sense in many instances (Goodyer, 1981; Liebman, Hoenig, & Berger, 1976; Mullins & Olson, 1990). It is difficult to conceptualize any successful treatment of children that does not involve some work with parents and families. The work of Minuchin and colleagues (1975) with patients with a variety of so-called psychosomatic conditions has emphasized a view of the patient's physical symptoms as serving a particular function within the family system. They suggested that a focus of the family on the child's physical symptoms may detour the family from important areas of conflict, and serve to preserve familial homeostasis. They have also described specific patterns of family interaction including enmeshment, parental overprotection, familial rigidity, and poor conflict resolution and conflict avoidance (Minuchin et al., 1975; Minuchin, Rosman, & Baker, 1978). A family systems approach to patients with somatization has been described by Mullins and Olson (1990). Wood (1993) has critically examined earlier conceptualizations of family systems issues in such patients and makes a sophisticated attempt to integrate biological and psychosocial models. Unfortunately, despite the great interest in family therapy, research regarding its efficacy in pediatric somatization is lacking.

Close collaboration with the primary care physician or referring specialist is extremely important. Many somatizing children have been seen by multiple physicians, with each physician having little knowledge of what others may have recommended. In most circumstances, the medical care of somatizing children should be consolidated with a single primary physician or team leader. This improves communication, and also decreases the risk of treatment efforts being diluted or confused. Work with adults with somatization disorder has demonstrated that something as simple as a consultation letter from the consulting psychiatrist to the primary care physician outlining ways of approaching such patients was effective in improving patient satisfaction with healthcare and in reducing healthcare expenditures (Smith, Monson, & Ray, 1986). An extension of that work to somatizing patients with a lifetime history of six to twelve unexplained physical symptoms demonstrated an improvement of physical functioning and a significant cost-offset for patients receiving the treatment intervention (Smith, Rost, & Kashner, 1995).

For some persistently somatizing patients, regularly scheduled office visits to the primary care physician may be of benefit, as patients are able to see the physician without the requirement that they be sick. The physician can become an important attachment figure for many chronically somatizing patients and their family members. Helping primary care providers to remember this is exceedingly important, as patients and families may fear that involvement in treatment with a mental health professional will jeopardize their relationship with the referring health care provider. Without the continued involvement of the referring health care professional, many patients and families will feel "dis-missed" or "passed on," which serves to maintain the stigma often associated with somatization.

Equally important is close communication with the school, particularly with patients for whom school absenteeism or school refusal is an issue. School officials might benefit from a better understanding of the patient's difficulties. Moreover, it should be made clear to all those involved that medical excuses for missed school on the basis of somatization are not acceptable. This requires close collaboration between the treating mental health professional, the primary care physician, the parents, and the school. It is sometimes necessary to communicate to the patient that absence from school without the approval of the collaborative treatment team and an appropriate medical excuse will be viewed as truancy, and that the school will take action accordingly. In many instances, a thoughtful letter to the school can benefit treatment efforts, particularly when the primary care physician and the school understand that medical excuses for any absences need to come from that physician alone, thus circumventing the tendency to "doctor shop," particularly for medical excuses.

Pharmacological Treatments

There are no available studies in the literature regarding the use of psychotropic medication in the treatment of children and adolescents with somatization per se. Nevertheless, many such patients suffer from concomitant anxiety, depression, or other psychiatric difficulties that may be amenable to treatment with medication. Antidepressant medication has been found to reduce somatic symptoms in depressed adults, and anxiolytic medications such as benzodiazepenes and antidepressants alleviate somatic symptoms in patients suffering from anxiety disorders, including panic disorder (see Kellner, 1991).

Clinical experience suggests that there are many young patients who benefit from the use of psychotropic medication in the relief of medically unexplained physical symptoms, particularly recurrent complaints of pain or fatigue. In those patients who may experience physical symptoms associated with emotional arousal and anxiety, a short course of anxiolytic medication might be beneficial. The use of a benzodiazepine over the short term may be very helpful in demonstrating to the patient and family that many of their physical symptoms are the result of anxiety and symptoms of emotional arousal rather than the product of a serious physical disease. Other patients appear to respond well to antidepressant medications, such as tricyclic antidepressants and selective serotonin reuptake inhibitors (SSRIs). The SSRIs may be especially useful in anxious patients and in patients with comorbid anxiety and depression. They are generally well tolerated, but should be begun at a low dose and gradually titrated upward, given the prevalence of anxiety and the sensitivity of many somatizing patients to side effects. Theoretically, SSRIs may benefit patients with obsessional illness worry, given their efficacy in the treatment of pediatric obsessive compulsive disorder (e.g., Riddle et al., 1992). In sum, comorbid psychiatric disorders should be treated aggressively, and the careful use of medication in such circumstances may be warranted. Controlled trials with children and adolescents with specific disorders are needed. The interested reader is referred to reviews by Kutcher, Reiter, and Gardner (1995) and Allen, Leonard, and Swedo (1995) for more detailed information regarding the treatment of pediatric anxiety disorders, and to Riddle (1995a; 1995b) for a more comprehensive review of recent developments in pediatric psychopharmacology.

Hospitalization

Although most somatizing children and adolescents are best managed on an outpatient basis, inpatient treatment may be beneficial in a number of circumstances, including cases involving refractory school refusal and persistent somatization where outpatient and other treatment options have been exhausted, or in cases of significant diagnostic uncertainty. Potential benefits of inpatient pediatric treatment of somatization in children and adolescents have been reported (Goodyer, 1985; Kotsopolous & Snow, 1986; Lemkuhl et al., 1989; Leslie, 1988; Maisami & Freeman, 1987). Inpatient treatment allows for close observation by skilled personnel, and greater control over the behavioral treatment of the patient (Delameter et al., 1983). The child is removed from the environment in which the symptoms developed, and inpatient staff can model alternative ways of dealing with the patient for family members and school personnel. Moreover, the improvement in functioning that can be orchestrated in an inpatient setting may help reassure family members that psychosocial treatment interventions are worthy of consideration, and may diminish family anxiety associated with the symptoms. Inpatient treatment that is truly multidisciplinary is necessary, and may be accomplished on a pediatric medical psychiatry inpatient unit (Campo & Raney, 1995). Rigorous discharge planning is essential, with many of the principles previously discussed being employed in formulating the discharge plan.

Course and Prognosis

The course and prognosis of pediatric somatization has been inadequately studied. There are few systematic longitudinal studies of pediatric somatization. Furthermore, available studies vary in the types of patients selected and the diagnoses applied, as well as in the length of time of follow-up. Follow-up assessments have been limited and not systematic across most studies. It is also significant that most studies have looked at the presence or absence of the original symptom as the sole outcome measure. Other outcomes such as functional status or psychiatric status also should be assessed (Campo & Fritsch, 1994).

Follow-up studies of children and adolescents with recurrent abdominal pain show that 25 to 50 percent continue to experience some degree of abdominal discomfort in adulthood (Apley & Hale 1972; Christensen & Mortensen, 1975; Liebman, 1978; Stickler & Murphy, 1979; Stone & Barbero, 1970). In a recent follow-up study that examined RAP patients five to six years after original assessment, former RAP patients reported significantly higher levels of abdominal discomfort, other somatic symptoms, and functional disability than did formerly healthy controls (Walker, Garber, Van Slyke, & Greene, 1995). In addition, former RAP patients were reported by parents to have higher levels of internalizing emotional symptoms such as anxiety and depression than former well patients in the study, and RAP patients had significantly higher levels of mental health service utilization. There was also a trend suggesting that former RAP patients visited medical clinics more frequently in the year prior to the follow-up assessment.

In patients with pseudoneurologic or conversion symptoms, significant clinical improvement or complete recovery has been reported in 50 to 100 percent of such patients (Goodyer, 1981; Goodyer & Mitchell, 1989; Grattan-Smith et al., 1988; Kotsopolous & Snow, 1986; Lehmkuhl et al., 1989; Leslie, 1988; Maisami & Freeman, 1987; Proctor, 1958; Spierings et al., 1990; Turgay, 1990).

The variables that predict later outcome are currently unknown, and although multiple somatic symptoms and greater chronicity of somatization have been reported to predict poor outcomes (Ernst, Routh, & Harper, 1984; Grattan-Smith et al., 1988; Robins & O'Neal, 1953), other studies do not support this (Goodyer & Mitchell,

1989; Lehmkuhl et al., 1989; Walker et al., 1991). Conversion symptoms or pseudoneurologic symptoms may be especially predictive of later functional impairment (Goodyer & Mitchell, 1989; Robins & O'Neal, 1953). Given the relative lack of reliable information relating to prognosis in pediatric somatization, it is especially difficult to determine what role treatment plays in influencing outcome.

Collaborative Treatment

Given that somatization is relatively common in the pediatric medical setting, mental health professionals need to take an active role in the education of health care professionals, especially in primary care settings. This would include help in identifying appropriate screening measures for psychiatric disorder, and in familiarizing primary care professionals with how important it is to incorporate psychological issues and concerns fully in the assessment process of patients with common physical symptoms such as recurrent abdominal pain or headaches. Communicating a willingness to be available for telephone consultation is important, as physicians may be unsure about which of their patients may benefit from referral to a mental health professional.

Ideally, mental health professionals should strongly consider maintaining a physical presence in the primary care medical setting, or even in subspecialty clinics, as this allows for greater coordination of collaborative efforts. Further, a presence in the medical setting undermines the institutionalized dichotomy between mind and body that can be so stigmatizing and destructive in the treatment of somatization. True integration of mental health services within the medical setting allows a seamless integration of the medical and the psychiatric/psychological, potentially making assessment and treatment unified processes. An outline of the approach to the pediatric patient with somatization is provided in Table 7.2.

CASE ILLUSTRATION

Clinical Presentation

David presented for consultation at age 15, after reluctantly accepting a referral from a school counselor. David was an excellent student who was well liked by teachers and peers, though he had always been somewhat shy and socially inhibited. He had developed an ap-

Table 7.2. Suggestions for Professionals: An Approach to the Pediatric Patient with Somatization

- Acknowledge the reality of the patient's suffering and the family's concern
- Do not challenge the reality of the symptom(s)
- Communicate an unwillingness to prejudge the cause of the symptom(s)
- Be alert to undiagnosed physical disease, but remember the risks of excessive medical investigation
- Avoid diagnosis by exclusion alone; look for positive evidence of somatization
- Identify social or interpersonal reinforcers for the symptom(s)
- Begin psychiatric assessment early
- Consider the possibility of maltreatment
- Discuss the diagnosis frankly with patient and family
- Avoid communicating any sense of embarrassment regarding the diagnosis
- Take a rehabilitative approach; avoid the promise of a cure
- Minimize reinforcement of the sick role
- Identify and reward responsible, health promoting behavior
- Maintain a unified treatment approach, with clearly defined expectations for the patient, the family, and the professionals involved in collaborative care
- Emphasize the importance of school attendance; avoid homebound instruction
- Attempt to consolidate medical care with a single provider

parent viral illness shortly after returning to school in the fall, and appeared to recover, but shortly thereafter began to complain of a progression of fluctuating physical symptoms, including fatigue, abdominal discomfort, chest pain and headaches. School attendance became increasingly sporadic, and he stopped attending school altogether after several weeks. At the time of evaluation, he had not been back to school for three full weeks. He had been medically evaluated by his family doctor and a number of medical specialists, including a surgeon, a gastroenterologist, a cardiologist, and a neurologist. A number of investigations, including electrocardiogram, Holter monitoring, esophagogastroduodenoscopy, electroencephalogram, and magnetic resonance imaging of the head were unremarkable, as were the results of extensive blood laboratory examinations. The family and patient had been told that the doctors "couldn't find anything wrong," though the neurologist suggested that David's headaches might be a mixed presentation of migraine and tension headaches. The parents had become increasingly frightened that a serious disease had been missed. The patient began to worry that he might have a brain tumor or another type of cancer, though he doubted that he truly had a life-threatening illness. He became fearful of leaving the home, as he was concerned that he would develop physical symptoms away from his parents, whom he considered to be a source of comfort and support.

His parents were especially resentful of psychiatric referral, which they perceived as being "given the brush-off" by their family doctor. They had agreed to see a mental health professional a few months earlier, and he had diagnosed David as suffering from depression. David and his parents experienced this as insufficient to explain his difficulties, and considered his low mood to be a consequence rather than a cause of his physical suffering. The second referral was accepted only at the urging of the school.

Assessment Findings

The initial history revealed no prior history of mental health consultation other than the recent consultation that had resulted in a diagnosis of depression. An early history of a shy, inhibited temperament and difficulties with novelty was elicited, as well as a history of separation fears during the early school years. Following the presumed viral illness in the fall, he acknowledged a change in mood, with predominant dysphoria, increased irritability, an increased need for sleep, a slight decrease in appetite associated with a slight loss of weight, decreased enjoyment of his usual activities, and a decreased sense of motivation, all of which he considered to be consequences of his physical illness.

David reported that some of his physical symptoms occurred in discrete "spells," during which he would experience the abrupt onset of dizziness or lightheadedness variably associated with palpitations, chest pain, abdominal discomfort, the sensation of a lump in his throat, problems catching his breath, tremor, feeling warm, and sweating. He admitted feeling fearful during the "spells," which lasted from a few minutes to as long as an hour, and occurred several times per week. He denied any specific fears or obsessive-compulsive symptoms, though he was clearly perfectionistic. There was no evidence of any death wish, suicidality, psychosis, delirium, bipolar illness, conduct difficulties, or alcohol/substance abuse, and no history of maltreatment of any sort.

David lived at home with his parents and was their youngest child. An older sister had left home for college in the fall, and although David acknowledged missing her, he and his parents attempted to minimize any disruption to family life. The parents appeared to be concerned and caring, but suspicious of professionals. The family was described as quite "close," and the mother admitted that David had always had a special relationship with her. He was somewhat distant from his father, whom he considered somewhat coarse and poorly educated. The marital relationship between the parents was strained, and the mother complained openly about how disruptive it had been when the father had lost his job on an assembly line earlier in the year and was now at home. The maternal grandmother had died within the year, and the mother reported feeling somewhat "down" for a few months afterward, but insisted that she had "kept this to herself" and maintained that it had had little effect on David, who had not been especially close to the grandmother in her view. The family history was remarkable for a history of untreated and unrecognized panic anxiety and probable dysthymia in the mother, as well as migraine, and anxiety and probable obsessive-compulsive disorder in the father, who also acknowledged depressive symptoms following the loss of his job. There was a history of alcohol abuse in the paternal grandfather.

Available medical records were reviewed and the referring physician was contacted by telephone. The family physician was confident that a serious disease had not been missed, and felt that the patient's symptoms were related to anxiety and "stress," but had been reluctant to discuss this openly with the family for fear of alienating them.

Treatment Selection and Course

It was abundantly clear that beginning by attempting to reframe David's symptoms as being representative of psychiatric disorder would be met with significant resistance and in all likelihood would be unsuccessful from a practical standpoint. From a descriptive psychiatric perspective, he appeared to be a boy with a premorbid shy, behaviorally inhibited temperament, who had experienced separation anxiety earlier in life, and who had recently developed symptoms consistent with both panic disorder with agoraphobia and major depression. He nevertheless suffered from abdominal discomfort, headaches, and other physical symptoms that appeared to be quite real subjectively. Biological vulnerabilities included a family history of anxiety disorder and depression, and a personal history of migraine and functional abdominal pain, which are known to be associated with symptoms of both anxiety and depression. The development of his symptoms appeared to be related to several stresssors, including the death of the grandmother and the sister's leaving home, which appeared to stimulate separation concerns and emotional arousal throughout the family. From a systemic perspective, his symptoms appeared to provide a diversion for the parents from their own conflicts; their focus on David seemed to make it easier for them to avoid confronting the fact that they would soon be alone together.

It was clear that it would first be important to cement rapport with the patient and his family, and arrive at a shared working conceptualization of his difficulties. David and his parents appeared relieved that his symptoms were considered to be quite real and worthy of attention, and talked at some length about how they had felt misunderstood and dismissed by his doctors. They were angry at what they had viewed as David being treated as a "faker" or malingerer, and were pleased and surprised to learn that his problems were not uncommon. They were reassured that his presentation did not appear to signify a serious physical disease, and that review of the medical records was unremarkable.

The complexity of the mind-body relationship was discussed in several ways, first by informing them of the relationship between migraine and psychopathology, and later by a discussion of the physiology of emotional arousal and its mediation by the autonomic nervous system. His symptoms were reviewed, and the patient and family were asked to interrupt if anything presented in the review or the conceptualization of his problems appeared to be incorrect. The diagnoses of panic disorder and depression were discussed, but the reality of the physical suffering was not denied, and a false dichotomy between the physical and the emotional was avoided. Current stressors were discussed, and specific family issues were reviewed in a tentative manner, going as far as the family seemed capable of tolerating. A review of available treatments was presented, including self-management techniques that might allow the patient to achieve a greater degree of control over his body processes than he might think possible, cognitive-behavioral approaches, expressive psychotherapy, family therapy, and the use of medication.

A rehabilitative approach was proposed, and the importance of a schedule, regular exercise, and a return to school was emphasized. He was informed that the physical symptoms he experienced were often chronic in nature, but that by working as a team we could do our best to ensure that his symptoms would no longer control and limit his life. Expectations of David and his parents that a return to full function should only follow a "cure" were discouraged. It was agreed that the school would be contacted and prior absences excused providing that David agreed to return to school immediately, and that a single physician manage his medical care and the administration of any future school excuses. Additional medical investigations or referrals to medical subspecialists were discouraged, but it was stressed that a change in his status or the development of new symptoms would be taken seriously by the medical team. With the permission of the patient and the parents, a letter was sent to the school explaining David's condition, making explicit that the presenting symptoms were not a legitimate excuse for continued absenteeism, and identifying the physician who would be responsible for determining the legitimacy of any future school excuses.

David and his parents were initially resistant to conceptualizing his difficulties as representative of psychiatric disorder, but were agreeable to his learning some self-management techniques, such as relaxation training and self-monitoring as they grudgingly accepted that his symptoms might be related to stress. They also felt that talking regularly about his current life stress would be helpful, but were unwilling to consider other approaches, including suggestions that both parents might benefit from psychiatric evaluation and treatment, and that they might benefit from work as a couple or a family.

A few sessions of individual psychotherapy allowed training in relaxation and cognitive-behavioral approaches to his symptoms, and there was some initial decrease in physical complaints, but no significant resolution. David returned to school for a few days, but then abruptly refused to attend, complaining of persistence of his physical symptoms. As parental frustration peaked, David surprised everyone by coming into his session and announcing that he had "figured out what was wrong" after viewing a television program during which a woman discussed her struggle with panic disorder and its eventual successful treatment. He experienced this as a self-discovery, and seemed oblivious to the fact that the diagnosis had been previously made but rejected. He inquired about the use of medication, and agreed to a trial of sertraline after discussion of potential risks, benefits, and side effects. He was begun on 25 mg each morning, but experienced an increase in anxiety and feelings of restlesssness despite the relatively low dose. He agreed to continue the medication only after beginning clonazepam 0.25 mg given orally twice daily. The sertraline was increased over the next several months to 100 mgs per day, and the clonazepam was tapered and discontinued. His panic anxiety diminished and ultimately resolved, his mood showed significant improvement, and his physical symptoms showed gradual improvement. Although he continued to report intermittent abdominal discomfort and headaches, the intensity of the symptoms and his emotional reaction to them appeared to be significantly diminished.

While the medication was being initiated, other efforts took place, including greater involvement of the parents in treatment and liaison with the school to develop a schedule for a graduated return, which was successfully negotiated over the next several weeks. Individual therapy progressed over the next three months, with David talking more openly about his own concerns related to separation and his developing autonomy in relation to his family, particularly his mother. He worked hard to face his fears and restructured his thinking regarding his experience of physical symptoms of emotional arousal. He became more involved with his peers after returning to school, and resumed his previously solid academic performance, despite being forced to attend summer school to complete work necessary for academic promotion. The parents agreed to participate in limited family work as an adjunct to his individual sessions, but preferred to keep the focus on David and his physical symptoms. They remained resistant to outside referral for individual evaluation or couples therapy.

Termination and Follow-Up

David's parents abruptly announced that they felt he was "his old self" after ten meetings for combined individual and parent work, as well as medication follow-up. They expressed concerns about the costs of continued treatment, and felt it was no longer necessary. David felt he was doing significantly better, but seemed reluctant to discontinue his psychotherapeutic work. The potential negatives of discontinuing treatment were discussed, including the unresolved family issues, but it was agreed that moving to monthly medication management would not be unreasonable providing that David continued in school and maintained his social functioning. After several months of medication follow-up, David called to communicate that his family doctor would prescribe his sertraline at his parents' request. After an extended discussion with David and his parents, they were instructed regarding how they might recognize any deterioration in David's status in the future, and the treatment relationship was terminated with a transfer of responsibility to the family physician. Recommendations for future management were communicated to the primary care physician in a letter, as well as an offer to be available for future consultation.

Two years later, David is preparing to graduate from high school and is planning to attend college away from home. He had discontinued the sertraline after approximately one year of successful treatment. He had done reasonably well for several months, but anxiety and depressive symptoms recurred during his senior year in high school, which resulted in a resumption of the sertraline by the family physician and resolution of his symptoms. Interestingly, David did not become especially concerned about his physical symptoms, interpreting them as indicative of a return of his panic anxiety and depression. Significant family conflict persists. David has been arguing more with his parents, who have come to view him as increasingly defiant, despite continued excellent performance behaviorally and academically at school. He has become more social and active with his peers, and recently began to date. He is not in any formal treatment with a mental health professional, but continues to follow-up with his family physician and intermittently practices his relaxation exercises.

SUMMARY

Medically unexplained physical symptoms are common in children and adolescents, and are the source of great confusion for primary care physicians, medical subspecialists, mental health professionals, and affected children and families. Such symptoms may serve as a common presentation of psychiatric disorder in the pediatric setting, and may be responsible for costly, inappropriate, and potentially dangerous overutilization of health care services. Further research is required in this important area, which provides an important window into the complexities of the relationship between mind and body, and highlights the importance of multidisciplinary collaboration and cooperation. Pediatric psychologists and psychiatrists have much to contribute to clinical work in medical settings, and to the expansion of the current knowledge base. Developing empirically based models for intervention and consultation in primary care settings should become a priority for mental health professionals, and determining how interventions with somatizing children and adolescents might add value to health care and ultimately prove cost-effective may help undermine the artificial boundaries between physical and mental health.

REFERENCES

Achenbach, T. M., Conners, C. K., Quay, H. C., Verhulst, F. C., & Howell, C. T. (1989). Replication of empirically derived syndromes as a basis for taxonomy of child/adolescent psychopathology. *Journal of Abnormal Child Psychology, 17*, 299–323.

Allen, A. J., Leonard, H., & Swedo, S. E. (1995). Current knowledge of medications for the treatment of childhood anxiety disorders. *Journal of the American Academy of Child and Adolescent Psychiatry, 34*, 976–986.

American Psychiatric Association. (1987). *Diagnostic and statistical manual of mental disorders* (3rd ed., rev.; DSM-III-R). Washington, DC: Author.

American Psychiatric Association. (1994). *Diagnostic and statistical manual of mental disorders* (4th ed.; DSM-IV). Washington, DC: Author.

Apley, J. (1975). *The child with abdominal pain*. Oxford: Blackwell.

Apley, J. (1958). A common denominator in the recurrent pains of childhood. *Proceedings of the Royal Society of Medicine, 51*, 1023–1024.

Apley, J., & Hale, B. (1973). Children with recurrent abdominal pain: How do they grow up? *British Medical Journal, 3*, 7–9.

Apley, J., & Naish, N. (1958). Recurrent abdominal pains: A field survey of 1,000 school children. *Archives of Diseases of Children, 33*, 165–170.

Aro, H., & Taipale, V. (1987). The impact of timing of puberty on psychomatic symptoms among fourteen to sixteen year old Finnish girls. *Child Development, 58*, 261–268.

Aro, H., Paronen, O., & Aro, S. (1987). Psychosomatic symptoms among 14–16 year old Finnish adolescents. *Social Psychiatry, 22*, 171–176.

Aro, H., Hanninen, V., & Paronen, O. (1989). Social support, life events and psychosomatic symptoms among 14–16 year old adolescents. *Social Science and Medicine, 29*, 1051–1056.

Beidel, D., Christ, M. A. G., & Long, P. J. (1991). Somatic complaints in anxious children. *Journal of Abnormal Child Psychology, 19*, 659–670.

Belmaker, E. (1984). Nonspecific somatic symptoms in early adolescent girls. *Journal of Adolescent Health Care, 5*, 30–33.

Belmaker, E., Espinoza, R., & Pogrund, R. (1985). Use of medical services by adolescents with non-specific somatic symptoms. *International Journal of Adolescent Medicine and Health, 1*, 150–156.

Bergman, A. B., & Stamm, S. J. (1967). The morbidity of cardiac non-disease in school children. *New England Journal of Medicine, 276*, 1008–1013.

Bohman, M., Cloninger, C. R., von Knorring, A. L., & Sigvardsson, S. (1984). An adoption study of somatoform disorders: III. Cross-fostering analysis and genetic relationship to alcoholism and criminality. *Archives of General Psychiatry, 41*, 872–878.

Bolton, J., & Cohen, P. (1986). 'Escape with honour': The need for face-saving. *Bulletin of Anna Freud Centre, 9*, 19–33.

Bridges, K. W., & Goldberg, D. P. (1985). Somatic presentation of DSM-III psychiatric disorders in primary care. *Journal of Psychosomatic Research, 29*, 563–569.

Caldwell, T. A., & Stewart, R. S. (1981). Hysterical seizures and hypnotherapy. *American Journal of Clinical Hypnosis, 23*, 294–298.

Campo, J. V. (1995). Somatization disorder. In R. T. Ammerman & M. Hersen (Eds.), *Handbook of child behavior therapy in the psychiatric setting* (pp. 427–451). New York: John Wiley and Sons.

Campo, J. V., & Fritsch, S. L. (1994). Somatization in children and adolescents. *Journal of the American Academy of Child and Adolescent Psychiatry, 33*, 1223–1235.

Campo, J. V., & Raney, D. (1995). The pediatric medical-psychiatric unit in a psychiatric hospital. *Psychosomatics, 36*, 438–444.

Caplan, H. L. (1970). Hysterical "conversion" symptoms in childhood. Unpublished M.Phil. Thesis. University of London.

Carek, D. J., & Santos, A. B. (1984). Atypical somatoform disorder following infection in children—A depressive equivalent? *Journal of Clinical Psychiatry, 45*, 108–111.

Carlson, G., & Kashani, J. H. (1988). Phenomenology of major depressive disorder from childhood through adulthood: An analysis of 3 studies. *American Journal of Psychiatry, 145*, 1222–1225.

Christensen, M. F., & Mortensen, O. (1975). Long-term prognosis in children with recurrent abdominal pain. *Archives of Diseases of Children, 50*, 110.

Cloninger, C. R. (1994). Somatoform and dissociative disorders. In G. Winokur & P. J. Clayton (Eds.), *The Medical Basis of Psychiatry, 2nd edition* (pp. 169–192). Philadelphia: W.B. Saunders.

Cloninger, C. R., Reich, T., & Guze, S. B. (1975). The multifactorial model of disease transmission: III. Familial relationship between sociopathy and hysteria (Briquet's Syndrome). *British Journal of Psychiatry, 127*, 23–32.

Cloninger, C. R., Sigvardsson, S., von Knorring, A. L., & Bohman, M. (1984). An adoption study of somatoform disorders: II. Identification of Two Discrete Somatoform Disorders. *Archives of General Psychiatry, 41*, 863–871.

Creak, M. (1938). Hysteria in childhood. *British Journal of Childhood Diseases, 35*, 85–95.

Delamater, A. M., Rosenbloom, N., Conners, K., & Hertweck, L. (1983). The Behavioral treatment of hysterical paralysis in a ten-year-old boy: A case study.

Journal of the American Academy of Child Psychiatry, 1, 73–79.

Dubowitz, V., & Hersov, L. (1976). Management of children with non-organic (hysterical) disorders of motor function. *Developmental Medicine and Child Neurology, 18,* 358–368.

Elkins, G. R., & Carter, B. D. (1986). Hypnotherapy in the treatment of childhood psychogenic coughing: A case report. *American Journal of Clinical Hypnosis, 29,* 59–63.

Ernst, A. R., Routh, D. K., & Harper, D. C. (1984). Abdominal pain in children and symptoms of somatization disorder. *Journal of Pediatric Psychology, 9,* 77–86.

Fabrega, H. (1990). The concept of somatization as a cultural and historical product of western medicine. *Psychosomatic Medicine, 52,* 653–672.

Faull, C., & Nicol, A. R. (1986). Abdominal pain in six-year-olds: An epidemiological study in a new town. *Journal of Child Psychology and Psychiatry, 27,* 251–260.

Fenton, G. W. (1986). Epilepsy and hysteria. *British Journal of Psychiatry, 149,* 28–37.

Finney, J. W., Lemanek, K. L., Cataldo, M. F., Katz, H. P., & Fuqua, R. W. (1989). Pediatric psychology in primary healthcare: Brief targeted therapy for recurrent abdominal pain. *Behavior Therapy, 20,* 283–291.

Freud, S. (1962). The aetiology of hysteria. In J. Strachey (Ed.), *The standard edition of the complete psychological works of Sigmund Freud.* London: Hogarth Press.

Friedman, S. B. (1973). Conversion symptoms in adolescents. *Pediatric Clinics of North America, 20,* 873–882.

Gadow, K. D., & Sprafkin, J. (1994). *Manual for the Stony Brook Child Symptom Inventories.* Stony Brook, NY: Checkmate Plus, Ltd.

Gadow, K. D., & Sprafkin, J. (1995). *Adolescent supplement to the Child Symptom Inventories manual.* Stony Brook, NY: Checkmate Plus, Ltd.

Garber, J., Zeman, J., & Walker, L. S. (1990). Recurrent abdominal pain in children: Psychiatric diagnoses and parental psychopathology. *Journal of the American Academy of Child and Adolescent Psychiatry, 29,* 648–656.

Garber, J., Walker, L. S., & Zeman, J. (1991). Somatization symptoms in a community sample of children and adolescents: Further validation of the children's somatization inventory. *Psychological Assessment, A Journal of Consulting and Clinical Psychology, 3,* 588–595.

Garralda, M. E. (1996). Somatisation in children. *Journal of Child Psychology and Psychiatry, 47,* 13–33.

Garralda, M. E., & Bailey, D. (1987). Psychosomatic aspects of children's consultations in primary care. *Archives of Psychiatry and Neurological Sciences, 236,* 319–322.

Garrick, T., Ostrov, E., & Offer, D. (1988). Physical symptoms and self-image in a group of normal adolescents. *Psychosomatics, 29,* 73–80.

Gold, S. (1965). Diagnosis and management of hysterical contracture in children. *British Medical Journal, 1,* 21–23.

Goldberg, D. P., & Bridges, K. (1988). Somatic presentations of psychiatric illness in the primary care setting. *Psychosomatic Research, 32,* 137–144.

Goodwin, J., Simms, M., & Bergman, R. (1979). Hysterical seizures in 4 adolescent girls. *American Journal of Orthopsychiatry, 49,* 698–703.

Goodyer, I. M. (1981). Hysterical conversion reactions in childhood. *Journal of Child Psychology and Psychiatry, 22,* 179–188.

Goodyer, I. M. (1985). Epileptic and pseudoepileptic seizures in childhood and adolescence. *Journal of the American Academy of Child Psychiatry, 1,* 3–9.

Goodyer, I. M., & Mitchell, C. (1989). Somatic and emotional disorders in childhood and adolescence. *Journal of Psychosomatic Research, 33,* 681–688.

Goodyer, I. M., & Taylor, D. C. (1985). Hysteria. *Archives of Diseases of Children, 60,* 680–681.

Grattan-Smith, P., Fairley, M., & Procopis, P. (1988). Clinical features of conversion disorder. *Archives of Diseases of Children, 63,* 408–414.

Greene, J. W., Walker, L. S., Hickson, G., & Thompson, J. (1985). Stressful life events and somatic complaints in adolescents. *Pediatrics, 75,* 19–22.

Gross, M. (1979). Incestuous rape: A cause for hysterical seizures in 4 adolescent girls. *American Journal of Orthopsychiatry, 49,* 704–708.

Hodges, K., Kline, J. J., Barbero, G., & Flanery, R. (1984). Life events occurring in families of children with recurrent abdominal pain. *Journal of Psychosomatic Research, 28,* 185–188.

Hodges, K., Kline, J. J., Barbero, G., & Woodruff, C. (1985). Anxiety in children with recurrent abdominal pain and their parents. *Psychosomatics, 26,* 859–866.

Hodges, K., Kline, J. J., Barbero, G., & Flanery, R. (1985). Depressive symptoms in children with recurrent abdominal pain and in their families. *Journal of Pediatrics, 107,* 622–626.

Kashani, J. H., Lababidi, Z., & Jones, R. S. (1982). Depression in children and adolescents with cardiovascular symptomatology: The significance of chest pain. *Journal of the American Academy of Child Psychiatry, 21,* 187–189.

Kellner, R. (1986). *Somatization and hypochondriasis.* New York: Praeger.

Kellner, R. (1991). *Psychosomatic Syndromes and Somatic*

Symptoms. Washington, DC: American Psychiatric Press, Inc.

Klevan, J. L., & DeJong, A. R. (1990). Urinary tract symptoms and urinary tract infection following sexual abuse. *American Journal of Diseases of Children, 144*, 242–244.

Klonoff, E. A., & Moore, D. J. (1986). "Conversion reactions" in adolescents: A biofeedback-based operant approach. *Journal of Behavior Therapy & Experimental Psychiatry, 17*, 179–184.

Kotsopoulos, S., & Snow, B. (1986). Conversion disorders in children: A study of clinical outcome. *Psychiatric Journal of the University of Ottawa, 11*, 134–139.

Kowal, A., & Pritchard, D. (1990). Psychological characteristics of children who suffer from headache: A research note. *Journal of Child Psychology and Psychiatry, 31*, 637–649.

Kriechman, A. M. (1987). Siblings with somatoform disorders in childhood and adolescence. *Journal of the American Academy of Child and Adolescent Psychiatry, 26*, 226–231.

Kutcher, S., Reiter, S., & Gardner, D. (1995). Pharmacotherapy: Approaches and applications. In J. S. March (Ed.), *Anxiety disorders in children and adolescents* (pp. 341–385). New York: Guilford.

LaBarbera, J. D., & Dozier, J. E. (1980). Hysterical seizures: The role of sexual exploitation. *Psychosomatics, 21*, 897–903.

Larson, B. S. (1991). Somatic complaints and their relationship to depressive symptoms in Swedish adolescents. *Journal of Child Psychology and Psychiatry, 32*, 821–832.

Lask, B., & Fosson, A. (1989). *Childhood illness: The psychosomatic approach*. New York: John Wiley & Sons.

Last, C. G. (1991). Somatic complaints in anxiety disordered children. *Journal of Anxiety Disorders, 5*, 125–138.

Laybourne, P. C., & Churchill, S. W. (1972). Symptom discouragement in treating hysterical reactions of childhood. *International Journal of Child Psychotherapy, 1*, 111–123.

Lehmkuhl, G., Blanz, B., Lehmkuhl, U., & Braun-Scharm, H. (1989). Conversion disorder: Symptomatology and course in childhood and adolescence. *European Archives of Psychiatry and Neurological Sciences, 238*, 155–160.

Leslie, S. A. (1988). Diagnosis and treatment of hysterical conversion reactions. *Archives of Diseases of Children, 63*, 506–511.

Lewis, C. F., & Lewis, M. A. (1989). Educational outcomes and illness behaviors in participants in a child-initiated care system: A 12-year follow-up study. *Pediatrics, 84*, 845-850.

Liebman, W. H. (1978). Recurrent abdominal pain in children: A retrospective survey of 119 patients. *Clinical Pediatrics, 17*, 149–153.

Liebman, R., Honig, P., & Berger, H. (1976). An integrated treatment program for psychogenic pain. *Family Process, 15*, 397–405.

Linton, S. J. (1986). A case study of the behavioural treatment of chronic stomach pain in a child. *Behaviour Change, 3*, 70–73.

Lipowski, Z. J. (1988). Somatization: The concept and its clinical application. *American Journal of Psychiatry, 145*, 1358–1368.

Livingston, R. (1993). Children of people with somatization disorder. *Journal of the American Academy of Child and Adolescent Psychiatry, 32*, 536–544.

Livingston, R., & Martin-Cannici, C. M. (1985). Multiple somatic complaints and possible somatization disorder in prepubertal children. *Journal of the American Academy of Child Psychiatry, 24*, 603–607.

Livingston, R., Taylor, J. L., & Crawford, S. L. (1988). A study of somatic complaints and psychiatric diagnosis in children. *Journal of the American Academy of Child and Adolescent Psychiatry, 27*, 185–187.

Looff, D. H. (1970). Psychophysiologic and conversion reactions in children. *Journal of the American Academy of Child Psychiatry, 9*, 318–331.

Mai, F. M., & Merskey, H. (1980). Briquet's treatise on hysteria. *Archives of General Psychiatry, 37*, 1401–1405.

Maisami, M., & Freeman, J. M. (1987). Conversion reactions in children as body language: A combined child psychiatry/neurology team approach to the management of functional neurologic disorders in children. *Pediatrics, 80*, 46–52.

Maloney, M. J. (1980). Diagnosing hysterical conversion reactions in children. *Journal of Pediatrics, 97*, 1016–1020.

Mansdorf, I. J. (1981). Eliminating somatic complaints in separation anxiety through contingency management. *Journal of Behavior Therapy and Experimental Psychiatry, 12*, 73–75.

Masek, B., Russo, D. C., & Varni, J. W. (1984). Behavioral approaches to the management of chronic pain in children. *Pediatric Clinics of North America, 31*, 1113–1131.

McCauley, E., Carlson, G. A., & Calderon, R. (1991). The role of somatic complaints in the diagnosis of depression in children and adolescents. *Journal of the American Academy of Child and Adolescent Psychiatry, 30*, 631–635.

Mechanic, D. (1964). The influence of mothers on their children's health attitudes and behaviors. *Pediatrics*, 444–453.

Mikail, S. F., & von Baeyer, C. L. (1990). Pain, somatic

focus, and emotional adjustment in children of chronic headache sufferers and controls. *Social Sciences and Medicine, 31*, 51–59.

Miller, A. J., & Kratchwill, R. T. (1979). Reduction of frequent stomach ache complaints by time out. *Behavior Therapy, 10*, 211–218.

Minuchin, S., Baker, L., Rosman, B. L., Liebman, R., Milman, L., & Todd, T. C. (1975). A conceptual model of psychosomatic illness in children. *Archives of General Psychiatry, 32*, 1031–1038.

Minuchin, S., Rosman, B. L., & Baker, L. (1978). *Psychosomatic families: Anorexia nervosa in context*. Cambridge: Harvard University Press.

Mizes, J. S. (1985). The use of contingent reinforcement in the treatment of a conversion disorder: A multiple baseline study. *Journal of Behavior Therapy and Experimental Psychiatry, 16*, 341–345.

Mullins, L. L., & Olson, R. A. (1990). Familial factors in the etiology, maintenance, and treatment of somatoform disorders in children. *Family Systems Medicine, 8*, 159–175.

Offord, D. R., Boyle, M. H., Szatmari, P., Rae-Grant, N. I., Links, P. S., Cadman, D. T., Byles, J. A., Crawford, J. W., Blum, H. M., Byrne, C., Thomas, H., & Woodward, C. A. (1987). Ontario Child Health Study: II. Six-month prevalence of disorder and rates of service utilization. *Archives of General Psychiatry, 44*, 832–836.

Organista, P. B., & Miranda, J. (1991). Psychosomatic symptoms in medical outpatients: An investigation of self-handicapping theory. *Health Psychology, 10*, 427–431.

Oster, J. (1972). Recurrent abdominal pain, headache and limb pains in children and adolescents. *Pediatrics, 50*, 429–436.

Parsons, T. (1964). *Social structure and personality*. New York: Free Press.

Pennebaker, J. W., & Susman, J. R. (1988). Disclosure of traumas and psychosomatic processes. *Social Sciences and Medicine, 26*, 327–332.

Pilowsky, I. (1969). Abnormal illness behavior. *British Journal of Medicine and Psychiatry, 42*, 347–351.

Pilowsky, I., Bassett, D. L., Begg, M. W., & Thomas, P. G. (1982). Childhood hospitalization and chronic intractable pain in adults: A controlled retrospective study. *International Psychiatry in Medicine, 12*, 75–84.

Poikolainen, K., Kanerva, R., & Lonnquist, J. (1995). Life events and other risk factors for somatic symptoms in adolescence. *Pediatrics, 96*, 59–63.

Proctor, J. T. (1958). Hysteria in childhood. American Journal of Orthopsychiatry, *28*, 394–407.

Rauste-von Wright, M., & von Wright, J. (1981). A longitudinal study of psychosomatic symptoms in healthy 11–18 year old girls and boys. *Journal of Psychosomatic Research, 25*, 525–534.

Riddle, M. A. (Guest Ed.). (1995a, January). *Child and adolescent clinics of North America. Pediatric psychopharmacology I*. Philadelphia: Saunders.

Riddle, M. A. (Guest Ed.). (1995b, April). *Child and adolescent clinics of North America. Pediatric psychopharmacology II*. Philadelphia: Saunders.

Riddle, M. A., Scahill, L., King, R. A., Hardin, M. T., Anderson, G. M., Ort, S. I., Smith, J. C., Leckman, J. F., & Cohen, D. J. (1992). Double-blind, crossover trial of fluoxetine and placebo in children and adolescents with obsessive compulsive disorder. *Journal of the American Academy of Child & Adolescent Psychiatry, 31:6*, 1062–1069.

Riley, A. W., & Wissow, L. S. (1994). Recognition of emotional and behavioral and family violence in pediatric primary care. In J. Miranda, A. H. Hohmann, C. C. Attkisson, & D. B. Larson (Eds.), *Mental disorders in primary care* (pp. 206–238). San Francisco: Jossey Bass.

Rimsza, M. E., Berg, R. A., & Locke, C. (1988). Sexual abuse: Somatic and emotional reactions. *Child Abuse and Neglect, 12*, 201–208.

Rivinus, T. M., Jamison, D. L., & Graham, P. J. (1975). Childhood organic neurological disease presenting as psychiatric disorder. *Archives of Diseases of Children, 40*, 115–119.

Robins, E., & O'Neal, P. (1953). Clinical features of hysteria in children—with a note on prognosis: A two to seventeen year follow-up study of 41 patients. *Nervous Child, 10*, 246–271.

Robinson, J. O., Alverez, J. H., & Dodge, J. A. (1990). Life events and family history in children with recurrent abdominal pain. *Journal of Psychosomatic Research, 34*, 171–181.

Rock, N. (1971). Conversion reactions in childhood: A clinical study on childhood neuroses. *Journal of the American Academy of Child Psychiatry, 10*, 65–93.

Routh, D. K., & Ernst, A. R. (1984). Somatization disorder in relatives of children and adolescents with functional abdominal pain. *Journal of Pediatric Psychology, 9*, 427–437.

Rutter, M., Tizard, J., & Whitmore, K. (1970). *Education, health and behavior*. London: Longman Group.

Ryan, N. D., Puig-Antich, J., Ambrosini, P., Nelson, B., & Krawiec, V. (1987). The clinical picture of major depression in children and adolescents. *Archives of General Psychiatry, 44*, 854–861.

Sanders, M. R., Rebgetz, M., Morrison, M., Bor, W., Gordon, A., Dadds, M., & Shepherd, R. (1989). Cognitive-behavioral treatment of recurrent nonspecific abdominal pain in children: An analysis of generalization, maintenance, and side effects. *Journal of Consulting and Clinical Psychology, 57,* 294–300.

Sanders, M. R., Shepherd, R. W., Cleghorn, G., & Woolford, H. (1994). The treatment of recurrent abdominal pain in children: A controlled comparison of cognitive-behavioral family intervention and standard pediatric care. *Journal of Consulting and Clinical Psychology, 62,* 306–314.

Sank, L. I., & Biglan, A. (1974). Operant treatment of a case of recurrent abdominal pain in a 10-year-old boy. *Behavior Therapy, 5,* 677–681.

Scaloubaca, D., Slade, P., & Creed, F. (1988). Life events and somatization among students. *Journal of Psychosomatic Research, 32,* 221–229.

Schulman, J. L. (1988). Use of a coping approach in the management of children with conversion reactions. *Journal of the American Academy of Child and Adolescent Psychiatry,* 785–788.

Shapiro, E. G., & Rosenfeld, A. A. (1987). *The somatizing child.* New York: Springer-Verlag.

Shorter, E., Abbey, S. E., Gillies, L. A., Singh, M., & Lipowski, Z. J. (1992). Inpatient treatment of persistent somatization. *Psychosomatics. 33,* 295–301.

Silver, L. B. (1982). Conversion disorder with pseudoseizures in adolescence: A stress reaction to unrecognized and untreated learning disabilities. *Journal of the American Academy of Child Psychiatry, 5,* 508–512.

Simon, G. E. (1991). Somatization and psychiatric disorder. In L. J. Kirmayer & J. M. Robbins (Eds.), *Current concepts of somatization: Research and clinical perspectives* (pp. 37–62). Washington, DC: American Psychiatric Press.

Smith, G. R., Monson, R. A., & Ray, D. C. (1986). Psychiatric consultation in somatization disorder. *New England Journal of Medicine, 314,* 1407–1413.

Smith, G. R., Rost, K., & Kashner, T. M. (1995). A trial of the effect of a standardized psychiatric consultation on health outcomes and costs in somatizing patients. *Archives of General Psychiatry, 52,* 238–243.

Smith, T. W., Snyder, C. R., & Perkins, S. C. (1983). The self-serving function of hypochondriacal complaints: Physical symptoms as self-handicapping strategies. *Journal of Personality and Social Psychology, 44,* 787–797.

Spierings, C., Poels, P. J. E., Sijben, N., Gabreels, F. J. M., & Renier, W. O. (1990). Conversion disorders in childhood: A retrospective follow-up study of 84 patients. *Developmental Medicine and Child Neurology, 32,* 865–871.

Srinath, S., Bharat, S., Girimaji, S., & Seshadri, S. (1993). Characteristics of a child inpatient population with hysteria in India. *Journal of the American Academy of Child and Adolescent Psychiatry, 32,* 822–825.

Starfield, B., Katz, H., Gabriel, A., Livingston, G., Benson, P., Hankin, J., Horn, S., & Steinwachs, D. (1984). Morbidity in childhood—A longitudinal view. *New England Journal of Medicine, 310,* 824–829.

Stefansson, J. G., Messina, J. S., & Meyerowitz, S. (1976). Hysterical neurosis, conversion type: Clinical and epidemiological considerations. *Acta-Psychiatra Scandinavian, 53,* 119–138.

Steinhausen, H. C., Aster, M. V., Pfeiffer, E., & Gebel, D. (1989). Comparative studies of conversion disorders in childhood and adolescence. *Journal of Child Psychology and Psychiatry, 30,* 615–621.

Stevenson, J., Simpson, J., & Bailey, V. (1988). Research note: Recurrent headaches and stomachaches in preschool children. *Journal of Child Psychology and Psychiatry, 29,* 897–900.

Stickler, G. B., & Murphy, D. B. (1979). Recurrent abdominal pain. *American Journal of Diseases of Children, 133,* 486–489.

Stone, R., & Barbero, G. (1970). Recurrent abdominal pain in childhood. *Pediatrics, 45,* 732–738.

Thomson, A. P. J., & Sills, J. A. (1988). Diagnosis of functional illness presenting with gait disorder. *Archives of Diseases of Children, 63,* 148–153.

Turgay, A. (1980). Conversion reactions in children. *Psychiatric Journal of the University of Ottawa, 5,* 287–294.

Volkmar, R. R., Poll, J., & Lewis, M. (1984). Conversion reactions in children and adolescents. *Journal of the American Academy of Child and Adolescent Psychiatry, 23,* 424–430.

Walker, L. S., Garber, J., & Greene, J. W. (1991). Somatization symptoms in pediatric abdominal pain patients: Relation to chronicity of abdominal pain and parent somatization. *Journal of Abnormal Child Psychology, 19,* 379–394.

Walker, L. S., Garber, J., & Greene, J. W. (1993). Psychosocial correlates of recurrent childhood pain: A comparison of pediatric patients with recurrent abdominal pain, organic illness and psychiatric disorder. *Journal of Abdominal Psychology, 102,* 248–258.

Walker, L. S., Garber, J., & Greene, J. W. (1994). Somatic complaints in pediatric patients: A prospective study of the role of negative life events, child social and academic competence and parental somatic symptoms. *Journal of Consulting and Clinical Pathology, 62,* 1213–1221.

Walker, L. S., Garber, J., & Van Slyke, D. A. (1995). Do parents excuse the misbehavior of children with physical or emotional symptoms? An investigation of the pe diatric sick role. *Journal of Pediatric Psychology, 20,* 329–345.

Walker, L. S., Garber, J., Van Slyke, D. A., & Greene, J. W. (1995). Long term health outcomes in patients with recurrent abdominal pain. *Journal of Pediatric Psychology, 20,* 233–245.

Walker, L. S., & Greene, J. W. (1987). Negative life events, psychosocial resources, and psychophysiological symptoms in adolescents. *Journal of Clinical Child Psychology, 16,* 29–36.

Walker, L. S., & Greene, J. W. (1989). Children with recurrent abdominal pain and their parents: More somatic complaints, anxiety, and depression than other patient families? *Journal of Pediatric Psychology, 14,* 231–243.

Walker, L. S., & Greene, J. W. (1991). Negative life events and symptom resolution in pediatric abdominal pain patients. *Journal of Pediatric Psychology, 16,* 341–360.

Walker, L. S., McLaughlin, F. J., & Greene, J. W. (1988). Functional illness and family functioning: A comparison of healthy and somaticizing adolescents. *Family Process, 27,* 317–325.

Walker, L. S., & Zeman, J. L. (1992). Parental response to child illness behavior. *Journal of Pediatric Psychology, 17,* 49–71.

Warwick, H. M., & Salkovskis, P. M. (1985). Reassurance. *British Medical Journal, 290,* 1028.

Wasserman, A. L., Whitington, P. F., & Rivera, F. P. (1988). Psychogenic basis for abdominal pain in children and adolescents. *Journal of the American Academy of Child and Adolescent Psychiatry, 27,* 179–184.

Weiner, B. (1993). On sin versus sickness: A theory of perceived responsibility and social motivation. *American Psychologist, 48,* 957–971.

Weiner, H., & Fawzy, F. I. (1989). An integrative model of health, disease, and illness. In S. Cheren (Ed.), *Psychosomatic medicine: Theory, physiology, and practice, vol. 1* (pp. 9–44). Madison, CT: International Universities Press.

Williams, D. T., & Singh, M. (1976). Hypnosis as a facilitating therapeutic adjunct in child psychiatry. *Journal of the American Academy of Child Psychiatry, 15,* 326–342.

Williams, D. T., Spiegel, H., & Mostofsky, D. I. (1978). Neurogenic and hysterical seizures in children and adolescents: Differential diagnostic and therapeutic considerations. *American Journal of Psychiatry, 135,* 82–86.

Wood, B., Watkins, J. B., Boyle, J. T., Nogueira, J., Zimand, E., & Carroll, L. (1989). The "psychosomatic family" model: An empirical and theoretical analysis. *Family Process, 28,* 399–417.

Wood, B. (1993). Beyond the "psychosomatic family:" A biobehavioral family model of pediatric illness. *Family Process, 32,* 261–278.

Wooley, S. C., Blackwell, B., & Winget, C. (1978). A learning theory model of chronic illness behavior: Theory, treatment, and research. *Psychosomatic Medicine, 40,* 379–401.

World Health Organization. (1988). *International classification of diseases, 10th revision.* Geneva: Author.

Zuckerman, B., Stevenson, J., & Bailey, V. (1987). Stomachaches and headaches in a community sample of preschool children. *Pediatrics, 79,* 677–682.

CHAPTER 8

SLEEP

Jodi A. Mindell
Ronald E. Dahl

DESCRIPTION OF THE PROBLEM

Sleep problems are quite common in children and adolescents. It is important for pediatric psychologists and psychiatrists to have a thorough understanding of sleep and sleep disorders because (1) sleep disorders can be mistaken for psychiatric or psychological disorders, (2) medical and psychiatric disorders can cause sleep disturbances, and (3) both primary sleep disorders and sleep problems secondary to other disorders often present for psychological or psychiatric evaluation. The purpose of this chapter is to provide an understanding of the physiology of sleep and present a thorough review of the assessment and treatment of common pediatric sleep disorders.

Physiology and Development of Sleep

An overview of sleep stages, physiology, and development provides an essential background for understanding specific sleep disorders. Sleep stages are determined by three electrophysiologic measures: the electroencephalogram (EEG), the electromyogram (EMG), and electro-oculogram (EOG). The patterning of these measures (EEG, muscle tone, and eye movements) divides sleep into the broad categories of rapid eye movement (REM) sleep and non-REM sleep.

REM sleep is also called paradoxic sleep because it has aspects of both deep sleep and light sleep. Body and brain-stem functions appear to be in a deep sleep state (muscle tone drops dramatically and the regulation of temperature, blood pressure, heartrate, and respirations have increased variability), whereas higher cortical brain function appears active. Dreaming is closely associated with REM sleep and when a person is awakened from REM alertness returns relatively briskly. REM periods occur in cycles of approximately 60–90 minutes throughout the night. The longest REM periods and most intense REM activity occurs in the latter part of the sleep period, just prior to morning awakening.

In contrast, the deepest non-REM sleep occurs in the first 1 to 3 hours after falling asleep. Non-REM sleep is further subdivided into stages 1, 2, 3, and 4. Stages 3 and 4 (also called delta or slow-wave sleep) represent the deepest sleep in human beings. This deep delta sleep increases in proportion to how long one has been awake and further increases (and becomes even deeper) following sleep loss or chronic sleep disturbances (as a deep "recovery" sleep). Children have extremely large amounts of deep slow-wave sleep, which gradually decreases as they get older. During this deep sleep (usually 1 to 3 hours after going to sleep), it is extremely difficult to arouse a child, and if aroused, the child appears disoriented, confused, and cognitively slow. Confused partial arousals (including sleep walking, night terrors, and such) usually emerge from this state. ⟵

Knowledge of the patterning of these sleep stages is a component that is important in the evaluation and treatment of sleep disorders. Figure 8.1 shows a typical example of a young prepubertal child's sleep pattern. Stages 1, 2, 3, and 4 are shown as progressively lower steps on the vertical axis, with REM indicated with striped boxes at an intermediate level (indicating the paradoxic relationship to sleep depth). This child fell briefly into stage 1, descended to stage 2, and then to stages 3 and 4, where she remained for approximately 1 hour. Then, just before midnight, the child's sleep returned to lighter stage 2, and then a brief 30-second arousal before returning to stage 2, then quickly to another hour of deep stage 3 and 4, followed by the first REM period at about 1:00 A.M. REM periods subsequently reappeared approximately every 60 to 90 minutes throughout the night, with longer REM periods toward early morning.

Three key points are illustrated by this sleep pattern: (1) most of the slow-wave sleep occurs in the first 1 to 3 hours after sleep onset (thus, most slow-wave-related disorders such as sleep terrors, sleepwalking, and par-

tial arousals are likely to occur at this time of the night); (2) most of the REM sleep occurs in the second half of the night (thus REM-related disorders such as nightmares are more frequent in the early morning hours); and (3) short periods of wakefulness typically occur five to seven times a night from normal sleep (however, most children quickly return to sleep after a brief adjustment in position, covers, or pillows, with no memory of the awakening).

Age-related (developmental) processes also exert profound influences on sleep regulation. As can be seen in Figure 8.2, total sleep decreases from 16 hours a day in the newborn period to approximately 8 hours a night by age 18. At age 1, the average child sleeps approximately 11 hours a night, with another 2.5 hours of sleep obtained in two separate daytime naps. By age 3, the average child gets 10.5 hours of sleep each night, with one 1.5-hour nap. In the United States, a typical child ceases daytime naps at about 4 to 5 years of age. It is also important to emphasize that there is considerable individual variation in sleep requirements as well as cultural influences on sleep and napping behavior (for example, daytime naps continue through adulthood in some cultures).

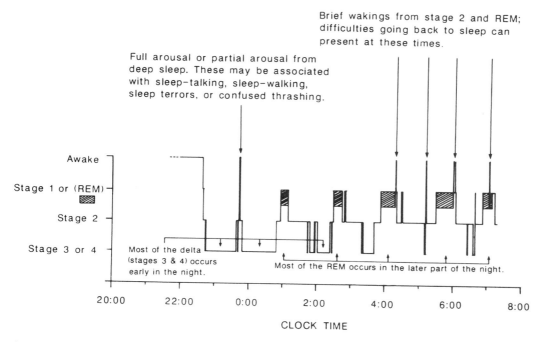

SLEEP PATTERN IN AN EARLY SCHOOL-AGE CHILD

Brief wakings from stage 2 and REM; difficulties going back to sleep can present at these times.

Full arousal or partial arousal from deep sleep. These may be associated with sleep-talking, sleep-walking, sleep terrors, or confused thrashing.

Awake

Stage 1 or (REM)

Stage 2

Stage 3 or 4

Most of the delta (stages 3 & 4) occurs early in the night.

Most of the REM occurs in the later part of the night.

20:00   22:00   0:00   2:00   4:00   6:00   8:00

CLOCK TIME

Figure 8.1. Typical sleep pattern in a child

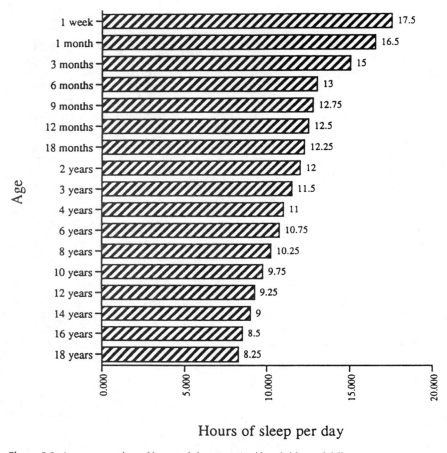

Figure 8.2. Average number of hours of sleep required by children of different ages

Maturation also results in changes in sleep stages with a gradual decrease in REM sleep and a significant drop-off in delta sleep, particularly during adolescence. Changes in sleep regulation during adolescence appear to be complex. There appears to be a significant increase in daytime sleepiness among adolescents—even if they obtain as much sleep as during prepuberty. Despite this evidence suggesting an increased physiologic need for sleep, there is substantial evidence that many adolescents frequently get significantly less sleep. The combination of early morning school schedules and late night social schedules results in many high school students often getting by on 6 to 7 hours (or less) of sleep per night during the school week. Adolescent behaviors on weekends and vacations, however, support the concept that their true sleep needs are much greater. There is also evidence that many of these adolescents have sig-

nificant daytime sleepiness and fatigue in the classroom. The effects of this relative sleep deprivation frequently seen during adolescence are not well understood, but from a clinical standpoint they may lead to significant problems with school performance, mood, and irritability. These topics are discussed further in the category of sleep/wake schedule disorders in adolescents.

Classification of Sleep Disorders

Before discussing any of the sleep disorders, it is important to mention the classification system of these disorders. Sleep disorders are basically classified into two major categories, the dyssomnias and the parasomnias, as delineated by the International Classification of Sleep

Disorders (ICSD; Diagnostic Classification Steering Committee, 1990). The dyssomnias include those disorders that result in difficulty either initiating or maintaining sleep, or involve excessive daytime sleepiness. The parasomnias, on the other hand, are disorders that disrupt sleep after it has been initiated and are disorders of arousal, partial arousal, or sleep stage transitions. They are disorders that intrude into the sleep process, but usually do not result in complaints of insomnia or excessive sleepiness. Note that these terms, as they are defined by the ICSD, differ slightly from their use in the fourth edition of the American Psychiatric Association's *Diagnostic and Statistical Manual of Mental Disorders* (DSM-IV; American Psychiatric Association, 1994). DSM-IV defines dyssomnias as those sleep disorders in which the predominant disturbance is in the amount, quality, or timing of sleep. The parasomnias are described as sleep disorders that involve abnormal behavioral or physiological events occurring in association with sleep, specific sleep stages, or sleep-wake transitions. Both methods of defining these terms, however, result in the same classification of disorders.

INCIDENCE AND PREVALENCE

Surveys have found that about 25 percent of children between the ages of 1 and 5 years experience some type of sleep disturbance (Bixler, Kales, Scharf, Kales, & Leo, 1976; Jenkins, Bax, & Hart, 1980; Lozoff, Wolf, & Davis, 1985; Richman, 1981; Richman, Stevenson, & Graham, 1975). These sleep disturbances come in many different forms. Salzarulo and Chevalier (1983) interviewed the families of 218 children, ages 2 to 15, referred for pediatric or child psychiatric consultation, and found that sleep talking was quite common (32 percent), followed by nightmares (31 percent), waking at night (28 percent), trouble falling asleep (23 percent), enuresis (17 percent), bruxism (10 percent), sleep rocking (7 percent), and night terrors (7 percent). In Dollinger's 1982 survey of mothers referring their children to a university clinic, the most common sleep problems (among 3- to 15-year-olds) were sleep talking (53 percent), restless sleep and bedtime refusal (both 42 percent), and refusing to go to sleep without a nightlight (40 percent). Other sleep problems included bad dreams (35 percent), difficulty in going to sleep (26 percent), crying out in sleep (16 percent), and nightmares (11 percent). Another study of healthy preadolescents, ages 8 to 10 years, found

that 43 percent of the children were experiencing a sleep problem that had lasted more than six months (Kahn et al., 1989). Looking at specific sleep disorders, parasomnias were present in 29 percent of the children, with enuresis (2 percent), sleepwalking (5 percent), and night fears (15 percent) reported.

ASSESSMENT APPROACHES

A thorough evaluation of sleep disorders follows a logical progression. The first step in evaluating a child or adolescent for a sleep disorder is the completion of a thorough sleep history. All aspects of the sleep-wake cycle need to be reviewed. Areas that need to be addressed include evening activities such as television watching, medications, intake of caffeinated beverages, bedtime, and bedtime routines. During the night, areas to be evaluated include latency to sleep onset, behaviors during the night, and the number and duration of nighttime awakenings. Details about abnormal events during sleep should be collected, such as night terrors, confusional arousals, respiratory disturbances, seizures, and enuresis. In the morning, waketime and sleepiness should be evaluated. It is also important to assess parental responses to nighttime arousals. Weekend as well as weekday schedules and symptoms should also be considered. During the day, sleepiness, naps, meals, caffeine intake, medications, and feelings of anxiety and depression should be reviewed. Medication intake should also be reviewed, as many medications can affect sleep (especially stimulants, asthma medications, anti-seizure drugs, and sedatives). A review of psychological symptoms during the day is also important. Symptoms of anxiety and depression are often linked to lack of sleep. For example, feelings of fatigue, irritability, and sluggishness may simply be the result of sleep deprivation. On the other hand, anxiety disorders and depression may cause sleep disturbances in some cases (see section below on sleep and psychiatric disorders).

Significant life events or stressors may be related to acute sleep problems and should also be assessed. Failure in school, death in the family, or a recent move can all contribute significantly to a sleep problem that resembles insomnia. A thorough evaluation should include questioning about school performance, social functioning, and family functioning. For example, a recent change in a family's financial status can result in sleep disturbances in children even if the parents do not believe that the child is aware of such problems. Often children, and especially adolescents, are much more aware of tensions in a family than parents are aware. Thus, it is important that a thorough evaluation of all aspects of sleep and daytime functioning be conducted.

The second step in the evaluation of sleep problems is the keeping of sleep diaries. A typical sleep diary includes information on the time of going to bed, latency to sleep onset, number and duration of nighttime awakenings, time of arising in the morning, total sleep time, and duration and time of naps. For the most useful information, two weeks of baseline sleep diaries should be kept. That way sleep patterns can clearly be delineated.

The third step is to determine which cases require formal sleep studies. In cases in which there is a concern about a specific underlying physiological problem, polysomnography (PSG) can be an essential component of assessment. Two specific areas where PSG studies are particularly important are to assess for sleep apnea (see below), and in unexplained excessive need for sleep, to rule out narcolepsy syndrome. Polysomnography typically consists of an overnight sleep study in which recordings of oxygen saturation, nasal and oral airflow, thoracic and abdominal respiratory movements, limb muscle activity, and electroencephalogram (EEG) are taken. As an adjunct to a PSG, a multiple sleep latency test (MSLT) is often conducted. This test, which is performed in two-hour intervals throughout the day following the overnight study, evaluates the client's level of daytime sleepiness. The MSLT consists of four or five 20-minute nap opportunities given at two-hour intervals. Measures of sleep latency are taken. If sleep occurs, the nap is terminated 15 minutes after sleep onset.

Given the breadth and scope of the different sleep disorders, differential diagnosis is important. The presenting complaints for many of the sleep disorders are similar, for example, "insomnia," excessive daytime sleepiness, or unusual behaviors during the night. Thus, it is important to conduct a thorough evaluation to fully assess which specific sleep disorder the child or adolescent is experiencing.

Differentiation between a sleep disorder and other medical or psychological problems is also important. A child with what looks like night terrors may actually be having seizures during sleep. In other cases, difficulties at bedtime may be symptomatic of a more general problem with noncompliance. Nighttime fears may be just one of many extensive fears in an extremely anxious child. In addition, delayed sleep phase syndrome should always be assessed before a diagnosis of school refusal is made. Given the similar characteristics of each disorder, it appears likely that sleep phase disorder may sometimes present as school refusal, especially among adolescents who constitute the majority of individuals with delayed sleep phase syndrome.

Furthermore, it is important to keep in mind that some children may have more than one sleep disorder or a sleep disorder that is associated with physical illness or another psychological disorder. For example, an adolescent may have narcolepsy and sleep apnea. Once one sleep disorder is identified, a thorough evaluation for all other sleep disorders should still be conducted. If not, sleep problems may continue.

INTERVENTION STRATEGIES

The approach to be taken in this section is to review the specific sleep disorders by classifying them into three general categories. The first category includes problems of "insomnia" or the sleepless child. The second includes excessive daytime sleepiness or hypersomnolence, including sleep apnea, narcolepsy, and schedule disorders. The final category consists of the parasomnias or abnormal behaviors associated with sleep, such as night terrors, sleepwalking, headbanging, and enuresis.

Insomnia/Sleepless Child

Insomnia in children usually presents itself as a child or adolescent with trouble going to bed, difficulties falling asleep, or frequent nighttime awakenings. These sleep disturbances will be discussed in this section. Insomnia occurs less frequently in children than adults, and is often the result of other factors such as negative sleep associations, adjustment problems, or other physiological sleep disturbances (for example, sleep apnea, delayed sleep phase syndrome).

Bedtime Problems

Resistance to going to bed is a very frequent complaint of parents of younger children. These sleep problems are referred to as limit-setting sleep disorders (Diagnostic Classification Steering Committee, 1990). Five to ten percent of the childhood population experience this sleep disorder. Bedtime struggles are often a source of considerable stress to both parents and children and often contribute to inadequate sleep for many family members. Some children with other psychological problems may also have difficulties at bedtime. For example, some children with attention-deficit/hyperactivity disorder (ADHD) or other disruptive behaviors may have difficulty settling at bedtime. Changes in medication regimens, including, surprisingly, a late afternoon stimulant dose can sometimes be beneficial with these children.

Parents of children who have bedtime difficulties often report that they are depressed, anxious, and are unhappy in their marriages (Durand & Mindell, 1990). Bedtime problems are usually alleviated once limits are set by the parent and are highly amenable to behavioral treatments such as graduated extinction (e.g., Adams & Rickert, 1989; Mindell & Durand, 1993; Richman, Douglas, Hunt, Lansdown, & Levere, 1985; Rickert & Johnson, 1988) and the establishment of bedtime routines (Weissbluth, 1982). Although hypnotic medications such as diphenhydramine (Benadryl) are commonly prescribed by many pediatricians, these drugs often result in a very limited, short-term improvement and development of tolerance to the drug, with little long-term benefit (Richman, 1985).

Bedtime problems can also be related to children's nighttime fears. These nighttime fears are the most common fears experienced by children, and are a normal developmental occurrence in young children. Many of these fears are learned through simple conditioning. For example, the bedroom may be a source of anxiety for some children, especially if the bedroom is the place where the child is sent as punishment. Also, in the middle of the night, if the child has a nightmare or awakens distressed, a parent typically comes into the room, turning on the light. Thus, a child may associate light with comfort and associate darkness with distress or nightmares. Some fears may be related to developmental stage, including separation anxiety and stranger anxiety. And others may be biologically based, such as being scared of the dark.

Although most children will outgrow their fears, a variety of therapeutic techniques can be utilized. Psychotherapy, especially with older children and adolescents, can be helpful (Connell, Persley, & Sturgess, 1987). This treatment may be quite useful when the nighttime fears are triggered by a traumatic event such as the death of a relative or friend. Guided imagery, relaxation training, and self-instruction can also be successful (Friedman & Ollendick, 1989; Graziano & Mooney, 1980, 1982; King, Cranstoun, & Josephs, 1989; Ollendick, Hagopian, & Huntzinger, 1991).

Difficulties Falling Asleep

Overlapping with bedtime problems and struggles, but somewhat distinct, are children who are compliant with bedtime routines but have persistent difficulties falling asleep. In some cases, parents can be relatively unaware of the magnitude of the problem when children remain quietly in their beds, but are unable to fall asleep. The differential diagnosis in this clinical situation includes sleep/wake schedule disorder, anxiety disorder, depression, and sleep onset association disorder. Many children worry or ruminate about distressing thoughts and images at bedtime, and this can become a habit. Often when children have worries or fears, they can avoid them during the day by distractions, activities, playing, etc.; but at night, they repeatedly dwell on distressing thoughts as they are trying to fall asleep. The increased arousal accompanying these negative cognitions can significantly inhibit the process of falling asleep. Treatment approaches are similar to those discussed under bed time problems (see Mindell, 1996). However, when a significant psychiatric disorder is diagnosed also, treatment of that disorder may result in improvement in any secondary sleep difficulties.

Nightwakings

As discussed above, studies suggest that approximately 30 percent of 1- and 2-year-olds have frequent nighttime arousals that disturb their parents. After age three, the prevalence decreases but does continue to be experienced by some children. There is further evidence that nighttime awakenings continue to be a problem in as many as 30 percent of children up to school age. Although medical problems (such as pain from an ear infection, allergy to cow's milk, colic, or the itching of atopic dermatitis) can contribute significantly to this problem in some children, the majority of cases result from behavioral and learned factors (Ferber, 1987). Many children fall asleep while being rocked, sucking on a pacifier, or drinking from a bottle. When these objects or circumstances are present, sleep is normal. However, when these objects or circumstances are not present, sleep is disturbed and can result in sleep-onset difficulties and/or frequent night wakings. To understand this disorder, it is important to realize that waking during the night is normal, and most children are able to return to sleep easily. These children are called "self-soothers." However, some children, known as "signallers," are unable to return to sleep until the conditions for sleep are reestablished. Behavioral interventions have been successful in treating sleep-onset association disorder (Jones & Verduyn, 1983; Milan, Mitchell, Berger, & Pierson, 1981; Schaefer, 1990; Seymour, Brock, During, & Poole, 1989). One method that is less stressful for parents is to intervene only at bedtime by implementing a behavioral program, involving a positive bedtime routine and graduated extinction. Once the child has been taught to self-soothe at bedtime, generalization occurs to reduce frequent night wakings (Mindell & Durand, 1993).

Adjustment Sleep Disorder

Some difficulties with sleeping are the result of a stressful event, difficulties in school, or an environmental change, and are referred to as representing an adjustment sleep disorder. It is often seen in children following a move, after the death of a relative, or before the first day of school. The duration of the sleep problem is often days, although some cases, often associated with ongoing stressors, may last as long as several months.

In general, treatment for an adjustment sleep disorder is not necessary, since the problem usually resolves naturally over time. If treatment is sought, primarily for longer-term sleep problems, psychological therapies typically focus on the disrupting events and encourage engaging in communication. With resolution of the precipitating event, the sleep problems typically dissipate, with sleep returning to normal.

Excessive Daytime Sleepiness/Hypersomnolence

Complaints of excessive sleepiness and/or increased needs for sleep occur occasionally in the older child and frequently in adolescents. A thorough and detailed history is an essential part of the evaluation of these complaints. It is important to characterize the nature of the sleepiness (that is, drifting off to sleep during boring activities versus sleep attacks), the frequency and duration of symptoms, and whether the symptoms are occurring at particular times of day or only during certain situations. A family history of increased sleep needs and sleepiness can be important in the consideration of narcolepsy and idiopathic central nervous system hypersomnolence. It is also essential to be aware of the wide individual variations in sleep needs. One perfectly normal child may require two more hours of sleep overnight than does a same-aged peer or sibling.

The approach to the sleepy child or adolescent consists of considering four basic categories of problems: (1) inadequate amounts of sleep, (2) disturbed nocturnal sleep, (3) increased sleep requirements despite adequate nocturnal sleep, and (4) circadian and scheduling disorders. The history and evaluation should be directed at characterizing the problem with respect to these categories.

Inadequate Amounts of Sleep

The most common cause of mild-to-moderate sleepiness in children and adolescents is an inadequate number of hours in bed. A combination of social schedules leading to late nights with early-morning school requirements can significantly compress the number of hours of sleep. The catch-up sleep of naps, weekends, and holidays can further contribute to the problem by leading to erratic schedules and even later nights. In taking a sleep history, it is important to ask specific questions concerning schedules. Many families will say the adolescent "usually" goes to bed at a certain time, but when asked for an exact time covering the previous few nights, a much later hour is reported. When assessing the amount of sleep, it is important to obtain details of bedtime (with lights out and the child or adolescent attempting to fall asleep), estimates of sleep latency, nighttime arousals, time of actually getting up in the morning versus time awakened, difficulty getting up, and the frequency, timing, and duration of daytime naps. It is also essential to get details of sleep/wake schedules on weekends as well as during the school week. When this type of specific information is obtained (either by interview or by having the family maintain a sleep diary), evidence of inadequate sleep is often evident.

When inadequate sleep is identified, recommendations to go to bed earlier are unlikely to lead to significant changes in behavior for many children and most adolescents. Often the primary role of the clinician is to help the entire family understand (and acknowledge the consequences resulting from) the inadequate sleep. Sleep deprivation frequently contributes to many factors that the family identifies as problems, including falling asleep in school, oversleeping in the morning, fatigue, and irritability. With respect to sleep (as in many areas of health), strategies of prevention and maintaining healthy habits make great common sense but have little salience in the decision-making processes of many adolescents until problems become severe. In cases in which the adolescent's school or social functioning is significantly impaired by the sleep problem, a strict behavioral contract (agreed upon by the family) can be essential. The contract should specify hours in bed (with only small deviations on the weekends) and target the specific behaviors contributing to bad sleep habits, such as specific late-night activities, erratic napping, oversleeping for school, and so on. The choice of rewards for successes and negative consequences for failures, as well as an accurate method of assessing compliance, are essential components of the contract.

Disturbed Nocturnal Sleep

When symptoms of sleepiness occur despite an adequate schedule of hours in bed, disruptions of sleep should be considered. Disturbances within sleep can be more difficult to assess by history alone. Although some families may report that the child or adolescent is waking frequently, in other cases the family may be unaware of subtle disruptions of sleep leading to daytime sleepiness. The use of drugs or alcohol is an important consideration in these cases. In addition to the obvious effects of late-night stimulants such as cocaine, there are also more complex drug/sleep interactions. Alcohol, for example, can facilitate sleep onset but can lead to decreased delta and REM sleep. Further, the withdrawal from stimulants, alcohol, and marijuana can produce transient but severe sleep disruptions. Caffeine is also a commonly used substance in the adolescent population in the form of caffeinated sodas, coffee, and tea. Elimination of caffeine can be an important step in treating symptoms of difficulty falling asleep, which can lead to daytime sleepiness. Prescription medications such as beta-adrenergic agonists for asthma or stimulants for attention deficit disorder can also result in significant sleep disruptions.

A few *specific* sources of daytime sleepiness should be considered in this age group (sleep-disordered breathing, narcolepsy, and sleep/wake schedule disorders) and are discussed in greater detail.

Sleep-Disordered Breathing

Obstructive sleep apnea syndrome (OSAS) involves repetitive episodes of upper airway obstruction during sleep, often causing a reduction in blood oxygen saturation (Guilleminault, Korobkin, & Winkle, 1981). In adults, the typical clinical picture of OSAS is obesity, hypersomnolence, and lethargy. In children, the clinical appearance is quite different (Brouillette, Fernback, & Hunt, 1982). The most common cause of OSAS in children is hypertrophy of adenoids and tonsils. When awake, many of these children have little difficulty breathing, however, with decreased muscle tone during sleep, the airway becomes smaller and airway resistance increases. This leads to more difficulties breathing. At its most severe, these apneic episodes result in nocturnal hypoxemia and bradycardia, with the potential outcome of pulmonary hypertension with cor pulmonale. More commonly, however, they result in frequent brief arousals from sleep, that increase the muscle tone to the neck and pharyngeal muscles, open the airway, and allow the child to resume breathing. Although the total number of

minutes of arousal during the night may be small, the repeated, chronic, but brief disruptions in sleep can lead to significant daytime symptoms in children, primarily excessive sleepiness. (A comparable image would be answering a wrong number on the telephone 15 to 30 times during the night.) It is important to note that the child is usually unaware of waking up, and the parents may only describe very restless sleep. Studies indicate that the most frequent symptoms reported by families were loud chronic snoring (or noisy breathing), restless sleep with unusual sleeping positions (attempts by the child to move and open the airway), a history of problems with tonsils, adenoids, and/or ear infections, and signs of inadequate nighttime sleep (e.g., Croft, Brockbank, Wright, & Swanston, 1990). Some children with sleep apnea may be excessively active during the day, rather than appearing sleepy. Some cases of children with attention-deficit/hyperactivity problems have been diagnosed with sleep apnea. For these children, treatment of the sleep apnea may result in improvement of the ADHD symptoms.

The average age at diagnosis for children with sleep apnea is seven years (Mauer, Staats, & Olsen, 1983), and it is more common in boys (Guilleminault & Anders, 1976). Certain categories of children are at high risk for sleep apnea, including those with maxofacial abnormalities, micrognathia, a history of cleft palates (particularly with pharyngeal flap repairs), and Down's syndrome. Children who are morbidly obese (greater than 150 percent ideal body weight) are also at increased risk for sleep apnea (Mallory, Fiser, & Jackson, 1989).

The diagnosis of OSAS can often be made clinically. Many pediatric otolaryngologists are experienced in assessing children with signs of snoring and disturbed sleep for evidence of adenoidal hypertrophy. It is important to understand that even moderate-sized adenoids and tonsils (which cause no problems when awake) may produce obstructive symptoms during sleep. Polysomnographic studies, though, can aid in the diagnosis and are often recommended. Unfortunately, however, sleep studies in children with the syndrome can be difficult to interpret, as there are few normative studies in this age group that include nighttime pulmonary monitoring. Even more important, some children show such brief apneas that they do not meet published criteria for obstructive sleep apneas. Nonetheless, some of these children are working so hard to breathe during sleep that over time, they show significant signs of disturbed sleep. Thus, sleep apnea in children can be difficult to diagnose, as children with relatively low apnea/hypopnea indices (which would fail to meet any criteria for OSAS) with convincing evidence of chronically disrupted sleep secondary to sleep-disordered breathing difficulties can be identified.

In children with sleep apnea, the most common form of treatment involves surgery to remove the airway obstruction (Croft et al., 1990). Tonsillectomy and/or adenoidectomy relieves symptoms in about 70 percent of all child cases. Other treatments are also recommended, including weight loss and the use of pharmacological agents. Furthermore, nasal continuous positive airway pressure (CPAP) has been found to be extremely successful in the treatment of obstructive sleep apnea in adults and has been suggested as an appropriate treatment for some children with sleep apnea (Guilleminault, Riley, Powell, Simmons, & Nino-Murcia, 1985).

Narcolepsy

Narcolepsy is a chronic disorder which is characterized by excessive sleepiness, often presenting itself as repeated episodes of naps or lapses into sleep of short duration throughout the day (Diagnostic Classification Steering Committee, 1990; Guilleminault, 1986, 1987; Mitler, Nelson, & Hajdukovic, 1987). Additional characteristics of narcolepsy are other abnormally timed elements of REM physiology such as muscle paralysis (cataplexy and sleep paralysis) and dream imagery (hypnogogic and hypnopopic hallucinations). Narcolepsy is not rare, affecting approximately 10 out of every 10,000 people in this country (a prevalence approximately that of multiple sclerosis). Narcolepsy appears to be a neurologic disorder with a strong genetic predisposition. Nearly all identified cases of narcolepsy have HLA-DR2 antigen. Family history of narcolepsy and/or excessive sleepiness can be helpful, though it is not found in many cases. Although traditionally the onset of narcolepsy is thought to be late adolescence and adulthood, there is increasing evidence that symptoms may begin in childhood (Dahl, Holtum, & Trubnick, 1994; Kotagal, Hartse, & Walsh, 1990).

The classic symptoms of narcolepsy include (1) sleep attacks, (2) cataplexy (the sudden loss of muscle tone without change of consciousness), (3) sleep paralysis (inability to move after waking up), and (4) hypnogogic hallucinations (dream-like imagery before falling asleep). These symptoms do not all occur together or consistently in many individuals with narcolepsy. Particularly in younger patients, signs of sleepiness may be the only symptom. Cataplexy, a symptom unique to narcolepsy, is typically provoked by laughter, anger, or sudden emotional changes. It may be as subtle as a slight weakness in

the legs, or as dramatic as a patient's falling to the floor limp and being unable to move. The duration of cataplexy typically lasts from a few seconds to several minutes, with complete and immediate recovery. Mild symptoms of cataplexy can be difficult to identify in children, and may be only evident in retrospect following the diagnosis. Likewise, hypnogogic hallucinations can be difficult to elicit from a child's history. To further complicate matters, these symptoms often wax and wane in individuals with narcolepsy.

Clinical experience from a pediatric sleep center was recently reviewed in 16 consecutive cases of polysomnographically proven narcolepsy cases with the onset of symptoms by age 13 years (Dahl et al., 1994). Only 1 of the 16 patients presented with the classic clinical tetrad of symptoms (sleepiness, cataplexy, hypnogogic hallucinations, and sleep paralysis). Behavioral and emotional disturbances were present in 12 of the 16 narcoleptic patients, with 4 patients appearing to have been misdiagnosed with a psychiatric disorder before recognition of the narcolepsy. Obesity appeared as an unexpected association in this case series, with 11 of the 16 narcoleptic patients found to be overweight at the time of diagnosis. The varied clinical presentations, polysomnographic findings, family history, and associated psychiatric symptoms were described with an emphasis on the importance of considering narcolepsy in the differential diagnosis of any child or adolescent with excessive sleepiness.

The diagnosis of narcolepsy requires evaluation in a sleep laboratory. Polysomnographic signs of narcolepsy include early REM periods near sleep onset, fragmented nighttime sleep, excessive daytime sleepiness in objective nap studies during the day, and sleep-onset REM periods in naps. In prepubertal children, this diagnosis can be very difficult to establish (Kotagal et al., 1990), and repeat studies may be necessary before reaching a final diagnosis.

Treatment of narcolepsy is generally focused on (1) education and counseling of the patient and family, (2) adherence to a regular schedule to obtain optimal sleep with good sleep habits (often including scheduled naps), (3) use of short-acting stimulant medication for treatment of daytime sleepiness, with drug holidays to avoid build-up of tolerance (Wittig, Zorick, Roehrs, Sickelsteel, & Roth, 1983), and (4) use of REM-suppressant medications (such as protriptyline) when symptoms of cataplexy are problematic (Reite, Nagel, & Ruddy, 1990). Unfortunately, most studies done on pharmacological treatments for narcolepsy involve adults, with few studies including children.

Idiopathic Hypersomnolence

Some children and adolescents have significantly increased sleep needs without evidence of the REM abnormalities seen in narcolepsy. This condition has been called idiopathic hypersomnolence. There is often a familial history of excessive sleep needs, and these individuals show clear objective sleepiness in nap studies despite having obtained what appears to be adequate amounts of nighttime sleep. These disorders are also frequently treated with stimulant medication when the diagnosis is definitively established and daytime functioning is impaired.

Kleine-Levin Syndrome

Symptoms of excessive somnolence, hypersexuality, and compulsive overeating were first described in adolescent boys by Kleine (1925) and Levin (1929). Mental disturbances (irritability, confusion, and occasional auditory or visual hallucinations) have also been reported in these cases.

This syndrome (with more than 100 published cases) occurs three times more frequently in males. Typically, symptoms begin during adolescence either gradually or abruptly, and in about half the cases the onset follows a flu-like illness or injury with loss of consciousness. Frequently, there is an episodic nature to the symptoms, with cycles lasting from 1 to 30 days. The syndrome usually disappears spontaneously during late adolescence or early adulthood.

Laboratory tests, imaging studies, EEGs, and endocrine measures do not appear to be helpful in making the specific diagnosis of Kleine-Levin syndrome. It is important to rule out other organic causes of similar symptoms such as a hypothalamic tumor, localized CNS infection, or vascular accident. The presence of neurologic signs, evidence of increased CNS pressure, abnormalities in temperature regulation, abnormalities in water regulation, or other endocrine abnormalities point to an organically based abnormality. A family history of bipolar illness or other signs suggesting an early-onset bipolar illness should also be considered in the differential. Although stimulant medication or use of lithium carbonate has been reported to be helpful in individual cases, there is no clear consensus on treatment (Billiard, 1989).

Delayed Sleep Phase Syndrome

A common event that occurs especially with adolescents is staying up late at night, which in some individuals may lead to a complete shift in their sleep-wake schedule. The end result is delayed sleep phase syndrome (DSPS), with symptoms of sleep-onset insomnia and extreme difficulty awakening at a desired time in the morning. Approximately 7 percent of adolescents are sleep phase delayed. DSPS often begins with a tendency to stay up late at night, sleeping late in the morning, and/or taking a late afternoon nap. This process often begins on weekends, holidays, or summer vacations. Problems become apparent when school schedules result in morning wake-up battles and difficulties getting to school (Carskadon, Anders, & Hole, 1988). Often these adolescents cope by taking afternoon naps and catching-up on their sleep on the weekends. Although some of these behaviors occur in many normal adolescents, in extreme cases the circadian system can become set to such a late time that even highly motivated adolescents can have difficulty shifting their sleep back to an earlier time. In some instances, attempts to correct the problem go against circadian principles. For example, an adolescent who has been going to bed at 2:30 A.M. and getting up at 11:30 during vacation tries to go to bed at 10:00 P.M. the Sunday night before the first day back at school and finds that her physiology is quite resistant to sleep. For a few days she may be able to manage to get up for school by overriding the system (despite inadequate sleep) but then takes a long nap after school. Despite numerous nights of trying to go to bed at 10:00 P.M. she is unable to consistently shift her temperature cycle and circadian system back to an earlier phase.

The treatment of delayed sleep phase syndrome consists of two parts. The first is to gradually align the sleep system to the desirable schedule (Czeisler et al., 1981). The second is to maintain that alignment. The process of alignment consists of gradual, small, consistent advances of 15 minutes a day in bedtime and wake-up time. It is often best to begin from the time the adolescent usually goes to sleep without difficulty. It is important during this process to avoid any naps and to be consistent across weekends and holidays. In severe cases, some adolescents on very late schedules respond more favorably to going around the clock with successive delays in bedtime. This process has been described as phase delay "chronotherapy." Since the biologic clock tends to run on a 25-hour cycle, individuals can often accommodate phase delays more easily than phase advances. Hence, the schedule changes can proceed with longer delays of 2 to 3 hours per day. Again, it is important that there are no naps during the chronotherapy. Upon waking up, engaging in some activity and, if possible, exposure to bright light such as walking outdoors can help facilitate the process. Although many children and adolescents do very well with this type of phase delay chronotherapy, the first weekend or vacation of returning to old habits can undo all the advances made. Particularly in the first 2 to 3 weeks following chronotherapy, a rigid wake-up time 7 days a week should be instituted. Later, if the child or adolescent wants to stay up late on an occasional weekend night, he may be able to do so but should not be permitted to sleep more than 1 or 2 hours later than his usual wake-up time for school. Strict behavioral contracts (worked out with the parents), with specific rewards for success and serious consequences for failures, are often essential in this type of intervention. It should be noted that some children and adolescents will be resistant to treatment. In those cases, psychological issues will need to be addressed.

Parasomnias

Parasomnia is the term given to one of a group of unusual behaviors emerging from sleep. These include sleep walking, night terrors, confused partial arousal, nightmares, and enuresis. Headbanging and bruxism are also addressed under this topic as other unusual sleep-related events in children.

Partial Arousals

Sleepwalking, sleeptalking, and sleep terrors are all variations of partial arousals from deep sleep, usually stages 3 and 4. As discussed earlier, most children have a very deep period of slow-wave sleep 1 to 3 hours after sleep onset. At the end of this very deep sleep period, the transition to lighter sleep, REM sleep, or a brief arousal is often accompanied by unusual transition behaviors. Many children, on close observation, mumble, grimace, or demonstrate some awkward movements during this transition. For children with parasomnias, these transition episodes can consist of talking, calm or agitated sleepwalking, confused partial arousals, and, at times, what appears to be panic-like events. During these episodes, the child remains essentially asleep and has no memory of the event in the morning. The episodes can last from seconds to 30 minutes, with most events lasting 2 to 10 minutes. Because many parents think the child is having a nightmare or dream, they often attempt to awaken and reassure the child. This can be very distressing for the parent, since the child often stares blankly, does not recognize the parents, and can appear incoherent. Sometimes children thrash about wildly, let out blood-curdling screams, and bolt away from parents.

The event usually terminates spontaneously with the child returning to deep sleep.

Partial arousals are quite common in younger children. Chronic sleepwalking occurs in approximately 1-6 percent of children, with as many as 20 percent of all children having at least one such episode (Anders, 1982; Soldatos & Lugaresi, 1987). Sleep terrors are less frequent, with estimates ranging from 1 to 6 percent (Broughton, 1968; DiMario & Emery, 1987; Soldatos & Lugaresi, 1987). The discrepancies among reported rates of partial arousals may be a result of the difficulty in measuring the occurrence of these events, which the children do not remember and the parents may not observe. Surveys are more likely to measure the rates at which these problems affect the parents rather than their true prevalence.

Most partial arousals are a developmental phenomenon, with resolution as the child gets older. As delta sleep drops off in adolescence, the frequency of all of these delta-related events decreases dramatically. Studies indicate a genetic component to these sleep disturbances, in that there is usually a family history. Although many times parents are concerned that their child is severely anxious or depressed and that these sleep behaviors are a manifestation of psychological difficulties, this is rarely the case (Auchter, 1990; Fisher & McGuire, 1990; Taboada, 1975). Partial arousals, however, can be exacerbated or induced by fever, sleep deprivation, and some medications, such as lithium, prolixin, and desipramine (Klackenberg, 1982b). Furthermore, the history of children with frequent night terrors or partial arousals often indicates that these events occur in conjunction with chaotic sleep schedules, on the nights of recovery sleep following sleep loss, in conjunction with a change in schedule (such as beginning earlier mornings for school or daycare), or following periods of stress.

There are a number of considerations in the clinical evaluation and treatment of these problems. The first is to clearly identify that the episode is in fact a partial arousal. A contrast between night terrors and nightmares is provided in Table 8.1. Occurrence during the first third of the night, a state of confusion and partial arousal, the duration of the event, lack of memory of the event in the morning, a quick return to deep sleep following the event, and an increase in the frequency of events following sleep loss (or being overly tired) all strongly support the diagnosis of partial arousals. Once the problem is identified, it is important to explain to the parents and the rest of the family what these episodes are and what they are not. Reassurance of the family is one of the most important roles of the clinician. The next step should be to address the adequacy of the child's sleep and sched-

Table 8.1. Characteristic Features of Partial Arousals and Nightmares

	PARTIAL AROUSALS	NIGHTMARES
Time of night	first 1/3 of night	last 1/2 of night
Behavior	variable	very little motor behavior
Level of consciousness	unarousable or very confused if awakened	fully awake
Memory of event	amnesia	vivid recall
Family history	yes	no
Potential for injury	high	low
Frequency	common	very common
Stage of sleep	deep NREM	REM

ule. Increasing the amount of sleep and introducing more consistency into the schedule of the child can result in a dramatic decrease in the frequency of events. In addition, it is important to identify disturbances in the quality of sleep (such as sleep-disordered breathing or frequent middle-of-the-night awakenings), as sleep disruptions may result in a relative sleep deficit, increased intensity of delta, and more frequent partial arousals. Furthermore, it is important to emphasize safety (Clore & Hibel, 1993). Gates should be erected across stairs, and all windows and doors should be locked and bolted so that the child or adolescent is unable to leave the house.

Beyond reassurance, changes in sleep schedules, and safety, other treatments can be recommended. Behavioral methods can be successful (Kellerman, 1979; 1980). Such methods include the use of positive reinforcement for not having a night terror, in order to counteract the potential reinforcement of parental attention that may accompany having a night terror, and relaxation training strategies. A few studies have also shown moderate success with hypnosis (Koe, 1989; Kramer, 1989). There was initial success with scheduled awakenings (Lask, 1988). Medications such as a bedtime dose of a benzodiazepine, such as clonazepam or diazepam, or of a tricyclic antidepressant, such as imipramine, significantly decrease delta sleep and temporarily improve the situation in the child with frequent night terrors (Cameron & Thyer, 1985; Fisher, Kahn, Edwards, & Davis, 1973; Glick, Schulman, & Turecki, 1971; Popoviciu & Corfariu, 1983; Reite, Nagel, & Ruddy, 1990). Often when the medication is stopped, however, there is rebound delta and an increase in partial arousals (Weissbluth, 1984). In some cases when night terrors or partial arousals are extremely frequent, occur repeatedly within a single night, or are severely disruptive to the family, medications can be an important temporary adjunct to treatment. In these situations, often so much tension and fear are associated with going to sleep that it is important to "break the cycle" of sleep deprivation, disturbed sleep, increased pressure for delta, and frequent night terrors. Short-term use of medication (such as 25 to 75 mg of imipramine at bedtime depending on the patient's size and weight) in these situations can help create a window for more lasting intervention. Be sure to wean the child off any medications that are prescribed. Sudden withdrawal from many of these medications can result in significant rebound effects that include increased sleep problems.

Nightmares

Nightmares, in contrast to night terrors and other partial arousal disturbances, are events related to REM sleep. Nightmares are quite common in children, occurring in about 10–50 percent of all children between the ages of 3 and 6 years. Following a gradual onset, nightmares typically decrease in frequency over time. A small percentage of children will continue to have nightmares throughout adolescence, and even possibly into adulthood. One of the first steps in assessing frequent nightmares is distinguishing them from night terrors (see Table 8.1). Since nightmares occur more frequently during REM, they are much more likely to happen in the second half of the night. Following awakening from a nightmare, the child is alert and often describes detailed scenes of frightening images. The child usually has difficulty going back to sleep and often wants to remain with the parents. (With night terrors, in contrast, the child often does not recognize the parent and returns quickly to a very deep sleep.) Another important distinction is that, in the morning, children frequently remember and talk about their nightmares, whereas children with night terrors usually have no memory of the night terror. Although these distinctions are relatively easy to make in the older child or adolescent, they can be difficult in a younger child with limited verbal abilities.

Nightmares usually involve fears of attack, falling, or death (Kales, Soldatos, & Caldwell, 1980). Stressful periods and traumatic events will exacerbate the occurrence of nightmares. For example, distressing or frightening events such as automobile accidents or death of a relative are associated with increased nightmares. Nightmares are also often associated with post-traumatic stress disorder, and thus evaluation for this anxiety disorder should be conducted. In addition, some medications are associated with nightmares, including some beta blockers and antidepressants. Other medications produce nightmares as withdrawal symptoms, such as alcohol, barbiturates, and benzodiazepines. All in all, though, we know little about the causes of nightmares in children.

Treatment strategies for nightmares focus on anxiety reduction techniques such as relaxation and imagery, often combined with other behavioral strategies such as systematic desensitization (Cavior & Deutsch, 1975), response prevention (Roberts & Gordon, 1979), or dream reorganization (Palace & Johnston, 1989). Dream reorganization involves both systematic desensitization with coping self-statements and guided rehearsal of mastery endings to dream content. However, for most families, reassurance that nightmares are part of normal child development is beneficial and all that is necessary. It is also important to decrease the likelihood that the child will be treated as though psychologically disturbed.

Enuresis

Enuresis is diagnosed when persistent bed-wetting occurs after 5 years of age. Estimates indicate that bed-wetting occurs in 30 percent of 4-year-olds, 10 percent of 6-year-olds, 5 percent of 10-year-olds, and 3 percent of 12-year-olds. The spontaneous rate of remission after age 6 is about 15 percent per year (DeJonge, 1973). Primary enuresis, referring to those who have had a continuous enuretic condition, comprises 70–90 percent of all cases of the disorder. Secondary enuresis, in which the child has had at least 3–6 months of dryness, accounts for the remaining 10–30 percent of all cases. In addition, boys are more likely to be enuretic (up to age 10, about 50 percent more likely).

Many studies have researched various aspects of enuresis, including diagnosis, assessment, and treatment. Enuresis is undoubtedly the most well-studied childhood sleep disorder. Several behavioral treatments have high proven success rates. The most popular and effective technique is the bell-and-pad system, which sounds a bell or buzzer when bedwetting occurs. This method was developed by Mowrer and Mowrer in 1938. Reported success rates for this technique have been as high as 75 percent (Forsythe & Redmond, 1974; Fraser, 1972), with the best results in children over 7 years of age (McClain, 1979). Other treatment approaches for enuresis include bladder training (McClain, 1979; Troup & Hodgson, 1971), response prevention and contingency management (Luciano, Molina, Gomez, & Herruzo, 1993), hypnosis (Olness, 1975), and dietary control, such as a reduction in caffeine intake (Bond, Ware, & Hoelscher,

1990). Typically, a comprehensive treatment program is utilized, incorporating a number of components such as bladder-stretching exercises, visual sequencing, a nightly waking schedule, positive practice, and an alarm activated by wetness.

In some cases of enuresis, tricyclic antidepressants may be prescribed. Imipramine can be successful in controlling enuresis in up to 70 percent of cases when taken regularly (Ambrosini, Bianchi, Rabinovich, & Elia, 1993; Bindeglas & Dee, 1978). However, upon withdrawal from the medication, few children stay dry. Because of imipramine's potential cardiotoxic effects and the high relapse rate following withdrawal, it is often not recommended for long-term use (Scharf & Jennings, 1988). Another drug that has been used with success is desmopressin (DDAVP), an analogue of the antidiuretic hormone vasopressin (e.g., Miller, Goldberg, & Atkin, 1989). Desmopressin has success rates similar to those for imipramine, but it also almost always leads to relapse following discontinuation. Approximately 70 percent of cases, though, have persistent resolution of bed-wetting when maintained on desmopressin, with minimal side effects. Given that desmopressin is much more expensive and has higher relapse rates than other treatments, it may be the treatment of choice when used on a short-term, or as needed, basis (e.g., overnight camp, staying at a friend's house). Overall, the results from the above studies indicate that enuresis is highly amenable to treatment and should be considered a treatable disorder.

Other Behaviors during Sleep

Many children fall asleep while rocking their bodies, rolling back and forth, or banging their heads. These behaviors are very common in infants, with 60 percent of 9-month-olds doing one of these behaviors. Until two years of age, 22 percent of children continue to engage in one of these behaviors, and they are seen in approximately 5 percent of children after two years. The behavior usually disappears by age 4 but can persist through adolescence and into adulthood. Persistence beyond 10 years of age is reported to be associated with mental retardation or psychopathology.

Most of these rhythmic movement disorders occur at the onset of sleep, beginning during the drowsiness prior to sleep onset. Many children have a recurrence of the behavior in the middle of the night during sleep stage transitions back to wakefulness. That is, these children also seem to headbang or rock in order to go back to sleep after waking up during the night. Furthermore, some studies have shown that many children continue the behavior into stage 2 sleep. Some children seem to use these rhythmic behaviors as a self-comforting behavior even when they are awake during times of rest. Episodes typically last 5 to 15 minutes, but many last as long as 1 to 4 hours. The activity is often more rapid than one would imagine, with an average frequency of 45 bangs/rocks per minute and a reported range of 19 to 121 bangs/rocks per minute.

Injuries are uncommon and typically treatment is not instituted because this behavior is usually benign and self-limiting, and thus dissipates on its own. Treatment approaches have included behavioral modification programs. Psychiatric and neurologic evaluations may be indicated for older children when headbanging persists beyond 3 years of age. Benzodiazepines and tricyclic antidepressant medications have also been reported to be helpful in some cases. One major concern, however, about this sleep disorder is that it can be disruptive to the family and can have psychosocial consequences in older children and adolescents.

The other common behavior that can occur during sleep is bruxism, which involves grinding or clenching the teeth during sleep. Bruxism occurs in over 50 percent of normal infants, with the average age of onset at 10 months. Bruxism may cause dental problems, such as abnormal wear of the teeth or periodontal tissue damage, and may also be related to headaches or jaw pain. Although bruxism is usually treated through dental approaches, it can be amenable to EMG-activated biofeedback (Kardachi, Bailey, & Ash, 1978; Kardachi & Clarke, 1977; Piccione, Coates, George, Rosenthal, & Karzmark, 1982) and stress management approaches (Casas, Beemsterboer, & Clark, 1982). Unfortunately, most studies conducted on treatment of bruxism involve adults, with few studies, if any, researching the efficacy of treatment programs for bruxism in children.

Sleep and Psychiatric Disorders

The relationship between child/adolescent sleep disorders and psychiatric disorders is a very complex topic which has been discussed in greater detail elsewhere (Dahl, 1995; Dahl, 1996a; Dahl, 1996b). There is strong evidence for a bi-directional relationship between the regulation of sleep/arousal and the regulation of emotions and behaviors in children. That is, disruption of sleep or inadequate sleep in a child is strongly associated with emotional and behavioral changes. On the other hand, most major disturbances of mood are also associated with disturbances of sleep. Causal evidence also

supports a bidirectional relationship since acute sleep deprivation can be shown to cause behavioral and emotional changes in most children, and likewise, traumatic emotional experiences can clearly cause at least transient disruptions in sleep. In addition, there is extensive neurobiologic overlap between the control of sleep/arousal and the control of mood and behavior (see Dahl, 1996).

From a more pragmatic clinical perspective there are at least three areas of child psychiatry where sleep appears to be a very important domain to consider, including depression, ADHD, and PTSD. Each of these topics will be discussed briefly.

Depression

Major depressive disorder (MDD) in children and adolescents is associated with frequent symptoms of sleep disturbance. In a clinical review paper, 75 percent of children and adolescents with MDD reported insomnia, with 30 percent of subjects describing severe insomnia (Ryan et al., 1987). In that study, about 25 percent of depressed adolescents reported the opposite problems with prominent complaints of hypersomnia. On the other hand, it is critical to point out that objective EEG studies in subjects drawn from these same clinical samples found very little objective evidence of disrupted sleep, even among the adolescents with the most severe complaints of insomnia (Dahl et al., 1990, 1991, 1996). Some of the EEG changes seen in adult depression were evident in some depressed children and adolescents; however, the magnitude of these changes were quite small from a clinical perspective. For example, although the depressed group showed significantly longer latencies to fall asleep, the difference from the normal controls was about 15 minutes (30 minutes in the depressed adolescents compared to 15 minutes in the controls). Subjectively, however, 30 percent of these depressed adolescents reported that it took them more than 3 hours to fall asleep. The discrepancies between subjective and objective sleep disturbances have been the source of speculation.

The overlap with sleep/wake schedule problems is also important to consider. Often one of the most pragmatic clinical issues is to regularize the sleep/wake schedule in these adolescents and in at least a small percentage of the patients the resultant increase in sleep can produce improvements in mood, and often greater ability to implement other treatment approaches such as cognitive/behavioral therapy. These topics have been discussed in greater detail elsewhere (see Dahl, 1992).

Attention-Deficit/ Hyperactivity Disorder

The area of attention deficit disorders also reveals a picture of large subjective sleep disturbances which contrast with controlled studies showing small or infrequent sleep changes (Busby & Pivik, 1981; Greenhill et al., 1983; , Kaplan et al., 1987). There is evidence that sleep deprivation can clearly exacerbate ADHD symptoms, particularly irritability, distractibility, and difficulties with focused attention (Dahl et al., 1991b; Dahl et al., 1995; Guilleminault et al., 1982). More recent data has also suggested that children with ADHD may have high rates of LS/PLMS (Picchietti & Walters, in press). From a pragmatic clinical perspective, it is worth noting that attempts to increase or improve nighttime sleep can help in the management of daytime symptoms of ADHD and should be considered in treatment plans—particularly when the history suggests inadequate or insufficient sleep.

Post-Traumatic Stress Disorder

Post-traumatic stress disorder in children has also been associated with a variety of sleep problems, including recurrent nightmares, difficulty falling asleep, and fragmented night sleep (Sadeh, 1996; Wolfson, in press). Chronic sleep disruption in some traumatized children may also contribute to other daytime symptoms of mood and attentional difficulties. Treatment directed at the sleep problem (which may include psychotherapy, behavioral interventions, and in some cases medications) can be an important adjunct to treatment. These issues are discussed in more depth in other publications (Sadeh, 1996; Uhde, 1994; Wolfson, in press).

CASE ILLUSTRATION

Clinical Presentation

Troy was an 8-year-old boy who was seen by the first author for problems involving difficulty falling asleep at night, difficulty waking in the morning, and excessive daytime sleepiness. His mother reported that Troy had a long history of difficulty falling asleep at night, but his problem started becoming significantly worse one year prior to coming for treatment. When we saw him he was going to bed at approximately 10:15 P.M. and taking 45 to 60 minutes to fall asleep. On school days, his mother would wake him at 7:15 and it would take him at least a half-hour to get out of bed. On

weekends or during school vacations, Troy would not go to bed until at least 11:00 and would still require 30 minutes to fall asleep. He would usually get up around 8:30 A.M. on these days. Between the time when he would get into bed and finally fall asleep, Troy would repeatedly come out of his room calling for his mother. His mother sometimes gave him hydroxyzinepamoate (Vistaril) or acetaminophen (Tylenol) for Troy's "insomnia," especially on Sunday evenings.

Given Troy's sleep schedule, it was not unexpected that he was so sleepy during the day. His sleepiness had been getting progressively worse during the past year. During the past six months, Troy was falling asleep at inappropriate times, such as in school, while watching television, and while riding the bus. Troy had even fallen asleep in school while taking a test. His school work was being affected by his sleepiness and his performance in school was rapidly declining.

Further questioning about Troy's sleep revealed that he had a long-term history of being a "noisy breather" and a restless sleeper. He experienced infrequent nightmares and talked in his sleep on occasion. Troy denied any symptoms consistent with narcolepsy, such as cataplexy, hypnogogic hallucinations, or sleep paralysis.

In addition to Troy's sleep problems, Troy had some behavior problems during the day, including overactivity, impulsivity, and distractability. He had been seen by a psychologist for these difficulties when he was 5 years old, and had recently begun seeing the same therapist again. His teachers were concerned about possible learning difficulties and a potential diagnosis of attention deficit/hyperactivity disorder. A complete evaluation by the school was being scheduled for these latter problems.

Troy lived alone with his mother. His medical history was unremarkable. His mother had also been evaluated in the past for sleep problems. At the time, she was diagnosed with a disorder of initiating and maintaining sleep due to psychophysiological factors. She was successfully treated with sleep hygiene and sleep restriction.

Assessment Findings

Troy's history of difficulty falling asleep at night, late bedtime, difficulty waking in the morning, and excessive sleepiness during the day were consistent with insufficient sleep syndrome and delayed sleep phase syndrome. Sleep diary data, kept for two weeks, also indicated these problems. Such a sleep disorder was also consistent with his mother's long-term history of insomnia and successful treatment. A psychological assessment did not indicate any significant problems with anxiety or depression, although Troy clearly had difficulties with attention and was highly active.

However, there was a concern that an underlying sleep disrupter was also contributing to Troy's sleep problems, especially given his mother's report that Troy was a noisy breather and a restless sleeper. Thus, an overnight polysomnogram (PSG) was conducted. The PSG results indicated that Troy did experience an insignificant number of snore arousals during sleep. It did not appear that this problem was interfering with his ability to fall asleep at night but may have been a contributor to his daytime sleepiness.

Treatment Selection and Course

Following the overnight study, the results and impressions were discussed in detail with Troy and his mother. A number of treatment recommendations were made. For the snore arousals, it was suggested that Troy be evaluated by an ENT specialist to assess for any obstruction due to enlarged tonsils or adenoids. It was clear from the history that Troy was sleep deprived and had delayed sleep phase syndrome. To alleviate these sleep problems a number of behavioral recommendations were made. First, a regular bedtime routine was established that included plenty of quality time with his mother. Second, approximately 5–10 minutes after Troy was to go to bed, his mother was to check on him, in a rather neutral manner, to eliminate Troy's getting out of bed and seeking his mother's attention. Third, a sleep restriction schedule was implemented. Beginning on the first night, Troy was to go to bed at 11:15. Following three nights of this regimen, he would go to bed 15 minutes earlier. His mother was to continue with this 15 minutes earlier every third night schedule until Troy was going to bed at 10:00. He was to maintain this schedule on weekdays and weekends. In addition, every morning Troy was to be awakened at 7:15 and get out of bed immediately. He was also to spend as much time as possible in the early morning outside in bright sunlight. This schedule was chosen, rather than using the more typical chronotherapy of moving ahead around the clock, because Troy was not going to bed in the early morning hours. Therefore, we believed that such a procedure was not necessary and he would be able to move backward, as long as it was in small increments. In addition, sleep hygiene and sleep restriction had been successfully conducted by his mother for her sleep problems. Thus she was more likely to be invested in the treatment plan and more likely to insist on Troy's compliance.

Termination and Follow-Up

Troy was followed for several months after the initial treatment suggestions were made. The ENT specialist did not recommend a tonsillectomy or adenoidectomy. Because Troy's snore arousals were mild, no further intervention was suggested, although it was recommended that he continue to be monitored for sleep apnea. Troy initially did well on the new sleep schedule, rotating to a more regular bedtime and being less sleepy during the day. However, after a month of initial success, Troy began having difficulties again, as he was not maintaining the strict sleep schedule. On weekends, he began returning to his previous sleep patterns, which affected his weekday sleep. Once this was understood by Troy and his mother, Troy again began to do well. Troy's daytime behavior problems, however, persisted and he continued to have difficulties in school, although he was now not falling asleep. His mother was encouraged to proceed with the school testing and to continue to see a psychologist for Troy's behavior problems.

SUMMARY

Sleep disorders are commonly experienced by children and adolescents. Many people believe that the primary factors contributing to sleep disturbances are psychological in nature; however, in many cases, sleep problems do not appear to be the result of underlying psychopathology, but are best understood as physiologically or behaviorally based. In addition, many sleep problems are highly amenable to treatment. Unfortunately, they are often under-diagnosed and under-treated.

In sum, given the prevalence of these problems in the child and adolescent population, it is important for all pediatric psychologists and psychiatrists to be knowledgeable about sleep and sleep disorders. This information is essential whether or not the patient is going to be treated directly or is going to be referred for specialized services. We all spend approximately one-third of our lives sleeping, or trying to sleep; therefore, we should understand as much as we can about it.

REFERENCES

Abe, K., Ohta, M., Amatomi, M., & Oda, N. (1982). Persistence and predictive value of behaviours of 3-year-olds: A follow-up study at 8 years. *Acta Paedopsychiarica, 48,* 185–191.

Adams, L. A., & Rickert, V. I. (1989). Reducing bedtime tantrums: Comparison between positive routines and graduated extinction. *Pediatrics, 84,* 756–761.

Ambrosini, P. J., Bianchi, M. D., Rabinovich, H., & Elia, J. (1993). Antidepressant treatments in children and adolescents: II. Anxiety, physical and behavioral disorders. *Journal of the Academy of Child and Adolescent Psychiatry, 32,* 483–493.

American Psychiatric Association. (1994). *Diagnostic and statistical manual of mental disorders* (3rd ed.). Washington, DC: Author.

Anders, T. F. (1982). Neurophysiological studies of sleep in infants and children. *Journal of Child Psychology and Psychiatry and Allied Disciplines, 23,* 75–83.

Auchter, U. (1990). Anxiety in children: An investigation on various forms of anxiety. *Acta Paedopsychiatrica, 53,* 78–88.

Billiard, M. (1989). The Kleine-Levin Syndrome. In M. H. Kryger, T. Roth, & W. C. Dement (Eds.), *Principles and Practice of Sleep Medicine,* Philadelphia: W. B. Saunders Co.

Bindeglas, P. M., & Dee, G. (1978). Enuresis treatment with imipramine hydrochloride: A 10-year follow-up study. *American Journal of Psychiatry, 135,* 1549–1552.

Bixler, E. O., Kales, J. D., Scharf, M. B., Kales, A., & Leo, L. A. (1976). Incidence of sleep disorders in medical practice: A physician survey. *Sleep Research, 5,* 62.

Bond, T., Ware, J. C., & Hoelscher, T. J. (1990). Caffeine and enuresis: A case report. *Sleep Research, 19,* 195.

Broughton, R. J. (1968). Sleep disorders: Disorders of arousal? *Science, 159,* 1070–1078.

Brouillette, R. T., Fernback, S. K., & Hunt, C. E. (1982). Obstructive sleep apnea in infants and children. *Journal of Pediatrics, 100,* 31–40.

Busby, K., & Pivik, R. T. (1981). Sleep patterns in hyperkinetic and normal children. *Pediatrics, 4,* 366–371.

Cameron, O. G., & Thayer, B. A. (1985). Treatment of pavor nocturnus with alprazolam. *Journal of Clinical Psychiatry, 46,* 504.

Carskadon, M. A., Anders, T. F., & Hole, W. (1988). Sleep disturbances in childhood and adolescence. In H. E. Fitzgerald, B. M. Lester, and M. W. Yogman (Eds.), *Theory and research in behavioral pediatrics* (vol. 4). New York: Plenum.

Casas, J. M., Beemsterboer, P., & Clark, G. T. (1982). A comparison of stress-reduction behavioral counseling and contingent EMG biofeedback with an arousal task. *Behaviour Research and Therapy, 20,* 9–15.

Cavior, N., & Deutsch, A. (1975). Systematic desensitization to reduce dream induced anxiety. *Journal of Nervous and Mental Disease, 161,* 433–435.

Clore, E. R., & Hibel, J. (1993). The parasomnias of childhood. *Journal of Pediatric Health Care, 7,* 12–16.

Connell, H. M., Persley, G. V., & Sturgess, J. L. (1987). Sleep phobia in middle childhood—A review of six cases. *Journal of the American Academy of Child and Adolescent Psychiatry, 26,* 449–452.

Croft, C. B., Brockbank, M. J., Wright, A., & Swanston, A. R. (1990). Obstructive sleep apnea in children undergoing routine tonsillectomy and adenoidectomy. *Clinical Otolaryngology, 15,* 307–314.

Czeisler, C. A., Richardson, G. S., Coleman, R. M., Zimmerman, J. C., Moore-Ede, M. C., Dement, W. C., & Weitzman, E. D. (1981). Chronotherapy: Resetting the circadian clocks of patients with the delayed sleep phase syndrome. *Sleep, 4,* 1–21.

Dahl, R. E. (1992). Child and adolescent sleep disorders. In D. M. Kaufman (Ed.), *Child and adolescent neurology for psychiatrists.* Baltimore, MD: Williams and Wilkins.

Dahl, R. E. (1995). Sleep in behavioral and emotional disorders. In R. Ferber and M. Kryger (Eds.), *Principles and practices of sleep medicine in the child* (2nd ed.). Philadelphia: W. B. Saunders.

Dahl, R. E. (1996). The regulation of sleep and arousal: Development and psychopathology. *Development and Psychopathology, 16,* 3–29.

Dahl, R. E. (1996). Sleep and child psychiatry. In R. E. Dahl (Ed.), *Child and Adolescent Psychiatric Clinics of North America: Child and Adolescent Sleep Disorders* (pp. 543–548). Philadelphia: W. B. Saunders.

Dahl, R. E., Matty, M. K., Birmaher, B., Al-Shabbout, M., Williamson, D. E., & Ryan, N. D. (in press). Sleep onset abnormalities in depressed adolescents. *Biological Psychiatry.*

Dahl, R. E., Bernisal-Broadbent, J., Scanlon-Holdford, S., Lupo, M., Sampson, H. A., & Al-Shabbout, M. (1995). Sleep disturbance in children with atopic dermatitis. *Archives of Pediatrics and Adolescent Medicine, 149,* 856–860.

Dahl, R. E., Holtum, J., & Trubnick, L. (1994). A clinical picture of child and adolescent narcolepsy. *Journal of the American Academy of Child and Adolescent Psychiatry, 6,* 834–841.

Dahl, R. E., Pelham, W. E., & Wierson, M. (1991b). The role of sleep disturbances in attention deficit disorder symptoms: A case study. *Journal of Pediatric Psychology, 16,* 229–239.

Dahl, R. E., Puig-Antich, J., Ryan, N. D., Cunningham, S., Nelson, B., & Klepper, T. (1990). EEG sleep in adolescent with major depression. *Journal of Affective Disorders, 19,* 63–75.

Dahl, R. E., Ryan, N. D., Birmaher, B., Al-Shabbout, M., Williamson, D. E., Neidig, M., Nelson, B., & Puig-

Antich, J. (1991a). EEG sleep measures in prepubertal depression. *Psychiatry Research, 38*, 201–214.

DeJonge, G. A. (1973). Epidemiology of enuresis: A survey of the literature: Bladder control and enuresis. *Clinical and Developmental Medicine, 48/49*, 39–46.

Diagnostic Classification Steering Committee. (1990). *The international classification of sleep disorders: Diagnostic and coding manual.* Rochester, MN: American Sleep Disorder Association.

DiMario, F. J., & Emery, E. S. (1987). The natural history of night terrors. *Clinical Pediatrics, 26*, 505–511.

Dollinger, S. L. (1982). On the varieties of childhood sleep disturbance. *Journal of Clinical Child Psychology, 11*, 107–115.

Durand, V. M., & Mindell, J. A. (1990). Behavioral treatment of multiple childhood sleep disorders: Effects on child and family. *Behavior Modification, 14*, 37–49.

Ferber, R. (1987). The sleepless child. In C. Guilleminault (Eds.), *Sleep and its disorders in children.* New York: Raven Press.

Fisher, B., & McGuire, K. (1990). Do diagnostic patterns exist in the sleep behaviors of normal children? *Journal of Abnormal Child Psychology, 18*,179–186.

Fisher, C., Kahn, E., Edwards, A., & Davis, D. M. (1973). A psychophysiological study of nightmares and night terrors: The suppression of stage 4 night terrors with diazepam. *Archives of General Psychiatry, 28*, 252–259.

Forsythe, W. I., & Redmond, A. (1974). Enuresis and spontaneous cure rate: Study of 1129 enuretics. *Archives of Disease in Childhood, 49*, 259–263.

Fraser, M. S. (1972). Nocturnal enuresis. *Practitioner, 208*, 203–211.

Friedman, A. G., & Ollendick, T. H. (1989). Treatment programs for severe night-time fears: A methodological note. *Journal of Behavior Research and Experimental Therapy, 20*, 171–178.

Glick, B. S., Schulman, D., & Turecki, S. (1971). Diazepam (Valium) treatment in childhood sleep disorders: A preliminary investigation. *Diseases of the Nervous System, 32*, 565–566.

Graziano, A., & Mooney, K. (1980). Family self-control instruction for children's nighttime fear reduction. *Journal of Consulting and Clinical Psychology, 48*, 206–213.

Graziano, A., & Mooney, K. (1982). Behavioral treatment of "nightfears" in children: Maintenance of improvement at 2 1/2- to 3-year follow-up. *Journal of Consulting and Clinical Psychology, 50*, 598–599.

Greenhill, L., Puig-Antich, J., Goetz, R., et al. (1983). Sleep architecture and REM sleep measures in children with ADHD. *Sleep, 6*, 91–96.

Guilleminault, C. (1986). Narcolepsy. *Sleep, 9*, 99–291.

Guilleminault, C. (1987). Narcolepsy and its differential diagnosis. In C. Guilleminault (Ed.), *Sleep and its disorders in children* (pp. 181–194). New York: Raven Press.

Guilleminault, C., & Anders, T. F. (1976). Sleep disorders in children. *Advances in Pediatrics, 22*, 151–174.

Guilleminault, C., Korobkin, R., & Winkle, R. (1981). A review of 50 children with obstructive sleep apnea syndrome. *Lung, 159*, 275–287.

Guilleminault, C., Riley, R., Powell, N., Simmons, F. B., & Nino-Murcia, G. (1985). Obstructive sleep apnea syndrome in adolescents: Diagnosis and treatment [Abstract]. *Sleep Research, 14*, 159.

Guilleminault, C., Winkle, R., & Korobkin, R., et al. (1982). Children and nocturnal snoring: Evaluation of the effects of sleep related respiratory resistance and daytime functioning. *European Journal of Pediatrics, 139*, 165–172.

Hall, M., Dahl, R. E., Dew, M. A., & Reynolds, C. F. (1996). Sleep patterns following major negative life events. *Directions in Psychiatry, 15*, 1–7.

Jenkins, S., Bax, M., & Hart, H. (1980). Behavior problems in preschool children. *Journal of Child Psychology and Psychiatry, 21*, 5–17.

Jones, D. P. H., & Verduyn, C. M. (1983). Behavioral management of sleep problems. *Archives of Disease in Childhood, 58*, 442–444.

Kahn, A., Van de Merckt, C., Rebuffat, E., Mozin, M. J., Sottiaux, M., Blum, D., & Hennart, P. (1989). Sleep problems in healthy preadolescents. *Pediatrics, 84*, 542–546.

Kales, J. D., Kales, A., Soldatos, C. R., Caldwell, A. B., Charney, D. S., & Martin, E. D. (1980). Night terrors: Clinical characteristics and personality patterns. *Archives of General Psychiatry, 37*, 1406–1410.

Kales, J. D., Soldatos, C. R., & Caldwell, A. B. (1980). Nightmares: Clinical characteristics and personality patterns. *American Journal of Psychiatry, 137*, 1197–2001.

Kaplan, B. J., McNichol, J., Conte, R. A., et al. (1987). Sleep disturbance in pre-school aged hyperactive and non-hyperactive children. *Pediatrics, 80*, 839–841.

Kardachi, B. J., Bailey, J. O., & Ash, M. M. (1978). A comparison of biofeedback and occlusal adjustment on bruxism. *Journal of Periodontology, 49*, 367–372.

Kardachi, B. J., & Clarke, N. G. (1977). The use of biofeedback to control bruxism. *Journal of Periodontology, 48*, 639–642.

Kataria, S., Swanson, M. S., & Trevathon, G. E. (1987). Persistence of sleep disturbances in preschool children. *Behavioral Pediatrics, 110*, 642–646.

Kellerman, J. (1979). Behavioral treatment of night terrors in a child with acute leukemia. *Journal of Nervous and Mental Disease, 167*, 182–185.

Kellerman, J. (1980). Rapid treatment of nocturnal anxiety in children. *Journal of Behavior Therapy and Experimental Psychiatry, 11*, 9–11.

King, N., Cranstoun, F., & Josephs, A. (1989). Emotive imagery and children's night-time fears: A multiple baseline design evaluation. *Journal of Behavior Therapy and Experimental Psychiatry, 20*, 125–135.

Klackenberg, G. (1982a). Sleep behavior studied longitudinally: Data from 4–16 years on duration, night-awakening and bed sharing. *Acta Paediatrica Scandinavia, 71*, 501–506.

Klackenberg, G. (1982b). Somnambulism in childhood: Prevalence, course and behavioral correlations. *Acta Paediatrica Scandinavia, 71*, 495–499.

Kleine, W. (1925). Peiordische schlafsucht. *Monatsschr Psychiatr Neurol, 57*, 285–298.

Koe, G. G. (1989). Hypnotic treatment of sleep terror disorder: A case report. *American Journal of Clinical Hypnosis, 32*, 36–40.

Kotagal, S., Hartse, K. M., & Walsh, J. K. (1990). Characteristics of narcolepsy in preteenaged children. *Pediatrics, 85*, 205–209.

Kramer, R. L. (1989). The treatment of childhood night terrors through the use of hypnosis–A case study: A brief communication. *The International Journal of Clinical Hypnosis, 4*, 283–284.

Lask, B. (1988). Novel and non-toxic treatment for night terrors. *British Medical Journal, 297*, 592.

Levin, M. (1929). Narcolepsy and other varieties of morbid somnolence. *Archives of Neurology and Psychiatry, 22*, 1172–1200.

Lozoff, B., Wolf, A. W., & Davis, N. S. (1985). Sleep problems seen in pediatric practice. *Pediatrics, 75*, 477–483.

Luciano, M. C., Molina, F. J., Gomez, I., & Herruzo, J. (1993). Response prevention and contingency management in the treatment of nocturnal enuresis: A report of two cases. *Child and Family Behavior Therapy, 15*, 37–51.

Mallory, G. B., Fiser, D. H., & Jackson, R. (1989). Sleep-associated breathing disorders in morbidly obese children and adolescents. *Journal of Pediatrics, 115*, 892–897.

Mauer, K. W., Staats, B. A., & Olson, K. D. (1983). Upper airway obstruction and disordered nocturnal breathing in children. *Mayo Clinic Proceedings, 58*, 349–353.

McClain, L. G. (1979). Childhood enuresis. *Current Problems in Pediatrics, 9*, 1–36.

Milan, M. A., Mitchell, Z. P., Berger, M. I., & Pierson, D. F. (1981). Positive routines: A rapid alternative to extinction for elimination of bedtime tantrum behavior. *Child Behavior Therapy, 3*, 13–25.

Miller, K., Goldberg, S., & Atkin, B. (1989). Nocturnal enuresis: Experience with long-term use of intranasally administered desmopressin. *Journal of Pediatrics, 114*, 723–726.

Mindell, J. A., & Durand, V. M. (1993). Treatment of childhood sleep disorders: Generalization across disorders and effects on family members. *Pediatric Psychology, 18*, 731–750.

Mindell, J. A. (1996). Treatment of child and adolescent sleep disorders. In R. E. Dahl (Ed.), *Child and Adolescent Psychiatric Clinics of North America: Child and Adolescent Sleep Disorders* (pp. 741–751). Philadelphia: W. B. Saunders.

Mitler, M. M., Nelson, S., & Hajdukovic, R. (1987). Narcolepsy: Diagnosis, treatment, and management. *Psychiatric Clinics of North America, 10*, 593–606.

Mowrer, O. H., & Mowrer, W. M. (1938). Enuresis—A method for its study and treatment. *American Journal of Orthopsychiatry, 8*, 436–459.

Ollendick, T. H., Hagopian, L. P., & Huntzinger, R. M. (1991). Cognitive-behavior therapy with nighttime fearful children. *Journal of Behavior Therapy and Experimental Psychiatry, 22*, 113–121.

Olness, K. (1975). The use of self-hypnosis in the treatment of childhood nocturnal enuresis: A report on 40 patients. *Clinical Pediatrics, 14*, 273–279.

Palace, E. M., & Johnston, C. (1989). Treatment of recurrent nightmares by the dream reorganization approach. *Journal of Behavior Therapy and Experimental Psychiatry, 20*, 219–226.

Picchietti, D. L., & Walters, A. S. (in press). Restless legs syndrome and periodic limb movement disorder in children and adolescents: Comorbidity with attention deficit/hyperactivity disorder. In R. E. Dahl (Ed.), *Child and adolescent psychiatric clinics of North America: Child and adolescent sleep disorders*. Philadelphia: W. B. Saunders.

Piccione, A., Coates, T. J., George, J. M., Rosenthal, D., & Karzmark, P. (1982). Nocturnal biofeedback for nocturnal bruxism. *Biofeedback and Self-Regulation, 7*, 405–419.

Popoviciu, L., & Corfariu, O. (1983). Efficacy and safety of midazolam in the treatment of night terrors in children. *British Journal of Clinical Pharmacology, 16*, 97–102.

Reite, M. L., Nagel, K. E., & Ruddy, J. R. (1990). *Concise guide to evaluation and management of sleep disorders.* Washington, DC: American Psychiatric Press.

Richman, N. (1981). A community survey of characteristics of one to two year olds with sleep disruptions. *Journal of the American Academy of Child Psychiatry, 20*, 281–291.

Richman, N. (1985). A double-blind drug trial of treatment in young children with waking problems. *Journal of Child Psychology and Psychiatry, 4,* 591–598.

Richman, N., Douglas, J., Hunt, H., Lansdown, R., & Levere, R. (1985). Behavioral methods in the treatment of sleep disorders—A pilot study. *Journal of Child Psychology and Psychiatry, 26,* 581–590.

Richman, N., Stevenson, J. E., & Graham, P. J. (1975). Behavior problems in three-year-old children: An epidemiological study in a London borough. *Journal of Child Psychology and Psychiatry, 12,* 5–33.

Rickert, V. I., & Johnson, C. M. (1988). Reducing nocturnal awakening and crying episodes in infants and young children: A comparison between scheduled awakenings and systematic ignoring. *Pediatrics, 81,* 203–212.

Roberts, R. N., & Gordon, S. B. (1979). Reducing childhood nightmares subsequent to a burn trauma. *Child Behavior Therapy, 1,* 373–381.

Ryan, N. D., Puig-Antich, J., Rabinovich, H., et al. (1987). The clinical picture of major depression in children and adolescents. *Archives of General Psychiatry, 44,* 854–860.

Sadeh, A. (1996). Stress, trauma, and sleep in children. In R. E. Dahl (Ed.), *Child and Adolescent Psychiatric Clinics of North America: Child and Adolescent Sleep Disorders* (pp. 685–700). Philadelphia: W. B. Saunders.

Salzarulo, P., & Chevalier, A. (1983). Sleep problems in children and their relationships with early disturbances of the waking-sleeping rhythms. *Sleep, 6,* 47–51.

Schaefer, C. E. (1990). Treatment of night wakings in early childhood: Maintenance of effects. *Perceptual and Motor Skills, 70,* 561–562.

Scharf, M. B., & Jennings, S. W. (1988). Childhood enuresis: Relationship to sleep, etiology, evaluation, and treatment. *Annals of Behavioral Medicine, 10,* 113–120.

Seymour, F. W., Brock, P., During, M., & Poole, G. (1989). Reducing sleep disruptions in young children: Evaluation of therapist-guided and written information approaches: A brief report. *Journal of Child Psychology and Psychiatry, 30,* 913–918.

Soldatos, C. R., & Lugaresi, E. (1987). Nosology and prevalence of sleep disorders. *Seminar in Neurology, 7,* 236–242.

Taboada, E. L. (1975). Night terrors in a child treated with hypnosis. *American Journal of Clinical Hypnosis, 17,* 270–271.

Troup, C., & Hodgson, N. (1971). Nocturnal functional bladder capacity in enuretic children. *Journal of Urology, 105,* 129–132.

Uhde, T. W. (1994). Anxiety disorders. In M. H. Kryger, T. Roth, & W. C. Dement (Eds.), *Principles and practices of sleep medicine* (2nd ed.). Philadelphia: W. B. Saunders.

Weissbluth, M. (1982). Modification of sleep schedule with reduction of night waking: A case report. *Sleep, 5,* 262–266.

Weissbluth, M. (1984). Is drug treatment of night terrors warranted? *American Journal of Diseases in Children, 138,* 1086.

Wittig, R., Zorick, F., Roehrs, T., Sickelsteel, J., & Roth, T. (1983). Narcolepsy in a 7-year-old child. *Journal of Pediatrics, 102,* 725–727.

Wolfson, A. R. (1996). Sleeping patterns of children and adolescents: Developmental trends, disruptions, and adaptations. In R. E. Dahl (Ed.), *Child and Adolescent Psychiatric Clinics of North America: Child and Adolescent Sleep Disorders* (pp. 549–568). Philadelphia: W. B. Saunders.

CHAPTER 9

ELIMINATION DISORDERS

Michael W. Mellon
H. Patrick Stern

DESCRIPTION OF DISORDERS

Consistent with the theme of this volume, we present a biobehavioral perspective of the childhood elimination disorders, functional enuresis, and encopresis. Although traditionally conceptualized as medical or psychiatric disorders, recent advances in assessment and treatment highlight the importance of understanding the childhood elimination disorders through the interaction of physiological mechanisms within the context of behaviorism and child development. This model is lucidly described and exemplified in Meyers' (1991) "Mini-Series On: Interactive Models in Behavioral Medicine." As such, the childhood functional elimination disorders may represent a prototypical example of how the collaboration between pediatric psychologists and medical professionals leads to the optimal assessment and treatment of these relatively common, yet troublesome, disorders.

Enuresis generally refers to accidental wetting after the age of 5 years, occurring with a frequency of twice a week for at least 3 consecutive months, or indicates that the presence of wetting episodes produces considerable distress and impairment in social, academic (occupational), or other important areas of the child's functioning (American Psychiatric Association, 1994). *Diurnal enuresis* refers to daytime wetting and is distinguished from nocturnal enuresis, which applies to children who only bedwet. This distinction is relevant because of a significantly higher incidence of medical problems such as urinary tract infection and abnormal urodynamics in diurnal enuresis (Arnold & Ginsberg, 1973; Jarvelin, Huttunen, Seppanen, Seppanen, & Moilanen, 1990). Children with daytime wetting often require further medical evaluation and treatment. The focus of this chapter is nocturnal enuresis without daytime wetting.

Bedwetting has been associated with problems of emotional and social adjustment among enuretic children, though the nature of this association remains unclear. The association appears to be greatest in girls, in diurnal enuretics, and in secondary enuretics, but it is important to emphasize that psychiatric disturbance is present in only a minority of enuretic children (Essen & Peckham, 1976; Kaffman & Elizur, 1977; Rutter, Yule, & Graham, 1973; Stromgren & Thomsen, 1990). Experimental studies have demonstrated that enuretic children treated for bedwetting improve more than untreated controls on measures of self-concept and peer relations (Baker, 1969; Lovibond, 1964; Moffatt, Kato, & Pless, 1987). Continued recommendations to parents by health professionals to wait for their child to "outgrow" the disorder may now be considered inappropriate due to the potential psychosocial consequences of continued bedwetting and the availability of effective treatment options.

Of the numerous etiological explanations for bedwetting, none is completely adequate in explaining the problem. The two leading etiological hypotheses are (a) deficiency in nocturnal secretion of antidiuretic hormone, and (b) absence of learned muscular responses needed to inhibit micturition during sleep (see review by Houts, 1991). Clearly, while enuresis may be viewed as a physical problem with behavioral and psychological consequences, this does not necessarily imply that effective treatment consists of medication therapy. On the contrary, the most effective treatment for bedwetting is some form of urine alarm (Houts et al., 1994). As with other physical problems such as obesity and diabetes, enuresis may be best conceptualized as a biobehavioral problem in which physiological mechanisms may be altered by changes in behavior through the use of learning and conditioning principles.

Functional childhood encopresis refers to the repeated involuntary passage of feces into clothing, occurring at least once per month for at least three months, past the mental and chronological age of four years, and not due to organic causes of fecal incontinence such as Hirschsprung's Disease (American Psychiatric Association, 1994). The *retentive* versus *nonretentive* distinction, which refers to children whose soiling is accompanied by chronic constipation and those who soil without retention, reflects the treatment utility of this dichotomy. A history of painful defecation, fecal impaction, severe withholding and fecal soiling is documented in a large retrospective study of children who presented with fecal soiling (Partin, Hamill, Fischel, & Partin, 1992). Treatments that ignore the high base-rate of retention and constipation, and fail to target this problem accordingly, will most likely lead to a poor outcome.

Normal bowel function, which involves a complex interaction between physiology and learned motor responses and fecal contingencies, is achieved in 98 percent of children by age four (Bellman, 1966). Because of space limitations, the reader is referred to Whitehead and Schuster (1985) for an in-depth account of normal bowel function and physiology. For present purposes, however, it is important to understand that bowel continence is maintained through a complex balance between the interaction of retentive and expulsive forces governed by reflexive processes and voluntary motor responses (Mellon & Houts, 1995).

From a biobehavioral perspective, functional encopresis results when the voluntary mechanisms of defecation are disrupted through multiple influences: physiological predisposition to constipation (Stern et al., 1995), dysfunctional defecation dynamics (Loening-Baucke & Cruikshank, 1986; Wald, Chandra, Gabel, & Chiponis, 1987), and a conditioned aversion response to painful defecation maintained through negative reinforcement (Partin et al., 1992; Mellon & Houts, 1995). Once physiological function is disrupted, the passage of feces at inappropriate times and places in the form of large stools or overflow soiling occurs. Treatments based on unitary medical and behavioral theories are, at best, only marginally effective because they either fail to acknowledge the learning history that maintains the soiling for the former, and the problem of severe and chronic constipation for the latter. As with enuresis, the collaboration between psychologists and physicians leads to the optimal assessment and treatment of functional encopresis.

EPIDEMIOLOGY

Although the reported prevalence of enuresis varies (DeJonge, 1973), it is conservatively estimated that about 7 percent of all 8-year-old children wet their beds, with most of them doing so every night of the week (Essen & Peckham, 1976; Fergusson, Horwood, & Shannon, 1986; Jarvelin, Vikevainen-Tervonen, Moilanen, & Huttunen, 1988; Verhulst et al., 1985). Less than 10 percent of these children have some sort of physical abnormality of the urinary tract (American Academy of Pediatrics Committee on Radiology, 1980; Jarvelin et al., 1990; Kass, 1991; Redman & Seibert, 1979; Rushton, 1989; Stansfeld, 1973). Bedwetting appears to have a strong genetic component, and enuretic children may show signs of delayed maturation of the nervous system (Jarvelin, 1989; Jarvelin et al., 1991). Up to age 11 years, more than twice as many males as females suffer from enuresis.

Epidemiological studies indicate that the prevalence of enuresis declines with age and this has contributed to the belief among professionals and parents that children will outgrow the problem (Haque et al., 1981; Shelov et al., 1981). Although the spontaneous remission rate is estimated to be 16 percent per year, cessation of bedwetting without treatment can take several years (Forsythe & Redmond, 1974). Moreover, as many as 3 percent of all enuretic children may continue with enuresis into adulthood (Forsythe & Redmond, 1974; Levine, 1943; Thorne, 1944).

Estimates of the prevalence of nonorganically based childhood encopresis have been quite variable and range from 0.5 percent to 10 percent, with most figures ranging between 2 percent and 3 percent. This variability is related to the contention that estimates from clinic-referred populations tend to be higher than those from nonreferred samples. Encopresis is more common in males, with male/female estimates ranging from 6:1 (Levine, 1982) to 2:1 (Bellman, 1966).

There is ample evidence that the prevalence of encopresis tends to diminish with age. Bellman (1966), for example, reported a sharp decline in prevalence from 8.1

percent to 2.8 percent between the ages of 3 and 4 years old. Consistent with Bellman's findings, Rutter, Tizzard, and Whitmore (1970) have noted that the prevalence of encopresis gradually levels off to 0.75 percent between the ages of 10 and 12 years old. As might be expected from gender differences, prevalence levels off to 0.3 percent for females and 1.2 percent for males. Similar to that of enuresis, such figures suggest that most children will eventually outgrow soiling, although the detrimental psychosocial effects of accepting this passive approach appear to be significantly greater.

Regarding taxonomic distinctions, it has been estimated that more than 75 percent of encopretics are retentive versus nonretentive (Levine, 1975). The distinction between retentive and nonretentive encopresis is probably the most useful in terms of treatment implications as well as etiology of soiling.

ASSESSMENT APPROACHES

Medical Issues

The goal of medical assessment for the elimination disorders is to identify physical causes for bedwetting or soiling. We consider the following components of medical assessment to represent the standard of practice for so-called functional childhood enuresis and encopresis. Psychologists who fail to secure a minimally appropriate medical assessment prior to proceeding to treatment may prevent the child from receiving needed and effective medical interventions. Physical complications may occur. In the case of monosymptomatic bedwetting, about 3 percent to 5 percent of cases will exhibit physical pathologies. For encopresis, incidence of physical causes of soiling is much higher.

With *nocturnal enuresis*, physical diseases such as nephritis and diabetes cause the incomplete processing of urine and result in the excessive voiding and overproduction of urine which can promote or prolong bedwetting. All children presenting with either day and/or night wetting need to have a complete physical and a urinalysis and culture. A careful history that includes questioning about excessive fluid intake, dramatic changes in weight, and family history of diabetes or kidney problems can help determine if more extensive tests are required, such as a renal sonogram or voiding cystourethrogram.

Laboratory examination of the urine and a culture can be performed quickly and at low cost in many outpatient settings. It is estimated that 5 percent of boys and 10 percent of girls presenting with enuresis have urinary tract infections (Stansfeld, 1973). Surprisingly, a child can have urinary tract infection without the symptoms of a burning sensation while urinating or fever. If left untreated, these infections can cause progressive renal damage and reduce functional bladder capacity, which can make bedwetting more difficult to treat. Fortunately, most urinary tract infections can be treated with 7 to 10 days of broad-spectrum antibiotics (Margileth, Pedreira, Hirschman, & Coleman, 1976). Of those children who are successfully treated for urinary tract infections, about 40 percent will stop bedwetting when the infection is cleared (Schmitt, 1982). In most cases, however, the infection may be simply associated with the bedwetting, rather than a cause (Shaffer, 1985), and the bedwetting will still have to be treated once the infection has been eliminated.

We have found reviewing the history of caffeine ingestion and assessing for the presence and extent of constipation to be useful in enhancing general treatment effectiveness. In a study of children who presented with enuresis and a concomitant history of constipation, simply treating the constipation led to a significant reduction in bedwetting in the majority of subjects (O'Regan, Yazbeck, Hamberger, & Schick, 1986). Although its contribution to enuresis is not well documented in the research literature, common sense dictates the elimination of caffeine from the bedwetters diet because it is a diuretic.

In the absence of significant clues that indicate a physical cause of enuresis such as a history of kidney disease, diurnal wetting, or current signs of urinary tract infection, the medical community does not support the routine use of invasive diagnostic procedures such as cystoscopy and intravenous pyelogram (American Academy of Pediatrics Committee on Radiology, 1980). The availability and lowered cost of less-invasive procedures such as ultrasonography or urodynamic studies support their use in screening for organic pathologies when warranted, which is estimated to occur in only 2 percent to 5 percent of monosymptomatic bedwetters. When ultrasound exams identify anatomic abnormalities, urological consultation is indicated. Children who have demonstrable physical defects, such as meatal stenosis or urethral stricture, are generally treated surgically. However, surgical correction of these structural defects does not correct the concomitant bedwetting in the majority of cases (Arnold & Ginsberg, 1973).

For *functional encopresis*, the principal aims of medical assessment are to identify the physiological variables influencing the soiling by differentiating organic from functional encopresis. In addition, determining the need for a course of purgatives and whether dysfunctional defecation dynamics exist are goals of the medical assessment. Researchers have noted that an organic cause may be found in 2 percent to 15 percent of children presenting with encopresis (Liebman, 1979; Schmitt, 1984). Organic problems are more common in retentive than nonretentive encopresis (Schmitt, 1984). Physical disorders that can result in soiling and need to be ruled out include Hirschsprung's disease (Ravitch, 1958), congenital hypothyroidism, and anorectal anomalies (Hendren, 1978; Leape & Ramenofsky, 1978). Although these disorders present with similar symptomatic behavior, their proper management is quite different from that of functional encopresis and is beyond the scope of this chapter.

Most professionals agree that a thorough medical history and complete physical with rectal exam should be performed to exclude organic involvement and determine the causes of soiling. Professionals have emphasized different areas in the history but all do agree that it should include a review of medications that could result in constipation and overflow soiling (Sondheimer, 1985; Suberman, 1976), as well as a description of the frequency and type of accidents. The complete physical usually includes a routine check of all systems, examination of stool for occult blood, and in the case of females, a urinalysis because of a high incidence (2.72 percent to 20 percent) of urinary tract infection caused by soiling and fecal bacterial infiltration (Sondheimer, 1985). At a minimum, the physical exam involves palpation of the abdomen for fecal masses and digital examination of the anus for rectal stenosis (Liebman, 1979; Nisley, 1976). In addition, the exam should include checking for the presence of an anterior ectopic anus (Leape & Ramenofsky, 1978), and inspection of the anus for fissures which may be causing or exacerbating soiling by encouraging the child to withhold stools for fear of pain (Fleischer, 1976; Mercer, 1967; Schmitt, 1984). Use of an abdominal x-ray (KUB) has been shown to provide a more accurate determination of whether retention or physical anomalies are present and possibly overlooked by history, rectal exam, and abdominal palpation. Abdominal x-rays can be reliably scored for degree of stool retention (Barr, Levine, Wilkinson & Mulvihill, 1979; Levine, 1975).

When physical causes have been suspected, a number of additional procedures have been used, including barium and gastrograffin enemas, and rectal biopsy. Gastrograffin enemas are used when prior examination leads to suspicion of physiological abnormalities because the procedure is less likely to worsen fecal impaction than when barium is used, and may actually help with evacuation of the bowel. Liebman (1979) reported that in a sample of 123 children with bowel problem onset before one year old, barium enema was diagnostic in 2 of 3 cases of Hirschsprung's disease.

Further, more invasive procedures such as suction biopsy or a full-thickness surgical biopsy of the rectal wall may be used to verify a diagnosis of Hirschsprung's disease (Fitzgerald, 1975; Liebman, 1979). Levine (1982), however, has cautioned that even with this method misdiagnosis is possible, because an apparent decrease in ganglionic cells may be due to the chronic stretching of the rectal wall that can occur in functional encopresis.

Contemporary assessment efforts have focused upon dysfunctional defecation dynamics assessed by anorectal manometry, and suggest a possible etiological role and a role in maintenance of the problem (Loening-Baucke & Cruikshank, 1986; Wald, Chandra, Chiponis & Gabel, 1986; Whitehead & Schuster, 1985). The anorectal manometric abnormalities that have been described in encopretics with constipation are decreased relaxation response of the internal anal sphincter with rectal distention (Abrahamian & Lloyd-Still, 1984; Loening-Baucke, 1984), decreased sensitivity of rectum and sigmoid colon (Goligher & Hughes, 1951; Loening-Baucke, 1984), and abnormal contraction of the external anal sphincter during defecation (Loening-Baucke & Cruikshank, 1986; Wald et al., 1986). Controlled studies have also demonstrated that treatment resistance was related to severe constipation, abnormal contraction of the external anal sphincter and pelvic floor during defecation, and inability to defecate 100 ml balloons (Loening-Baucke, 1989; Loening-Baucke, Cruikshank, & Savage, 1987). Loening-Baucke (1990) and Wald and associates (1987) found that children trained to produce normal defecation patterns through biofeedback were more successful with traditional cathartic and laxative protocols.

Psychological and Psychiatric Issues

Barring medical problems as a cause of bedwetting, the treatment of choice for *nocturnal enuresis* includes some version of urine alarm therapy. However, this treatment requires a large investment of time and effort not only from the child, but also the parent(s). An in-depth clinical interview of the parents and child will determine whether they are able to implement a rather demanding treatment, and help identify any associated psychopathology. Factors that have been associated with bedwetters who will successfully complete treatment and maintain those gains include information about history of enuresis, prior treatments, parental attitudes and beliefs, family and home environment, behavioral problems, and the child's current wetting pattern. The presence of relevant psychiatric symptoms or significant psychosocial stressors in the family may make a stronger argument for considering the use of pharmacological treatment to manage the bedwetting. Until psychosocial stressors can be reduced to sub-clinical levels or eliminated, behavioral treatment is unlikely to be effectively implemented.

A thorough history of a child's wetting pattern will reveal whether their wetting occurred after a period of nighttime continence (6 months to a year), which is referred to as secondary enuresis. Medical or emotional factors may have been involved. If the onset of bedwetting has coincided with stressful events or the presence of psychiatric symptoms, it may be useful to initially focus attention on minimizing current stressful events or treating psychiatric problems prior to implementing urine alarm treatment.

Carefully reviewing prior behavioral and pharmacological interventions will often identify the reasons those treatments failed and how problems in treatment might be resolved in the future. Often, previous failure with the urine alarm is due to inadequate parental instruction and preparation. Often, parents were not properly instructed to awaken the child, and they did not realize the treatment can require 16 weeks of effort to be successful. Frequent and careful monitoring during treatment can prevent repeating a disappointing experience. Previous drug treatment failures are the norm rather than the exception, and parents can be reassured that the continued bedwetting is not due to inadequate parenting.

Because some research has suggested that extremely noncompliant children are more likely to experience relapse following successful treatment (Dische et al., 1983; Sacks & DeLeon, 1973), a screening questionnaire such as the Child Behavior Checklist (CBCL) (Achenbach & Edelbrook, 1983) can identify children who need additional attention. Children with externalizing behavioral problems (Externalizing T score of greater than 70) are likely to be noncompliant with any parental requests, let alone the significant demands of waking to the urine alarm in the middle of the night. Likewise, internalizing behavior problems such as significant levels of anxiety and depression may interfere with the enuretic child's capacity to handle the rigors of urine alarm treatment. A clinical decision has to be made whether to train parents in contingency management prior to beginning behavioral treatment for enuresis. Failure to identify child noncompliance and internalizing problems prior to urine

alarm treatment can lead to a poor outcome. Such a poor outcome will only further contribute to a child's already lowered sense of confidence and self-efficacy that is typically associated with bedwetting.

Parental attitudes and beliefs have implications for those families that enter treatment. A large survey of parents of bedwetters (Haque et al., 1981) indicated that as many as 35 percent dealt with the enuresis by punishing the child when bedwetting occurred. Butler, Brewin, and Forsythe (1986) found that a greater perceived burden on the mother and attributing the cause of bedwetting to the child were associated with greater parental intolerance as assessed by Morgan and Young's (1975) Tolerance for Enuresis Scale, and this has been predictive of treatment dropout. Informing parents that bedwetting is a deficit in physical learning rather than a willful act can lead to the family support necessary before behavioral treatment is implemented.

Because of the genetic contribution to enuresis, the problem of bedwetting may be a common experience within the family. Young and Morgan (1973) reported a relationship between treatment dropout and positive family history of enuresis, and Fielding and Doleys (1989) have suggested that these findings may be indicative of complacency or poor motivation in these families. The potentially large demands of behavioral treatment can be disrupted by a lack of motivation for complete implementation and noncooperation in the family. We use a behavioral contracting approach designed to increase cooperation and understanding of each family member's responsibilities with treatment. If the family is unable to agree to the goals of treatment, it does not begin.

Assessment of family stress and disturbance and the physical home environment is important because they have been associated with slow response to treatment, treatment failure and relapse. Couchells, Johnson, Carter, and Walker (1981) reported that families seeking help for bedwetting are more likely to be experiencing stress than those families who do not seek treatment. Family disturbances and high maternal anxiety have been associated with slow response to treatment (Morgan & Young, 1975). Dische, Yule, Corbett, and Hand (1983) reported that marital discord, mental or physical handicap of family members, poor maternal coping skills, and unusual family living arrangements were predictors of behavioral treatment failure and relapse.

Having the parents complete the Locke-Wallace Marital Adjustment Test (MAT) (Locke & Wallace, 1959) may indicate significant marital distress (MAT scores below 85 for either spouse) that could interfere with urine alarm treatment. Among single parents, typically mothers, the Beck Depression Inventory (BDI) (Beck, Rush, Shaw, & Emery, 1980) may identify significant parental distress (scores above 15) that may require therapeutic attention prior to starting behavior therapy for enuresis. Finally, the Symptom Checklist (SCL-90-R) (Derogatis, 1977) is useful in screening for significant levels of global psychiatric distress. Clinically significant elevations in any of the above areas of psychological functioning would allow the health care provider to judge whether prior marital or family therapy is necessary to prevent a negative outcome when behavior therapy is used for enuresis.

A 2-week baseline of wetting frequency should be established. Parents can complete record forms that include wet or dry nights, the size of the wet spot, and whether the child spontaneously awakened to void in the toilet. As a general rule of thumb, the more frequently the child wets, the longer it will take for the child to stop bedwetting. As such, it is important to determine if a child is a multiple wetter (i.e., wets more than once per night). This may not be apparent until urine alarm treatment begins, as there is often only one large wet spot in the morning. Multiple wetters typically require more time to reach the success criterion of 14 consecutive dry nights, and informing parents accordingly will contribute to realistic expectations about progress and avoid discouragement and possible dropout.

Behavioral assessment for *functional encopresis* includes both a clinical interview with parents and children and direct observations and records of relevant target behaviors. The aims of the assessment are to determine if appropriate toileting behaviors are present or need to be learned, to identify parental and child responses (including any psychopathology) that may be maintaining soiling, and to evaluate parental motivation for compliance with the treatment regimen. The latter issue is particularly important, considering the evidence that links parental compliance with remission of soiling (Levine & Bakow, 1976).

The interview should include a review of developmental milestones and previous attempts at toilet training. Information about failed attempts at toilet training or treatment for soiling may reveal problems with parental responses, such as placing excessive pressure on the child to have bowel movements, delivering inconsistent or excessive punishment for soiling accidents, and failing to attend to appropriate toileting behavior. As in the case of assessment for enuresis, some evaluation of marital discord and inconsistent parental expectations of the child is needed. Often, these latter problems need to be remediated before a treatment program can be successfully implemented. In those families where there has been

a history of ineffective treatment, it is usually beneficial to assist parents to view the soiling as a response the child cannot control rather than one that the child does deliberately. Occasionally, soiling may be part of a general response class of oppositional behavior or other psychopathology, and this can be assessed through broad band behavior checklists like the CBCL (Achenbach & Edelbrock, 1983). Our preference is to screen for psychopathology with the CBCL due to its time-saving quality (i.e., mailed out before initial visit and quickly scored) and address any identified psychiatric problems during the diagnostic interview. Finally, an accurate count of the child's underpants is needed to prevent hiding of soiled pants.

An interview with the child can assess whether or not the child experiences the need to have a bowel movement. Among retentive encopretics, it is not uncommon for the child to report that he or she does not feel the urge to defecate. Reports of fear of the toilet and of painful bowel movements may indicate a need for gradual exposure and in vivo desensitization procedures. Finally, because many behavioral interventions rely on use of tangible reinforcers to promote proper toileting practice, an inventory of rewards and pleasant events for the child should be completed.

Behavioral observations by the clinician and parents are needed to individualize a treatment program. Direct observation of the child's toileting behavior is instructive and should include how the child undresses, approaches the toilet, executes the Valsalva maneuver, and whether the child wipes completely. Information about the frequency and type of the accidents is needed to establish a baseline of at least two weeks for measuring progress (Doleys, 1983). Parents can be instructed to keep daily records of both soiling accidents and bowel movements in the toilet to create a topography of each behavior. The frequency of soiling and bowel movements (BMs) in the toilet, the size of the accident or appropriate BMs, the consistency of the stool (i.e., whether the stool was loose or hard, smooth or grainy), and time and place accidents or appropriate BMs occurred should be included in the record. Records also need to indicate the number of self-initiated bathroom visits and BMs in the toilet, as well as parental response to accidents. Recording the time of day that bowel activity (either accidents or appropriate toileting) typically occurs is necessary to establish times for scheduled toileting practice. For those interventions that require manipulation of diet, it is important to have parents record complete details of the child's food intake.

Similar to enuresis, this assessment process is a continual one of monitoring the effects of encopresis treatment. Both researchers and clinicians have found it helpful to view treatment as a single case design where functional analysis of appropriate toileting behavior and soiling accidents leads to systematic interventions based on recorded frequencies of those two classes of behavior. Fortunately, as in the case of enuresis, the relevant variables (i.e., "wet versus dry," or "soiled versus unsoiled") are highly salient and can be measured reliably when parents are properly instructed.

TREATMENT STRATEGIES

In accordance with the suggested outline for this book, we have contrasted behavioral and medical treatments for nocturnal enuresis and functional encopresis. However, it appears clear that the optimal management of the elimination disorders requires close multidisciplinary collaboration, as well as an appreciation of the importance of integrating physical and psychological conceptualizations of the problems presented. As will be delineated in both the medical and psychological sections, singular medical or behavioral treatments are considered to be inadequate. Therefore, the greatest emphasis is placed upon combined behavioral and medical treatments.

Psychological and Behavioral Treatments

More than 50 years of controlled clinical trials and a recent quantitative review of treatments clearly indicates that some version of urine alarm treatment is the treatment of choice for medically and psychosocially uncomplicated bedwetting if long-term cure is the outcome goal (see review by Houts, Berman, & Abramson, 1994). However, as indicated in the section on psychological assessment of enuresis, the use of pharmacological treatment to manage bedwetting may be appropriate in the presence of significant levels of psychosocial stressors in the family. This clinical decision regarding matching treatment to patient circumstances is best made in the context of collaboration between pediatric psychologists and physicians; this is the authors' current practice.

For simple, uncomplicated *nocturnal enuresis*, the authors' preference is for multicomponent treatments that have been demonstrated to positively influence the problems of speed of treatment response and relapse in urine alarm therapy by adding other behavioral procedures to the basic urine alarm treatment. Fourteen years of systematic research by Dr. Arthur C. Houts and his students at the University of Memphis has led to the de-

velopment and modification of one such multicomponent treatment called Full Spectrum Treatment. For a complete review of other behavioral treatments for enuresis, see the summary by Scott, Barclay, and Houts (1992).

Full Spectrum Treatment (FST) was designed to provide parents and children with an inexpensive, easy-to-use, and effective treatment for uncomplicated nocturnal enuresis. Families are provided with a detailed manual complete with support materials. Treatment has been demonstrated to be most effective if delivered by a trained professional (Houts, Whelan, & Peterson, 1987). The treatment components are (a) basic urine alarm treatment, (b) cleanliness training, (c) retention control training, and (d) overlearning. For basic urine alarm treatment, we prefer the newer urine alarm devices (e.g., Palco Wet Stop®, Palco Labs, 8030 Soquel Avenue, Santa Cruz, CA 95062) that are worn on the body and have been found to be more reliable than the older devices that required use of a bedpad and free-standing alarm box. Most of these newer alarm devices are turned off by removing the urine-sensitive probe from the child's underwear and drying it off, because the moisture completes the micro-circuit.

With *basic urine alarm treatment*, children are instructed to follow the rule of getting out of bed and standing up before turning off the alarm. Basic urine alarm treatment leads to the complete cessation of bedwetting in 70 percent to 75 percent of children (Doleys, 1977; Houts et al., 1994). However, a quarter of children fail to stop wetting because they either do not become sensitized to awaken to the alarm, or they become discouraged by the demands of treatment or the length of time required to notice improvement. Of greater concern with basic urine alarm treatment is that as many as 41 percent of children who stopped bedwetting will subsequently relapse (Doleys, 1977). This problem has lead some investigators to emphasize relapse prevention (Houts, Peterson, & Whelan, 1986).

The steps involved in *cleanliness training* are displayed in a wall chart ("Daily Steps to A Dry Bed") that is kept in the child's room. The chart also allows the child and parents to record the patient's progress with either a *wet* or *dry* for each night of training. Lovibond (1964) indicated that basic urine alarm training will fail if the child is not required to awaken to the alarm. To preclude the child from learning not to respond to the alarm by not waking completely and going back to sleep, parents are instructed to have the child go through with the full procedure of remaking the bed even if the sheets are not wet. We have further recommended to parents that they have their child both wash his or her face and do math problems that are not committed to rote memory to assure the child is alert.

Retention control training is a daily activity done while the child is awake, and will typically take 2 to 3 weeks to complete. The child is given money for holding his or her urine for increasing amounts of time in a step-by-step fashion up to 45 minutes. Houts, Peterson, and Whelan (1986) discovered that this procedure speeds the acquisition of the inhibitory response (i.e., pelvic floor contraction or "Kegel" exercise) believed to be conditioned by the urine alarm procedure. In clinical practice, the first author has found that repeating retention control training if the frequency of wets increases after a period of progress will halt the regression.

Investigators have reduced relapse for certain categories of enuretics in basic urine alarm treatment by employing intermittent alarm schedules (Finley, Rainwater, & Johnson, 1982). FST uses a simpler procedure called *overlearning* (Young & Morgan, 1972) to prevent relapse. Overlearning was initiated after the child attained the first success criterion of 14 consecutive dry nights. At this point, the child would be required to consume 16 ounces of water during the hour before bedtime and this would continue until the child achieved the second success criterion of 14 more consecutive dry nights. Although this procedure produced a 50 percent reduction in the relapse rate for FST, it was also observed that the children who failed to achieve the second success criterion also failed to recover from the relapse induced by the overlearning procedure (Houts, Peterson, & Whelan, 1986). This has led the University of Memphis research group to the successful modification of the overlearning procedure.

The *modified form of overlearning* requires the child to gradually increase in a stair-step way the amount of water ingested just prior to bedtime. The first step is to determine the maximum amount of water ingested by the child and this is based on a formula for functional bladder capacity: 1 ounce for each year of age plus 2 ounces (Berger, Maizels, Moran, Conway, & Firlit, 1983). Children then begin the overlearning procedure by drinking 4 ounces of water 15 minutes before bedtime. If they remain dry for two consecutive nights at 4 ounces, the amount increases by 2 ounces to 6 ounces. The amount of water continues to increase by 2 ounces for each consecutive two-day period the child remains dry until the child's maximum amount is reached. If a wet occurs at any time, the amount is reduced to that of the previous dry night and continues at that amount for five days. If the child is still dry, the amount increases again according to the above schedule until the maximum is reached and 14 more consecutive dry nights are achieved during the overlearning procedure. The results from this modified procedure suggest that the rate of relapse can be reduced up to yet another 50 percent, making the average relapse rate for FST between 10 percent and 15 percent rather than the typical 41 percent for urine alarm treatment alone.

Although the average success rate of FST is an impressive 70 percent, the University of Memphis research group has continued to experiment with adding a nightly waking schedule in an effort to improve outcome. Unfortunately, this procedure has not contributed to increased efficacy of FST (Whelan & Houts, 1990). In addition, delivery of FST via didactic videotape in order to reduce costs for families (Houts, Whelan, & Peterson, 1987) was disappointingly less effective than live delivery.

Perhaps the most significant problem of FST and other multicomponent treatment approaches that incorporate the urine alarm is *delayed response*. In FST, most children reach the first goal of 14 consecutive dry nights in approximately 8 weeks of treatment. The second success criterion of 14 more consecutive dry nights during overlearning will require approximately an additional 4 weeks. Some children will not attain the first goal even after 12 weeks of treatment, which is often frustrating to the child and parents.

We have dealt with the problem of delayed responding by keeping the child and parents focused on the often subtle signs of progress: (a) reduction of wet nights over baseline, (b) reduction in wet nights in which the child needed assistance to wake to the alarm, (c) reduction in multiple wets per night, (d) reduction in the size of the wet spot, and (e) an increase in the interval between bedtime and the first wetting episode. Providing regular follow-up and supportive therapy to the child and parents facilitates continued compliance with treatment.

Children who are multiple wetters are especially likely to overproduce urine and be delayed responders. These children may be appropriate candidates for combined behavioral and pharmacological treatments, although the research on this approach is limited to two investigations. Although both studies (Philpott & Flasher, 1970; Sukhai, Mol, & Harris, 1989) suggested an improvement over basic urine alarm treatment alone, the latter is more appealing because of less side effects associated with the use of desmopressin (DDAVP) versus the imipramine used in the former. Our elimination disorders clinic is uniquely poised to collaborate on this treatment approach. We believe that desmopressin addresses the problem of overproduction of urine and multiple wetting that contributes to slow responding to FST and increased risk for dropout. Further research is needed to systematically explore the efficacy of this approach. The case example for enuresis that we will present will not only highlight the apparent effectiveness of combined desmopressin and FST, but also demonstrates how interdisciplinary collaboration can optimize the assessment and treatment of nocturnal enuresis.

In the following sections on behavioral and medical treatments for *functional encopresis*, the reader is cautioned against drawing firm conclusions about what represents the treatment of choice for encopresis. The treatment outcome literature for functional encopresis is limited by the fact that approximately 1 percent of published reports are randomized trials that compared two or more interventions and 91 percent involve case studies or simple pre-post group designs (Houts & Abramson, 1990). It is our tentative assertion that treatments emphasizing the combined use of cathartics and laxatives, complex behavioral interventions, and biofeedback represent approaches with the most promising outcome data.

We believe that functional encopresis represents a "biobehavioral" problem that is best treated through the collaboration of physicians and pediatric psychologists. This conclusion is based upon the evidence that between 75 percent (Levine, 1975) and 95 percent (Christopherson & Rapoff, 1983) of clinic-referred children with soiling are classified as retentive encopretics. Further, 63 percent have a history of painful defecation that began in infancy that led to the pain-avoidance response of external anal sphincter contraction during defecation, and this continued response maintains the constipation (Partin et al., 1992). Treatment of functional encopresis, therefore, must address the physiological aspects of constipation, fecal impaction, and frequent soiling. It must also address the pain-avoidance response and retention that interfere with normal defecation. We acknowledge that a small minority of children presenting with encopresis are not retentive and would not require cathartic and laxative therapies. A flat plate abdominal x-ray must be done to be sure retention does not exist.

In general, behavioral treatments have focused on teaching prerequisite skills for toileting and/or on changing contingencies of reinforcement so that soiling cannot be maintained and appropriate toileting can occur. Specific behavioral procedures that have been used are toileting skills training (Crowley & Armstrong, 1977); discrimination training (Olness, McParland, & Piper, 1980); overcorrection, negative reinforcement and punishment for soiling (Ayllon, Simon, & Wildman, 1975; Rolider & Van Houten, 1985); positive reinforcement for sitting on the toilet (Neale, 1963); positive reinforcement for defecation in the toilet (*Type I Reinforcement*) (Keehn, 1965); and positive reinforcement for clean underwear (*Type II Reinforcement*) (Pedrini &

Pedrini, 1971). Some of these methods have been used alone (e.g., biofeedback, reinforcement for clean underwear, and negative reinforcement). More frequently, as individual cases required, they have been combined into treatment packages, and this latter trend has produced greater efficacy. Overall, Houts and Abramson (1990) estimate that behavioral treatments resulted in an upper bound estimate (defined as percent cured minus percent relapsed) of 63 percent permanently cured. Simple behavioral methods are estimated to have resulted in 59 percent being permanently cured in contrast to 67 percent being permanently cured for complex behavioral programs. This manner of organizing the literature certainly suggests that combined behavioral procedures are more effective than when used in isolation. Obviously, randomized controlled studies are needed to develop a reliable behavioral treatment package.

Various behavioral procedures have been used in conjunction with cathartics and/or diet modification. These treatment packages have been based upon the assumption that reinforcement and punishment procedures to produce appropriate bowel habits will be ineffective if longstanding constipation and fecal impaction of the colon and rectum are left untreated. Doleys (1983) indicated that approaches that combine reinforcement with cathartics are more effective when they involve Type I reinforcement. Houts & Abramson (1990) estimated that combining cathartics with Type I reinforcement leads to an upper bound estimate of 72 percent permanently cured versus 48 percent that employ Type II reinforcement. Interestingly, when laxatives alone or laxatives with purgatives have been used with a combination of Type I and Type II reinforcement, results have been less promising, with overall estimates of 62 percent permanently cured. Houts and Abramson (1990) also noted that, compared to those protocols that used initial evacuation with enemas, those that did not use evacuation resulted in lower estimates of permanent cure (85 percent versus 30 percent). This trend is consistent with the recommendation of Parker and Whitehead (1983), who have advocated the use of water enemas over laxatives, because enemas clean out the colon and rectum more immediately and thoroughly. The authors have employed a fading schedule of soap suds enemas for children with severely impacted colons.

Several investigations have included dietary fiber increases alone or together with laxatives in combination with behavioral interventions (Hein & Beerends, 1978; Houts, Mellon, & Whelan, 1988; Houts & Peterson, 1986; Sluckin, 1981; Taitz, Wales, Urwin, & Molnar, 1986; Wakefield, Woodbridge, Steward, & Croke, 1984). The use of diet modifications instead of laxatives was prompted by reports of laxative dependency and patterns of passive defecation related to long-term use of cathartics (Schaefer, 1979). Overall, these dietary manipulation treatments appear to be less effective than those involving laxatives, with an upper bound estimate for permanent cure of 60 percent (Houts & Abramson, 1990).

The overall effectiveness of interventions that combined cathartic and behavioral treatments can be estimated to have an upper bound estimate of permanent cure of 66 percent. Whereas this overall estimate is somewhat lower than for other types of treatment strategies, the studies reviewed by Houts & Abramson (1990) suggested that addition of cathartics to certain types of multifaceted behavioral interventions results in substantial gains over use of behavioral intervention alone. Specifically, a combination of cathartics and enema with Types I and II reinforcement, and a combination of laxatives and diet with support for parents have been quite successful. At the very least, Type I reinforcement should be included in combined cathartic/behavioral treatments.

Several investigators have documented the increased risk of failing conventional cathartic/laxative treatment when abnormal defecation dynamics exist. These investigators have also shown that retraining encopretic children to make the appropriate response through biofeedback leads to greater treatment efficacy in as many as six one-hour sessions, and is complementary to a conventional cathartic/laxative regimen (Loening-Baucke, 1990; Wald et al., 1987). Biofeedback training most likely assists with the neuromuscular responses involved in defecation and may shorten the length of time it takes to achieve a resolution of soiling problems compared to the conventional approaches previously described.

Although the evidence is only suggestive, given the current empirical findings, the authors cautiously speculate that combining the biofeedback training of anorectal response competency with cathartics (or laxatives) and diet manipulation, as well as behavioral treatment that includes Type I reinforcement, may prove to represent the ideal treatment for functional encopresis. The aim of such treatment would be to immediately and completely evacuate the bowel and to ensure that future constipation is prevented through the use of a high-fiber diet and laxatives. Biofeedback training of anorectal musculature would lead to more efficient control of the physiological responses needed to attain continence, and behavioral intervention would establish regular toileting habits.

Pharmacological Treatments

Medication therapy for *nocturnal enuresis* began in the early 1960s when imipramine (brand name Tofranil)

was found to reduce urinary incontinence in adult psychiatric patients treated for depression (MacLean, 1960). The 1970s saw the introduction of a bladder antispasmodic medication known as oxybutynin chloride (brand name Ditropan). This drug has been shown to reduce spasms of the bladder and to increase bladder capacity, in addition to being a treatment for bedwetting (Buttarazzi, 1977; Thompson & Lauvetz, 1976). Finally, a synthetic version of the naturally occurring hormone known as vasopressin was introduced to the United States from Europe in the late 1980s. Desmopressin (brand name DDAVP) is currently taken intranasally to treat excessive urine production by stimulating the kidney to concentrate urine so that the bladder capacity during sleep is not exceeded. A quantitative review by Houts and associates (1994) reported that although pharmacological treatments produce a better outcome than no treatment, these gains are nearly lost at follow-up, and barely exceeded the spontaneous remission rate.

Because of the numerous and potentially dangerous side effects of imipramine (see Werry, Dowrick, Lampen, & Vamos, 1975), and indications that oxybutynin chloride may not be more efficacious than the spontaneous cure rate of 16 percent, the authors believe desmopressin (DDAVP) represents the most viable pharmacological treatment for nocturnal enuresis. Imipramine, which has a slightly lower efficacy than DDAVP, might be worth considering in cases resistant to all other treatments, or in children with the added diagnosis of depression. The toxicity of the drug in overdose must be emphasized to the family. A recent review of all controlled trials of DDAVP indicated that only 24.5 percent of patients achieve short-term dryness and only 5.7 percent remained dry after stopping treatment (Moffatt, Harlos, Kirshen, & Burd, 1993). Houts and associates (1994) report a more promising figure of 21 percent remaining dry by follow-up. However, these figures are far less impressive than the 45 percent lasting cure for behavioral treatments using the urine alarm alone. Therefore, the use of DDAVP for anything more than the management of bedwetting until the child spontaneously remits is not supported by current scientific knowledge.

The available research regarding pharmacologic treatments for *functional encopresis* may be decades behind that of nocturnal enuresis. However, a recent report by Stern et al. (1995) presents the interesting finding that plasma levels of the gastrointestinal hormones pancreatic polypeptide and motilin may be involved in the chronic constipation often seen with encopretics. The implication is that hormone corrective therapy may play a role in the management of constipation symptoms of functional encopresis. More basic research will be required to determine whether the hormone anomalies are a result or a cause of chronic constipation, and if pharmacologic treatment can be developed.

Pharmacological or medical treatments for functional encopresis have involved use of purgatives and laxatives (Berg & Jones, 1964; Loening-Baucke & Younoszai, 1982), dietary manipulation (Loening-Baucke & Cruickshank, 1986), and pharmacological compounds assumed to affect the musculature involved in defecation (Gavanski, 1971). Typically, these interventions include regular toileting of the child once any fecal impaction has been removed. The overall effectiveness of medical approaches indicate that the upper bound estimate of permanent cure was 59 percent (Houts & Abramson, 1990). In comparison to other treatment options that have been researched, in most cases medical intervention alone may not be the treatment of choice. Nevertheless, the assumption that some treatment may be necessary for cleansing the encopretic of fecal retention should not be discarded because initial evacuation may be necessary before another treatment can be successful.

CASE ILLUSTRATIONS

Enuresis

Clinical Presentation

J. L. is a 12-year-old male who originally presented to our clinic because of diurnal (3–4 times per week) and nocturnal enuresis (6–7 times per week), constipation, recent parental divorce, and inconsistent academic achievement. J. L. was being cared for by his mother and paternal grandparents on different nights of the week because of his mother's unusual work schedule. His father had limited contact with J. L.

Assessment Findings

His physical exam and laboratory workup revealed significant levels of stool retention throughout the colon and a normal urinalysis and urine culture. J. L. was treated with a fading course of rectal suppositories and increased dietary fiber for constipation, elimination of caffeine, and desmopressin (DDAVP) for the enuresis. J. L.'s diurnal enuresis remitted within 2 weeks of treatment and his bedwetting was reduced to 1–2 times per week at 40 mcg. of DDAVP. J. L. was also provided

with individual and family therapy to address the issues of divorce and poor school performance.

Treatment Selection and Course

J. L. continued to have intermittent success with the DDAVP but would frequently relapse to pretreatment levels of bedwetting once the medication was discontinued. J. L. also began complaining of headaches, which the family attributed to DDAVP. It was also determined that J. L. was ingesting many caffeinated beverages. It was recommended that caffeine be eliminated and the headaches resolved. Full Spectrum Training would also be implemented in combination with a systematic titration of DDAVP to manage the multiple wetting exhibited by J. L. who was also encouraged to continue on his high-fiber diet to control constipation. The combination FST and DDAVP would be monitored in our clinic every 2 weeks, with J. L. decreasing his DDAVP to 30 mcg. as FST was initiated.

By the 4th week of treatment and at 20 mcg. of DDAVP, J. L. had achieved 8 out of 14 dry nights and was complying well with all aspects of FST. DDAVP was then reduced to 10 mcg. before bed and J. L. was encouraged to carry out all aspects of treatment, and to be patient with his progress. J. L. had achieved 11 out of 14 dry nights by the 6th week of treatment with DDAVP remaining at 10 mcg. before bed. Compliance was still excellent and DDAVP was discontinued.

By the 8th week of treatment, J. L. had nearly relapsed with only one dry night in the past 2 weeks. He was also having multiple wets nearly every other night. It was reported that J. L. was not waking to the alarm and that he was discouraged. J. L. was quite sleepy during the day as a new school year had just begun and he had not yet adhered to his new bedtime schedule. J. L. had also begun to have large diameter and every-other-day bowel movements. Although his abdominal exam was unremarkable for constipation, an abdominal x-ray revealed significant constipation. J. L. was encouraged to get to bed earlier, given therapeutic support to adhere to all aspects of FST, and a temporary course of soap suds enemas was initiated for constipation. DDAVP was not started pending compliance with the new treatment plan.

J. L.'s wetting once again improved by the 10th week of treatment with 6 out of 14 dry nights. It was also reported that he was having difficulty with anger management related to continued struggles with his parent's divorce. Individual therapy was initiated with the pediatric psychologist to work on anger control and improve compliance with enuresis treatment. The decision was made not to resume DDAVP.

J. L. continued to make steady progress by the 12th week of treatment, with 7 out of 14 dry nights. J. L. continued to have some trouble waking to the alarm and had occasional multiple wets per night. It was also reported that J. L. was drinking approximately 32 ounces of water within the 5 hours prior to bedtime and would sweat profusely throughout the day. He was screened for urine concentrating ability in the morning and his specific gravity was negative for diabetes insipidus. J. L. was encouraged to continue with treatment and be patient with progress. By the 14th week of treatment J. L. continued to make progress with 9 out of 14 dry nights and there was no plan to restart DDAVP unless another regression in treatment occurred. If he does regress, we would begin the DDAVP with the goal of controlling the multiple wetting.

Termination and Follow-Up

This case is currently ongoing. Although J. L. represents a patient with many risk factors associated with a poor outcome with the urine alarm (i.e., multiple wetting, constipation, psychosocial stressors, non-optimal living arrangements, etc.), he is continuing to make steady progress. The collaboration between a physician and pediatric psychologist has enabled us to target medical and behavioral issues together that have arisen in J. L.'s care. Without this type of collaboration, J. L. may have received either psychological or medical interventions only, or an uncoordinated combination that we believe would not have been beneficial. We will continue to serve this patient, evaluate our progress, and adjust treatment accordingly until J. L.'s bedwetting has ceased.

Encopresis

Clinical Presentation

K. D. is a 6-year-old male who presented with fecal soiling (2–3 times per day) since infancy, intermittent constipation, and both diurnal and nocturnal enuresis. K. D. was also previously diagnosed with attention deficit disorder and had been on 20 mg. of methylphenidate per day for a year. K. D. also exhibited oppositional-defiant behavior at home. K. D.'s parents divorced the previous year and he was living with his mother, 5-year-old sister,

and the maternal grandmother. His mother indicated that K. D. often refused to sit on the toilet to attempt a bowel movement. If cajoled to use the toilet, K. D. would often back-up to the toilet to pass stool while standing.

Assessment Findings

The physical assessment was remarkable for a palpable colon, asthma, and uncoordinated fine-motor movements. Laboratory results indicated a normal urinalysis and culture. An abdominal x-ray (KUB) indicated abnormally large amounts of stool throughout the colon. K. D.'s mother did not remember the last time he had a bowel movement in the toilet, and he would often have 2–3 small accidents each day after school or early evening. K. D. would have approximately one large fecal accident each week.

Treatment Selection and Course

Because the encopresis was the most bothersome problem for K. D., it was prioritized for treatment. K. D. was started on 2 ounces of mineral oil, a fading course of bisacodyl (brandname Dulcolax) suppositories, increased dietary fiber and scheduled toileting. A clinic follow-up visit 2 weeks later revealed poor compliance with all aspects of treatment and continuation of soiling, with a frequency of 2 accidents per day. K. D. and his mother were then scheduled to meet with the pediatric psychologist to address problems with treatment compliance. Daily soap suds enemas were implemented to vigorously treat the fecal retention.

Behavioral treatment initially involved the use of stickers on the soiling record, candy for each BM in the toilet, and prompts to use the toilet after dinner. K. D. was also instructed on how to sit on the toilet with a platform to support his feet. Two weeks later K. D. had only had 3 accidents, but was only having BM's in the toilet with the enema. The next step involved the use of tokens for each self-initiated BM in the toilet to be cashed in for a special toy. At this point, K. D.'s mother missed her next two appointments.

Two months later, K. D.'s mother called regarding guidance with educational programming at school and requested that the pediatric psychologist attend a meeting. K. D.'s mother had since been married and a more stable home environment established. It was reported that K. D. was still soiling with the same frequency and would not cooperate with scheduled toileting. K. D. was found on physical exam to have a palpable colon and by history was having frequent large-diameter bowel movements. Recommendations for daily soap suds enemas, 2 ounces of mineral oil, scheduled toileting and incentive program were made. Tokens in the form of $5 bills were made with K. D.'s name on them. He would have to earn 4 of them (one for each self-initiated BM) to get a toy of his choice. During the next 2 weeks of treatment, K. D. only had one soiling accident and 3 self-initiated BM's in the toilet. He continued to have adequate evacuation in the toilet with the enemas.

Termination and Follow-Up

Assessment of treatment effectiveness is ongoing and will be adjusted to meet the multiple needs that K. D. presents. Again, the collaboration between the pediatric psychologist and physician has allowed for the continuation of K. D.'s treatment even under the influence of multiple psychosocial complications. The immediate goal of treatment is the continued balance between the bowel laxatives, mineral oil and dietary changes, and the use of Type I reinforcement to establish habitual and effective self-initiated bowel evacuation.

These cases were purposely selected because the authors felt they represented examples of the complicated and multiple needs of children presenting with enuresis or encopresis. We did not report an example of a simple "cure" in order to highlight how multidisciplinary collaboration can be a resource for the multiple "real-life" needs of children that professionals often see in their clinics. We believe that this biobehavioral model cannot only address the multiple needs of children with elimination disorders and their families, but also serve as a model of wellness and illness health care throughout childhood.

SUMMARY

The functional elimination disorders of children present a challenge to clinicians and researchers in the fields of medicine and psychology. Both enuresis and encopresis can be conceptualized as biobehavioral problems that require a new kind of thinking for both disciplines. On the one hand, clinicians and researchers need to understand the basic physiology of micturition and defecation if they are to solve these problems. On the other hand, and because of the functional nature of the problems, they also need to understand principles of conditioning and learning if they are to provide psychosocial interventions that restore basic physiological mechanisms to their proper functioning.

Although multicomponent treatments that include the urine alarm are effective for the majority of nocturnal bedwetters, further clinical evaluations combining this approach with desmopressin for the multiple wetter are warranted. Similarly, the effectiveness of cathartics, dietary manipulation, and behavior therapy (i.e., Type I reinforcement) may be greatly enhanced by the use of anorectal manometry to teach the physiological response that will assure regular and efficient bowel evacuation. This biobehavioral approach to these problems is likely to lead to new knowledge about how changes in human behavior at the socially influenceable level can alter the function of organ systems at the biochemical and neuromuscular level.

REFERENCES

Abrahamian, F. P., & Lloyd-Still, J. (1984). Chronic constipation in childhood: A longitudinal study of 186 patients. *Journal of Pediatric Gastroenterology and Nutrition, 3*, 460–467.

Achenbach, T. M., & Edelbrock, C. (1983). *Manual for the child behavior checklist*. Burlington, VT: Department of Psychiatry, University of Vermont.

American Academy of Pediatrics: Committee on Radiology. (1980). Excretory urography for evaluation of enuresis. *Pediatrics, 65*, 644–645.

American Psychiatric Association. (1994). *Diagnostic and statistical manual of mental disorders* (4th ed.). Washington, DC: Author.

Arnold, S. J., & Ginsberg, A. (1973). Enuresis, incidence and pertinence of genitourinary disease in healthy enuretic children. *Urology, 2*, 437–443.

Ayllon, T., Simon, S. J., & Wildman, R. W. (1975). Instructions and reinforcement in the elimination of encopresis: A case study. *Journal of Behavior Therapy and Experimental Psychiatry, 6*, 235–238.

Baker, B. L. (1969). Symptom treatment and symptom substitution in enuresis. *Journal of Abnormal Psychology, 74*, 42–49.

Barr, R. G., Levine, M. D., Wilkinson, R. H., & Mulvihill, D. (1979). Chronic and occult stool retention: A clinical tool for its evaluation in school aged children. *Clinical Pediatrics, 18*, 674–686.

Beck, A. T., Rush, A. J., Shaw, B. F., & Emery, G. (1980). *Cognitive therapy of depression*. New York: Guilford Press.

Bellman, M. (1966). Studies on encopresis. *Acta Pediatrica Scandinavica* (Suppl. 170), 7–151.

Berg, I., & Jones, K. V. (1964). Functional fecal incontinence in children. *Archives of Disease in Childhood, 39,* 465–472.

Berger, R. M., Maizels, M., Moran, G. C., Conway, J. J., & Firlit, C. F. (1983). Bladder capacity (ounces) equals age (years) plus 2 predicts normal bladder capacity and aids in diagnosis of abnormal voiding patterns. *The Journal of Urology, 129,* 347–349.

Butler, R. J., Brewin, C. R., & Forsythe, W. I. (1986). Maternal attributions and tolerance for nocturnal enuresis. *Behaviour Research and Therapy, 24,* 307–312.

Buttarazzi, P. J. (1977). Oxybutynin chloride (Ditropan) in enuresis. *The Journal of Urology, 118,* 46.

Christophersen, E. R., & Rapoff, M. A. (1983). Toileting problems of children. In C. E. Walker & M. C. Roberts (Eds.), *Handbook of clinical child psychology* (pp. 593–615). New York: Wiley.

Couchells, S. M., Johnson, S. B., Carter, R., & Walker, D. (1981). Behavioral and environmental characteristics of treated and untreated enuretic children matched with nonenuretic controls. *The Journal of Pediatrics, 99,* 812–816.

Crowley, C. P., & Armstrong, P. M. (1977). Positive practice, overcorrection, and behavior rehearsal in the treatment of three cases of encopresis. *Journal of Behavior Therapy and Experimental Psychiatry, 8,* 411–416.

DeJonge, G. A. (1973). Epidemiology of enuresis: A survey of the literature. In I. Kolvin, R. C. MacKeith, & S. R. Meadow (Eds.), *Bladder control and enuresis,* (pp. 39–46). London: William Heinemann.

Derogatis, L. R. (1977). *SCL-90: Administration, scoring & procedures manual for the revised version.* Baltimore: Clinical Psychometric Research.

Dische, S., Yule, W., Corbett, J., & Hand, D. (1983). Childhood nocturnal enuresis: Factors associated with outcome of treatment with an enuresis alarm. *Developmental Medicine and Child Neurology, 25,* 67–80.

Doleys, D. M. (1977). Behavioral treatments for nocturnal enuresis in children: A review of the recent literature. *Psychological Bulletin, 84,* 30–54.

Doleys, D. M. (1983). Enuresis and encopresis. In T. H. Ollendick & M. Hersen (Eds.), *Handbook of child psychopathology* (pp. 201–226). New York: Plenum Press.

Essen, J., & Peckham, C. (1976). Nocturnal enuresis in childhood. *Developmental Medicine and Child Neurology, 18,* 577–589.

Fergusson, D. M., Horwood, L. J., & Shannon, F. T. (1986). Factors related to the age of attainment of nocturnal bladder control: An 8 year longitudinal study. *Pediatrics, 78,* 884–890.

Fielding, D., & Doleys, D. M. (1989). Elimination problems: Enuresis and encopresis. In E. J. Mash & L. G. Terdal (Eds.), *Behavioral assessment of childhood disorders* (pp. 586–623). New York: The Guilford Press.

Finley, W. W., Rainwater, A. J., & Johnson, G. (1982). Effect of varying alarm schedules on acquisition and relapse parameters in the conditioning treatment of enuresis. *Behaviour Research and Therapy, 20,* 69–80.

Fitzgerald, J. F. (1975). Encopresis, soiling, constipation: What's to be done? *Journal of Pediatrics, 56,* 348–349.

Fleisher, D. R. (1976). Diagnosis and treatment of disorders of defecation in children. *Pediatric Annals, 5,* 71–101.

Forsythe, W. I., & Redmond, A. (1974). Enuresis and spontaneous cure rate: Study of 1129 enuretics. *Archives of Disease in Childhood, 49,* 259–263.

Gavanski, M. (1971). Treatment of non-retentive secondary encopresis with imipramine and psychotherapy. *Canadian Medical Association Journal, 104,* 46–48.

Goligher, J. D., & Hughes, E. S. (1951). Sensibility of the colon and rectum. *Lancet, 1,* 543–548.

Haque, M., Ellerstein, N. S., Gundy, J. H., Shelov, S. P., Weiss, J. C., McIntire, M. S., Olness, K. N., Jones, D. J., Heagarty, M. C., & Starfield, B. H. (1981). Parental perceptions of enuresis: A collaborative study. *American Journal of Diseases of Childhood, 135,* 809–811.

Hein, H. A., & Beerends, J. J. (1978). Who should accept primary responsibility for the encopretic child?: A successful pediatric program based on dietary control, bowel training, and family counseling. *Clinical Pediatrics, 17,* 67–70.

Hendren, W. H. (1978). Constipation caused by anterior location of the anus and its surgical correction. *Journal of Pediatric Surgery, 13,* 505–512.

Houts, A. C. (1991). Nocturnal enuresis as a biobehavioral problem. *Behavior Therapy, 22,* 133–151.

Houts, A. C., & Abramson, H. (1990). Assessment and treatment for functional childhood enuresis and encopresis: Toward a partnership between health psychologists and physicians. In S. B. Morgan and T. M. Okwumabua (Eds.), *Child and adolescent disorders: Developmental and health psychology perspectives* (pp. 47–103). Hillsdale, NJ: Lawrence Erlbaum.

Houts, A. C., Berman, J. S., & Abramson, H. (1994). Effectiveness of psychological and pharmacological treatments for nocturnal enuresis. *Journal of Consulting and Clinical Psychology, 62,* 737–745.

Houts, A. C., Mellon, M. W., & Whelan, J. P. (1988). Use of dietary fiber and stimulus control to treat retentive encopresis: A multiple baseline investigation. *Journal of Pediatric Psychology, 13,* 435–445.

Houts, A. C., & Peterson, J. K. (1986). Treatment of a retentive encopretic child using contingency management and diet modification with stimulus control. *Journal of Pediatric Psychology, 11,* 375–383.

Houts, A. C., Peterson, J. K., & Whelan, J. P. (1986). Prevention of relapse in Full-Spectrum home training for primary enuresis: A components analysis. *Behavior Therapy, 17*, 462–469.

Houts, A. C., Whelan J. P., & Peterson J. K. (1987). Filmed vs. live delivery of Full-Spectrum home training for primary enuresis: Presenting the information is not enough. *Journal of Consulting and Clinical Psychology, 55*, 902–906.

Jarvelin, M. R. (1989). Developmental history and neurological findings in enuretic children. *Developmental Medicine and Child Neurology, 31*, 728–736.

Jarvelin, M. R., Huttunen, N., Seppanen, J., Seppanen, U., & Moilanen, I. (1990). Screening of urinary tract abnormalities among day and nightwetting children. *Scandinavian Journal of Urology and Nephrology, 24*, 181–189.

Jarvelin, M. R., Moilanen, I., Kangas, P., Moring, K., Vikevainen-Tervonen, L., Huttunen, N. P., & Seppanen, J. (1991). Aetiological and precipitating factors for childhood enuresis. *Acta Pediatrica Scandinavia, 80*, 361–369.

Jarvelin, M. R., Vikevainen-Tervonen, L., Moilanen, I., & Huttunen, N. P. (1988). Enuresis in seven-year-old children. *Acta Paediatrica Scandinavia, 77*, 148–153.

Kaffman, M., & Elizur, E. (1977). Infants who become enuretics: A longitudinal study of 161 kibbutz children. *Monographs of the Society for Research in Child Development, 42*, (2, Serial no. 170), 1–54.

Kass, E. J. (1991). Approaching enuresis in an uncomplicated way. *Contemporary Urology, 3*, 15–24.

Keehn, J. D. (1965). Brief case-report: Reinforcement therapy of incontinence. *Behaviour Research & Therapy, 2*, 239.

Leape, L. L., & Ramenofsky, M. L. (1978). Anterior ectopic anus: A common cause of constipation in children. *Journal of Pediatric Surgery, 13*, 627–630.

Levine, A. (1943). Enuresis in the navy. *American Journal of Psychiatry, 100*, 320–325.

Levine, M. D. (1975). Children with encopresis: A descriptive analysis. *Pediatrics, 56*, 412–416.

Levine, M. D. (1982). Encopresis: Its potentiation, evaluation, and alleviation. *Pediatric Clinics of North America, 29*, 315–330.

Levine, M. D., & Bakow, H. (1976). Children with encopresis: A study of treatment outcome. *Pediatrics, 58*, 845–852.

Liebman, W. M. (1979). Disorders of defecation in children: Evaluation and management. *Postgraduate Medicine, 66*, 105–110.

Locke, H. J. & Wallace, K. M. (1959). Short marital adjustment and prediction tests: Their reliability and validity. *Marriage and Family Living, 21*, 251–255.

Loening-Baucke, V. A. (1984). Sensitivity of the sigmoid colon and rectum in children treated for chronic constipation. *Journal of Pediatric Gastroenterology and Nutrition, 3*, 454–459.

Loening-Baucke, V. A. (1989). Factors determining outcome in children with chronic constipation and faecal soiling. *Gut, 30*, 999–1006.

Loening-Baucke, V. A. (1990). Modulation of abnormal defecation dynamics by biofeedback treatment in chronically constipated children with encopresis. *Journal of Pediatrics, 116*, 214–222.

Loening-Baucke, V. A., & Cruikshank, B. M. (1986). Abnormal defecation in chronically constipated children with encopresis. *Journal of Pediatrics, 108*, 562–566.

Loening-Baucke, V. A., Cruikshank, B., & Savage, C. (1987). Defecation dynamics and behavior profiles in encopretic children. *Pediatrics, 80*, 672–679.

Loening-Baucke, V. A., & Younoszai, M. K. (1982). Abnormal anal sphincter response in chronically constipated children. *Journal of Pediatrics, 100*, 213–218.

Lovibond, S. H. (1964). *Conditioning and enuresis*. Oxford: Pergamon.

MacLean, R. E. G. (1960). Imipramine hydrochloride (Tofranil) and enuresis. *American Journal of Psychiatry, 117*, 551.

Margileth, A. M., Pedreira, F. A., Hirschman, G. H., & Coleman, T. H. (1976). Urinary tract bacterial infections: Office diagnosis and management. *Pediatric Clinics of North America, 23*, 721–734.

Mellon, M. W., & Houts, A. C. (1995). Elimination disorders. In R. T. Ammerman & M. Hersen (Eds.), *Handbook of child behavior therapy in the psychiatric setting* (pp. 341–366). New York: Wiley-Interscience.

Mercer, R. D. (1967). Constipation. *Pediatric Clinics of North America, 14*, 175–185.

Meyers, A. W. (1991). Biobehavioral interactions in behavioral medicine. *Behavior Therapy, 22*, 129–131.

Moffatt, M. E. K., Harlos, S., Kirshen, A. J., & Burd, L. (1993). Desmopressin acetate and nocturnal enuresis: How much do we know? Pediatrics, 92, 420–425.

Moffatt, M. E. K., Kato, C., & Pless, I. B. (1987). Improvements in self-concept after treatment of nocturnal enuresis: Randomized controlled trial. *The Journal of Pediatrics, 110*, 647–652.

Morgan, R. T. T., & Young, G. C. (1975). Parental attitudes and the conditioning treatment of childhood enuresis. *Behaviour Research & Therapy, 13*, 197–199.

Neale, D. H. (1963). Behaviour therapy and encopresis in children. *Behaviour Research & Therapy, 1*, 139–149.

Nisley, D. D. (1976). Medical overview of the management of encopresis. *Journal of Pediatric Psychology, 4*, 33–34.

Olness, K., McParland, F. A., & Piper, J. (1980). Biofeedback: A new modality in the management of children with fecal soiling. *Journal of Pediatrics, 96*, 505–509.

O'Regan, S. O., Yazbeck, S., Hamberger, B., & Schick, E. (1986). Constipation a commonly unrecognized cause of enuresis. *American Journal of Disabilities in Childhood, 140*, 260–261.

Parker, L., & Whitehead, W. (1983). Treatment of urinary and fecal incontinence in children. In D. C. Russo & J. W. Varni (Eds.), *Behavioral pediatrics: Research and practice* (pp.143–174). New York: Plenum Press.

Partin, J. C., Hamill, S. K., Fischel, J. E., & Partin, J. S. (1992). Painful defecation and fecal soiling in children. *Pediatrics, 89*, 1007–1009.

Pedrini, B. C., & Pedrini, D. T. (1971). Reinforcement procedures in the control of encopresis: A case study. *Psychological Reports, 28*, 937–938.

Philpott, M. G., & Flasher, M. C. (1970). The treatment of enuresis: Further clinical experience with imipramine. *The British Journal of Clinical Practice, 24*, 327–329.

Ravitch, M. M. (1958). Pseudo Hirchsprung's disease. *Annals of Surgery, 147*, 781–795.

Redman, J. F., & Siebert, J. J. (1979). The uroradiographic evaluation of the enuretic child. *The Journal of Urology, 122*, 799–801.

Rolider, A., & Van Houten, R. (1985). Treatment of constipation-caused encopresis by a negative reinforcement procedure. *Journal of Behavior Therapy and Experimental Psychiatry, 16*, 67–70.

Rushton, H. G. (1989). Nocturnal enuresis: Epidemiology, evaluation, and currently available treatment options. *The Journal of Pediatrics, 114*, 691–696.

Rutter, M., Tizzard, J., & Whitmore, K. (Eds.). (1970). *Education, health, and behavior*. London: Longman.

Rutter, M., Yule, W., & Graham, P. (1973). Enuresis and behavioral deviance. In I. Kolvin, R. C. MacKeith, & S. R. Meadow (Eds.), *Bladder control and enuresis*, (pp. 137–147). London: William Heinemann.

Sacks, S., & DeLeon, G. (1973). Case histories and shorter communications: Conditioning of two types of enuretics. *Behaviour Research & Therapy, 11*, 653–654.

Schaefer, C. E. (1979). *Childhood encopresis and enuresis: Causes and therapy*. New York: Van Nostrand Reinhold.

Schmitt, B. D. (1984). Encopresis. *Primary Care, 11*, 497–511.

Schmitt, B. D. (1982). Nocturnal enuresis: An update on treatment. *Pediatric Clinics of North America, 29*, 21–37.

Scott, M. A., Barclay, D. R., & Houts, A. C. (1992). Childhood enuresis: Etiology, assessment, and current behavioral treatment. In M. Hersen, R. M. Eisler, & P. M. Miller (Eds.) *Progress in Behavior Modification* (pp. 84–117). Sycamore, IL: Sycamore Publishing.

Shaffer, D. (1985). Enuresis. In M. Rutter & L. Hersov (Eds.), *Child and adolescent psychiatry: Modern approaches* (pp. 465–481). Oxford: Blackwell Scientific Publications.

Shelov, S. P., Gundy, J., Weiss, J. C., McIntire, M. S., Olness, K., Staub, H. P., Jones, D. J., Haque, M., Ellerstein, N. S., Heagarty, M. C., & Starfield, B. (1981). Enuresis: A contrast of attitudes of parents and physicians. *Pediatrics, 67*, 707–710.

Sluckin, A. (1981). Behavioural social work with encopretic children, their families and the school. *Child Care, Health, and Development, 7*, 67–80.

Sondheimer, J. M. (1985). Helping the child with chronic constipation. *Contemporary Pediatrics*, March, 12–22.

Stansfeld, J. M. (1973). Enuresis and urinary tract infection. In I. Kolvin, R. C. MacKeith, & S. R. Meadow, (Eds.), *Bladder control and enuresis* (pp. 102–103). London: William Heinemann.

Stern, H. P., Stroh, S. E., Fiedorek, S. C., Kelleher, K., Mellon, M. W., Pope, S. K., & Rayford, P. L. (1995). Increased plasma levels of pancreatic polypeptide and decreased plasma levels of motilin in encopretic children. *Pediatrics, 96*, 111–117.

Stromgren, A., & Thomsen, P. H. (1990). Personality traits in young adults with a history of conditioning-treated childhood enuresis. *Acta Psychiatrica Scandinavia, 81*, 538–541.

Suberman, R. I. (1976). Constipation in children. *Pediatric Annals, 5*, 32–48.

Sukhai, R. N., Mol, J., & Harris, A. S. (1989). Combined therapy of enuresis alarm and desmopressin in the treatment of nocturnal enuresis. *European Journal of Pediatrics, 148*, 465–467.

Taitz, L. S., Wales, J. K. H., Urwin, O. M., & Molnar, D. (1986). Factors associated with outcome in management of defecation disorders. *Archives of Disease in Childhood, 61*, 472–477.

Thompson, I. M., & Lauvetz, R. (1976). Oxybutinin in bladder spasm, neurogenic bladder, and enuresis. *Urology, 8*, 452–454.

Thorne, F. C. (1944). The incidence of nocturnal enuresis after age of 5 years. *American Journal of Psychiatry, 100*, 686–689.

Verhulst, F. C., van der Lee, J. H., Akkerhuis, G. W., Sanders-Woudstra, J. A. R., Timmer, F. C., & Donkhorst, I. D. (1985). The prevalence of nocturnal enuresis: Do DSM III criteria need to be changed? A brief research report. *Journal of Child Psychology and Psychiatry, 26*, 989–993.

Wakefield, M. A., Woodbridge, C., Steward, J., & Croke, W. M. (1984). A treatment programme for faecal incontinence. *Developmental Medicine & Child Neurology, 26*, 613–616.

Wald, A., Chandra, R., Chiponis, D., & Gabel, S. (1986). Anorectal function and continence mechanisms in childhood encopresis. *Journal of Pediatric Gastroenterology and Nutrition, 5,* 346–351.

Wald, A., Chandra, R., Gabel, S., & Chiponis, D. (1987). Evaluation of biofeedback in childhood encopresis. *Journal of Pediatric Gastroenterology and Nutrition, 6,* 554–558.

Werry, J. S., Dowrick, P. W., Lampen, E. L. & Vamos, M. J. (1975). Imipramine in enuresis: Psychological and physiological effects. *Journal of Child Psychology and Psychiatry, 16,* 289–299.

Whelan, J. P., & Houts, A. C. (1990). Effects of waking schedule on primary enuretic children treated with Full-Spectrum Home Training. *Health Psychology, 9,* 164–176.

Whitehead, W. E., & Shuster, M. M. (1985). *Gastrointestinal disorders: Behavioral and physiological basis for treatment.* New York: Academic Press.

Young, G. C., & Morgan, R. T. T. (1972). Overlearning in the conditioning treatment of enuresis: A long-term follow-up study. *Behaviour Research & Therapy, 10,* 419–420.

Young, G. C., & Morgan, R. T. T. (1973). Rapidity of response to the treatment of enuresis. *Developmental Medicine and Child Neurology, 15,* 488–496.

CHAPTER 10

DEVELOPMENTAL DISABILITIES

Marc J. Tassé
Michael G. Aman
Johannes Rojahn
Richard A. Kern

DESCRIPTION OF DISORDERS

Developmental disabilities are defined in Public Law 100-146 of 1987 as any severe and chronic mental or physical disability of a person that is manifested before the person attains the age of twenty-two years. This disability, which is likely to continue indefinitely, results in substantial functional limitations in three or more of the following areas of activity: self-care, receptive and expressive language, learning, mobility, self-direction, capacity for independent living, and economic self-sufficiency. This disability also reflects the person's need for a combination of special interdisciplinary or generic care/treatment, or other services that are of lifelong or extended duration and are individually planned and coordinated. Four major developmental disabilities are mental retardation, autism, cerebral palsy, and epilepsy (Baroff, 1991). In order to allow a thorough presentation within the constraints of a single chapter, we will limit our presentation and discussion of developmental disabilities primarily to mental retardation and autism.

Mental Retardation

The definition and classification of mental retardation has evolved over the years from a metaphorical description to a more function-based description (Blatt, 1987). Function-based definitions preclude issues of etiology and instead place emphasis on observable and measurable characteristics (i.e., intellectual functioning and adaptive behavior).

The American Association on Mental Retardation (AAMR) has led the way in defining mental retardation. It published its first official definition in 1921, and in 1959 the AAMR departed from the traditional exclusive use of IQ by incorporating adaptive behavior into its definition and classification system (Heber, 1959, 1961).

The definition and classification of mental retardation is essential in the process of establishing eligibility for services. In 1992, the AAMR's committee on terminology and classification published the AAMR's ninth edition of its manual on definition and classification (Luckasson et al., 1992). Luckasson and associates' (1992) manual represents a clear departure from previous manuals and systems of classification with its inclusion of systems of supports. Some, such as Schalock and colleagues (1994), have described this willful departure from current definitions as typifying an existing paradigm shift in the field of mental retardation.

American Association on Mental Retardation Definition (Luckasson et al., 1992)

In their ninth manual, the AAMR broadened its title from "Classification in mental retardation" to include the notion of supports in "Mental retardation: Definition, classification and systems of supports." The diagnosis and classification process of the new definition is structured in a multidimensional schema where mental retardation

> . . . refers to substantial limitations in present functioning. It is characterized by significantly subaverage intellectual functioning, existing concurrently with related limitations in two or more of the following applicable adaptive skill areas: communication, self-care, home-living, social skills, community use, self-direction, health and safety, functional academics, leisure, and work. Mental retardation manifests itself before age 18. (page 5)

Luckasson and associates (1992) define "significantly subaverage intellectual functioning" as 70–75 or less on an individually-administered IQ test. Previously, "Significant subaverage intellectual functioning" had been defined by the AAMR as being ". . . approximately IQ 70 or below" (Grossman, 1983; page 1). Although never stated clearly in Luckasson and associates' (1992) manual, the decision to use "70–75" was motivated by a desire to account for a 5-point error variance resulting from current standardized IQ tests. Controversy has arisen because of this apparent change in the IQ criterion and some other aspects of the new definition (MacMillan, Gresham, & Siperstein, 1993; Reiss, 1994a; Schalock et al., 1994).

Salient Aspects of Luckasson et al. (1992) Definition

Mental retardation is assessed using a multidimensional approach, and Luckasson and associates (1992) emphasize the involvement of a multidisciplinary team throughout this process. The four identified dimensions are:

I. Intellectual functioning and adaptive behavior
II. Psychological/emotional considerations
III. Physical health/etiological considerations
IV. Environmental considerations (home/school/work)

The Diagnostic and Statistical Manual (DSM) of the American Psychiatric Association and the International Classification of Diseases (ICD) of the World Health Organization have historically incorporated the AAMR's definition into their respective systems of diagnosis and classification. The AAMR establishes a three-step process to be applied to diagnosis, classification, and assessment of the individual's needs:

Step 1. Establish a diagnosis of mental retardation. The person has mental retardation if present functioning is below 70 to 75 IQ and this intellectual impairment results in limitations in two or more adaptive skills. These deficits must occur before the age of 18 years. In an effort to minimize importance placed on the intellectual functioning, levels of mental retardation (mild, moderate, severe, and profound), which were based solely on IQ, have been completely eliminated in Luckasson and associates' (1992) manual. If the individual meets the criteria for mental retardation in step 1, steps 2 and 3 must be completed for an acceptable assessment of the individual's level of functioning and need for support services.

Step 2. Describe the individual's strengths, weaknesses, and assessed need for supports based on the multidimensional schema. Strengths and weaknesses are identified in terms of intellectual functioning and from the applicable ten adaptive skills. During step 2, the individual's psychological and emotional health is assessed. This is where any mental health diagnosis (DSM-IV or ICD-10) or challenging behavior is recorded.

Step 3. Make a complete evaluation of the individual's interaction with the different applicable environments (home/school/work). During this evaluation, a profile is constructed of the individual's level of needed supports for all four dimensions and in all applicable environments. The level of need for supports is translated into four levels of intensity:

   i. Intermittent: episodic, punctual, of short duration.
   ii. Limited: similar to intermittent in nature, but somewhat more durable.
   iii. Extensive: regular in nature and of on-going duration.
   iv. Pervasive: constant, multi-level, life/health maintaining, typically extensive in scope.

Other Classifications

There currently exist three authoritative definitions and systems of classification of mental retardation (AAMR, DSM-IV, ICD-10). We noted previously that the DSM and ICD systems have historically adopted the AAMR definition of mental retardation, but this practice changed somewhat with the tenth revision of the ICD (ICD-10; World Health Organization, 1992) and the fourth revision of the DSM (DSM-IV; American Psychiatric Association, 1994). Currently, the three systems of diagnosis and classification differ slightly from one another with regard to their description and criteria for defining mental retardation. Table 10.1 illustrates these three systems.

Autistic Disorder

Autistic disorder was first identified by a child psychiatrist named Leo Kanner (1943). Kanner described eleven children under his care and termed their shared syndrome as "early infantile autism." He described these children with autism as being characterized by a preference for aloneness, accompanied by a disinterest in people, an obsessive desire for sameness in their environment, impairments in social communication, and a fascination with objects (Kanner, 1943, 1944). Autistic disorder is most frequently identified by the age of 2 to 3 years (Lotter, 1967). Concurrent to Kanner's work, Hans Asperger reported on a group of children very similar to Kanner's group. Originally available only in German, Asperger's work was long ignored and then gradually gained recognition following the work of Lorna Wing (Wing, 1981). Asperger syndrome has come to be viewed as a mild variant of autistic disorder in relatively bright children (Gillberg & Gillberg, 1989).

Autistic disorder (DSM-IV) or Infantile Autistic Disorder (ICD-10) was first included in these diagnostic systems about 15 years ago under the category of pervasive developmental disorders. The DSM-IV's diagnostic criteria of autistic disorder focus on three main areas of functioning social skills, communication skills, and interests and activities. The diagnostic criteria

Table 10.1. AAMR, DSM-IV, and ICD-10 Definitions of Mental Retardation

AAMR (LUCKASSON ET AL., 1992)	DSM-IV (APA, 1994)	ICD-10 (WHO, 1992)
IQ: 70–75 or lower	IQ: approximately 70 or lower	IQ: approximately 69 or lower
No levels of mental retardation.	Mild: 50–55 to approximately 70. Moderate: 35–40 to 50–55. Severe: 20–25 to 35–40. Profound: below 20–25.	Mild: approximately 50 to 69. Moderate: approximately 35 to 49. Severe: approximately 20 to 34. Profound: below 20.
Concurrent limitations in at least two of the applicable ten adaptive skills: communication, self-care, home living, social skills, community use, self-direction, health and safety, functional academics, leisure and work.	Concurrent impairments in at least two of the following areas: communication, self-care, home living, social skills, community use, self-direction, health and safety, functional academics, leisure and work.	Diminished ability to adapt to daily living demands of the normal environment.
		Extent of behavioral impairment: .0 no, or minimal impairment of behavior .1 significant impairment of behavior requiring attention or treatment .8 other impairments of behavior .9 without mention of impairment of behavior
Mental retardation manifests before age 18 years.	The onset is before age 18 years.	Manifested during the developmental period.

contained in the DSM-IV (American Psychiatric Association, 1994) for autistic disorder are as follows:

A. A total of six (or more) items from (1), (2), and (3), with at least two from (1), and one each from (2) and (3):
   1. Qualitative impairment in social interaction, as manifested by at least two of the following:
      a. marked impairments in the use of multiple nonverbal behaviors such as eye-to-eye gaze, facial expression, body postures, and gestures to regulate social interaction
      b. failure to develop peer relationships appropriate to developmental level
      c. a lack of spontaneous seeking to share enjoyment, interest or achievements with other people (e.g., by a lack of showing, bringing, or pointing out objects of interest)
      d. lack of social or emotional reciprocity
   2. Qualitative impairments in communication as manifested by at least one of the following:
      a. delay in, or total lack of, the development of spoken language (not accompanied by an attempt to compensate through alternative modes of communication such as gesture or mime)
      b. in individuals with adequate speech, marked impairment in the ability to initiate or sustain a conversation with others
      c. stereotyped and repetitive use of language or idiosyncratic language
      d. lack of varied, spontaneous, make-believe play or social imitative play appropriate to developmental level
   3. Restricted repetitive and stereotyped patterns of behavior, interests and activities, as manifested by at least two of the following:
      a. encompassing preoccupation with one or more stereotyped and restricted patterns of interest that is abnormal either in intensity or focus
      b. apparently inflexible adherence to specific, nonfunctional routines or rituals
      c. stereotyped and repetitive motor mannerisms (e.g., hand or finger flapping or twisting, or complex whole-body movements)
      d. persistent preoccupation with parts of objects
B. Delays or abnormal functioning in at least one of the following areas, with onset prior to age three years: (1) social interaction, (2) language as used in social communication, or (3) symbolic or imaginative play.
C. The disturbance is not better accounted for by Rett's Disorder or Childhood Disintegrative Disorder. (American Psychiatric Association, 1994; pp. 70–71)

Areas of behavioral disturbance that are typically observed at various ages of development in the autistic child are presented in Table 10.2.

Children with autism are frequently characterized by mental retardation (estimated 75 percent co-morbidity). However, some children with autism have demonstrated remarkable talents or skills (Hermelin & O'Connor, 1990; Kanner, 1943, 1944; Waterhouse, 1988; Young & Nettelbeck, 1994). Individuals who possess these exceptional skills are commonly referred to as autistic-savants (the term idiot-savants was dropped due to its pejorative connotation). Autistic-savants have demonstrated that they are capable of numerous accomplishments, including piano recitals, calendar calculations, mathematical calculations, artistic paintings or drawings, and feats of memory.

Included among the pervasive developmental disorders are also Rett's disorder, childhood disintegrative disorder, Asperger's disorder, and pervasive developmental disorder not otherwise specified. We will only briefly describe these other pervasive developmental disorders. *Rett's disorder* is characterized by a regression of motor ability, deceleration of head growth, the development of stereotypic hand gestures, loss of social engagement early in the course, language impairment, and psychomotor retardation following a normal period of development during at least the first five months of an infant's life (APA, 1994). Rett's disorder is of unknown etiology and has been diagnosed only in girls. Most children with Rett's disorder function in the severe to profound range of mental retardation. *Childhood disintegrative disorder* is similar to Rett's disorder in that it is characterized by a period of normal early infant development. However, unlike Rett's disorder, childhood disintegrative disorder is diagnosed equally in boys and girls and the period of normal development is more prolonged. Typically, onset occurs after at least two years of normal development (American Psychiatric Association, 1994). Regression may include loss of previously acquired language, adaptive skills, bowel and bladder control, play or motor skills. *Asperger's disorder* is characterized by impairments in reciprocal social interactions, stereotypic interests in specific topics, preference for routines, good language ability but some language peculiarities such as a superficially perfect language that may at times seem too formal and an inability to maintain a conversation, poor nonverbal communication skills, and some motor clumsiness or stereotypes. Children with Asperger's disorder present no significant deficits in intellectual and adaptive skills, but have marked impairment in social skills (American Psychiatric Association, 1994). The main clinical challenge is

Table 10.2. Areas of Disturbance Observed in Autistic Children

AGE	SENSORY-MOTOR	SPEECH-LANGUAGE	RELATION TO PEOPLE OBJECTS AND EVENTS
0 – 6 months	- quiet or fussy - persistent rocking - startled or non-responsive to stimuli - unusual sleep cycle	- no vocalization - crying, not related to needs	- no anticipatory social responses (absent or delayed in smiling response) - poor or absent eye-contact - fails to respond to mother's attention and crib toys
6 - 12 months	- sleeping and eating cycles fail to develop - uneven motor development - difficulty with transition to table foods - failure to hold objects or attachment to unusual objects - appears to be deaf - preoccupation with fingers - over or underreaction to sensory stimuli	- babbling may stop - does not imitate sounds, gestures, or expressions	- unaffectionate: difficult to engage in baby games - does not wave "bye-bye" - no interest in toys - flicks objects away
12 – 24 months	- sleep cycle problems - loss of previously acquired skills - sensitivity to stimuli - seeks repetitive stimulation - stereotyped behavior - mannerisms (e.g., hand-flapping, object twirling)	- no speech or occasional words - stops talking - gestures do not develop - repeats sounds non-communicatively	- withdrawn - no separation distress - unusual use of toys (e.g., spins, flicks, lines up objects)
24 – 36 months	- sleep cycle problems continue - refuses to do things which he appears capable of doing - delay in self-care skills - unusual sensitivity to stimuli and mannerisms persist - hypoactivity or hyperactivity	- mute or intermittent talking - echolalia (e.g., repeats TV commercials) - specific cognitive abilities (e.g., good rote memory, puzzle skills) - leads adult by hand to communicate needs	- does not play with others - prefers to be alone - unusual use of toys continues
36 – 60 months	- continued disturbances in above areas with the exception that sensitivity to stimuli and mannerisms may decrease	- no speech - echolalia - pronoun reversal - abnormal tone and rhythm in speech - unusual thoughts	- continued disturbances in above areas with the exception that may become more social - upset by changes in environment or routine

From Freeman, B. J., & Ritvo, E. R. (1989). The syndrome of autism: Establishing the diagnosis and principles of management. *Pediatric Annals, 13*, 284–295. Reprinted with permission.

making a differential diagnosis between autistic disorder (high functioning with no mental retardation) and Asperger's disorder. Szatmari (1991) found three substantive differences between the two syndromes: social responsiveness, communication, and imaginative play. Children with Asperger's disorder are more socially responsive to their parents and engage in more social behavior with peers, exhibit less echolalia and idiosyncratic speech although their speech may be perseverative or repetitive, and children with Asperger's disorder do exhibit imaginary play (Szatmari, 1991). Pervasive developmental disorder (PDD) not otherwise specified (including atypical autism) is used when a child presents deficits in the three broad areas of PDD (social interaction, communication, and behavior and interests) but does not meet the diagnostic criteria for a specific PDD (American Psychiatric Association, 1994).

EPIDEMIOLOGY

Prevalence and Incidence

Prevalence estimates for mental retardation as a global category are not very reliable. Since mental retardation is caused and shaped by many different factors, as presented below, it may be of interest to review epidemiological figures reported for specific etiologies. For example, the incidence of Down syndrome, the most frequent etiology of mental retardation associated with cytogenetic abnormalities has been reported to be 0.1 percent in the total population between 1960 and 1989 (Staples, Sutherland, Haan, & Clisby, 1991). Fragile X syndrome is the second most prevalent chromosomal condition responsible for mental retardation. It is estimated that fragile X may account for as much as 10 percent of all cases of mental retardation. Mental retardation caused by the fragile X chromosome occurs in approximately 0.06 percent of all children. Fetal alcohol syndrome, another leading cause of mental retardation, has been estimated to be responsible for 8 percent of all individuals with mild mental retardation. Estimates from studies conducted in the United States indicated that the prevalence of fetal alcohol syndrome ranged between 1 in 28 to 1 in 750 births depending on the sampled population (Burd & Martsolf, 1989).

Autism is a behaviorally defined syndrome with multiple etiologies (Gillberg, 1990). Recent studies suggest that autism is much more prevalent than previously believed. Estimates have ranged as high as 12 cases per 10,000 births (Gillberg, Schaumann, & Steffenburg, 1991), but the number is more typically reported to be around 2–5 cases per 10,000 births (American Psychiatric Association, 1994). Asperger's syndrome, often described as "high functioning" autism, has been reported in a recent total population study to occur in at least 40 of every 10,000 children or in 0.4 percent (Ehlers & Gillberg, 1993). Rett's syndrome, another relatively rare form of pervasive developmental disorder, which occurs exclusively in females, has been reported as occurring in approximately 1 of every 10,000 girls (Hagberg, 1985; Kerr & Stephenson, 1986; cited in Van Acker, 1991).

Prevalence of Mental Retardation at Different Levels of Severity[1]

Mental retardation is not equally distributed across levels of severity. Mild mental retardation is much more

prevalent than profound mental retardation. Prevalence of mental retardation decreases as the level of functioning decreases. Taking a theoretical perspective of an assumed normal distribution of IQ in the general population, 2.14 percent of the general population should have IQ scores between 69 and 55 (i.e., the group of people with mild mental retardation); only 0.13 percent fall below three standard deviations (which includes moderate to profound mental retardation) (Isaac & Michael, 1978). This also means that 94.3 percent of all persons with mental retardation should fall into the mild range, while only 5.7 percent should fall in the moderate, severe, and profound range of mental retardation.

Empirical epidemiological studies in mental retardation are few and most of them were conducted in Europe and Canada, where compulsory national health service registries exist. Such actuarial data systems greatly simplify epidemiological research but the extent to which their results can be generalized to other countries is debatable. In addition, international findings differ from one another. This is probably not due to actual differences in the distribution of mental retardation in these parts of the world but rather a factor of the methodological differences between these studies. Nevertheless, empirical studies clearly show a lower prevalence of severe and profound mental retardation as opposed to milder forms. However, a more gradual slope has been observed than that suggested by the theoretical normal distribution of intellectual functioning. For instance, in a Swedish survey of 8- to 12-year-old children with mental retardation, the proportion of more severe forms of mental retardation (defined as IQs < 50) was almost 30 percent of the total population with mental retardation (Hagberg, Hagberg, Lewerth, & Lindberg, 1981). This discrepancy between empirically derived figures and theoretical sample distribution parameters exists. Diseases and accidents may contribute disproportionately in enhancing the prevalence of the more severe than milder levels of mental retardation.

Prevalence as a Function of Age

The prevalence of mental retardation is not equally distributed across all age levels. The prevalence of mild mental retardation increases steadily from birth to adolescence, while severe forms of mental retardation remain relatively stable during childhood and adolescence. The reason for this increase in the prevalence of mild mental retardation is probably mainly due to a matter of case identification rather than actual change in "true prevalence." Mild forms of mental retardation are often overlooked in early childhood and become more apparent as

---

[1]The authors recognize that the new AAMR definition of mental retardation has forsaken classification into different levels of severity according to IQ scores as was previously common (mild, moderate, severe, and profound mental retardation). Nevertheless, it has been used in this context because the authors feel that a classification into levels of severity is useful for illustrative purposes.

the child grows older or progresses through a more cognitively challenging environment (e.g., school). Severe and profound mental retardation often coincide with birth defects that are identified at birth and change very little as a function of age. These varied prevalence rates across age also support the widely held notion that a relatively larger proportion of cases with mild mental retardation are a function of adverse environmental factors, while those with severe/profound mental retardation tend to result from inborn factors. An adverse environment may also have a cumulative negative effect on the initially relatively unimpaired organism, thus resulting in mild mental retardation.

Figure 10.1 shows integrated prevalence estimates along the chronological age range from three different surveys: Denmark (Dupont, 1989), England (Kushlick & Cox, 1973), and Scotland (Innes, Kidd, & Ross, 1968). All three surveys relied on registers and census data of the general population as case-finding methods for mental retardation. This figure demonstrates a steep rise of registered cases with mental retardation until it reaches a peak between the ages of 20 and 25, after which a slow decline sets in. The increase is probably a reflection of the increased need for services as a child matures. The declining prevalence in early adulthood has been attributed to an increased mortality rate for people with mental retardation.

Gender Ratio

Mental retardation is slightly more prevalent in males than in females. Gender ratio estimates vary depending on the survey. A ratio of 1.3 males to 1 female has been found to be a stable statistic in Danish registries (Dupont, 1989). Part of the discrepancies between sexes can be attributable to chromosomal etiologies of mental retardation. For instance, fragile X syndrome is manifested more frequently in males than females (1.5:1). However, in conditions in which the chromosomal contribution is unclear, a differential sex prevalence may also exist. Rett's disorder for instance, occurs only in females. On the other hand, there are approximately three to four times more males than females among reported cases of autism (Ritvo & Freeman, 1984).

Associated Conditions

People with mental retardation are often afflicted with concurrent physical handicaps, particularly cerebral palsy, seizure disorders, and sensory handicaps. Cerebral palsy is a nondegenerative neuromuscular disorder of movement and balance (see Baroff, 1991) that may be associated with mental retardation but does not cause mental retardation. All these concurrent handicaps are generally more likely to occur as the level of functioning

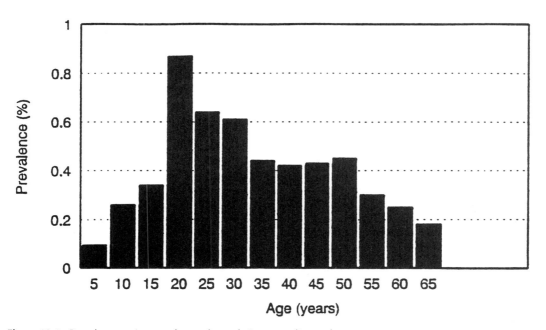

Figure 10.1. Prevalence estimates of mental retardation according to three surveys

decreases. Kiely (1987) reviewed the epidemiological literature and compared the results from three published studies. She found that seizure disorders in lower-functioning groups (i.e., IQ < 40) were consistently more frequent than in higher-functioning groups. In the low-functioning group, seizure disorders were observed among 8 percent to 36 percent, while they occurred in only 5 percent to 18 percent of those with mild mental retardation. A similar trend was seen with cerebral palsy. Between 16 percent to 23 percent of the lower-functioning groups had cerebral palsy, while only 4 percent to 7 percent of the group with mild mental retardation presented with cerebral palsy.

ASSESSMENT APPROACHES

Medical Issues

Medical evaluation of the person with developmental disabilities or mental retardation is aimed at identifying conditions that either cause or exacerbate the disability or that may co-occur with it. Because of the lack of understanding of the biological causes of mental retardation and autism, medical evaluation often cannot uncover an etiology. This, unfortunately, is particularly true for cases of mild mental retardation (Schaefer & Bodensteiner, 1992). Nevertheless, advances in several fields have resulted in the identification of etiologic factors for impairment in many individuals thought previously to be undiagnosable.

Etiology

Mental retardation. The causes of mental retardation are varied. Mental retardation may be explainable by a single factor, an interaction of multiple causal factors (50 percent of cases; McLaren & Bryson, 1987), or it may be of unknown etiology. In general, causes are grouped into prenatal, perinatal, and postnatal influences.

Prenatal causes of mental retardation involve cerebral damage that may have resulted from hereditary disorders (e.g., Lesch-Nyhan, PKU, Tay-Sachs), chromosomal abnormalities (e.g., Down, Klinefelter, fragile X syndromes), or insults to the fetus during development (e.g., maternal drug abuse, fetal alcohol syndrome, intrauterine infections). Prenatal causes account for less than 30 percent of cases (Scott & Carran, 1987). Mental retardation may also result from perinatally transmitted diseases communicated from mother to infant (e.g., sexually

transmitted diseases) or trauma during a difficult delivery (e.g., head injury, hypoxia). Postnatal causes of mental retardation occur in the individual's environment and may impede development or cause brain damage (e.g., traumatic head injury, poisons or toxins, degenerative diseases). Psychosocial factors are the most prevalent postnatal cause of developmental disabilities. Formerly referred to as cultural-familial mental retardation, psychosocial factors most frequently result in mild levels of mental retardation when operative (Aman, Hammer, & Rojahn, 1993). Baroff (1991) identifies psychosocial risk factors within an impoverished social environment that may be lacking in nutritional diet, stimulation, and an adult presence responsible for providing care and learning experiences. For a more exhaustive review of the many etiologies of mental retardation, the reader should consult Baroff (1991), Matson and Mulick (1991), and Thapar, Gottesman, Owen, O'Donovan, and McGuffin (1994).

Autism. The exact cause or causes of autism remain unknown. What can be ruled out are psychological trauma, bad parenting, physical abuse, and separation anxiety (Ritvo & Freeman, 1984). Much of the current research and speculation revolves around the functioning of the brain and its neurochemistry. Most researchers and clinicians agree that the causal factors are most probably of a neurological nature and affect cerebral functioning (Morgan, 1986; Ritvo & Freeman, 1984; Rutter & Schopler, 1987). Research efforts to elucidate the causes of autism are still ongoing. Although the exact causes of autism elude us, promising treatment intervention programs exist that can improve the quality of life of many children with autism.

Medical History

Evaluation begins with the person's medical history, starting with the prenatal period. Maternal age and health during pregnancy, use of alcohol, medications, or illicit drugs, exposure to teratogens, and the occurrence of any untoward events such as preterm labor or vaginal bleeding should be ascertained, since all of these have been associated with suboptimal outcome for the fetus and with later impairment in the child (Allen, 1993). The individual's gestational age at birth, the need for resuscitation in the delivery room or for intensive care in the post-partum period, and the presence of infection, jaundice, birth defects, or neurologic, cardiac, or respiratory problems also should be investigated, since these, too, are associated with later developmental disabilities (Menke, McClead, & Hansen, 1991).

The person's health history since infancy should be obtained, with particular focus on the existence of any significant illnesses or injuries, such as meningoencephalitis (Baraff, Lee, & Schriger, 1993) or head trauma (Michaud, Duhaime, & Batshaw, 1993), which could damage the central nervous system and cause mental retardation post-natally. Information on the presence of any defects commonly associated with mental retardation, such as seizure disorders, cerebral palsy, visual or auditory deficits, feeding problems, communication disorders, psychiatric conditions, or behavioral disorders, should be sought, as they often exert significant effects on the individual's adaptive outcome (Batshaw, 1993). Many neurodevelopmental disorders, such as Down's syndrome (Roizen, 1989), have characteristic constellations of physical problems such as congenital heart malformations or atlanto-axial subluxation accompanying them, and the occurrence and the severity of these defects should be investigated. Finally, the presence of any other chronic medical problems, such as diabetes, asthma, or hypertension, should be ascertained; while these conditions may be unrelated to the etiology of the individual's mental retardation, they can impact profoundly on overall health (Minihan & Dean, 1990).

Information on the person's family medical and developmental history, particularly on the existence of relatives with congenital defects, genetic syndromes, or developmental disabilities, should be pursued, since it can often direct diagnostic efforts toward hereditary causes of mental retardation. Data on the person's social background should also be obtained, since psychosocial or socioeconomic factors may not only determine the family resources, both financial and intellectual, for assisting the individual with mental retardation or autism to maximize his/her potential, but may even contribute to severity of impairment (Rowitz, 1991).

Developmental history should be assessed, focussing on the person's acquisition of milestones in communication, motor, language, social, and adaptive skills. Parents' concerns about their child's skills should be ascertained; several studies have shown that parental suspicion of a disability can be a sensitive indicator of developmental pathology (Coplan, Gleason, Ryan, Burke, & William, 1982; Glascoe, Altemeier, & Maclean, 1989). In a general-pediatric ambulatory clinic or office setting, standardized screening instruments of developmental functioning should be used (Levy & Hyman, 1993).

Physical Examination

A physical examination should be performed. This exam should look especially at the person's somatic growth (height, weight, height × weight, and head circumference); it should also focus on the presence of any congenital anomalies or dysmorphic features, neurocutaneous signs, organomegaly, or eye abnormalities (Levy & Hyman, 1993). A useful approach is to examine the person's body by anatomic region and then, if anomalies are found, to return to those organ systems likely to have associated defects. For example, if dystrophic fingernails are observed, other structures derived from the same embryologic precursor (in this case, the ectoderm), such as the hair, the skin, and the teeth, should be examined (Aase, 1990).

Hearing should be assessed in any child with a suspected language delay. The cause of a hearing deficit can be related to the underlying cause of developmental disabilities, as in the cases of congenital infections with organisms such as cytomegalovirus or in the genetic syndromes that involve dysmorphic craniofacial features (Levy & Hyman, 1993). A variety of testing procedures, including brainstem auditory-evoked potentials, behavioral audiometry, and traditional audiometry, are available to assess children of differing cognitive levels and cooperation (Nozza & Fria, 1990).

Vision also should be assessed in the developmentally disabled child. Significant visual defects of various types occur frequently in persons both with idiopathic mental retardation (Woodruff, 1977; Woodruff, Cleary, & Bader, 1980) or with developmental deficits such as cerebral palsy (Maino, 1979), congenital anomaly syndromes, genetic or metabolic disorders, or infection (Menacker, 1993). Significant visual deficit obviously affects the acquisition of gross- and fine-motor skills; it also may have a role in the development of higher cognitive functions. Several methods of assessment have been devised to test the visual acuity of children unable to respond to the traditional Snellen charts, including visual evoked potential recording, preferential looking techniques, and the electroretinogram (Menacker, 1993).

Laboratory Testing

Laboratory studies of various sorts may be obtained. These include chromosomal and molecular-genetic analyses, metabolic testing, and assays for toxic substances.

Chromosomal analysis is becoming increasingly useful in determining an underlying diagnosis for developmental disabilities. Progress in cytogenetic techniques such as banding (Punnett & Zakai, 1990), special stains and cultures, and breakage studies, as well as in molecular genetic techniques such as fluorescent in-situ hybridization, gene dosage measurements, and restriction fragment length polymorphisms (Schaefer & Boden-steiner, 1992), have made it possible to identify structural abnormalities in chromosomes with a precision and at a resolution previously impossible. These techniques can reveal the presence of small chromosomal changes such as insertions or deletions, ring portions, marker regions, and breakage points, that can be associated clinically with developmental disabilities or mental retardation. An obvious example is the fragile X syndrome, that is associated with a fragile site at Xq27.3 on the X-chromosome (Webb, 1991). This and other X-linked syndromes may account for up to 20 percent of moderate to severe mental retardation in males (Opitz, 1991).

The new genetic techniques have demonstrated the existence of so-called "contiguous gene syndromes"—multisystem disorders apparently caused by the operation of aberrant genes located in close physical proximity to each other on the chromosome (Schmickel, 1986). A number of contiguous gene syndromes have been identified, including Angelman syndrome, Prader-Willi syndrome, Langer-Giedion syndrome, Beckwith-Wiedemann syndrome, and Smith-Magenis syndrome, and many more are under investigation (Punnett & Zakai, 1990). Ultimately, many of the syndromes of multiple congenital anomalies may prove to be the result of contiguous abnormal genes, rather than of single-gene alterations, as was previously believed.

Biochemical studies to rule out inborn errors of metabolism may also be done in selected persons. Many studies of the etiology of mental retardation report a 3–7 percent incidence of such disorders (Schaefer & Boden-steiner, 1992). However, routine testing for metabolic disease in all individuals with mental retardation or autism is neither helpful diagnostically nor cost-effective. It must be recognized that most cases of inborn metabolic error manifest themselves in their severe forms in the first hours to weeks of life, long before neurodevelopmental disabilities become apparent; the symptoms that they induce such as vomiting, seizures, metabolic acidosis, or coma, often bring affected infants to medical attention independent of any developmental concerns.

While there are a number of these conditions that have milder forms with insidious onsets and episodic patterns of symptoms during childhood, there are still others, notably the storage diseases, which typically first appear in older infants and children (Applegarth, Dimmick, & Toone, 1989). Neurodevelopmental symptoms caused by these types of disorders are often non-specific, but associated findings like cataracts, dysmorphic facial features, hepatosplenomegaly, or a patient's tendency to develop severe vomiting, seizures, mental deterioration, or unusual body odors during intercurrent illnesses, can point toward these diagnoses (Applegarth, Dimmick, & Toone, 1989).

If a child outside the newborn period is suspected of having an inborn error of metabolism, a good battery of diagnostic tests would include serum electrolytes, fasting blood glucose, blood ammonia, blood lactate and pyruvate, serum amino acid quantitation, urinalysis, and urinary amino and organic acid screens. These studies can help to indicate the presence of amino- or organo-acidopathies, disorders of carbohydrate metabolism, and urea-cycle disorders. If the child is suspected of having a storage disease or a disorder of peroxisomal or mitochondrial function, biochemical analyses of skin, liver, or skeletal muscle may be necessary to make a diagnosis (Applegarth, Dimmick, & Toone, 1989).

Testing for the presence of lead in blood should be done on all children as a part of basic health screening, but especially on children with developmental disabilities. Lead intoxication, even at low levels, can cause cognitive, behavioral, and language skill deficits both in children who were exposed to lead *in utero* (Bellinger, Leviton, Waternaux, Needleman, & Rabinowitz, 1987) and in those exposed during childhood (Needleman, Schell, Bellinger, Leviton, & Allred, 1988; Needleman & Gastsonis, 1990). These findings led the United States' Centers for Disease Control in 1991 to revise its definition of the "acceptable" maximum level of lead in blood from 25 micrograms/dL to 10 micrograms/dL (U.S. Department of Health and Human Services, 1991).

Adequacy of blood iron levels also should be assessed. Iron deficiency, as demonstrated by a hemoglobin level of less than 100 gm/L, has been shown to be associated with cognitive delay in infants. This delay may persist for years after dietary iron supplementation has corrected the hematologic deficit (Lozoff, Jimenez, & Wolf, 1991). In addition, iron deficiency often coexists with low-level lead intoxication (U.S. Department of Health and Human Services, 1991), so that both conditions must be investigated and, if necessary, treated concurrently.

Radiologic Imaging

Brain imaging procedures can provide valuable diagnostic information in many patients. While children with neurodevelopmental problems may either lack definable brain abnormalities or have nonspecific ones, others can have lesions that permit the diagnosis of conditions such as genetic or teratogenic malformations, congenital infections, traumatic or ischemic encephalopathies, vascular accidents, inborn errors of metabolism, or neurodegenerative diseases (Mantovani, 1994). A variety of modalities is available. Cranial ultrasound, done through the open anterior fontanelles of newborn infants, is used to identify brain injuries, such as intraventricular hemorrhage or periventricular leukomalacia, that are associated with later developmental disabilities (Hope et al., 1988; Mantovani & Powers, 1991). Ultrasound also may be used to prospectively monitor infants at risk for brain injury, such as those undergoing extracorporeal membrane oxygenation (ECMO) (Matamoros, Anderson, McConnell, & Bolam, 1989), who have central nervous system infections (Cleveland, Herman, Dot, & Kushner, 1987), or who have had ventricular shunts placed to relieve hydrocephalus (Holt, 1989).

Computerized axial tomography (CT) and magnetic resonance imaging (MRI) are used to detect architectural changes in the brain, including brain malformation, such as holoprosencephaly, hydrocephalus, agenesis of the corpus callosum, and Dandy-Walker syndrome (Nickel, 1992; Barkovich, Gressens, & Evrard, 1992), and brain damage, such as hypoxic-ischemic encephalopathy (Byrne, Welch, Johnson, Darrah, & Piper, 1990), cerebral (Rorke & Zimmerman, 1992), or periventricular (Johnson et al., 1987) infarction, and metabolic or neurodegenerative disorders (Kendall, 1992). In conjunction with clinical history and physical and neurodevelopmental findings, these modalities can help to identify the type and timing of these changes, differentiating between those of prenatal origin and those of perinatal or of neurodegenerative cause (Mantovani, 1994). MRI has sufficient resolution to allow delineation of neuronal migration defects like schizencephaly, heterotopias, or cortical dysgenesis (Barnes, 1992).

So-called "functional" brain imaging techniques such as positron emission tomography (PET), single photon emission computed tomography (SPECT), and magnetic resonance or near-infrared spectroscopy are so far in only limited use in the area of pediatric diagnostic radiology (Mantovani, 1994). However, these techniques already have begun to reveal subtle neuroanatomic and neurometabolic derangements in autism, which for so long seemed to have no identifiable pathologic correlates (Schifter et al., 1994).

The question of which patients with neurodevelopmental problems to image has not been answered definitively. Neuroimaging techniques obviously are indispensable for diagnosing brain malformations and lesions. They have been less useful, however, in predicting outcome through clinical-radiologic correlation; brain anatomy still must be distinguished from brain function (Levene, 1990). Cranial ultrasound has become a routine part of the care of high-risk neonates, and has been shown to provide reliable prognostic information regarding at least some major disabilities like cerebral palsy (Van de Bor, Ouden, & Guit, 1992; Roth, Baudin, & McCormick, 1993). Correlation of ultrasound findings with less severe problems, however, has not been as high (Roth et al., 1993). Likewise, efforts to relate MRI or CT findings to specific prognoses have invariably been compromised by unexpected outcomes (Roth et al., 1993).

Still, the identification of cerebral damage or dysgenesis can provide useful clinical information, as well as logical closure and at least a partial indication of cause to the family of a developmentally disabled child (Blackman, McGuinness, Bale, & Smith, 1991). MRI imaging, the modality of choice, therefore should be done in most children with neurodevelopmental impairment, especially those with mental retardation or motor deficits of unknown cause, with sudden unexplained declines in developmental skills, with disproportionally large or small head circumferences in comparison with height and weight, with focal neurologic deficits, with multiple congenital anomalies, or with neurocutaneous signs.

Psychological and Psychiatric Issues

Aside from establishing a diagnosis, the primary clinical purpose of testing and assessing the behavior of people with mental retardation and autism is to determine their strengths and weaknesses. This in turn can be used to enhance the individual's autonomy and maximize access to the most beneficial supports, placements, and treatments. Assessment is also an important component of clinical outcome research.

People with developmental disabilities often represent a difficult group to assess. Many of the assessment strategies for other clinical populations are based strongly on the notion that the client can communicate symptoms verbally. Cognitive deficits are associated with comprehension impairments. The individual may not understand the clinician's questions during a physical exam. Hence, more so than with other populations, clinicians dealing with people with mental retardation or autism will resort to a *multimodal strategy*. This means that different information sources are used to develop a converging picture that will accurately reflect the individual's developmental status. These multimodal strategies often include be-havior observations under natural or contrived condi-tions, rating scale information obtained from third-party informants, such as parents, teachers or others familiar with the client, and standardized tests. For a more de-tailed discussion of assessment in mental retardation, the reader is referred to Aman et al. (1993) and Reiss (1994b). For more in-depth information on psychologi-cal assessment of autism, the reader should consult Mat-son (1994) and Schopler and Mesibov (1988). In the present context, we will only briefly highlight some of the more important issues.

Systematic Behavior Observation

Direct behavior observation is a particularly well-suited strategy for collecting information on individuals with mental retardation or autism because it relies ex-clusively on trained observers. During observations the observer classifies targeted behavior (e.g., aggression, self-injurious behaviors) into predefined behavior cate-gories in an ongoing fashion.[2]

One of the advantages of observational techniques is that they can be adapted to virtually any need. They are also quite easy to interpret and their use does not hinge on elaborate statistical assumptions. Systematic obser-vational techniques are often used in addition and sub-sequent to interviews with parents or teachers (depending on the setting of observations). A more comprehensive account of observational methodologies can be found in Rojahn and Schroeder (1991).

Intelligence Tests

Since intelligence is a key element in diagnosing mental retardation, intelligence tests have long played an important role with this population. The most widely used intelligence tests for individuals with limited cog-nitive abilities are the Wechsler intelligence scales and the Stanford-Binet. *The Wechsler Preschool and Pri-mary Scale of Intelligence—Revised* (WPPSI-R; Wech-

[2]Standardized observation systems do exist (e.g., Schroeder, Rojahn, & Mulick, 1978), but they are less common in mental retardation than in other clinical populations (e.g., conduct disorders, ADHD). The reason may be that this population is very heterogeneous and their behavior highly idiosyncratic.

sler, 1991), for instance, was developed for children be-tween the ages of 3 years and 7 years. It contains 12 sub-tests and is considered a downward extension of the *Wechsler Intelligence Scale For Children—III* (WISC-III; Wechsler, 1992). The WISC-III, which has 13 sub-tests, covers the age range between 6 years and 16 years. *The Stanford Binet Intelligence Scale, Fourth Edition*, which consists of 15 subtests, was developed for the age ranges between 2 and 23 years (Thorndike, Hagen, & Sattler, 1986).

Traditional intelligence tests, such as the ones just mentioned, were normed and standardized on develop-mentally typical populations. Intelligence becomes in-creasingly more difficult to test reliably as a person's cognitive abilities decrease. IQ scores beyond the fourth standard deviation below the mean (severe and profound mental retardation) are often suspect and should be treated with great caution. Another important aspect in testing intelligence is that people with mental retardation frequently have motor and sensory limitations as well as deficient communication skills. Intelligence test scores are fraught with potential problems and for these reasons a score on any intelligence test must be interpreted by properly-trained psychologists only (Luckasson et al., 1992). For an authoritative and in-depth treatment of in-telligence tests for children with special needs the reader is referred to Sattler (1992).

Adaptive Behavior Scales

Concurrent with cognitive deficits, a limitation in adaptive and functional skills is an essential component for the classification of people with mental retardation (American Psychiatric Association, 1994; Luckasson et al., 1992; World Health Organization, 1992). Among the most popular instruments are the *Vineland Adaptive Behavior Scales* (Sparrow, Balla, & Cicchetti, 1984), the *AAMR Adaptive Behavior Scales: Residential and Community II* (Nihira, Leland, & Lambert, 1992), and the *Scales of Independent Behavior* (Bruininks, Wood-cock, Weatherman, & Hill, 1984). Currently, in light of the AAMR's (Luckasson et al., 1992) and DSM-IV's (American Psychiatric Association, 1994) operational definition of adaptive behavior, which is divided into ten specific adaptive skills, there exists no single standard-ized assessment instrument that is capable of assessing these ten skill areas. Work toward providing clinicians with such a tool is underway (see Schalock et al., 1994; B. Bryant, personal communication, October, 1994). For a critical and comprehensive review of existing scales of adaptive behavior the reader should consult Reschly (1990).

Assessment of Psychopathology and Harmful Behavior

One of the greatest concerns for people with mental retardation or autism is their propensity for emotional problems and problem behaviors. While exact figures on the prevalence of psychiatric disorders are not available, some data suggest that people with mental retardation may be particularly vulnerable (Nezu, Nezu, & Gill-Weiss, 1992; Reiss, 1994b). Destructive behaviors, such as aggressive physical attacks on other people and chronic self-injurious behaviors, pose a serious problem. Besides the personal discomfort that presumably accompanies emotional problems and destructive behavior, they are also major obstacles to a person's development toward independence and community integration. Assessment of these behaviors is important for programmatic reasons.

Many instruments have become available in recent years. The most widely used broad-range psychopathology scales include the *Aberrant Behavior Checklist* (Aman, Singh, Stewart, & Field, 1985), the *Reiss Scales for Children's Dual Diagnosis* (Reiss & Valenti-Hein, 1990), and the *Strohmer-Prout Behavior Rating Scale* (Strohmer & Prout, 1989). Other, narrow-band instruments focus on specific conditions. Examples of these are the *Self-Report Depression Questionnaire* (Reynolds & Baker, 1989), the *Behavior Problems Inventory* (Rojahn, Polster, Mulick, & Wisniewski, 1989), and the *Preschool Behavior Questionnaire* (Behar, 1977; Aman & Rojahn, 1994). It is important to note that some of these instruments are specifically geared to a limited range of cognitive functioning (e.g., *Strohmer-Prout Behavior Rating Scale*) or to a certain chronological age range (e.g., *Preschool Behavior Questionnaire*).

An important step in the process of planning any behavioral intervention is the functional analysis of the target behavior. Functional analysis refers to the technology of determining the motivational factors maintaining a given behavior. Ideally, a functional analysis is based on the actual experimental testing of specific hypotheses concerning the environmental conditions that maintain the target behavior. Hypotheses are derived from unstructured behavior observations and interviews of people familiar with the client. Behavior motivation rating scales would be much more economical; however, ratings of motivational variables have proven unreliable.

TREATMENT STRATEGIES

Psychological and Behavioral Treatments

Mental Retardation

Although mental retardation is functionally defined, which would open the possibility of contemplating "cure" (Blatt, 1987), this controversy will not be addressed. Rather, it is sufficient to reiterate Luckasson and associates (1992) when they comment that with appropriate supports (e.g., psychological/behavioral interventions) the level of functioning of a person with mental retardation will generally improve. Treatment strategies applied to mental retardation have focused on teaching skills or reducing maladaptive behavior, which would contribute to ameliorating the individual's condition.

Behavior management. Behavior interventions have been applied to promoting a wide array of behavioral skills (e.g., toilet training, social skills communication, anger management). Components of programs aimed at shaping or increasing behaviors should always start with thorough functional and task analyses. To teach a new behavior, a procedure of behavior chaining (forward or backward) may be used. Another important component of the behavior intervention is the reinforcement schedule. Generally, the density of reinforcements should be higher in the early phases of skill teaching, and the reinforcement schedule should be varied or intermittent as the skill is mastered. For a more extensive presentation of this topic, the reader should consult Foxx (1982a), LaVigna and Donnellan (1986), Matson (1990), and Matson and Mulick (1991).

A second focus of behavioral interventions has been on reducing challenging behaviors. Some of the more problematic behaviors reported in the literature are self-injurious behavior, aggression, and stereotyped behavior. Not all techniques employed in behavior reduction include punitive or aversive measures. A good example of a non-aversive behavioral intervention whose primary goal is behavior suppression are the differential reinforcement techniques. These techniques include differential reinforcement of other (i.e., non-maladaptive) behavior, alternative behavior, and incompatible behavior. Carr and Durand (1985) presented an effective technique that they termed "functional communication training," that works essentially like a differential reinforcement of alternate behavior technique. It should be emphasized that a functional analysis (previously presented) will maximize the effectiveness of any behavioral intervention and will permit the establishing of the "function" of the maladaptive behavior. The reader interested in this general area can consult Cipani (1989), Konarski, Favell, and Favell (1993), and Thompson and Gray (1994).

Prevention. We will briefly present two early intervention programs that attempt to prevent mental retardation in at-risk populations. Since a significant proportion of cases of mental retardation are associated with poverty, many prominent programs have been geared toward reducing the prevalence of psychosocial mental retardation. Many of these early intervention programs were set up as a result of an impetus from the Kennedy era of the 1960s. Two such intervention/prevention programs in the United States are Head Start and the Milwaukee Project.

Head Start. This early intervention program was first started in the mid-1960s during the U.S. government's "War on Poverty." Head Start was not specifically funded to reduce the prevalence of mental retardation. Rather, it was established to combat the detrimental effects of poverty and cultural deprivation on the cognitive functioning of young children (Peters, 1980). Much of the focus of Head Start has been to provide four types of services: social services, health services, parent involvement, and education. The health and social service components are an attempt to reduce health-related factors (e.g., lead poisoning, malnutrition) that may contribute to mental retardation. The enriched preschool programming was set up with the hope of countering the stimulus-poor home environment of these children. Much of the Head Start rationale, which is centered on countering scholastic failure and poor development of cognitive functioning, espouses the view that cognitive functioning is highly malleable during the first 5 years of life. The Head Start program is generally packed into one preschool year. Some have criticized the optimism of the Head Start movement in thinking that any significant impact can be achieved in only one year (Garber, 1988).

The Head Start program has always been able to sustain the popular vote, and this has been reflected in increases in funding by almost 70 percent between the early 1980s and 1992 (Hood, 1993). It has not escaped criticism concerning certain of its aspects. Washington (1985) is critical of Head Start's lack of cultural diversity in staffing and curricula content and its cultural deficit approach to program implementation, although studies have shown decreases in certain long-term social factors (e.g., teenage pregnancy, delinquency, unemployment) often associated with poverty (Seitz, Rosenbam, & Apfel, 1985). However, gains in cognitive functioning seem to be of relatively small magnitude (Locurto, 1991; Westinghouse Learning Corporation, 1969) and are not sustained over time (Herrnstein & Murray, 1994).

Milwaukee Project. The Milwaukee Project emanated from similar concerns that spawned the Head Start movement. The Milwaukee Project was, however, specifically geared to the prevention of mental retardation and the fight against cultural-familial mental retardation (Garber, 1988). This project emphasizes an intensive educational program for children as early as a few months old. The intervention program starts with a 1:1 teacher to infant ratio and moves gradually to small group formats as the child progresses in age and skills. Garber (1988) reported two essential focal points of the program: rehabilitation aimed at the parent and early infant stimulation. The parents in Garber's study had mild mental retardation, and rehabilitation consisted of training skills that better enabled the parent to provide economically for the family. During the parent's habilitation, the child participates in enriched stimulation activities that take part at the Infant Stimulation Center. The activities in the Milwaukee Project (Garber, 1988) shift from socio-emotional development to perceptual-motor development and finally to cognitive-language development as the child progresses from infancy to early childhood.

In Garber's (1988) report of comparative data between a control group and an experimental group that completed the Milwaukee curriculum, he presented data demonstrating a reversal of decline in cognitive performance for the experimental group. Gains were reported for the treatment group in the areas of learning performance and language development.

It is important to note, however, that Garber (1988) did not use random procedures in allocating his subjects to the control and experimental groups. Gilhousen and colleagues (Gilhousen, Allen, Lasater, & Farrell, 1990) expressed skepticism of the positive effects reported in the Milwaukee Project. Gilhousen et al. (1990) concluded that a minimal difference (less than 10 IQ points) was found between the experimental and control group, and no difference was found in reading achievement.

Large amounts of money are spent in early intervention programs (Hood, 1993), and it appears that a long-lasting impact with regard to correlates of mental retardation (IQ and adaptive skills) remains to be unequivocally established. This is not surprising, however, in light of the brevity of intervention typically used thus far.

Autism

Behavioral principles dealing with promoting adaptive skills and reducing maladaptive behavior in children with mental retardation apply equally to children with autism. Several treatment approaches have emerged over the 50 years since Kanner (1943) first described autism. Generally, behavioral approaches have been most popular in guiding development of treatment packages for children with autism.

Rutter (1985) has identified basic goals that should be included in treatment involving children with autism. His basic goals include the following three components: (a) the promotion of normal development (cognitive functioning, language development, and social skills), (b) the reduction of challenging behaviors (stereotyped behavior, self-injurious behavior, non-compliance), and (c) the alleviation of family distress.

Behavioral principles have heavily influenced two major treatment programs for children with autism which incorporate Rutter's (1985) basic goals of effective treatment for autism: (a) the UCLA young autism project, and (b) the Treatment and Education of Autistic and Communication-handicapped CHildren (TEACCH). Both of these programs consist of intense training that includes the involvement of professionals and parents of the children with autism. We have come a long way since the days of Bettelheim's (1967) "refrigerator parents."

The UCLA Young Autism Project. This project was established by O. Ivar Lovaas in 1970 at UCLA. The main component involves intense one-on-one training for approximately 40 hours per week (Lovaas, 1987). Parents are intricately involved in the training program, which is carried out in the homes, school, or community of the children, with the collaboration of a team of undergraduate students and supervision from graduate students.

Lovaas (1987) devised this program so that it would commence at an age no older than 46 months. Early enrollment into the UCLA program appears to be a bid to take full advantage of the early years of high neuroplasticity of the child. The UCLA young autism project utilizes discrete trials to shape and augment prosocial behavior. During the first phase of the program, treatment focuses on teaching compliance, simple imitation, and appropriate toy play while simultaneously intervening to suppress self-stimulation and non-compliant behavior.

Phase two of the project involves teaching expressive speech, early abstract language, and social play with peers. The third and final phase incorporates teaching the expression of emotions, functional academic skills (reading, writing, arithmetic), and more complex cognitive abilities, such as vicarious learning or cause-effect learning.

After approximately 15 years of program operation and data collection, Lovaas presented the results of the UCLA young autism project. Lovaas (1987) reported on 19 experimental subjects who went through at least two years of the intensive treatment program. Of the 19 autistic children in the treatment group, 9 (47 percent) successfully entered and completed normal first grade and had a mean IQ of 107 (IQ range: 94–120); 8 (42 percent) were enrolled in aphasia classes, with a measured IQ ranging from IQ 56 to 95 (mean = 70); and the remaining 2 children (11 percent) were enrolled in autistic/mental retardation classes (IQ < 30). These impressive results, which seem to be maintained (McEachin, Smith, & Lovaas, 1993), have nonetheless attracted some skepticism regarding the selection criteria, pre- and post-treatment measures, and diagnostic criteria of the experimental group. Interested readers are strongly urged to read Schopler, Short, and Mesibov (1989) and Lovaas, Smith, and McEachin (1989) to familiarize themselves with these issues. Replications of the UCLA young autism project remain to be completed.

TEACCH. The TEACCH program was founded in North Carolina in 1966 by Eric Schopler. TEACCH's comprehensive classroom and residential programs are geared toward individualized treatment inspired from behavioral principles (Reichler & Schopler, 1976). Schopler's work was also heavily influenced by psychoeducational principles that emphasize parent involvement on an equal footing with a multidisciplinary treatment team. Much like Lovaas's program, Schopler maximizes treatment generalization and carry-over by enlisting parents as co-therapists. In the TEACCH program, parents are trained in behavior management principles and their role within their child's treatment evolves from trainee to trainer to emotional support and, finally, to social advocate (Mesibov, Schopler, & Sloan, 1983).

The TEACCH-accredited classroom is typically in public schools in classes of no greater than 8 pupils. TEACCH classrooms are self-contained and separate from mainstream classrooms; however, children with autism in the TEACCH program can take part in appropriate regular classroom activities (McHale & Gamble, 1986). The teaching staff in these classrooms is carefully selected and extensively trained by TEACCH professionals.

The TEACCH curriculum is intricately influenced by the individualized assessment procedure (discussed further in this chapter) with input from teacher observations and parent information. Olley (1986) presents a typical four-step process of developing an individualized treatment plan in a TEACCH program. The four-steps comprise (a) obtaining detailed information from individual assessment of the child's skills (both through naturalistic observations and informant-based questionnaires), (b) interviewing the parents and obtaining their personal views regarding their child's skills and the parents' desired results, (c) assimilating the information obtained in the previous two steps and incorporating this information into specific curriculum objectives, and (d) based on these objectives, designing a training curriculum (Olley, 1986). Much of the curriculum selected is based not only on functional academic skills, but also on more general daily living skills, with a general curriculum strategy focused on exploiting the child's strengths while working on skill deficits.

A literature search of Educational Resources Information Center (ERIC) and psycLIT databases (10/17/94) failed to turn up a review of the TEACCH program from a source independent of a TEACCH center.

Comments. Both the UCLA young autism project and TEACCH place significant importance on acquiring and promoting language skills, which are fundamental in facilitating social interactions (Lovaas, 1977). However, since some autistic children, due to underlying biological/physiological deficits, are incapable of acquiring spoken language (Rutter, 1985), sign language or communication tools (e.g., Bliss board, picture systems) are incorporated into these programs as substitutes for verbal language. A second important variable in all of the early intervention programs discussed is age. The younger the child is entered into an intervention program, the greater the potential for gain.

In recent years, we have also seen a rapid proliferation of interest and debate over a procedure called "facilitated communication." Facilitated communication (FC) will only be briefly mentioned, and only because of the popular attention and media hype that it has drawn over the last few years.

FC entails the use of a typing device (any keyboard or other commercialized FC device) along with the close involvement of a trained "facilitator," who provides physical hand-over-hand or hand-over-forearm support (Biklen et al.,1991). FC found its origins with people who have cerebral palsy, who required some physical support in order to guide their movements toward the keyboard. FC was introduced into the field of developmental disabilities by Douglas Biklen, professor of special education at Syracuse University. People with autism who had been previously assessed as functioning at the profound level of mental retardation were reported to be typing with high levels of literacy via FC (Biklen, 1990).

The contention regarding FC centers on the ownership of the produced messages. A large number of empirical studies have demonstrated a strong facilitator influence (knowingly or not) in the production of FC messages (Eberlin, McConnachie, Ibel, & Volpe, 1993; Moore, Donovan, & Hudson, 1993; Szempruch & Jacobson, 1993; Wheeler, Jacobson, Paglieri, & Schwartz, 1993). In other words, it appears that the facilitators, not the persons with autism, were producing the messages. The question of propriety of the typed words is especially crucial in cases where serious allegations and accusations of abuse have been directed at parents and direct-care workers through FC.

At the time of this writing, we are not aware of any sound research that supports the validity of FC. Several professional organizations have officially argued against the use of FC. The American Academy of Child and Adolescent Psychiatry ("Professional organizations offer resolutions on FC," 1994), the American Association on Mental Retardation ("AAMR board approves policy on FC," 1994), the American Psychological Association (B. L. Baker, personal communication, 8 June 1994), and the American Speech-Language-Hearing Association (Asha, 1995) have drafted resolutions cautioning their respective membership as to the absence of scientific support for the validity of FC.

Pharmacological Treatments

Rationale for Pharmacotherapy

Generally speaking, psychotropic medications are given with one of three objectives in mind. The first of these is the management of well-defined disorders, such as the prescription of neuroleptics ("antipsychotics") for true psychosis, antidepressants for major depression, and so forth. Unfortunately, there can be difficulties in recognizing and diagnosing such psychiatric disorders in people who have more severe forms of mental retardation (Reiss, 1994b). The second common objective is the suppression of behavior problems or symptoms, which do not in themselves comprise a DSM-IV diagnosis. Examples may be verbal or physical aggression, self-injury, unruly behavior, and so forth. The third objective of pharmacotherapy is "chemical restraint," which is effectively a crisis intervention procedure for dealing with dangerous or violent behavior on a temporary basis until more appropriate therapies can be put into place.

Although disorder-specific prescribing should be the ideal for which clinicians strive, limitations in our knowledge base, as alluded to above, have confined the amount of this treatment in the mental retardation and autism fields. However, there is growing recognition of the need to rationalize prescribing, and this has led to apparent increases in disorder-specific prescribing. Traditionally, symptom suppression has accounted for the brunt of pharmacotherapy in mental retardation and this is probably still the case today. Problems such as self-injury, aggression, shouting/screaming, and so forth are common, often serious, and only infrequently part of a well-recognized syndrome or disorder. Chemical restraint is becoming quite uncommon and is usually subject to a number of review procedures and checks in most progressive treatment settings. Listed below are some of the common conditions and symptoms for which pharmacotherapy is given.

Autism

There is, as aforementioned, a strong association between autism and the presence of mental retardation. Aman, Van Bourgondien, Wolford, and Sarphare (1994) recently surveyed over 800 clients with autism and found that psychotropic drugs were a common mode of treatment (30.5 percent of clients were so treated). In decreasing order of prevalence, the most common groups of medication were neuroleptics, stimulants, sedative/hypnotics, antidepressants, antihypertensives, and mood stabilizers.

Neuroleptics. Although thioridazine (Mellaril) is the most commonly prescribed drug for behavioral management in autism (Aman et al., 1994), there is little, if any, research on its use with this population. In contrast, haloperidol (Haldol, Serenace) has been assessed in several well-controlled studies (Anderson et al., 1984; Campbell et al., 1982; Cohen et al., 1980). These have shown significant drug-induced reductions in stereotypic behavior, social withdrawal, and hyperactivity, and there were significant combined effects of haloperidol and contingent reinforcement on language acquisition. Chlorpromazine (Largactil, Thorazine) was not found to

be helpful in patients with autism and was found to cause significant sedation (Campbell et al., 1972), whereas early studies reported benefits with trifluoperazine (Stelazine) (Fish, Shapiro, & Campbell, 1966) and fluphenazine (Prolixin) (Engelhardt, Polizos, Waizer, & Hoffman, 1973).

Fenfluramine (Pondimin, Ponderax). This drug, which is structurally related to the amphetamines, has been extensively studied in recent years. Fenfluramine became of interest because it is known that children with autism tend to have higher than average levels of serotonin in blood, and fenfluramine is a serotonin depleting agent. Early studies suggested that this agent had marked effects on cognitive/social development and social relatedness (Aman & Kern, 1989). However, subsequent and better controlled studies indicated mild or null effects in these areas. The most common findings observed across studies include reduced activity level, reduced stereotypic behavior, and possibly increased social relatedness (Aman & Kern, 1989). There is little reason to believe that fenfluramine (or any other drug for that matter) improves IQ in children with autism. This agent should be used conservatively because there is at least a theoretical risk that it may have a neurotoxic effect on certain serotonergic systems in the brain (Aman & Kern, 1989).

Psychostimulant drugs. The stimulants methylphenidate (Ritalin) and dextroamphetamine (Dexedrine) are the most commonly prescribed psychotropic drugs for children (typically given for Attention Deficit Hyperactivity Disorder; ADHD), and they are prescribed to about 12 percent of children with autism. Given that they are well established for managing ADHD, and given the high prevalence of hyperactive symptoms in autism, they would appear to be promising agents for such children. Early studies of these drugs in children with autism were generally negative or suggestive of marginal improvement (Aman, 1982), although more recent reports indicate a more positive role (Birmaher, Quintana, & Greenhill, 1987; Strayhorn, Rapp, Donina, & Strain, 1988). Psychostimulant medication clearly benefits some youngsters with autism, although the likelihood of a beneficial response does not appear to be as high as in children with ADHD and normal IQ.

Other agents. Other treatments are often given on a trial-and-error basis or in relation to other symptoms that occur in conjunction with the autism (see below). Agents that have been given include tricyclic antidepressants [e.g., tricyclic antidepressants such as imipramine

(Tofranil) for depressive symptoms or hyperactivity], clonidine (Catapres) for hyperactivity, and naltrexone (Trexan) for symptoms of autism, for self-injury and stereotypy. In the past, there has been some advocacy of certain vitamin combinations for treating these children (Rimland, Callaway, & Dreyfus, 1978). Researchers have reviewed this evidence and found both a theoretical rationale and the experimental support for vitamin therapy to be lacking (Aman & Singh, 1988; Kozlowski, 1992).

Attention-Deficit/Hyperactivity Disorder (ADHD)

ADHD is the most common behavioral disorder in children of average intellectual ability, and this also appears to be the case in youngsters with mental retardation.

Stimulant medication. This group includes methylphenidate, dextroamphetamine, and pemoline (Cylert), but only the first two have been assessed in controlled studies with appropriately selected children. Recent group studies with methylphenidate (given in doses of 0.3 to 0.6 mg/kg) indicated significant improvement in overactivity, attention-related behavior, and on-task behavior (Aman, Kern, McGhee, & Arnold, 1993a; Aman, Marks, Turbott, Wilsher, & Merry, 1991; Handen, Breaux, Gosling, Ploof, & Feldman, 1990; Handen et al., 1992; Varley & Trupin, 1982). One study of dextroamphetamine and methylphenidate in children with fragile X syndrome and ADHD found negligible to modest evidence of stimulant-induced improvements (Hagerman, Murphy, & Wittenberger, 1988). Hence, there is a sound empirical basis for concluding that stimulants can and do reduce problematic behavior in some children with mental retardation and ADHD. However, the results of at least one study suggest that the stimulants may be much less effective in children with more severe mental retardation (e.g., severe and profound retardation) and some children with low to moderate functional handicaps as well (Aman et al., 1991).

Fenfluramine. As previously mentioned, studies of fenfluramine were inspired by work with this drug (in youngsters with autism) that suggested improvements in attention and overactivity. One group study and a case report have now been reported suggesting a possible role for fenfluramine in individuals with mental retardation and ADHD. Parent and teacher ratings indicated improvements on conduct, activity level, and attention span (Aman, Kern, McGhee, & Arnold, 1993a; Gadow & Pomeroy, 1990), and there were also improvements on certain cognitive tasks (Aman, Kern, McGhee, & Arnold, 1993b).

Other drugs. Neuroleptic drugs were the first agents shown to have a role in managing ADHD in children of average intellectual ability (Campbell, Gonzalez, Ernst, Silva, & Werry, 1993), but they are not well studied for this purpose in mental retardation or autism (Aman & Singh, 1980). Some early studies suggested a possible role for neuroleptic drugs (Burk & Menolascino, 1968; Ucer & Kreger, 1969), but it is difficult to be enthused about the possibility of long-term therapy in light of the possibility of developing tardive dyskinesia (see side effects).

Antidepressant drugs (e.g., imipramine) are often the second line of treatment if stimulants fail in ADHD children of average intellectual ability. We are not aware of any studies of antidepressants in children with ADHD and mental retardation, although they would certainly be worth a trial. Other drugs sometimes used clinically include buproprion (Wellbutrin) and clonidine (Catapres), although there are virtually no data with these agents in such children.

Self-Injury

Self-injury is a relatively common and potentially serious problem in people with mental retardation or autism and, not surprisingly, it has frequently been the target of drug treatment.

Neuroleptics. These have frequently been used as a treatment for self-injury. Thioridazine has been studied the most and has the most supportive data for a therapeutic role, whereas the data on chlorpromazine are not promising (Aman, 1993). Limited data are available on haloperidol, but it may also be helpful in managing such persons (Aman, 1993).

Opiate antagonists. One popular theory maintains that a dysfunction of the endogenous opiate system may be responsible for the appearance and maintenance of self-injury in some individuals (Sandman, 1991). There are now numerous studies looking at the effects of two opiate blockers, naloxone (Narcan) and naltrexone (Trexan), in people with self-injury, although most of these have had very small numbers of subjects (see Aman, 1993).

About half of the studies have reported symptom suppression, but frequently the reductions have been quite small (Aman, 1993). One recent large-scale study failed to find any reduction in self-injury (Campbell, Anderson et al., 1993). Only naltrexone is currently a viable treatment among the opiate blockers, as it alone is available in oral form, is a relatively pure opiate antagonist, and has a sufficiently long half-life to be practical in the clinical context (Sandman, 1991). Nalrexone is worthy of consideration in clients with self-injury, although any therapeutic effect must be established on a case-by-case basis.

Beta blockers. Recently there has been interest in the possible role of beta blockers, such as propranolol (Inderal) and nadolol for managing acting-out problems such as aggression and self-injury. The preliminary data from these uncontrolled studies suggest that these agents may have some therapeutic role to play (Arnold & Aman, 1991). Further trials appear to be indicated.

Other. There has also been considerable interest in the idea that self-injury may be caused by underlying depression or obsessive compulsive disorder in some clients with mental retardation or autism. Because of this there have been very small trials of various antidepressant drugs, such as clomipramine (Anafranil), trazodone (Desyrel), and the newer serotonin specific reuptake inhibitors (SSRIs) [e.g., fluoxetine (Prozac)]. To date, a number of optimistic case reports have appeared in the literature, but systematic group studies are lacking.

Aggression

Neuroleptics. Traditionally, the neuroleptics such as thioridazine, chlorpromazine, and haloperidol have featured most predominantly here (Aman, 1987; Aman & Singh, 1980). It is unlikely that they have any specific effect on aggression per se, and it is possible that these drugs tend to dampen all behavior in general. Early studies did show reductions in impulsive, aggressive, and tantrum behavior, but many of these studies were flawed methodologically (Aman & Singh, 1980).

Beta blockers. Recently there has been an upsurge in the use of these drugs, which have a role in dampening autonomic hyperarousal. Arnold and Aman (1991) reviewed 10 reports of the use of propranolol and nadolol in managing aggression, rage, and self-injury in people with developmental disabilities. All of these comparisons indicated reductions in hostile behavior, but the research methodology was usually weak.

Lithium carbonate. There is also a small group of studies that suggest that this drug may reduce assaultive, aggressive, and destructive behavior in some patients (see Aman & Singh, 1991). Again, the methodology is weak in several of these studies. The use of lithium in controlling aggressive behavior deserves further evaluation in better designed studies.

Anxiety

To the best of our knowledge, there are no published studies of anxiolytic medication in people with mental retardation chosen for high levels of anxiety. Very clearly, the interest of care providers and the scientific community has been in acting-out problems. However, anxiolytic drugs like the benzodiazepines (e.g., diazepam [Valium], alprazolam [Xanax]) probably act in much the same way in people with mental retardation as in the general population. One group has reported that some clients with high levels of self-injury and stereotypic behavior tend to react paradoxically (i.e., with hyperexcitability) to the anxiolytics (Barron & Sandman, 1985). Occasionally, antianxiety drugs have been utilized to reduce acting-out behavior, but the result has often been an increase in problem behavior (Aman & Singh, 1991).

Other Disorders and Symptoms

There simply is not enough research available to guide us in the treatment of all psychiatric disorders that occur in mental retardation. For the most part, existing evidence indicates that clinicians are safe in prescribing similar drugs for like conditions in the psychiatric literature. Hence, a rational approach is to use antidepressants for major depression, neuroleptics ("antipsychotics") for schizophrenia and other psychoses, lithium carbonate for bipolar disorder, and so forth. However, there can be problems in ascertaining the existence of such disorders, especially as the degree of developmental handicap increases (Einfeld & Aman, 1995; Reiss, 1994b).

Side Effects

By definition, any biologically active substance like behavior modifying medication must also be capable of producing side effects. Suffice it to say here that side effects with these drugs can run the gamut from those that are merely an inconvenience to those that are life threatening. Of the drugs discussed, neuroleptics, lithium carbonate, propranolol, and antidepressants are all capable of causing serious and potentially lethal side effects. Neuroleptics have received a great deal of attention because, when used chronically, they have a significant risk of causing tardive dyskinesia, a potentially irreversible movement disorder. They can also, although rare in incidence, cause neuroleptic malignant syndrome which in its early stages is a flu-like condition that, if untreated can result in death. It is, of course, important to be aware of the potential risks when considering pharmacotherapy. What is most important is to be as informed as possible, so that the relevant care providers can weigh the costs (and risks) of using psychotropic medication against the costs of not using such treatment. As more and more information becomes available, the decision will grow easier to make.

CASE ILLUSTRATION

Clinical Presentation

The client, M.G., was a boy of 10 years 8 months who was referred by his mother for possible inclusion in an ongoing study of methylphenidate (Ritalin) and fenfluramine (Pondimin) in children with mental retardation and hyperactivity (ADHD). On testing with the Stanford-Binet Intelligence Scale: Fourth Edition, M.G. was found to have an IQ of 70. At initial contact, he was receiving methylphenidate given in doses of 15 mg before school and 10 mg at noon. He was also taking l-hyoscyamine sulfate (Levsin) sustained release preparation, a long-acting antihistamine, for chronic nocturnal enuresis. M.G. was attending a class for children with developmental disabilities, but he was mainstreamed for music, art, and gym classes. The etiology of his developmental handicap was unknown. M.G. had an unremarkable birth and medical history. The parents were well educated; the father worked as a teacher and the mother was a nurse. The household appeared to be well organized, with no apparent signs of psychosocial distress.

Assessment Findings

M.G.'s behavior was assessed by means of standardized behavior rating scales that were completed by his parents and teacher. While he was still taking methyl-

phenidate (Ritalin), he was somewhat overactive and inattentive, although not extremely so. On ceasing methylphenidate for a week, his scores on the Hyperactivity subscales of the Aberrant Behavior Checklist (ABC) and Conners Teacher Questionnaire were very high. Attention Problem and Motor Excess subscale scores were also very high on the Revised Behavior Problem Checklist (RBPC), another rating scale completed by his parents. M.G. also received moderately high scores on the Irritability subscale of the ABC and on the Conduct Problem subscales of the RBPC and Conners Teacher Rating Scale (Conners, 1969), indicating some management and acting-out problems. On laboratory measures completed for the study in which M.G. was participating, he had very high recordings on a measure of seat activity, taken while he performed automated cognitive tasks. He also had a relatively low amount of on-task performance and a high rate of irrelevant hand activity (recorded with direct observations of behavior) while performing an arithmetic task used as an academic probe. Clinical interview with M.G.'s mother revealed symptoms that were consistent with a DSM-III-R diagnosis of ADHD. As M.G. met study criteria, he was invited to join the controlled evaluation.

Treatment Selection and Course

The protocol for this study entailed a comparison of placebo, methylphenidate (0.4 mg/kg/day), and three doses of fenfluramine (1.0, 1.5, and 2.0 mg/kg/day), with the sequence determined randomly for each subject. Each of these conditions was to be given for two weeks. A baseline of one week of known placebo preceded the sequence of experimental medications. Because of the possibility of interaction effects, we would only admit M.G. to the study if the l-hyoscyamine tablets were discontinued, and his parents readily agreed to this. All medications were given on a double blind basis (i.e., neither the parents, M.G.'s teachers, nor study personnel knew when each of the conditions would be given). The actual sequence that M.G. received was as follows: (1) fenfluramine medium dose (21.8 mg, given in the morning and evening); (2) placebo (given in the morning and evening); (3) methylphenidate (11.6 mg) given in the morning and placebo given in the evening; (4) fenfluramine high dose (29.0 mg, given in the morning and evening); and (5) fenfluramine low dose (14.5 mg, given in the morning and evening).

During the placebo baseline, M.G.'s bedwetting increased markedly, suggesting that the l-hyoscyamine had provided some symptomatic relief. His sleep pattern improved (as he began to fall asleep earlier), and M.G.'s appetite increased to a more normal level. His mother described him as having his old "sparkle" in his eyes, but he grew more argumentative at school and his rating scale scores related to attention span and activity level deteriorated both at home and at school.

In the first treatment condition, M.G.'s mother reported that he seemed sedated and "spaced out." He slept exceptionally well and was described as very cooperative. His mother felt that the quality of his school work and of his cursive writing declined. Curiously, M.G.'s father felt that he seemed "more intelligent" if given ample time to perform. Parent and teacher ratings completed during this phase showed a steep decrease in overactivity, no change in attention span, and a marked increase on the Lethargy/Social Withdrawal subscale of the ABC. This appears to be a further reflection of the side effects reported by M.G.'s mother. In light of M.G.'s unwanted sedation, the study director confidentially broke the medication code and removed the high-dose fenfluramine condition from the planned medication sequence. The identity of the eliminated condition and the reasons for doing this were not disclosed until M.G. completed the study.

During the second treatment phase (placebo), M.G.'s mother described him as having increases in activity level, talkativeness, temper tantrums, and emotional liability. Appetite also improved. He was noticeably more active on visiting the laboratory for routine cognitive testing and side effects monitoring. Parent and teacher behavior ratings showed increases in overactivity (both raters), inattention (teacher only), and irritability (parent only).

With methylphenidate (given in the morning only), M.G. was described by his mother as having good behavior between 9:00 A.M. and 1:00 P.M., but becoming difficult to manage in the afternoon. The quality of his homework, which he did in the evening, was poor. Behavior ratings showed moderate improvements in overactivity and irritability and a slight improvement in attention span.

The high-dose fenfluramine condition was skipped, and M.G. received low-dose fenfluramine in his final treatment phase. M.G.'s mother described him as calm and controlled much of the time and as having a "more likeable" personality. He slept longer in the morning, a change perceived by his parents as an improvement, as M.G. characteristically had had mild insomnia. He also had nasal congestion, decreased appetite, and, his mother felt, poorer coordination during this treatment phase. Both parent and teacher ratings suggested fairly marked

improvements in overactivity, and the mother's ratings indicated substantial improvements on the Irritability subscale of the ABC.

The study director, a psychologist, and the study's pediatrician met with M.G.'s mother on the final day of the study. In general, the parent and teacher ratings showed mild to moderate improvements with both methylphenidate and low-dose fenfluramine. Because fenfluramine has a much longer half-life, improvements were evident throughout the day, whereas they were present for only about 4 to 5 hours with methylphenidate. The cognitive tests generally indicated better performance with methylphenidate and low-dose fenfluramine, although there were a few variables in which performance was best with placebo. On discussion, M.G.'s mother, the psychologist, and the pediatrician concluded that it would be best to continue with methylphenidate given at a dose of 10 mg in the morning and 5 mg at midday. Methylphenidate was chosen over fenfluramine largely because of evidence from animal research that indicated a theoretical risk of neurotoxic effects on the brain from fenfluramine (Aman & Kern, 1989) (an issue that all parents were versed in prior to participating). M.G.'s mother and the researchers also felt that findings were sufficiently positive that low-dose fenfluramine should be regarded as a back-up treatment for M.G. should he become unable to use methylphenidate in the future.

There are two interesting aspects to this case. The first is that M.G.'s parents wanted him to join the study even though he was apparently deriving some benefit from his previous methylphenidate regimen. In the past we have found that many parents are attracted to a study like this, because it affords them a "second opinion" or a chance to evaluate the long-term treatment that their child is already receiving. Formal research studies should be capable of providing a far more detailed analysis of medication effects than is possible in routine assessments done in most medical practices. In the case of this study, data were collected on four fronts: (a) parent behavior ratings on standardized scales; (b) teacher ratings on similar scales; (c) a battery of cognitive tests; and (d) an extensive side effects checklist, plus heart rate, blood pressure, and weight monitoring. The second is that M.G. derived (or appeared to derive) equal or nearly equal benefit from 15 mg/day of methylphenidate after the study was completed as he had from 25 mg/day he was taking upon entry into the study. We have found that the drug-free baseline is quite helpful for preparing children so that they have a chance of benefitting from relatively low doses of medication. In some instances we have admitted children on very high doses of methylphenidate only to find that they do better at lower levels.

M.G. appeared to show equal behavioral gains with less medication, but he had a decline in side effects, particularly in his difficulty falling asleep at night.

Clinicians in private practice settings sometimes have difficulty accessing computerized assessment instruments or conveniently carrying out placebo-controlled drug trials. However, they can utilize the monitoring techniques of studies like this to guide their decision making. Having parents and teachers fill out a short behavior inventory such as the Conners Rating Scale (available both in parent and teacher forms; Conners, 1969) at the time of initial referral and then at weekly or bi-weekly intervals of baseline behavioral observations of the child in natural settings, and comparison data to see if and when a given medication (or a given dose or schedule of it) is improving target misbehaviors.

Clinicians can also make use of other treatment modalities besides medications. They can request the involvement of the school-based behavior management specialists that many systems now employ to help teachers find new classroom strategies for improvement of a child's school performance and for modification of his or her problem behavior. They also can link families with counseling agencies that provide parents with training in behavior management techniques.

SUMMARY

We presented mental retardation and autism, two forms of developmental disabilities. Mental retardation is functionally defined as a significant deficit in intellectual functioning with concurrent limitations in two or more adaptive skills, and is manifested before 18 years of age. Autism is a severe disability that appears in the first few years of a child's life and is lifelong. Children with autism experience limitations in communication and social interactions and exhibit restricted and repetitive patterns of behavior.

The prevalence of mental retardation is estimated at approximately 3 percent (APA, 1994) of the general population. The etiology can be of either organic/genetic or psychosocial origin, with the majority of cases of mental retardation (89 percent) being in the mild range of retardation (IQ 55 to 70). The prevalence of autism is estimated at approximately four or five cases in every 10,000 births. Its etiology remains unknown; however, a neurological basis is strongly suspected.

Assessment and identification of the more severe levels of mental retardation are frequently done at birth or during the first few weeks of life. The milder levels of

mental retardation may go undiagnosed until the commencement of school. Milder cases of mental retardation are more often of a psychosocial etiological nature than cases of severe mental retardation, which most likely result from a pre- or perinatal insult.

Autism is characterized by marked impairments and is diagnosed during the early stages of development. Diagnosis of autism may be made within the first three years of the child's life. Early intervention programs are available for both forms of developmental disabilities. Head Start and the Milwaukee Project are early intervention programs that strive to curb the negative effects of an impoverished home environment. We also presented two intervention programs for children with autism, the UCLA young autism project and TEACCH. Both programs emphasize early intervention and active parental participation in the intervention. The UCLA young autism program specifically targets young children before the ages of three or four years. TEACCH is a school-based program that involves children of all school ages.

We presented the different psychological, psychiatric, and psychopharmacological interventions currently in use with individuals with mental retardation and autism. Behavioral and pharmacological interventions are useful primarily to help control concomitant psychopathology, physical disorders, and/or inappropriate behavior in individuals with developmental disabilities.

REFERENCES

AAMR board approves policy on Facilitated Communication. (1994, September/October). *AAMR News & Notes, 7*, (5), 1.

Aase, J. M. (1990). *Diagnostic dysmorphology*. New York: Plenum Medical Book Co.

Allen, M. C. (1993). The high-risk infant. *Pediatric Clinics of North America, 40*, 479–490.

Aman, M. G. (1982). Stimulant drug effects in the developmental disorders and hyperactivity: Toward a resolution of disparate findings. *Journal of Autism and Developmental Disorders, 12*, 385–398.

Aman, M. G. (1987). (Guest editorial). Overview of pharmacotherapy: Current status and future directions. *Journal of Mental Deficiency Research, 31*, 121–130.

Aman, M. G. (1993). Efficacy of psychotropic drugs for reducing self-injurious behavior in the developmental disabilities. *Annals of Clinical Psychiatry, 5*, 171–188.

Aman, M. G., Hammer, D., & Rojahn, J. (1993). Mental retardation. In T. H. Ollendick & M. Hersen (Eds.), *Hand-*

book of child and adolescent assessment (pp. 321–345). Boston: Allyn & Bacon.

Aman, M. G., & Kern, R. A. (1989). Review of fenfluramine in the treatment of the developmental disabilities. *Journal of the American Academy of Child and Adolescent Psychiatry, 28*, 549–565.

Aman, M. G., Kern, R. A., McGhee, D. E., & Arnold, L. E. (1993a). Fenfluramine methylphenidate in children with mental retardation and ADHD: Clinical and side effects. *Journal of the American Academy of Child and Adolescent Psychiatry, 32*, 851–859.

Aman, M. G., Kern, R. A., McGhee, D. E., & Arnold, L. E. (1993b). Fenfluramine and methylphenidate in children with mental retardation and attention deficit hyperactivity disorder: Laboratory effects. *Journal of Autism and Developmental Disorders, 23*, 491–506.

Aman, M. G., Marks, R. E., Turbott, S. H., Wilsher, C. P., & Merry, S. N. (1991). The clinical effects of methylphenidate and thioridazine in intellectually subaverage children. *Journal of the American Academy of Child and Adolescent Psychiatry, 30*, 246–256.

Aman, M. G., & Rojahn, J. (1994). The psychometric characteristics of the Preschool Behavior Questionnaire in preschoolers with developmental handicaps. *Journal of Developmental and Physical Disabilities, 6*, 1–15.

Aman, M. G., & Singh, N. N. (1980). The usefulness of thioridazine for treating childhood disorders: Fact or folklore? *American Journal of Mental Deficiency, 84*, 331–338.

Aman, M. G., & Singh, N. N. (1988). Vitamin, mineral, and dietary treatments. In M. G. Aman & N. N. Singh (Eds.), *Psychopharmacology of the developmental disabilities* (pp. 168–196). New York: Springer-Verlag.

Aman, M. G., & Singh, N. N. (1991). Pharmacological intervention. In J. L. Matson & J. A. Mulick (Eds.), *Handbook of mental retardation* (2nd ed., pp. 347–372). New York: Pergamon Press.

Aman, M. G., Singh, N. N., Stewart, A. J., & Field, C. J. (1985). The Aberrant Behavior Checklist: A behavior rating scale for the assessment of treatment effects. *American Journal of Mental Deficiency, 89*, 485–491.

Aman, M. G., Van Bourgondien, M. E., Wolford, P. C., & Sarphare, G. (1994). *Psychotropic and anticonvulsant drugs in subjects with autism: Prevalence and patterns of use.* Manuscript submitted for publication, Massey University, New Zealand.

American Psychiatric Association. (1994). *Diagnostic and statistical manual of mental disorders (fourth edition): DSM-IV.* Washington, DC: Author.

American Speech-Language-Hearing Association (1995). Position statement: Facilitated communication. *Asha, 37*, 22.

Anderson, L. T., Campbell, M., Grega, D. M., Perry, R., Small, A. M., & Green, W. H. (1984). Haloperidol in the treatment of infantile autism: Effects on learning and behavioral symptoms. *American Journal of Psychiatry, 141*, 1195–1202.

Applegarth, D. A., Dimmick, J. E., & Toone, J. R. (1989). Laboratory detection of metabolic disease. *Pediatric Clinics of North America, 36*, 49–65.

Arnold, L. E., & Aman, M. G. (1991). Beta blockers in mental retardation and developmental disorders. *Journal of Child and Adolescent Psychopharmacology, 1*, 361–373.

Baraff, L. J., Lee, S. I., & Schriger, D. L. (1993). Outcomes of bacterial meningitis in children: A meta-analysis. *Pediatric Infectious Disease Journal, 12*, 389–394.

Barkovich, A. J., Gressens, P., & Evrard, P. (1992). Formation, maturation, and disorders of brain neocortex. *American Journal of Neuroradiology, 13*, 423–446.

Barnes, P. D. (1992). Imaging of the central nervous system in pediatrics and adolescence. *Pediatric Clinics of North America, 39*, 743–776.

Baroff, G. S. (1991). *Developmental disabilities: Psychosocial aspects.* Austin, TX: Pro-ed.

Barron, J., & Sandman, C. A. (1985). Paradoxical excitement to sedative-hypnotics in mentally retarded clients. *American Journal of Mental Retardation, 90*, 124–129.

Batshaw, M. L. (1993). Mental retardation. *Pediatric Clinics of North America, 40*, 507–521.

Behar, L. B. (1977). The Preschool Behavior Questionnaire. *Journal of Abnormal Child Psychology, 5*, 265–275.

Bellinger, D., Leviton, A., Waternaux, C., Needleman, H., & Rabinowitz, M. (1987). Longitudinal analysis of prenatal and postnatal lead exposure in early cognitive development. *New England Journal of Medicine, 316*, 1037–1043.

Bettelheim, B. (1967). *The empty fortress: Infantile autism and the birth of the self.* New York: The Free Press.

Biklen, D. (1990). Communication unbound: Autism and praxis. *Harvard Educational Review, 60*, 291–314.

Biklen, D., Morton, M. W., Saha, S. N., Duncan, J., Gold, D., Hardardottir, M., Kerna, E., O'Connor, S., & Rao, S. (1991). "I amn not a utistivc on thje typ" ("I'm not autistic on the typewriter"). *Disability, Handicap, and Society, 6*, 161–180.

Birmaher B., Quintana, H., & Greenhill, L. (1987). Methylphenidate treatment of hyperactive autistic children. *Journal of the American Academy of Child and Adolescent Psychiatry, 27*, 248–251.

Blackman, J. A., McGuiness, G. A., Bale, J. F., & Smith, W. L. (1991). Large postnatally acquired porencephalic cysts: Unexpected outcomes. Journal of Child Neurology, 6, 58–64.

Blatt, S. (1987). The conquest of mental retardation. Austin, TX: Pro-ed.

Bruininks, R. H., Woodcock, R. W., Weatherman, R. F., & Hill, B. K. (1984). *Scales of Independent Behavior.* Allen, TX: DLM/Teaching Resources.

Burd, L., & Martsolf, J. T. (1989). Fetal alcohol syndrome: Diagnosis and syndromal variability. *Physiology and Behavior, 46,* 39–43.

Burk, H. W., & Menolascino, F. J. (1968). Haloperidol in emotionally disturbed mentally retarded individuals. *American Journal of Psychiatry, 124,* 1589–1591.

Byrne, P., Welch, R., Johnson, M. A., Darrah, J., & Piper, M. (1990). Serial MRI in neonatal hypoxic-ischemic encephalopathy. *Journal of Pediatrics, 117,* 694–700.

Campbell, M., Anderson, L. T., Cohen, I. L., Perry, R., Small, A. M., Green, W. H., Anderson, L., & McCandless, W. H. (1982). Haloperidol in autistic children: Effects on learning, behavior, and abnormal involuntary movements. *Psychopharmacology Bulletin, 18,* 110–112.

Campbell, M., Anderson, L. T., Small, A. M., Adams, P., Gonzalez, N. N., & Ernst, M. (1993). Naltrexone in autistic children: Behavioral symptoms and attentional learning. *Journal of the American Academy of Child and Adolescent Psychiatry, 32,* 1283–1291.

Campbell, M., Fish, B., Korein, J., Shapiro, T., Collins, P., & Koh, C. (1972). Lithium and chlorpromazine: A controlled crossover study of hyperactive severely disturbed young children. *Journal of Autism and Childhood Schizophrenia, 2,* 234–263.

Campbell, M., Gonzalez, N. M., Ernst, M., Silva, R. R., & Werry, J. S. (1993). Antipsychotics (neuroleptics). In J. S. Werry & M. G. Aman (Eds.), *Practitioner's guide to psychoactive drugs for children and adolescents* (pp. 269–296). New York: Plenum Medical Books.

Carr, E. G., & Durand, V. M. (1985). Reducing behavior problems through functional communication training. *Journal of Applied Behavior Analysis, 18,* 111–126.

Cipani, E. (1989). *The treatment of severe behavior disorders: Behavior analysis approaches.* Washington, DC: American Association on Mental Retardation.

Cleveland, R. H., Herman, T. E., Dot, R. F., & Kushner, D. C. (1987). Evolution of neonatal herpes encephalitis as demonstrated by cranial US with CT correlation. *American Journal of Perinatalogy, 4,* 215–219.

Cohen, I. L., Campbell, M., Posner, D., Small, A. M., Triebel, D., & Anderson, L. T. (1980). Behavioral effects of haloperidol in young autistic children: An objective analysis using a within-subjects reversal design. *Journal of the American Academy of Child Psychiatry, 19,* 665–677.

Conners, C. K. (1969). A teacher rating scale for use in drug studies with children. *American Journal of Psychiatry, 126,* 152–156.

Coplan, J., Gleason, J. R., Ryan, R., Burke, M. G., & Williams, M. L. (1982). Validation of an early language milestone scale in a high risk population. *Pediatrics, 70,* 677–683.

Dupont, A. (1989). 140 years of Danish studies on the prevalence of mental retardation. *Acta Psychiatrica Scandinavia, 79,* 105–112.

Eberlin, M., McConnachie, G., Ibel, S., & Volpe, L. (1993). Facilitated communication: A failure to replicate the phenomenon. *Journal of Autism and Developmental Disorders, 23,* 507–530.

Ehlers, S., & Gillberg, C. (1993). The epidemiology of Asperger syndrome. A total population study. *Journal of Child Psychology and Psychiatry, 8,* 1327–1350.

Einfeld, S. L., & Aman, M. G. (1995). Issues in the taxonomy of psychopathology in children and adolescents with mental retardation. *Journal of Autism and Developmental Disorders, 25,* 143–167.

Engelhardt, D. M., Polizos, P., Waizer, J., & Hoffman, S. P. (1973). A double-blind comparison of fluphenazine and haloperidol. *Journal of Autism and Childhood Schizophrenia, 3,* 128–137.

Fish, B., Shapiro, T., & Campbell, M. (1966). Long-term prognosis and the response of schizophrenic children to drug therapy: A controlled study of trifluoperazine. *American Journal of Psychiatry, 123,* 32–39.

Foxx, R. M. (1982a). *Increasing behaviors of severely retarded and autistic persons.* Campaign, IL: Research Press.

Gadow, K. D., & Pomeroy, J. C. (1990). A controlled case study of methylphenidate and fenfluramine in a mentally retarded, hyperactive child. *Australia and New Zealand Journal of Developmental Disabilities, 16,* 323–334.

Garber, H. L. (1988). *The Milwaukee Project: Preventing mental retardation in children at risk.* Washington, DC: American Association on Mental Retardation.

Gilhousen, M. R., Allen, L. F., Lasater, L. M., & Farrell, D. M. (1990). Veracity and vicissitude: A critical look at the Milwaukee Project. *Journal of School Psychology, 28,* 285–299.

Gillberg, C. (1990). Autism and pervasive developmental disorders. *Journal of Child Psychology and Psychiatry, 31,* 99–119.

Gillberg, C., & Gillberg, C. (1989). Asperger syndrome— some epidemiological considerations: A research note. *Journal of Child Psychology and Psychiatry, 30,* 631–638.

Gillberg, C., Schaumann, H., & Steffenburg, S. (1991). Is

autism more common now than 10 years ago? *British Journal of Psychiatry, 158*, 403–409.

Glascoe, F. P., Altemeier, W. A., & MacLean, W. E. (1989). The importance of parents' concerns about their child's development. *American Journal of Diseases of Children, 143*, 955–958.

Grossman, H. J. (1983). *Classification in mental retardation.* Washington, DC: American Association on Mental Deficiency.

Hagberg, B. (1985). Rett syndrome: Swedish approach to analysis of prevalence and cause. *Brain and Development, 7*, 277–280.

Hagberg, B., Hagberg, G., Lewerth, A., & Lindberg, U. (1981). Mild mental retardation in Swedish school children. *Acta Paediatrica Scandinavia, 70*, 441–444.

Hagerman, R. J., Murphy, M. A., & Wittenberger, M. D. (1988). A controlled trial of stimulant medication in children with the fragile X syndrome. *American Journal of Medical Genetics, 30*, 377–392.

Handen, B. L., Breaux, A. M., Gosling, A., Ploof, D. L., & Feldman, H. (1990). Efficacy of methylphenidate among mentally retarded children with attention deficit hyperactivity disorder. *Pediatrics, 86*, 922–930.

Handen, B. L., Breaux, A. N., Janosky, J., McAuliffe, S., Feldman, H., & Gosling, A. (1992). Effects and non-effects of methylphenidate in children with mental retardation and ADHD. *Journal of the American Academy of Child and Adolescent Psychiatry, 31*, 455–461.

Heber, R. (1959). A manual on terminology and classification in mental retardation. *American Journal of Mental Deficiency, 64* (Monograph Supplement).

Heber, R. (1961). A manual on terminology and classification in mental retardation (second edition). *American Journal of Mental Deficiency, 66* (Monograph Supplement).

Hermelin, B., & O'Connor, N. (1990). Factors and primes: A specific numerical ability. *Psychological Medicine, 20*, 63–169.

Herrnstein, R. J., & Murray, C. (1994). *The bell curve: Intelligence and class structure in American life.* New York: The Free Press.

Holt, P. J. (1989). Posthemorrhagic hydrocephalus. *Journal of Child Neurology, 4*, S23–S31.

Hood, J. (1993, February 19). What's wrong with Head Start. *The Wall Street Journal.*

Hope, P. L., Gould, J. J., Howard, S., Hamilton, P. A., Costello, A. M., & Reynolds, E. O. (1988). Precision of ultrasound diagnosis of pathologically verified lesion in the brains of very preterm infants. *Developmental Medicine and Child Neurology, 30*, 457–471.

Innes, G., Kidd, C., & Ross, H. S. (1968). Mental subnormality in North-East Scotland. *British Journal of Psychiatry, 114*, 35–41.

Isaac, S., & Michael, W. B. (1987). *Handbook in research and evaluation* (10th ed.). San Diego, CA: EDITS.

Jacobson, J. W., & Mulick, J. A. (1992). A new definition on MR or a new definition of practice? *Psychology in Mental Retardation and Developmental Disabilities, 18*, 9–14.

Johnson, M. A., Pennock, J. M., Bydder, G. M., Dubowitz, L. M. J., Thomas, D. J., & Young, I. R. (1987). Serial MR imaging in neonatal cerebral injury. *American Journal of Neuroradiology, 8*, 83–92.

Kanner, L. (1943). Autistic disturbances of affective contact. *The Nervous Child, 2*, 417–450.

Kanner, L. (1944). Early infantile autism. *Journal of Pediatrics, 25*, 211–217.

Kendall, B. E. (1992). Disorders of lysosomes, peroxisomes, and mitochondria. *American Journal of Neuroradiology, 13*, 621–653.

Kerr, A., & Stephenson, J. B. P. (1986). A study of the natural history of Rett syndrome in 23 girls. *American Journal of Medical Genetics, 24*, 77–83.

Kiely, M. (1987). The prevalence of mental retardation. *Epidemiological Review, 9*, 194–218.

Konarski, E. A., Favell, J. E., & Favell, J. E. (1993). *Manual for the assessment and treatment of the behavior disorders of people with mental retardation.* Morganton, NC: Western Carolina Center Foundation.

Kozlowski, B. W. (1992). Megavitamin treatment of mental retardation in children: A review of effects on behavior and cognition. *Journal of Child and Adolescent Psychopharmacology, 2*, 307–320.

Kushlick, A., & Cox, G. (1973). The epidemiology of mental handicap. *Developmental Medicine and Child Neurology, 15*, 748–759.

LaVigna, G. W., & Donnellan, A. M. (1986). *Alternatives to punishment: Solving behavior problems with non-aversive strategies.* New York: Irvington Publishers, Inc.

Levene, M. I. (1990). Cerebral ultrasound and neurological impairment: Telling the future. *Archives of Diseases in Childhood, 65*, 469–471.

Levy, S. E., & Hyman, S. L. (1993). Pediatric assessment of the child with developmental delay. *Pediatric Clinics of North America, 40*, 465–477.

Locurto, C. (1991). Beyond IQ in preschool programs? *Intelligence, 15*, 295–312.

Lotter, V. (1967). Epidemiology of autistic conditions in young children: II. Some characteristics of the parents and children. *Social Psychiatry, 1*, 124–137.

Lovaas, O. I. (1977). *The autistic child: Language devel-*

opment through behavior modification. New York: John Wiley & Sons, Inc.

Lovaas, O. I. (1987). Behavioral treatment and normal educational and intellectual functioning in young autistic children. *Journal of Consulting and Clinical Psychology, 55,* 3–9.

Lovaas, O. I., Smith, T., & McEachin, J. J. (1989). Clarifying comments on the young autism study: Reply to Schopler, Short, & Mesibov, *Journal of Consulting and Clinical Psychology, 57,* 165–166.

Lozoff, B., Jimenez, E., & Wolf, A. W. (1991). Long-term developmental outcome of infants with iron deficiency. *New England Journal of Medicine, 325,* 687–694.

Luckasson, R., Coulter, D. L., Polloway, E. A., Reiss, S., Schalock, R. L., Snell, M. E., Spitalnik, D. M., & Stark, J. A. (1992). *Mental retardation: Definition, classification, and systems of supports* (9th ed.). Washington, DC: American Association on Mental Retardation.

MacMillan, D. L., Gresham, F. M., & Siperstein, G. N. (1993). Conceptual and psychometric concerns about the 1992 AAMR definition of mental retardation. *American Journal on Mental Retardation, 98,* 325–335.

Maino, J. H. (1979). Ocular defects associated with cerebral palsy. *Review of Optometry, 116,* 69–72.

Mantovani, J. F. (1994). Brain imaging in children with neurodevelopmental disorders. *Infants and Young Children, 7,* 60–68.

Mantovani, J. F., & Powers, J. A. (1991). Brain injury in premature infants: Patterns on cranial ultrasound, their relationship to outcome and the role of developmental intervention in the NICU. *Infants and Young Children, 4,* 20–32.

Matamoros, A., Anderson, J. C., McConnell, J., & Bolam, D. L. (1989). Neurosonographic findings in infants treated by ECMO. *Journal of Child Neurology, 4,* 552–561.

Matson, J. L. (1990). *Handbook on behavior modification with the mentally retarded.* New York: Plenum Press.

Matson, J. L. (1994). *Autism in children and adults: Etiology, assessment, and intervention.* Pacific Grove, CA: Brooks/Cole.

Matson, J. L., & Mulick, J. A. (1991). *Handbook of mental retardation.* New York: Pergamon Press.

McEachin, J. J., Smith, T., & Lovaas, O. I. (1993). Long-term outcome for children with autism who received early intensive behavioral treatment. *American Journal on Mental Retardation, 97,* 359–372.

McHale, S. M., & Gamble, W. C. (1986). Mainstreaming handicapped children in public school settings: Challenges and limitations. In E. Schopler & G. B. Mesibov (Eds.), *Social behavior in autism* (pp. 191–212). New York: Plenum Press.

McLaren, J., & Bryson, S. E. (1987). Review of recent epidemiological studies of mental retardation: Prevalence, associated disorders, and etiology. *American Journal on Mental Retardation, 92,* 243–254.

Menacker, S. J. (1993). Visual function in children with developmental disabilities. *Pediatric Clinics of North America, 40,* 659–674.

Menke, J. A., McClead, R. E., & Hansen, N. B. (1991). Perspectives on perinatal complications associated with mental retardation. In J. L. Matson & J. A. Mulick (Eds.), *Handbook of mental retardation* (2nd ed). New York: Pergamon Press.

Mesibov, G. B., Schopler, E., & Sloan, J. L. (1983). Service development for adolescents and adults in North Carolina's TEACCH program. In E. Schopler & G. B. Mesibov (Eds.), *Autism in adolescents and adults.* New York: Plenum Press.

Michaud, L. J., Duhaime, A. C., & Batshaw, M. L. (1993). Traumatic brain injury in children. *Pediatric Clinics of North America, 40,* 553–565.

Minihan, P. M., & Dean, D. H. (1990). Meeting the needs for health services of persons with mental retardation living in the community. *American Journal of Public Health, 80,* 1043–1048.

Moore, S., Donovan, B., & Hudson, A. (1993). Facilitator-suggested conversational evaluation of facilitated communication. *Journal of Autism and Developmental Disorders, 23,* 541–551.

Morgan, S. B. (1986). Early childhood autism: Changing perspectives. *Journal of Child and Adolescent Psychology, 3,* 3–9.

Needleman, H. L., Schell, M. A., Bellinger, D., Leviton, A., & Allred, E. N. (1988). The long-term effects of exposure to low doses of lead in childhood. *New England Journal of Medicine, 322,* 83–88.

Needleman, H. L., & Gatsonis, C. A. (1990). Low-level lead exposure and the IQ of children: A meta-analysis of modern studies. *Journal of the American Medical Association, 263,* 673–678.

Nezu, C. M., Nezu, A. M., & Gill-Weiss, M. J. (1992). *Psychopathology in persons with mental retardation.* Champaign, IL: Research Press.

Nickel, R. E. (1992). Disorders of brain development. *Infants and Young Children, 5,* 1–11.

Nihira, K., Leland, H., & Lambert, N. N. (1992). *Adaptive Behavior Scales: Residential and Community* (2nd edition). Austin, TX: Pro-ed.

Nozza, R. J., & Fria, T. J. (1990). The assessment of hearing and middle-ear function in children. In C. D. Bluestone, S. E. Stool, & M. D. Scheetz, (Eds.), *Pediatric otolaryngology* (2nd ed.). Philadelphia: W.B. Saunders Company.

Olley, G. (1986). The TEACCH curriculum for teaching social behavior to children with autism. In E. Schopler & G. B. Mesibov (Eds.), *Social behavior in autism*. New York: Plenum Press.

Opitz, J. M. (1991). Special issue: X-linked mental retardation. *American Journal of Medical Genetics, 38*, 173–180.

Peters, D. L. (1980). Social science and social policy and the care of young children: Head Start and after. *Journal of Applied Developmental Psychology, 1*, 7–27.

Professional organizations offer resolutions on FC (1994, Summer/Fall). *The IARET Newsletter, 6*, 8.

Punnett, H. H., & Zakai, E. H. (1990). Old syndromes, new cytogenetics. *Developmental Medicine and Child Neurology, 32*, 824–831.

Reichler, R. J., & Schopler, E. (1976). Developmental therapy: A program model for providing individual services in the community. In E. Schopler & R. J. Reichler (Eds.), *Psychopathology and child development*. New York: Plenum Press.

Reiss, S. (1994a). Issues in defining mental retardation. *American Journal on Mental Retardation, 99*, 1–7.

Reiss S. (1994b). *Handbook of challenging behavior: Mental health aspects of mental retardation*. Worthington, OH: IDS Publication Corporation.

Reiss, S., & Valenti-Hein, D. (1990). *Reiss Scales for Children's Dual Diagnosis: Test manual*. Worthington, OH: IDS Publishing Corporation.

Reschly, D. J. (1990). Adaptive behavior. In A. R. Thomas & J. Grimes (Eds.), *Best practices in school psychology* (2nd ed., pp. 29–42). Washington, DC: National Association of School Psychologists.

Reynolds, W. M., & Baker, J. A. (1989). Assessment of depression in persons with mental retardation. *American Journal on Mental Retardation, 93*, 93–103.

Rimland, B., Callaway, E., & Dreyfus, P. (1978). The effects of high doses of vitamin B_6 on autistic children: A double-blind crossover study. *American Journal of Psychiatry, 135*, 472–475.

Ritvo, E. R., & Freeman, B. J. (1984). A medical model of autism: Etiology, pathology, and treatment. *Psychiatric Annals, 13*, 298–305.

Rojahn, J., Polster, L. M., Mulick, J. A., & Wisniewski, J. J. (1989). Reliability of the Behavior Problems Inventory. *Journal of the Multihandicapped Person, 2*, 283–293.

Rojahn, J., & Schroeder, S. R. (1991). Behavioral assessment. In J. L. Matson (Ed.), *Handbook of mental retardation* (2nd ed., pp. 240–259). New York: Plenum.

Roizen, N. (1989). Down syndrome preventive medicine check list. *Down Syndrome Papers and Abstracts for Professionals, 12*, 1–8.

Rorke, L. B., & Zimmerman, R. A. (1992). Prematurity, postmaturity and destructive lesions. *American Journal of Neuroradiology, 13*, 517–536.

Roth, S. C., Baudin, J., & McCormick D. C. (1993). Relation between ultrasound appearance of the brain of very preterm infants and neurodevelopmental impairment at eight years. *Developmental Medicine and Child Neurology, 35*, 755–768.

Rowitz, L. (1991). Social and environmental factors and developmental handicaps in children. In J. L. Matson & J. A. Mulick (Eds.), *Handbook of mental retardation* (2nd ed). New York: Pergamon Press.

Rutter, M. (1985). The treatment of autistic children. *Journal of Child Psychology and Psychiatry, 26*, 193–214.

Rutter, M., & Schopler, E. (1987). Autism and pervasive developmental disorders: Concepts and diagnostic issues. *Journal of Autism and Developmental Disorders, 17*, 159–186.

Sandman, C. A. (1991). The opiate hypothesis in autism and self-injury. *Journal of Child and Adolescent Psychopharmacology, 1*, 237–248.

Sattler, J. M. (1992). *Assessment of children. Revised and updated third edition*. San Diego: Author.

Schaefer, G. B., & Bodensteiner, J. B. (1992). Evaluation of the child with idiopathic mental retardation. *Pediatric Clinics of North America, 39*, 929–943.

Schalock, R. L., Stark, J. A., Snell, M. E., Coulter, D. L., Polloway, E. A., Luckasson, R., Reiss, S., & Spitalnik, D. M. (1994). The changing conception of mental retardation: Implications for the field. *Mental Retardation, 32*, 181–193.

Schifter, T., Hoffman, J. M., Hatten, H. P., Hanson, M. W., Coleman, R. E., & DeLong, G. R. (1994). Neuroimaging in infantile autism. *Journal of Child Neurology, 9*, 155–161.

Schmickel, R. D. (1986). Contiguous gene syndrome: A component of recognizable syndromes. *Journal of Pediatrics, 109*, 231–241.

Schopler, E., & Mesibov, G. B. (1988). *Diagnosis and assessment in autism*. New York: Plenum Press.

Schopler, E., Short, A., & Mesibov, G. B. (1989). Relation of behavioral treatment to "normal functioning": Comments on Lovaas. *Journal of Consulting and Clinical Psychology, 57*, 162–164.

Schroeder, S. R., Rojahn, J., & Mulick, J. A. (1978). Ecobehavioral organization of developmental day care for the chronically self-injurious. *Journal of Pediatric Psychology, 3*, 81–88.

Scott, K. G., & Carran, D. T. (1987). The epidemiology and prevention of mental retardation. *American Psychologist, 42*, 801–804.

Seitz, V., Rosenbaum, L., & Apfel, N. (1985). Effects of

family support intervention: A ten year follow-up. *Child Development, 56*, 376–391.

Sparrow, S. S., Balla, D. A., & Cicchetti, D. V. (1984). *Vineland Adaptive Behavior Scales.* Circle Pines, MN: American Guidance Service.

Staples, A. J., Sutherland, G. R., Haan, E. A., & Clisby, S. (1991). Epidemiology of Down syndrome in South Australia, 1960–1989. *American Journal of Human Genetics, 49*, 1014–1024.

Strayhorn, J. M., Rapp, N., Donina, W., & Strain, P. S. (1988). Randomized trial of methylphenidate for an autistic child. *Journal of the American Academy of Child and Adolescent Psychiatry, 27*, 244–247.

Strohmer, D. C., & Prout, H. T. (1989). *Strohmer-Prout Behavior Rating Scale manual.* Schenectady, NY: Genium.

Szatmari, P. (1991). Asperger's syndrome: Diagnosis, treatment, and outcome. *Psychiatric Clinics of North America, 14*, 81–93.

Szempruch, J., & Jacobson, J. W. (1993). Evaluating the facilitated communications of people with developmental disabilities. *Research in Developmental Disabilities, 14*, 253–264.

Thapar, A., Gottesman, I. I., Owen, M. J., O'Donovan, M. C., & McGuffin, P. (1994). The genetics of mental retardation. *British Journal of Psychiatry, 164*, 747–758.

Thompson, T., & Gray, D. B. (1994). *Destructive behavior in developmental disabilities: Diagnosis and treatment.* Thousand Oaks, CA: SAGE Publications, Inc.

Thorndike, R. L., Hagen, E. P., & Sattler, J. M. (1986). *Technical manual, Stanford-Binet Intelligence Scale: Fourth Edition.* Chicago: Riverside.

Ucer, E., & Kreger, K. C. (1969). A double-blind study comparing haloperidol with thioridazine in emotionally disturbed, mentally retarded children. *Current Therapeutic Research, 11*, 278–283.

U.S. Department of Health and Human Services (1991). *Preventing Lead Poisoning in Young Children.* Public Health Service Centers for Disease Control Statement.

Van Acker, R. V. (1991). Rett syndrome: A review of current knowledge. *Journal of Autism and Developmental Disabilities, 21*, 381–406.

Van de Bor, M., Ouden, L. D., & Guit, G. L. (1992). Value of cranial ultrasound and MRI in predicting neurodevelopmental outcome in preterm infants. *Pediatrics, 90*, 196–199.

Varley, C. K., & Trupin, E. W. (1982). Double-blind administration of methylphenidate to mentally retarded children with attention deficit disorder: A preliminary study. *American Journal of Mental Deficiency, 86*, 560–566.

Washington, V. (1985). Head Start: How appropriate for minority families in the 1980s? *American Journal of Orthopsychiatry, 55*, 577–589.

Waterhouse, L. (1988). Extraordinary visual memory and pattern perception in an autistic boy. In L. K. Obler & D. Fein (Eds.), *The exceptional brain.* New York: Guilford Press.

Webb, T. (1991). Molecular genetics of Fragile X: A cytogenetics viewpoint. Report of the Fifth International Symposium on X-linked Mental Retardation. *Journal of Medical Genetics, 28*, 814–817.

Wechsler, D. (1991). *Wechsler Preschool and Primary Scale of Intelligence* (Revised). San Antonio, TX: The Psychological Corporation.

Wechsler, D. (1992). *Wechsler Intelligence Scale for Children* (3rd edition). San Antonio, TX: The Psychological Corporation.

Westinghouse Learning Corporation. (1969). *The impact of Head Start: An evaluation of the effects of Head Start on children's cognitive and affective development.* Springfield, VA: U.S. Department of Commerce.

Wheeler, D. L., Jacobson, J. W., Paglieri, R. A., & Schwartz, A. A. (1993). An experimental assessment of facilitated communication. *Mental Retardation, 31*, 49–60.

Woodruff, M. E., Cleary, T. E., & Bader, D. (1980). The prevalence of refractive and ocular anomalies among 1242 institutionalized mentally retarded persons. *American Journal of Optometry and Physiologic Optics, 57*, 70–84.

Woodruff, M. E. (1977). Prevalence of visual and ocular anomalies in 168 non-institutionalized mentally retarded children. *Canadian Journal of Public Health, 68*, 225–232.

World Health Organization (1992). *The ICD-10 classification of mental and behavioural diseases: Clinical descriptions and diagnostic guidelines.* Geneva: World Health Organization.

Young, R. L., & Nettelbeck, T. (1994). The "intelligence" of calendrical calculators. *American Journal on Mental Retardation, 99*, 186–200.

CHAPTER 11

ATTENTION-DEFICIT/ HYPERACTIVITY DISORDER

Gary Vallano
Gregory T. Slomka

DESCRIPTION OF DISORDER

Introduction

The designation attention-deficit/hyperactivity disorder (ADHD) is itself a partial description of the hallmark features of this disorder. Inattention, hyperactivity, and impulsivity are considered the core features of ADHD as outlined in the *Diagnostic and Statistical Manual of Mental Disorders, Fourth Edition* (DSM-IV; American Psychiatric Association, 1994). Following the listing of diagnostic criteria for ADHD, the DSM-IV describes three subtypes of the disorder: the *predominantly inattentive type*, the *predominantly hyperactive-impulsive type*, and the *combined type* (see Table 11.1). The DSM-IV has provided clinicians and researchers with a framework with which to more consistently diagnose ADHD and to communicate this information to other mental health care providers, patients, families, other professionals, and third-party payment providers.

However, a brief historical perspective of this disorder illustrates the diagnostic complexity that extends beyond the descriptive bounds of the current system. Barkley (1990) provides an historical overview of ADHD that outlines this issue. Briefly, the early association of the core features of inattention, impulsivity, and hyperactivity with identifiable physical disorders such as cen-

tral nervous system trauma, infection, or toxicity in some children led to them being labeled as "brain damaged" children. However, the lack of a clearly identifiable organic cause in the majority of children with similar behavioral features led to the concepts of "minimal brain damage" and "minimal brain dysfunction." Finally, the increased focus on the behavioral descriptors of hyperactivity (Laufer & Denhoff, 1957; Stewart, Pitts, Craig, & Dieruf, 1966) and further exploration in the areas of attention and impulse control (Douglas, 1972) have led to the development of our current classification of the disorder. Therefore, children with a variety of organic disorders that result in behavioral difficulties similar to the core features of ADHD, children with other psychiatric or learning difficulties that are associated with inattention, impulsivity, or hyperactivity, or children with primary difficulties in the areas of motor activity, impulsivity, or attention may descriptively be difficult to distinguish on initial presentation. In other words, children who suffered a serious closed head injury, have been exposed to toxic levels of lead, have a learning disorder, an anxiety disorder, or a variety of other difficulties may present with the primary

Table 11.1. DSM-IV Diagnostic Criteria for Attention-Deficit/Hyperactivity Disorder

A. Either (1) or (2):

  (1) six (or more) of the following symptoms of **inattention** have persisted for at least 6 months to a degree that is maladaptive and inconsistent with developmental level:

  Inattention

   (a) often fails to give close attention to details or makes careless mistakes in schoolwork, work, or other activities
   (b) often has difficulty sustaining attention in tasks or play activities
   (c) often does not seem to listen when spoken to directly
   (d) often does not follow through on instructions and fails to finish schoolwork, chores, or duties in the workplace (not due to oppositional behavior or failure to understand instructions)
   (e) often has difficulty organizing tasks and activities
   (f) often avoids, dislikes, or is reluctant to engage in tasks that require sustained mental effort (such as schoolwork or homework)
   (g) often loses things necessary for tasks or activities (e.g., toys, school assignments, pencils, books, or tools)
   (h) is often easily distracted by extraneous stimuli
   (i) is often forgetful in daily activities

  (2) six (or more) of the following symptoms of **hyperactivity-impulsivity** have persisted for at least 6 months to a degree that is maladaptive and inconsistent with developmental level:

  Hyperactivity

   (a) often fidgets with hands or feet or squirms in seat
   (b) often leaves seat in classroom or in other situations in which remaining seated is expected
   (c) often runs about or climbs excessively in situations in which it is inappropriate (in adolescents or adults, may be limited to subjective feelings of restlessness)
   (d) often has difficulty playing or engaging in leisure activities quietly
   (e) is often "on the go" or often acts as if "driven by a motor"
   (f) often talks excessively

  Impulsivity

   (g) often blurts out answers before questions have been completed
   (h) often has difficulty awaiting turn
   (i) often interrupts or intrudes on others (e.g., butts into conversations or games)

B. Some hyperactive-impulsive or inattentive symptoms that caused impairment were present before age 7 years.

C. Some impairment from the symptoms is present in two or more settings (e.g., at school [or work] and at home).

D. There must be clear evidence of clinically significant impairment in social, academic, or occupational functioning.

E. The symptoms do not occur exclusively during the course of a Pervasive Developmental Disorder, Schizophrenia, or other Psychotic Disorder and are not better accounted for by another mental disorder (e.g., Mood Disorder, Anxiety Disorder, Dissociative Disorder, or a Personality Disorder).

Code based on type:

  314.01 Attention-Deficit/Hyperactivity Disorder, Combined Type: if both Criteria A1 and A2 are met for the past 6 months

  314.00 Attention-Deficit/Hyperactivity Disorder, Predominately Inattentive Type: if Criterion A1 is met but Criterion A2 is not met for the past 6 months

  314.01 Attention-Deficit/Hyperactivity Disorder, Predominately Hyperactive-Impulsive Type: if Criterion A2 is met but Criterion A1 is not met for the past 6 months

  Coding note: For individuals (especially adolescents and adults) who currently have symptoms that no longer meet full criteria, "In Partial Remission" should be specified.

From the Diagnostic and Statistical Manual of Mental Disorders (4th ed., pp. 83–85) by the American Psychiatric Association, 1994, Washington, D.C.: Author. Copyright 1994 by the American Psychiatric Association. Reprinted by permission.

symptoms of inattention, impulsivity, and hyperactivity. It may not be possible to descriptively sort out this heterogeneous group until a thorough diagnostic assessment is completed.

Given our understanding of the historical evolution of this disorder and the diversity in our conceptualization of the core tenets of inattention, impulsivity, and hyperactivity, further description of the disorder must be considered a general overview at best, and *individualized* diagnostic assessment and treatment will be the more critical factor. One of the most concise and practical descriptions of this disorder found in the DSM-III (American Psychiatric Association, 1980), states that the child displays signs of developmentally inappropriate inattention, impulsivity, and hyperactivity.

> The signs must be reported by adults in the child's environment, such as parents and teachers. Because the symptoms are typically variable, they may not be observed by the clinician. When the reports of teachers and parents conflict, primary consideration should be given to the teacher reports because of greater familiarity with age-appropriate norms. Symptoms typically worsen in situations that require self-application, as in the classroom. Signs of the disorder may be absent when the child is in a new or a one-to-one situation. The number of symptoms specified is for children between the ages of eight and ten, the peak age range for referral. In younger children, more severe forms of the symptoms and a greater number of symptoms are usually present. The opposite is true of older children, (p. 43).

This description along with the DSM-IV criterion that "There must be clear evidence of clinically significant impairment in social, academic, or occupational functioning" (p. 84) provide a significantly informative description of what we now call attention-deficit/hyperactivity disorder.

The initial sentence in the DSM-III description not only outlines the three core features of inattention, impulsivity, and hyperactivity, it focuses on the issue of developmentally inappropriate behavior for mental and chronological age. Children with ADHD need to be assessed in the context of normal development. Each of the core features will vary greatly across different age ranges. Difficulties in our ability to discern between inappropriate and appropriate levels of attention, impulse control, and motor activity in children around the age of 2 to 3 years make diagnosis exceedingly difficult in preschool children, except in extreme cases or in retrospect. Parents are all too familiar with the concept of the "terrible two's," and their ability to distinguish ADHD in their child and bring them to treatment at this age is understandably limited. Similarly, parents typically have a limited frame of reference for age-appropriate behavior given their limited exposure to large numbers of similarly aged children. Therefore, teachers who will see 20 to 30 or more same-aged children each year may find it easier to identify those with significant difficulties. This, in addition to the increasing demands on attention, impulse control, and motor activity present in an academic setting, may account for the peak age-range of referral between the ages of eight and ten, and the greater reliance on teachers' reports for diagnosing this disorder.

Adolescents frequently do not display the overtly disruptive symptoms of hyperactivity and impulsivity that commonly result in many of these children being referred for assessment and treatment. More subtle symptoms of internal restlessness, socially inappropriate behavior, and academic underachievement are more likely to be their presenting symptoms (Evans, Vallano, & Pelham, 1995). Therefore, the concept of "developmentally inappropriate" is a complex and crucial component in the understanding of ADHD in children and adolescents.

The fact that symptoms are environmentally variable frequently misleads parents and professionals alike. Many parents have felt that their child could not have ADHD because they can watch cartoons or play video games for hours without difficulty. Unfortunately, some professionals have been misled by this same variability of symptom presentation. Children with ADHD will not necessarily be symptomatic in a physician's office during a brief visit (Sleator & Ullmann, 1981). Therefore, the need to explore the child's behavior is in typical tasks that require self-application, such as those in the classroom, is equally or more important than their behavior in the office setting.

Finally, the need to explore the severity of the symptoms and the nature of the functional impairment is critical. It is not difficult to argue that the media and lay press have a definite (and possibly negative) impact on our patients and their families as a result of the stories they choose to report. For example, in an article titled "The drugging of America's children" (Black, 1994), the title alone should emphasize the need for the professional to effectively communicate why treatment is indicated for the individual patient. If we are unable to clearly identify the significant difficulties that are occurring in daily functioning for the patient, we leave the door open for serious questions as to the appropriateness and necessity of our treatment interventions. Therefore, only those patients whose symptoms of inattention, impulsivity, and hyperactivity are significant enough to cause problematic impairment in daily life functioning warrant the diagnosis and subsequent interventions for the treatment of ADHD.

Neurobiological Factors

Attention-deficit/hyperactivity disorder, like learning disabilities, may arise from a variety of biologically determined etiologies. Hereditary factors may account for up to 50 percent of the variance expressed in hyperactivity (Goodman & Stevenson, 1989). Exposure to a variety of early insults to central nervous system (CNS) integrity correlate with the expression of an eventual ADHD phenotype. Abnormalities in a variety of neuro-transmitter systems (dopaminergic and noradrenergic) are likely implicated (Zametkin & Rappaport, 1987). Additionally, metabolic imaging studies implicate basal forebrain abnormalities in a number of cases (Lou et al., 1989; Zametkin et al., 1990). While increasing interest focuses upon theorized disruptions in pre-frontal and subcortical neural systems (Barkley, 1990), the attribution of acquired or developmental perturbations at this level of the cerebral substrate remains conjectural, but nonetheless a relevant area for future investigation. It is essential to recognize that psychosocial factors also influence the expression of ADHD symptoms. As summarized by Pennington (1991), psychosocial factors may produce a phenocopy of the disorder in the absence of any primary neurogenic etiology, and may influence the secondary expression of behavior problems commonly seen in association with ADHD.

Diagnostic Heterogeneity

ADHD within early DSM nosologies was initially described as a condition in which manifestations of excessive motor activity, impulsivity-distractibility, and attentional problems were exhibited. As was previously discussed, the current DSM-IV recognizes the heterogeneity associated with ADHD, and the behavioral criteria utilized for classification permit the identification of subtypes based on the prominence of any associated hyperactive-impulsive characteristics. The concept of ADHD herein will be broadened to recognize not only the heterogeneity of primary ADHD characteristics, but their comorbidity with a variety of other conditions.

In a review of multiple studies of the associated behavioral characteristics inherent in hyperactive-impulsive type ADHD vs. primarily inattentive ADHD populations, Dykman and Ackerman (1991) conclude that ADHD youngsters with prominent hyperactive-impulsive characteristics exhibit more problems related to impulse control and aggressive-defiant characteristics (i.e., *externalizing* behavior disorder traits). In contrast, ADHD-Inattentive Type youngsters express greater overanxious, dysthymic-depressed, and interpersonal withdrawal symptoms (i.e., *internalizing* behavior disorder characteristics). Additionally, Barkley (1991) summarizes data implicating dissociations between ADHD subtypes which suggest that ADHD without hyperactivity may represent a primary deficit in focus (executive dimensions of attention), whereas ADHD with hyperactivity may represent primarily deficits in response inhibition and sustained attention. Thus, ADHD subtypes appear dissociable along dimensions of both behavioral characteristics and cognitive abilities.

Although there is acceptance of the dissociation of ADHD subtypes along the dimensions of primary symptom attributes (i.e., with and without hyperactivity), efforts continue to delineate more specific subsyndromes based upon other behavioral characteristics. Current DSM-IV nosology advocates that other relevant findings associated with ADHD presentations be described and ranked in the diagnostic formulation based on the multi-axial criteria for other specific disorders (i.e., by the listing of any comorbid disorders). The high rate of aggressive-disruptive behavior posed by many youngsters with ADHD has led a number of investigators to question whether a third category of primary ADHD should be considered (Loney , 1987; Shaywitz & Shaywitz, 1988). Further investigation of the validity of a separate ADHD-plus or "aggressive" subtype continues.

It is further necessary to recognize ADHD within the continuum of other developmental disorders of childhood. The onset of primary symptom manifestations occurs early in the course of development. Thus, multifactoral influences upon both general adaption as well as learning and academic adjustment must be anticipated. ADHD complicity is manifest across the distribution of intellectual functioning, thus, its attributes are identifiable in gifted as well as intellectually limited youngsters. It is further recognized that there is a disproportionate expression of ADHD in other children with developmental learning disorders. In addition, there are a number of developmental, medical, and neurological conditions of childhood that can result in symptom manifestations consistent with the diagnosis of ADHD. ADHD must therefore be recognized as a heterogenous group of conditions which vary in their expression as a function of primary subtype, the age and developmental level of the individual being examined, and comorbidity with other conditions. As with other developmental disorders, it is necessary to further consider other psychosocial variables as potentially contributory. Therefore, a flexible, multi-variate method of assessment for purposes of differential diagnosis and treatment planning is necessary.

ADHD and Academic Performance

The association between ADHD and academic underachievement is not an issue open to debate. Marginal academic achievement has been identified in upward of

80 percent of this population (Anderson et al., 1987). Prospective studies have indicated disproportionate rates of school failure and drop-out (Barkley et al., 1990; Gittelman et al., 1985; Weiss & Hechtman, 1986). While the distribution of general intellectual abilities has not been found to be at variance with normative expectations, inconsistencies remain prominent in outcome studies summarizing IQ results in ADHD populations (Wikler et al., 1970). Barkley's (1990) review indicated 7- to 15-point lower scores between IQ's of affected individuals and control groups.

It is not uncommon to confront performances on standardized achievement tests at levels fully one standard deviation below normative expectations (Barkley, 1990). In addition to academic vulnerabilities, morbidity in the form of specific learning disabilities has been identified rather consistently in 10 percent to 27 percent of cases of ADHD (other studies have suggested highly divergent prevalences, with 9 percent to 63 percent identified across varied studies) (Fiore et al., 1993). Anderson et al. (1987) reported comorbidity of learning disabilities at 80 percent for a sample of 11-year-olds with ADHD. Estimates of ADHD in learning disabled populations span 26 percent to 41 percent (Silver, 1981) to 80 percent (Safer & Allen, 1976).

While scholastic achievement and academic adjustment problems remain well recognized, their etiology may reflect primary and/or secondary ADHD effects. Variable attentional capacity, impulsivity and motor restlessness, core behavioral characteristics associated with many ADHD presentations, impose obvious limitations upon academic skill acquisition. Further burden may be expressed secondary to the experience of reciprocal effects of a repeated pattern of academic failure.

In addition to these primary behavioral effects, specific externalizing or disruptive behavior problems associated with any conduct or oppositional disorder diagnoses have additional burdens associated with them, namely disadvantageous psychosocial adjustment and a distinct predisposition toward language-mediated cognitive inefficiencies. Similarly, confounds associated with internalizing behavior disorder complicity, such as over-anxious or depressive symptomatology, could interfere with performance on tasks involving non-verbal conceptual abilities, cognitive flexibility, and new learning potentials. Thus, ramifications of academic dysfunction are frequently multifactorally determined.

Given the high degree of overlap and the complexity of the disorders, it is often difficult to differentiate ADHD from learning disorders per se. Epstein and colleagues (1991) comment on the "blurring of boundaries" within differential criteria associated with ADHD subtypes and learning disabilities. As such, a comprehensive methodology for interdisciplinary assessment should be available in order to provide for more accurate differential diagnosis.

Attention as a Cognitive Construct

It must be recognized that "attention" as a construct relates to a variety of cognitive processes. Attentional development has been characterized by Kinsbourne (1992) as a set of processes inherently linked to the development of diverse higher cognitive functions. Age-appropriate development of attentional faculties permits incremental increases in "processing capacity" that in turn facilitate the ability to selectively decode increasing amounts of information, allocate or deploy processing strategies, and monitor ongoing performances. Development of attention may be dependent upon the ability to coordinate the activities of multiple neural centers, which evolve as a function of cerebral maturation and the effects of experience. Increasing capacity to flexibly display and sustain attention therefore represents an ongoing maturational demand that remains crucial over the course of cognitive development.

A variety of concepts have been borrowed from cognitive psychology and developmental neuropsychology to build models of linkage between attention and higher cognitive functioning. Concepts such as limited processing capacity, selective attention, distinctions between automatic vs. effortful processing, and so on, have been introduced over time. At the same time, advances have been made in further elucidating the neurological substrate of attentional mechanisms.

A number of theoretical models of attentional mechanisms linked to neuroanatomic correlates have been advanced. The work of Posner (1987), which delineated a hierarchically distributed neural network model, and Mirsky (1987) and Mirsky et al. (1991), which linked empirically derived components of attention to cortical and subcortical neural systems, are exemplary. As the Mirsky model offers a link to clinical assessment methodologies, its practical applications are discussed.

The Mirsky model provides an opportunity to assess aspects of attentional functioning from a multi-dimensional perspective. Traditionally, the practitioner has been limited to observational data (i.e., standardized behavioral assessment methodologies such as direct observation, questionnaires, and behavior rating scales), as well as indirect methods of inferring attentional dysfunction from performances on psychometric measures such as the Freedom from Distractibility factor from the Wechsler Scales (specifically, the Arithmetic, Digit Span, and Coding Subtests). It is crucial to bear in mind that the Wechsler Scales were neither created nor validated as measures of attentional functioning. In fact, the discriminate validity of this methodology for purposes of identifying ADHD complicity has been called into question (Cohen, Becker, & Campbell, 1990; Wielkiewicz, 1990). Clearly a theoretically driven model for the assessment of attentional mechanisms from the perspective of cognitive or information processing models would offer a valuable heuristic device for understanding not only the functional implications of attentional dysfunction, but furthering the understanding of subtypes of attentional disorders.

Mirsky advanced a model based on four factors incorporating the ability to (1) focus attention, (2) sustain attention, (3) shift attention in a flexible and adaptive fashion, and (4) encode information within working memory. Subsequent validation for a multi-component model of attentional functioning has been offered by Shum, McFarland, and Bain (1990).

Practitioners have borrowed upon this model and adopted specific neuropsychological tests to provide multivariate descriptions of attentional functioning. The attentional battery utilized in the Developmental Neuropsychology Program at Allegheny Neuropsychiatric Institute is exemplary (see Figure 11.1).

When combined with measures of general intellectual and academic ability (a typical psychoeducational battery) and the assessment of sensory, motor, higher cognitive and memory measures, one can attempt to dis-

FOCUS	Numbers, Letter Span Tests Word Span Sentence Recall
SUSTAIN	Cancellation Tasks ☐ Simple Visual ☐ Complex Visual ☐ Lexical Visual Search Tasks ☐ Structured ☐ Disorganized Continuous Performance Test Matching Familiar Figures Test
SHIFT	Trail B WISC III Coding Symbol Digit Modalities Test Wisconsin Card Sorting Test

ENCODE	Wide Range Assessment of Memory and Learning
	☐ Visual Memory
	   Visual
	☐ Design Memory
	   Visual
	☐ Verbal Memory
	   Verbal
	☐ Story Recall
	   Verbal

Figure 11.1 Factors reflecting attentional and cognitive assessments to measure attentional abilities

sociate the relative contribution of attentional dysfunction from other sources of variance. It remains important to recognize that until broader validation of such attentional batteries is achieved, such avenues of assessment serve only as paradigms for appreciating the potential cognitive ramifications of attentional dysfunction upon adaption.

Neuropsychological Risk Factors

Recognition of the linkage between ADHD and disproportionately high rates of developmental learning problems has led to the examination of other domains of cognitive functioning beyond attentional capacity. As a result, a variety of neuropsychological investigations of attentional disorders have been undertaken. Overviews provided by Barkley (1990), Pennington (1991), and DuPaul and Stoner (1994) highlight the broad array of neurocognitive deficits that can be exhibited in populations manifesting ADHD characteristics. At the level of elementary sensory-perceptual functions, examination is typically confounded by the effects of the limited capacity to focus or sustain attention more so than any deficits in sensory integration, per se. Motor function measures have, however, often yielded a high proportion of vulnerabilities that suggest underlying neuromaturational delays. These include inefficiencies of a standard deviation or more on motor speed and dexterity measures. A number of soft neurological signs (motor) have also been appreciated in children with ADHD.

In terms of higher-level cognitive faculties, indices suggestive of specific non-verbal information processing problems have not been found to be prevalent. In contrast, multiple associations have been identified between ADHD and select language processing inefficiencies (Baker & Cantwell, 1990). Higher rates of not only expressive language deficits, but also select receptive language problems have been identified (Zentall & Gohs, 1984). Evidence of central auditory processing vulnerabilities has also been identified (Riccio et al. 1994; Shapiro & Herod, 1994).

The examination of higher-level cognitive inefficiencies in this population appears to reveal metacognitive inefficiencies more so than modality specific information processing problems. For example, inefficient performances on a task involving visual analysis skills may be secondary to inefficient visual search strategies. In Douglas's (1983) review of memory performance in ADHD, there was no evidence of primary memory problems. Rather, it was suggested that strategy inefficiencies, or problems in integrating or organizing information for purposes of incorporation in working memory were more likely contributory.

The demonstration of inefficient strategy integration in combination with behavioral evidence of weak self-monitoring and frequent inhibitory control problems has led to speculation that more generalized executive function deficits may be expressed in ADHD populations. Indeed, preliminary data from Chelune et al. (1986) implicating significant differences in performance on the Wisconsin Card Sorting Test, a neuropsychological measure of executive functioning, combined with metabolic imaging studies (Lou et al., 1989; Zametkin et al., 1990) suggest anterior brain system disintegrity in ADHD. Follow-up studies using the Wisconsin Card Sorting Test and other presumed measures of frontal lobe integrity did not, however, yield consistent corroborative findings. Thus, while metacognitive deficiencies and strategy deficiencies are frequently identified in children exhibiting learning disabilities, many youngsters with ADHD also may exhibit similar problems (Conte, Kinsbourne, Swanson, Zirk, & Samuels, 1986). While the ontogeny of such deficits remains incompletely understood, and one cannot presume association to a specific cerebral substrate when motivational and/or developmental or psychological process disorders offer equally parsimonious explanations for such deficits, advancing the understanding of the functional ramifications of such deficiencies is viewed as crucial.

Thus, while no definitive pattern of neuropsychological disintegrity emerges, given (1) the heterogeneity of this disorder, (2) the fact attention is mediated at multiple levels within the cerebral substrate, and (3) the fact a variety of conditions have been associated with anomalies in attentional function, this ambiguous state of affairs is not surprising.

EPIDEMIOLOGY

Children with ADHD are the patients most commonly referred to mental health professionals who provide services for the pediatric age group (Ross & Ross, 1982). The prevalence of the disorder is estimated at between 3 percent and 5 percent of school-age children (American Psychiatric Association, 1994). Given the prevalence of this disorder, approximately one child in every average classroom with a size of 20 to 30 students will have ADHD. The referral patterns suggest that a significant portion of the mental health dollars spent for the treatment of children and adolescents will be for ADHD and associated difficulties. With regard to socioeconomic status (SES), there appears to be a small but not significant variability in the prevalence of ADHD across SES (Trites, 1979). Information regarding gender ratio indicates that it is four times more common in boys than girls in the general population, and nine times more common in clinic based samples (American Psychiatric Association, 1994). Available outcome information indicates that a significant number of children diagnosed with ADHD will continue to experience significant difficulties in adolescence and adulthood (Hechtman & Weiss, 1983). In summary, ADHD is a common condition that occurs in a significant number of children and adolescents and frequently continues to be problematic into adulthood. Therefore, thorough assessment and comprehensive treatment of ADHD are paramount in both the medical and the mental health setting.

ASSESSMENT APPROACHES

The assessment of ADHD will include a thorough evaluation from a variety of disciplines. The extent of the assessment will depend on the individual child or adolescent's history. The following is a general review that will apply to most children, but the assessing professional will need to individually tailor the assessment based on the information obtained during the course of the evaluation and treatment of the patient. It is important to remember that assessment remains an ongoing component of the treatment process and does not end following the initial one or two sessions with the child and family.

Medical Issues

Given the advent of managed care in the health care field, many children and adolescents will be referred by their primary care physician to the mental health provider or will be seen in medical settings. Therefore, a recent medical history and physical exam will have been completed prior to the initial visit for many patients. The results of this examination should be reviewed as part of a comprehensive assessment. If a recent medical history and physical exam have not been completed, the child or adolescent should be referred to his or her pediatrician or family physician as part of the initial assessment. As noted previously, a variety of medical conditions may present with behavioral features similar to those found in

ADHD. Those medical conditions that more commonly may present with symptoms of inattention, impulsivity, or hyperactivity will be discussed, but it is important to remember that the range of potential medical conditions associated with ADHD symptoms is broad, and that the differential diagnostic possibilities discussed in this chapter are by no means exclusive or exhaustive.

Hearing or vision difficulties may result in symptoms resembling those found in children with ADHD. Children who are having difficulty hearing their parents or teachers or seeing the material presented to them may appear off task or fidgety as a result of their deficits. Schools routinely screen vision and hearing, but this should be verified and not just assumed to have been completed. Children who live in older homes or have a history of pica are at increased risk for lead exposure, which may impact on their behavior and learning (Needleman et al., 1979). Strong consideration should be given to obtaining a serum lead level at the time of initial assessment. Absence seizures usually begin between the ages of 4 and 10 years. They are 1-second to 10-second lapses in attention that may occur multiple times per day. Children with absence seizures will have an interruption in their mental and physical activity. In addition to the history, an EEG will show characteristic synchronous 3-Hz spike and slow wave complexes. Also, partial complex seizures are associated with inattention, uncommunicative behavior, and automatisms (Kaufman, 1985). Children who present with a history of inattention and symptoms consistent with absence or partial complex seizures should be referred to a pediatric neurologist for further evaluation. Similarly, children with a history of CNS insult such as trauma, infection, or anoxia may require a more thorough neurologic and diagnostic evaluation when it is suspected that the insult may be resulting in symptoms of inattention, impulsivity, or hyperactivity.

Behavioral difficulties, declining academic performance, and a fidgety nervousness are common symptoms of hyperthyroidism. However, a thorough medical history and physical examination should distinguish children with hyperthyroidism from those with uncomplicated ADHD even before obtaining thyroid functions. A history of weight loss, temperature intolerance, tachycardia, goiter, skin changes, and ophthalmologic findings will assist in guiding further evaluation, as thyroid function tests are not part of the routine evaluation for ADHD. Those children in whom hyperthyroidism is suspected or identified should be referred to a pediatric endocrinologist for further evaluation and treatment.

Hyperactivity and other behavioral changes are not uncommon side effects in some medications used to treat the pediatric population. Medications such as phenobarbital and theophylline preparations may contribute to symptoms in this population. Therefore, a review of current medications and their side effects should be an integral part of the initial assessment. When clinically indicated, alternative medications may need to be considered if the behavioral side effects outweigh the clinical benefits of the medication.

In summary, a thorough medical history and physical examination should be part of any psychiatric assessment for ADHD. A variety of medical conditions and medications may result in features similar to those found in this disorder. However, given the frequency of uncomplicated ADHD, the majority of children with symptoms of ADHD will not have an undiagnosed medical condition especially by the time they come to the attention of the mental health provider.

Psychological and Psychiatric Issues

Utilizing current DSM-IV criteria, attention deficit disorders are characterized by the display of developmentally inappropriate combinations of inattention, impulsivity, and overactivity (American Psychiatric Association, 1994). It has been commonplace to assume that the behavioral inefficiencies characterized above represent deficits in rule-governed behaviors. Much of the effort in the differential diagnosis of attention deficit disorders has been directed at conceptualizing maladaptive behavior in terms of "excesses" and "deficits." It has become increasingly clear via subtype analysis that evaluation for "internalizing" behavior disorders is also necessary. A broad-based diagnostic formulation based on an assessment for both externalizing and internalizing disorders is important in planning treatment, not only for psychotherapeutic interventions, but also for pharmacotherapy. Response to medication may covary with the presence of internalizing symptoms. In addition to deficits in rule-governed behavior and risks associated with general emotional adjustment, it is further necessary to appreciate any associated cognitive dysfunction and its impact upon general adaption (Barkley, 1991). As attention deficit disorders are dissociable along dimensions of cognitive as well as behavioral limitations upon general adaption, flexible, multivariate assessment methodologies are required.

Behavioral Assessment

A variety of behavioral assessment methodologies have been available that rely principally upon observer ratings of the presence or absence, frequency or severity of recognizable patterns of ADHD characteristics. Within this context, screening measures have proven valuable as mechanisms for the identification of youngsters appropriate for further clinicodiagnostic evaluation. Other behavioral inventories provide greater breadth of coverage of ADHD-related behaviors, and enhance the psychometric validity of clinical decision making through the use of well-validated multi-dimensional child behavioral inventories, as well as more focused assessment protocols that offer further delineation of subtypes of ADHD. Highlighted in the discussion that follows are brief descriptions of relevant measures.

Conners Rating Scales (Goyette, Conners, & Ulrich, 1978; Conners 1990). The Conners Scales represent the most widely utilized methodology for the assessment of ADHD symptomatology. The instruments exist in abbreviated and standard forms in both parent and teacher versions. They consist of multivariate descriptors of child behavior rated on a Likert scale involving frequency/severity. The factor loadings on these tests permit multivariate descriptions of behavior and adjustment. More frequently, however, clinicians examine outcomes associated with the Hyperactivity Index Score or the Impulsive-Hyperactive Scale. Efficacy in discrimination of ADHD symptoms is well established, as is its sensitivity to objectifying the impact of pharmacological interventions. It must be recognized, however, that it dissociates primarily along dimensions of impulsivity and hyperactivity.

Edelbrock Child Assessment Profile (CAP) (Barkley, 1988). Edelbrock excerpted 12 items from the Teacher Version of the Child Behavior Checklist that loaded on the Inattentive and Overactive scales of this instrument. This brief rating scale completed by teachers or day program staff utilizing a three-point Likert scale has found widespread acceptance as a means of documenting clinical response to medication interventions. Physicians charting multiple baseline measures of treatment response may graph total obtained scores as a means of facilitating case monitoring. Barkley (1988) provides normative criteria that permit further use of the instrument to differentiate by gender along the dimensions of an Inattention as well as an Overactivity Scale. Thus, this brief screening methodology further offers at least coarse differentiation between attentional disorders with and without hyperactivity.

Attention Deficit Disorders Evaluation Scale (McCarney, 1989). These 46- and 60- item parent and teacher rating scales permit differential analysis of attention deficit disorder symptomatology utilizing an extension of the tripartite dimensions included in DSM-IV nosology (inattention, impulsivity, and hyperactivity). Ratings are based on a frequency scale with norm-referenced scoring as scaled scores based on both age and gender. The derived graphic profiles enhance its potential to offer confirmatory validity to DSM-IV subtyping, and parent as well as teacher rating forms make it a tool that is finding growing acceptance as an adjunct to formal DSM-IV differential diagnosis.

In contrast to these "focused" behavioral assessment methodologies designed to highlight ADHD symptom presentations, there are a variety of multisymptom measures that include some form of attention disorder index within a broader spectrum of other measures of child psychopathology.

Personality Inventory for Children (Wirt et al., 1984). This labor-intensive methodology for the third-party description of multisymptom child behavior problems would not characteristically be used as a methodology of choice in screening evaluations. It exists in three forms of varied lengths, with the shortest version involving 266 statements endorsed by a parent or caretaker in a true/false fashion. In addition to a Hyperactivity Scale, eight additional clinical and three developmental scales are included. When a comprehensive delineation of potential comorbidity associated with ADHD is required, this instrument offers broad coverage across major dimensions of child psychopathology (adjustment, overanxious, affective, and conduct disorders, as well as other forms of child psychopathology). Its developmental scales offer additional insights regarding functional ramifications of cognitive and academic dysfunction upon general adaption. Additionally, it offers three validity scales that aid in highlighting any potential "bias" that might influence rater responding, as well as an overall adjustment rating.

Child Behavior Checklist (Achenbach & Edelbrock, 1983; Achenbach, 1991). This instrument, like the Personality Inventory for Children, provides a multivariate description of child psychopathology, but does so more economically. The 112 items comprising the inventory

provide a total score that serves as an overall index of adjustment problems, as well as factor analytically derived subclassifications of child psychopathology. Factors scales vary as a function of age and gender over the course of childhood.

The value of the CBCL lies not mainly with its discriminant validity for identifying ADHD symptomatology, but in its potential to identify associated comorbidity. The derived profiles provide an index of both internalizing and externalizing behavior disorders. Thus, it is uniquely suited to discriminating any disruptive, aggressive, or disinhibited-dysocial behaviors from more overanxious, affective or social coping problems that may be seen in association with ADHD-Inattentive Type. In addition to a behavior problems checklist, the instrument includes a questionnaire format that provides an index of overall psychosocial adjustment. This rating scale also exists in a form adapted for completion by teachers. The factor structure of the derived attention scales aid in further discriminating between combined ADHD and the inattentive type.

Revised Behavior Problems Checklist (Quay & Peterson, 1983). This brief behavioral inventory also provides empirically derived clusters of behavioral pathology in children. Attention scales differentiate between an inattentive/immature cluster and a scale clustering mainly around problems associated with hyperactivity. Overviews of other behavioral assessment methodologies are discussed in DuPaul and Stoner (1994), as well as Barkley (1987).

Structured Interview Schedules

An alternative methodology to aid in differential diagnosis involves the utilization of structured interview schedules. These methodologies offer a standardized format to objectify and standardize clinical decision making. The ADHD Parent Interview (Barkley, 1990) surveys a variety of developmental and psychosocial factors in combination with assessment of targeted behavioral and adjustment issues. Other broad-focused child behavior interview schedules offer coverage of ADHD complicity in addition to other emotional and behavioral disorders, such as The Diagnostic Interview for Children—Parent Form (Costello et al., 1982). Semi-structured psychiatric interviews for children and adolescents have also been used. The practitioner must recognize, however, that many of these interview schedules may pre-date the current DSM-IV nosology pending updates and revisions.

Direct Observation

Additionally, a number of direct observational methods are available to provide context specific descriptors of the impact of adaptational skill inefficiencies in both structured (e.g., classroom) and more "open" settings (e.g., playgrounds and other social settings). These include the Classroom Observation of Conduct in ADD scale (Atkins, Pelham, & Licht, 1985), the ADHD Behavior Coding System (Barkley, 1990), and the CBCL-Direct Observation Form (Achenbach, 1986). Observational techniques also provide an opportunity to assess capacity to initiate and maintain behavior routines that hold adaptive significance (e.g., task preparation necessary for a classroom activity).

Overall levels of motor activity, talkativeness and intrusiveness, or disruptive behavior hold particular significance for social adaption. So, too, capacity to maintain rule-governed behaviors or proscriptions is critical. These latter behaviors are particularly relevant in the assessment of inhibitory controls. Reaction to behavioral consequences, particularly response to reinforcement schedules, are also of particular relevance. It is further essential to assess general social competence. In this regard, frequency as well as quality of relations with significant others is relevant. In addition, capacity to interpret social cues at age appropriate levels should be evaluated. Thus, presenting symptomatology and adaptive skill limitations dictate the focus of naturalistic observation.

Neuropsychological Assessment

The utilization of a neuropsychological test battery offers a unique means to expand upon the descriptive and explanatory power of more traditional psychoeducational measures (intelligence and achievement tests) in delineating specific adaptive competencies. Conners and Well (1986) summarize their application of a neuropsychological test battery with youngsters with ADHD, and report the empirical derivation of six distinct subgroups defined by unique patterns of neurocognitive performance. These findings highlight the functional utility of neuropsychological measures not only as a differential diagnostic tool to aid in identifying any comorbidity associated with ADHD, such as any developmental or acquired neurocognitive dysfunction, but also as a means to define unique attributes that could influence treatment.

It is possible to utilize a neuropsychological test battery as a heuristic for the purposes of further defining the functional correlates of any associated cognitive inefficiencies seen in this population. Examples of the utiliza-

tion of domain specific measures of neuropsychological functioning correlated with adaptational skill competencies follow. The implications of how domain specific descriptions of cognitive abilities might be useful in differential diagnosis and treatment planning are summarized in Table 11.1.

Thus, a limited neuropsychological test battery, when combined with traditional psychoeducational testing (intelligence and achievement testing), offers a unique opportunity to aid the process of differential diagnosis by (1) delineating patterns of attentional dysfunction at variance with normative expectations, (2) documenting comorbidity in the form of any acquired cerebral dysfunction or patterns of developmental learning disorder, and (3) elucidating functional ramifications of ADHD upon general problem solving skill proficiencies and other adaptive skill competencies, especially as they pertain to new learning. The ultimate goal of such assessment is the description of the structure and organization of cognitive abilities for a youngster at a particular point in time (Slomka & Tarter, 1993). Such a multi-modal assessment typically begins with a limited core battery sufficient to permit differential diagnosis. Specific areas of neurocognitive deficit are subsequently assessed in greater detail. This expanded portion of the battery should include repeatable measures of attentional functioning so the database can be utilized as a benchmark to evaluate response to treatment. Assessment is further directed at emotional, motivational, and psychosocial factors that may be contributory. Finally, an attempt is made to define etiology within the matrix of the developmental and psychosocial contexts in which the child presents. These steps reflect the "bio-behavioral systems" approach to neuropsychological assessment described by Taylor and Fletcher (1990).

TREATMENT STRATEGIES

Psychological and Behavioral Treatments

The multi-faceted nature of ADHD presentations requires the availability of a broad armamentarium of intervention strategies. As will be discussed, the effects of stimulant or other adjunctive pharmacological therapies may not provide broad-spectrum impact upon presenting problems. While improved primary attentional faculties as well as reductions in motor activity, aggression, and noncompliance may be experienced as a result of pharmacological treatments, residual cognitive, academic,

Table 11.1. Functional correlates of the neuropsychological examination

Sensory Perceptual Examination

- Examination of rudimentary perceptual processing abilities (auditory, visual, and tactual) can identify modality specific inefficiencies in information processing.
- Contrasting performances under unimodal, as compared to more complex processing demands, especially heteromodal processing tasks, provide a way to gauge complexity of information processing skills.

Psychomotor Performance

- Maturational lag in motor skill proficiencies is a common finding in youngsters with ADHD. To the degree such lag is expressed, the child is at an obvious disadvantage relative to normative expectations.
- Academically, deficits in motor proficiency are likely to be expressed in problems with graphomotor control, limitations in the legibility of writing, or reduced overall speed and efficiency associated with academic tasks requiring coordinated or integrated motor faculties.
- The identification of significant risk factors within any of these domains requires remediation and/or accommodation. More generalized motor awkwardness must be recognized for potential to impact self-esteem. Developing playground and sports-related skill proficiencies may help.
- Primary motor skill inefficiencies must be distinguished from secondary deficits in "executive functioning" (i.e., impairment due to impulsivity, variable task persistence, low frustration tolerance, or poor self-monitoring).

Spatial and Construction Abilities

- Documentation of significant non-verbal processing deficits requires the rule-out of nonverbal learning disability, a condition which can mimic aspects of attentional inefficiency.
- Deficits in this domain in combination with ADHD may manifest themselves in specific problems processing aspects of extrapersonal space. Discrete social skill deficits might be anticipated in such a scenario.
- If integrity is demonstrated on visual and spatial processing tasks, but deficits are identified on constructional tasks (part-to-whole assembly demands, or design copying tests), "executive function" deficits may be contributory (i.e., problems with motor organization and planning).

Language

- Receptive language disorders or central auditory processing problems may mimic characteristics of attentional dysfunction. As sequential information processing deficits can be seen in these conditions as well as ADHD, sensitivity to comorbidity with such conditions is essential in order to assure appropriate treatment planning.
- Limitations in comprehension monitoring skills require accommodations to modify the amount and complexity of auditory input (i.e., presenting directions to the child in a concrete, step-wise fashion).
- Written expression requires the mobilization and integration of multiple cognitive resources. Youngsters with ADHD complicity, especially those with distinct organizational skill deficits, may be particularly vulnerable in this area.

New Learning

- A limited apperceptive span places constraints on the amount of information that can be held in active working memory. "Monitoring" the pace at which new information is presented may prove helpful.
- Metacognitive weaknesses may culminate in weaknesses in organizing information for purposes of encoding in memory. Overt strategies that teach a child how to meaningfully organize information (eg., semantic clustering, mnemonic devices, etc.) are required in this scenario.

Complex Problem Solving

- Contrasts between a child's capacity to execute well-established problem-solving routines versus novel problem solving highlight possible deficits in "executive functions" that may require specific cognitive remediation techniques.
- Outcomes on measures involving cognitive flexibility (i.e., the capacity to carry out multi-step, sequenced cognitive operations) provide insights regarding overall levels of task complexity within which the child is likely to be successful. More specific vulnerabilities associated with on task vigilance, set-maintenance, and self-monitoring capacity can be exposed through the use of such measures.

---

and adaptational skill deficits may persist. Further, there are instances in which adverse clinical response or care-taker opinion contraindicate medication use. As such, it has been advocated that treatment begin with a standardized behavioral intervention (Hoza, Vallano, & Pelham, 1995). A baseline condition is then established and from this benchmark treatment interventions can be evaluated.

By far, the most empirically validated non-medical treatment methodologies applied to ADHD conditions involve behavioral therapies. Contingency management procedures involve primarily the use of positive reinforcement or consequences in order to shape desired adaptive behavior. Applications of behavior therapy techniques have proven effective in reducing hyperactivity and impulsivity, and in facilitating compliance, task maintenance, and general psychosocial adaption. As noted above, when combined with pharmacological strategies a multi-modal approach provides a means to treat diverse symptomatology. Advantages associated with behavioral therapies include cost effectiveness, adaptability across contexts in which children function, and the efficacy associated with training parents, teachers, and other caretakers as change agents. Further, these techniques have associated efficacy in dealing with co-morbid conditions. These include both conduct disorder and oppositional/defiant disorder, as well as the spectrum of internalizing disorders (i.e., anxiety and affective disorder complicity) that can also be manifest in the ADHD spectrum conditions.

Dinklage and Barkley (1992) cast the application of behavior therapies with ADHD children in perspective. Emphasizing the theoretical perspective that these youngsters have long been viewed as failing to respond to natural consequences, they characterized ADHD conditions as a "deficiency in the regulation and maintenance of behavior by its consequences which gives rise to problems with inhibiting, initiating or sustaining responses to tasks or stimuli, and adherence to rules or instructions, particularly in situations where consequences for such behaviors are delayed, weak or non-existent" (p. 290). Obviously, therapy modalities that exert greater controls over stimulus selectivity and reinforcement have intuitive appeal. Indeed, over the past 20 years they have proven most consistently efficacious as means for facilitating improved adaptive behavioral competencies in children. A number of reviews (Barkley, 1990; Hinshaw & Erhardt, 1990; Rapport, 1987; Werry & Wollerstein, 1989) have summarized the clinical efficacy of these interventions.

Behavioral Interventions

Treatment intervention is prefaced by multi-modal assessments to identify target symptoms, their relative frequency-intensity, and ecological specificity. Behavior problems and developmental concerns can then be aggregated and rank ordered. Specific treatment interventions are then matched with specific targeted behaviors. As was highlighted in the introduction, given the heterogeneity of ADHD presentations, a broad-based assessment methodology providing coverage of diverse symptoms that can be expressed differentially across contexts provides the foundation for treatment planning.

Contingency management programs. The applications of token economies, contingency contracting systems, response cost paradigms and time out from positive reinforcement represent the most common contingency management strategies utilized with children and adolescents. These interventions share in common attempts to shape behavior in a desired direction through modification of reinforcement hierarchies. Principals of operant conditioning have been applied to reduce or extinguish inappropriate or maladaptive behavior as well as in the facilitation of improved self-control. Most operant treatment programs require combinations of interventions so as to increase the expression of adaptive behavior and reduce undesirable behaviors:

1. *Differential reinforcement of low rates of behavior* is a strategy implemented when the frequency, and not necessarily the behavior itself, is inappropriate, such as a child excessively raising his or her hand to be recognized. In this reinforcement schedule, response is provided only after a predetermined length of time following the initial response.
2. *Differential reinforcement of other behavior* involves contingent reinforcement when an undesirable behavior has not been exhibited for a specified time period.
3. *Differential reinforcement of incompatible or alternative behavior* involves the selective reinforcement of behaviors that would preclude the child exhibiting other undesirable behavior or otherwise sustain redirected activity in other more acceptable forms of behavior.

Other strategies for reducing rates of inappropriate behavior include *response cost* procedures. Under these conditions the display of specific targeted unsanctioned behaviors results in a loss of reinforcement. Most often this involves a loss of a secondary reinforcer (points or tokens) or privileges. These procedures are clearly distinguishable from *punishment* wherein reduction in rates of unacceptable behavior are achieved via the imposition of aversive consequences. Such aversive consequences are certainly not sanctioned as appropriate in intervention plans for youngsters. There are, however, less aversive interventions, reprimands and over-correction procedures, which when necessary represent alternatives to punishment. *Reprimand*, for example, represents a verbal admonishment. In its use, the practitioner must remain aware of its limited utility especially if administered with frequency. *Over-correction* procedures involve either repeated positive practice (engagement in such activity precludes displays of targeted maladaptive behavior), or repeated acts of restitution. Utilization of any of the latter procedures requires careful supervision as they may be difficult to dissociate from "punishment."

Contingency management programming must also take into consideration the building of adaptive behavior and coping resources. Additional methodologies are available to shape desirable behaviors:

1. *Token Reinforcement Programs.* These strategies involve the delivery of immediate reinforcements under conditions in which desired behavior is being exhibited. These procedures characteristically involve secondary reinforcers appropriate to the age or developmental level of the subject. Accumulated tokens, points, or coins can be exchanged for selective primary reinforcers or privileges. Token economy systems have the potential to encompass not only social but academic competencies. These programs can be applied across the contexts in which similar behaviors are maintained, that is, across the varied environments in which a child functions. Home-based contingencies can be adapted to provide reinforcement for appropriate behavior at school. Such plans offer opportunities for parent/teacher interaction in cooperative treatment planning. They are also helpful as a means to foster adaptation to increased delay in reinforcement.

2. *Behavioral Contracting.* Contingency contracting involves active negotiation of a written agreement stipulating consequences that may be anticipated upon successful completion of targeted objectives or goals. Unlike the token economy, the subject must be capable of sustaining delays and gratification. The negotiations inherent in this system hopefully foster motivation, since the subject actively selects contingent reinforcers.

3. *Ignoring Inappropriate Behavior.* This tactic represents deliberate contingent withdrawal of attention. Such strategies are most effective for mild as compared to intense or high frequency behaviors.

Cognitive behavioral therapy techniques. In addition to the primary behavior therapies, a variety of self-control training strategies have been utilized with varying degrees of success. Interest in these interventions has been revived as a function of a conceptualization of ADHD as a deficit in "executive functions." These interventions fall more primarily under the rubric of cognitive-behavior therapies because of their emphasis on cognitive or self-control strategies, the inference being that such interventions may represent a means to accommodate for a central deficit in self-monitoring or self-reinforcement within ADHD populations. Such interventions typically include training in:

1. *Self-Instruction.* These strategies are typically directed at limiting impulsive responding and enhancing selective attention and task maintenance behaviors. They have demonstrated efficacy when combined with other more primary behavior therapy interventions (Barkley, 1989). Henshaw and Erhardt (1991) summarized the sequential strategies of cognitive training whereby, through a series of modeling techniques, a child progressively internalizes a self-guidance script. These techniques emphasize the importance of verbal mediation skills for the guidance and direction of ongoing behavior. Although these strategies hold strong intuitive appeal, adequacy as a unimodal treatment methodology remains in question. Generalization effects have been marginal.

2. *Self-Monitoring Skills.* Self-evaluation and self-monitoring skill development have been offered as strategies to facilitate "reflectivity" and as a means to mitigate against problems with impulsivity. They also represent an important component of a number of operant paradigms to reduce reliance upon externalized sources of behavioral monitoring. These include training in strategies that foster self-evaluation (e.g., observing video tapes, recognizing and recording instances of on-task or off-task behavior, etc). These activities can be matched with periods of time in which an independent rater as well as the child monitor prescribed periods of behavior. Braswell and Bloomquist (1991) provide further description of the operationalization of such strategies.

3. *Self-Reinforcement.* The logical extension of the previous two methodologies involves strategies in which the child not only monitors, but evaluates the quality of ongoing performance. Points or tokens are quantified in exchange for privileges or rewards for display of appropriate behaviors. Such strategies have been applied to building on-task vigilance, accuracy of performance, academic skills, and quality of peer interaction (Barkley, 1989). These strategies are also utilized when fading from behavioral monitoring provided by external sources (i.e., parents or teachers).

Other cognitive behavioral interventions involve integrative approaches toward self-instruction and problem solving. A number of such interventions combine self-monitoring, skill training, rehearsal of coping strategies and development of self-talk, as well as group-mediated problem solving experiences. These interventions have specifically focused on enhancement of social competence.

While much of the literature has been focused on treatment interventions for hyperactive-impulsive and combined ADHD, addressing high-frequency, aggressive-disruptive, oppositional, or off-task behavior, few investigations of standardized behavioral and/or cognitive behavioral treatment interventions with ADHD, Inattentive Type have been conducted. The effect of comorbidity in the form of anxiety- and/or mood-related symptomatology will require further investigation.

Highlighted in this discussion has been the expectation that heterogeneity in primary, secondary, and associated symptom manifestations tends to be the rule rather than the exception in ADHD populations. Pennington (1991) emphasizes that the child with ADHD is likely to be maturationally disadvantaged in comparison to age-mates. Thus, interventions may be required not only in areas of general psychosocial adaption, but also in a variety of other areas. Here, a broad range of social skill training programs hold potential applicability. In general, the older the child presenting for treatment, the more likely a complex symptom presentation can be anticipated (Cantwell, 1986). Thus, particularly in adolescence, the availability of broad-focused, heteromodal treatment interventions is required.

Pharmacological Treatments

Before initiating any pharmacologic treatment in children and adolescents, a thorough medical history and physical exam should be completed if not recently done. If the child is on medication, assuring that no adverse drug interactions are known with the proposed medication is necessary. The stimulants are the first line of pharmacologic intervention in the treatment of ADHD. The tricyclic antidepressants are the next most commonly used agents if stimulants are ineffective or contraindicated. The initial work-up prior to either of these classes of medications includes baseline height, weight, pulse, and blood pressure. Observations for any tics or involuntary movements should be completed prior to the initiation of these medications. If pemoline is being used, baseline liver functions should be obtained. If a tricyclic is being considered, a baseline EKG should be obtained (Dulcan, 1990; Ryan, 1990).

There is common agreement among most experts in the field that medication should only be used in combination with behavioral therapy (Barkley, 1990; Conners & Wells, 1986; Pelham & Murphy, 1986). The general

basic tenets of behavioral therapy are to clearly identify and label appropriate behaviors and positively reinforce them so they increase in frequency and to intervene to minimize inappropriate behaviors. Similarly, in a medication trial a clearly identified and individualized set of negative behaviors that are a result of the symptoms of inattention, impulsivity, or hyperactivity and a set of positive behaviors that are to be enhanced for that specific child should comprise the target symptoms of the medication trial. A baseline frequency of these behaviors should be established prior to initiating medication. Medication should be titrated based on maximizing the frequency of positive behaviors, minimizing the frequency of negative behaviors, and minimizing side effects. Although stepwise medication titration is the most common form of prescribing stimulants, randomized double blind placebo trials are the most comprehensive way to assess stimulant response. Please refer to Pelham (1993) or Pelham and Milich (1991) for a detailed description of this type of stimulant assessment.

Methylphenidate (Ritalin), dextroamphetamine (Dexedrine), and pemoline (Cylert) are widely used stimulants that are effective in about 75 percent of children with ADHD (Dulcan, 1990). Those children who do not respond to the initial stimulant trial have a significant likelihood of responding to a second stimulant (Elia, Borcherding, Rapoport, & Keysor, 1991). Dosing guidelines and side effect profiles of the stimulants are well established and outlined in a variety of resources such as Barkley (1990), Dulcan (1990), and Pelham (1993). In addition, a chapter entitled "*Use of Ritalin in the Practice of Pediatrics*" provides a concise overview for primary care providers (Fried, 1991).

Children who do not respond or cannot tolerate stimulants are typically treated with tricyclic antidepressants such as imipramine, desipramine, or nortriptyline (Biederman, Baldessarini, Wright, Knee, & Harmatz, 1989; Zametkin & Rapoport, 1987). In addition, children with a concurrent anxiety disorder or depression may benefit from both the antidepressant or anxiolytic effects of these medications and the behavioral effects (Pliszka, 1987).

Other antidepressants have been used in the treatment of ADHD—such as fluoxetine (Barrickman, Noyes, Kuperman, Schumacher, & Verda, 1991), bupropion (Simeon, Ferguson, & Van Wyck Fleet, 1986), and the monoamine oxidase inhibitors (Zametkin, Rapoport, Murphy, Linnoila, & Ismond, 1985)—but none have been as widely studied or extensively used for ADHD as the above agents. Clonidine has been used to treat children with ADHD, especially when a concurrent Tourette's

Disorder is present (Hunt, Capper, & O'Connell, 1990). Recently a similar agent, guanfacine, has been studied in an open trial with positive results (Hunt, Arnsten, & Asbell, 1995).

In summary, the stimulants remain the medications of first choice when treating ADHD in children and adolescents. The antidepressants provide the mental health provider with an effective alternative when necessary, and there are a variety of additional pharmacologic alternatives for treatment of refractory patients. These medications in combination with behavioral therapy are the mainstay of treatment for this disorder.

CASE ILLUSTRATION

Clinical Presentation

R.K. is an eight-year-old white male who presented to the outpatient clinic for assessment and treatment secondary to long-standing severe disruptive behaviors. His mother reported that as long as she could remember R.K. had been fidgety, had difficulty remaining seated, was inattentive, failed to finish tasks, was messy and disorganized, frequently interrupted others, and tended to blurt things out. In addition, over the last several years, he had become increasingly defiant, argumentative, quick tempered, spiteful, and disrespectful of authority, and his self-esteem appeared low.

Assessment Findings

During the course of the assessment R.K.'s mother endorsed significant symptoms of attention-deficit/hyperactivity disorder and oppositional defiant disorder. Functionally, she reported severe difficulties in school behavior and academics resulting in multiple suspensions and failing grades in several subjects. He was being rejected by many of his peers and was "kicked off" the soccer team. His sister was complaining that her friends did not want to come over to her house and play because of her brother's behavior, and his parents had been arguing more about how to discipline him. Aside from his irritable temper outbursts and low self-esteem, no other significant affective symptoms were reported. There was no history of other significant conduct disorder symptoms, anxiety, obsessions or compulsions, hallucinations or psychosis, motor or vocal tics, unusual eating or sleeping patterns, enuresis or encopresis, physical or sexual abuse, suicidal or homicidal ideation, or

other primary psychiatric disorder symptoms. His past treatment history included a year of individual play therapy with a therapist in private practice with minimal effectiveness on improving his behavior difficulties according to his mother. He was never hospitalized or treated with medication in the past.

Medically, he was a healthy boy with no acute medical problems. He had just received a reportedly unremarkable, but thorough physical examination by his pediatrician the week prior to assessment. His past medical history was remarkable for a "broken right arm" at age six after falling from a tree. He had no other history of significant medical problems. He was on no medications and was not allergic to any medications.

His family psychiatric history was remarkable for alcohol abuse in his biologic father and depression in his maternal grandmother and a maternal aunt. Otherwise, the family history was noncontributory.

His developmental history was essentially unremarkable. He met motor and language milestones at age-appropriate norms and had no difficulty with toilet training. His school history included generally average to slightly below average grades until this year. Reportedly, he was currently failing in math and science. He was in all regular education classroom placements.

As noted, he had few friends and was recently "kicked off" the soccer team secondary to his behavior. He lived at home with his mother, stepfather, and ten-year-old sister. Both parents worked. His mother was self-employed and worked primarily out of the home. Aside from increased arguing over his behavior, no significant marital difficulties were reported. His biologic father lived out of state and he would see him for two weeks during the summer and on major holidays when possible. No additional significant psychosocial stressors were reported. His parents reported inconsistent and ineffective attempts at managing his behavior. Primarily, they would "yell" at him or send him to his room. Frequently, they just gave in to him because it was easier than trying to get him to comply.

On mental status examination, R.K. was casually dressed and mildly disheveled. There were no dysmorphic features or abnormal movements noted. He was fidgety and easily distracted by extraneous noises throughout the evaluation. His speech flowed without difficulty and no articulation difficulties were noted. His vocabulary was somewhat below what would be expected for his age. He was spontaneous in his conversation and quite talkative. He denied significant depression, mania, anxiety, obsessions or compulsions, hallucinations or delusions, physical or sexual abuse, or other significant psychiatric symptoms. His insight into why he was being seen was fair at best. He said it was because "other kids get me into trouble and the teachers always blame me." He was alert throughout the evaluation and oriented to all spheres.

Given the above information, his school was contacted and his teacher described the most significant difficulties he had in the classroom. His work was generally incomplete or completed in a hurry with significant errors, and homework was frequently not turned in. He would call out in class without raising his hand and would leave his seat without permission. She also completed several standardized rating scales that reflected his difficulties as well. He was referred for testing to the school psychologist for further evaluation for a specific learning disorder. Test results indicated average intelligence with significantly below-average achievement in mathematics.

Treatment Selection and Course

After a thorough discussion focused on educating R.K. and his family about ADHD and the various treatment options that were available, several interventions were initiated. Parent behavioral training utilizing a group format interspersed with several individual sessions to develop a specific behavior program were the primary treatment recommendations. House rules were developed and some of the topics covered included chores, homework, and expectations of behavior when his sister's friends were visiting. A reward system specific to these rules was established and consequences were outlined for noncompliance. Additionally, after further consultation with his teacher, a daily report of his behavior in the classroom and his academic performance was developed. R.K., his teachers, and his parents were all responsible for certain aspects of this school-focused behavior program. Expectations of his behavior and academics were clearly outlined and this was incorporated into his reward system at home. Behavioral expectations were written down and closely tracked. Success was reinforced with a variety of reinforcers that R.K. helped identify and the parents could consistently provide him. Examples for him included extra television and video game time, half hour later bedtime, special play time with his mother, and an allowance for certain chores he completed. In addition, repeated noncompliance and aggression were managed with a time out. Additional negative behaviors resulted in loss of certain privileges or five-minute work chores. The program was

designed to assure his initial success by setting achievable goals and then gradually the expectations were increased.

Based on neurocognitive test results, specific recommendations were made to the school regarding individualized educational techniques that could be utilized, and R.K. was placed in a learning support classroom for mathematics. R.K. attended a social skills group that encouraged the use of more appropriate social interactions through group discussion, role play, modeling, and direct participation in supervised recreational and sports activities. He was also encouraged to participate in prosocial activities at school and in the community during the latter stages of his participation in this group. R.K. also underwent a trial of methylphenidate. Increased success on the above behavior programs at home and school, as well as changes on standardized rating scales completed by his parents and teachers, were noted. His dose was titrated by maximizing improvement on these measures while minimizing side effects. The greatest weight was placed on improvement on those measures that reflected his most significant problems with daily life functioning while at home and school.

Termination and Follow-Up

R.K. and his parents actively participated in the above treatment and a significant improvement in behavior and academics was reported. He continues on methylphenidate and his parents are still utilizing behavior programs. They have modified them to address more current issues. He continues to receive learning support in math and is maintaining a B average in school. Family arguments have decreased and his sister frequently has friends over to visit with only rare difficulty. He is on the soccer team and has joined the Boy Scouts. Overall, he is doing much better than he did on his initial presentation.

SUMMARY

Attention-deficit/hyperactivity disorder is one of the most commonly treated childhood psychiatric disorders at outpatient mental health care facilities. The etiology of the disorder is unknown. The core features and symptoms are descriptive in nature and include difficulties with attention, impulse control, and motor overactivity. These symptoms may vary across the developmental age of the patient and are often environmentally variable as well. A variety of medical conditions, learning disorders, and other psychiatric conditions may present with these core features. Therefore, initial assessment and diagnosis are important in distinguishing these other difficulties from ADHD in order to develop an appropriate and comprehensive treatment plan for the individual patient. The cooperative efforts of a variety of professionals are frequently required. The use of standardized rating scales and obtaining information from sources in addition to the patient and family is clearly important. Information from teachers is not only important in establishing the diagnosis, it is typically an integral part of treatment. The treatment focus should be on the individual areas of dysfunction resulting from difficulties with attention, impulse control, or overactivity. In general, behavior modification and pharmacotherapy with central nervous system stimulants are the mainstays of treatment. However, other treatment modalities and alternative pharmacologic agents are frequently utilized in conjunction with or as alternatives to these two primary interventions. Because of the chronicity of this disorder and the potential difficulties that continue in a significant number of children with ADHD into adolescence and adulthood, early, comprehensive, and continued treatment is recommended. Although there is no known "cure" for this disorder, appropriate treatment interventions can successfully ameliorate the difficulties these children experience in daily functioning.

REFERENCES

Achenbach, T. M. (1986). *Manual for the Child Behavior Checklist—Direct Observation Form*. Burlington, VT: University of Vermont, Department of Psychiatry.

Achenbach, T. M., & Edelbrock, C. S. (1983). *Manual for the Child Behavior Checklist and Revised Child Behavior Profile*. Burlington, VT: University of Vermont, Department of Psychiatry.

Achenbach, T. M. (1991). *Manual for the Child Behavior Checklist/4–18 and 1991 Profile*. Burlington, VT: University of Vermont, Department of Psychiatry.

American Psychiatric Association. (1980). *Diagnostic and statistical manual of mental disorders* (3rd ed.). Washington, DC: Author.

American Psychiatric Association. (1994). *Diagnostic and statistical manual of mental disorders* (4th ed.). Washington, DC: Author.

Anderson, J. C., Williams, S., McGee, R., & Silva, P. (1987). DSM-III disorders in preadolescent children. Prevalence in a large sample from the general population. *Archives of General Psychiatry, 44,* 69–76.

Atkins, M. S., Pelham, W. E., & Licht, M. H. (1985). A comparison of objective classroom measures and teacher ratings of attention deficit disorder. *Journal of Abnormal Child Psychology, 13,* 155–167.

August, G. J., & Garfinkel, G. D. (1989). Behavioral and cognitive subtypes of ADHD. *Journal of the American Academy of Child and Adolescent Psychiatry, 28,* 739–748.

Baker, L., & Cantwell, D. P. (1990). The association between emotional behavioral disorders and learning disorders in children with speech/language impairments. *Advances in Learning and Behavior Disabilities.*

Barkley, R. A. (1990). *Attention deficit hyperactivity disorder: A handbook for diagnosis and treatment*. New York: Guilford Press.

Barkley, R. A. (1989). Attention-deficit hyperactivity disorder. In E. J. Mash and R. A. Barkley (Eds.), *Treatment of childhood disorders* (pp. 39–72). New York: Guilford Press.

Barkley, R. A. (1988). Attention. In M. Tramontana & S. Hooper (Eds.), *Issues in child clinical neuropsychology* (pp. 145–176). New York: Plenum Press.

Barkley, R. A. (1987). Child behavior rating scales and checklists. In M. Rutter, A. H. Tuma, & I. J. Lann (Eds.), *Assessment and diagnosis in child psychopathology* (pp. 113–155). New York: Guilford Press.

Barkley, R. A., Dupaul, G. J., & McMurry, M. B. (1990). A comprehensive evaluation of attention deficit disorder with and without hyperactivity as defined by research criteria. *Journal of Consulting and Clinical Psychology, 58,* 775–789.

Barkley, R. A., Fisher, M., Edelbrock, C. S., & Smallish, L. (1990). The adolescent outcome of hyperactive children diagnosed by research criteria: An 8 year prospective follow-up study. *Journal of Child Psychology and Psychiatry, 42,* 937–947.

Barrickman, L., Noyes, R., Kuperman, S., Schumacher, E., & Verda, M. (1991). Treatment of ADHD with fluoxetine: A preliminary trial. *Journal of the American Academy of Child and Adolescent Psychiatry, 30,* 762–767.

Biederman, J., Baldessarini, R. J., Wright, V., Knee, D., & Harmatz, J. S. (1989). A double-blind placebo-controlled study of desipramine in the treatment of ADD. I. Efficacy. *Journal of the American Academy of Child and Adolescent Psychiatry, 28,* 777–780.

Black, A. (1994). The drugging of America's children. *Redbook*, Dec., 41–44, 50.

Braswell, L., & Bloomquist, M. L. (1991). *Cognitive-behavioral therapy with ADHD children: Child, family and school interventions*. New York: Guilford Press.

Cantwell, D. P. (1986). Attention deficit disorder in adolescents. *Clinical Psychology Review, 6*, 237–247.

Cantwell, D. P. (1986). Attention deficit and associated childhood disorders. In T. Millon & G. L. Kellerman (Eds.), *Contemporary directions in psychopathology* (pp. 403–428). New York: Guilford Press.

Chelune, G. J., Ferguson, W., Koon, R., & Dickey, T. O. (1986). Frontal lobe disinhibition in attention deficit disorder. *Child Psychiatry and Human Development, 16*, 221–232.

Cohen, M., Becker, M. G., & Campbell, R. (1990). Relationships among four methods of assessment of children with attention-deficit hyperactivity disorder. *Journal of School Psychology, 28*, 189–202.

Conners, C. K., & Wells, K. C. (1986). *Hyperkinetic children: A neuropsychosocial approach.* Beverly Hills: Sage Publications, Inc.

Conners, K. C. (1990). *Conners Rating Scales manual.* North Tonawanda, NY: Multi-Health Systems.

Conte, R., Kinsbourne, M., Swanson, J. M., Zirk, H., & Samuels, M. (1986). Presentation rate effects on paired associate learning by attention deficit disordered children. *Child Development, 57*, 681–687.

Costello, A. J., Edelbrock, C. S., Kalas, R., Kessler, M., & Klaric, S. (1982). *The NIMH Diagnostic Interview Schedule for Children (DISC).* Pittsburgh: Authors.

Douglas, V. L. (1983). Attention and cognitive problems. In M. Rutter (Ed.), *Developmental neuropsychiatry* (pp. 280–329). New York: Guilford Press.

Douglas, V. I. (1972). Stop, look, and listen: The problem of sustained attention and impulse control in hyperactive and normal children. *Canadian Journal of Behavioral Science, 4*, 259–282.

Dulcan, M. K. (1990). Using psychostimulants to treat behavioral disorders of children and adolescents. *Journal of Child and Adolescent Psychopharmacology, 1*, 7–20.

DuPaul, G. J., & Stoner, G. (1994). *ADHD in the schools.* New York: Guilford Press.

Dykman, R. A., & Ackerman, P. T. (1991). Attention deficit disorder and specific reading disability: Separate but often overlapping disorders. *Journal of Learning Disabilities, 24*, 96–103.

Elia, J., Borcherding, B. G., Rapoport, J. L., & Keysor, C. S. (1991). Methylphenidate and dextroamphetamine treatments of hyperactivity: Are there true nonresponders? *Psychiatry Research, 36*, 141–155.

Epstein, M. A., Shaywitz, S. E., Shaywitz, B. A., & Woolston, J. L. (1991). The boundaries of attention deficit disorder. *Journal of Learning Disabilities, 24*, 78–86.

Evans, S. E., Vallano, G., & Pelham, W. E. (1995). Attention deficit hyperactivity disorder. In V. B. Van Hasselt & M. Hersen (Eds.), *Handbook of adolescent psychopathology: A guide to diagnosis and treatment* (pp. 589–617). New York: Macmillan.

Fiore, T. A., Becker, E. A., & Nero, R. C. (1993). Educational interventions for students with Attention Deficit Disorder. *Exceptional Children, 60*, 163–173.

Fletcher, J. M. (1988). Brain-injured children. In E. J. Mash & L. G. Terdal (Eds.), *Behavioral assessment of childhood disorders* (Vol. 2) (pp. 451–490). New York: Guilford Press.

Fried, J. E. (1991). Use of Ritalin in the practice of pediatrics. In L. Greenhill & B. P. Osman (Eds.), *Ritalin: Theory and patient management* (pp. 131–140). New York: Mary Ann Liebert, Inc.

Gittelman, R., Mannuzza, S., Shenker, R., & Bonagura, N. (1985). Hyperactive boys almost grown up. *Archives of General Psychiatry, 42*, 937–947.

Goodman, R., & Stevenson, J. (1989). A twin study of hyperactivity-II. The etiological role of genes, family relationships and perinatal adversity. *Journal of Child Psychology and Psychiatry, 5*, 691–709.

Goyette, C. H., Conners, C. K., & Ulrich, R. F. (1978). Normative data for revised Conners parent and teacher rating scales. *Journal of Abnormal Child Psychology, 6*, 221–236.

Hechtman, L., & Weiss, G. (1983). Long-term outcome of hyperactive children. *American Journal of Orthopsychiatry, 53*, 532–541.

Hinshaw, S. P., & Erhardt, D. (1991). Attention deficit hyperactivity disorder. In P. C. Kendall (Ed.), *Child and adolescent therapy: Cognitive-behavioral applications* (pp. 98–130). New York: Guilford Press.

Herjanic, B., Brown, F., & Wheatt, T. (1975). Are children reliable reporters? *Journal of Abnormal Child Psychology, 3*, 41–48.

Hoza, B., Vallano, G., & Pelham, W. E. (1995). Attention-deficit/hyperactivity disorder. In R. T. Ammerman & M. Hersen (Eds.). *Handbook of child behavior therapy in the psychiatric setting* (pp. 181–198). New York: Wiley-Interscience.

Hunt, R. D., Arnsten, A. F. T., & Asbell, M. D. (1995). An open trial of guanfacine in the treatment of attention-deficit hyperactivity disorder. *Journal of the American Academy of Child and Adolescent Psychiatry, 34*, 50–54.

Hunt, R. D., Capper, L., & O'Connell, P. (1990). Clonidine in child and adolescent psychiatry. *Journal of Child and Adolescent Psychopharmacology, 1*, 87–102.

Kaufman, D. M. (1985). *Clinical neurology for psychiatrists* (2nd ed.). Orlando, FL: Grune & Stratton, Inc.

Kinsbourne, M. (1992). Development of attention and metacognition. In S. J. Segalowitz and I. Rapin (Eds.),

Handbook of neuropsychology (Vol. 7) (pp. 261–278). Amsterdam: Elsevier.

Laufer, M., & Denhoff, E. (1957). Hyperkinetic behavior syndrome in children. *Journal of Pediatrics, 50*, 463–474.

Loney, J. (1987). Hyperactivity and aggression in the diagnosis of attention deficit disorder. In B. B. Lahey & A. E. Kazdin (Eds.), *Advances in clinical child psychology*. New York: Plenum Press.

Lou, H. C., Henriksen, L., Bruhn, P., Borner, H., & Nielsen, J. B. (1989). Striatal dysfunction in attention deficit and hyperkinetic disorder. *Archives of Neurology, 46*, 48–52.

McCarney, S. B. (1989). *Attention Deficit Disorders Evaluation Scale–Home Version*. Columbia, MS: Hawthorne.

Mirsky, A. F. (1987). Behavioral and psychophysiological markers of disordered attention. *Environmental and Health Perspectives, 74*, 191–199.

Mirsky, A. F., Anthony, B. J., Duncan, C. C., Dhearn, M. B., & Kellam, S. G. (1991). Analysis of the elements of attention: A neuropsychological approach. *Neuropsychology Review, 2*, 109–145.

Needleman, H. L., Gunnoe, C., Leviton, A., Reed, R., Peresie, H., Maher, C., & Barrett, P. (1979). Deficits in psychologic and classroom performance of children with elevated dentine lead levels. *New England Journal of Medicine, 300* (March 29), 689–695.

Pelham, W. E. (1993). Pharmacotherapy for children with attention-deficit hyperactivity disorder. *School Psychology Review, 22*, 199–227.

Pelham, W. E., & Murphy, H. A. (1986). Attention deficit and conduct disorders. In M. Hersen (Ed.), *Pharmacological and behavioral treatment: An integrative approach* (pp. 108–148). New York: John Wiley and Sons.

Pelham, W. E., & Milich, R. (1991). Individual differences in response to ritalin in classwork and social behavior. In L. Greenhill & B. P. Osman (Eds.), *Ritalin: Theory and patient management* (pp. 203–221). New York: Mary Ann Liebert, Inc.

Pennington, B. F. (1991). *Diagnosing learning disorders. A neuropsychological framework*. New York: Guilford Press.

Pliszka, S. R. (1987). Tricyclic antidepressants in the treatment of children with attention deficit disorder. *Journal of the American Academy of Child and Adolescent Psychiatry, 26*, 127–132.

Posner, M. (1987). Structures and functions of selective attention. In T. Boll & B. K. Bryant (Eds.), *Clinical neuropsychology and brain function: Research, measurement, and practice* (pp. 169–202). Washington, DC: American Psychological Association.

Quay, H. C., & Peterson, D. R. (1983). *Interim Manual for the Revised Behavior Problem Checklist*. Unpublished manuscript, University of Miami.

Rappaport, M. D. (1987). Attention-deficit disorder with hyperactivity. In M. Hersen & V. B. Van Hasselt (Eds.), *Behavior therapy with children and adolescents* (pp. 325–361). New York: John Wiley and Sons, Inc.

Riccio, C. A., Hynd, G. W., Cohen, M. J., Hall, J., & Molt, L. (1994). Comorbidity of central auditory processing disorder and attention-deficit hyperactivity disorder. *Journal of the American Academy of Child and Adolescent Psychiatry, 33*, 849–857.

Ross, D. M., & Ross, S. A. (1982). *Hyperactivity: Research, theory, and action* (2nd ed.). New York: John Wiley and Sons, Inc.

Ryan, N. D. (1990). Heterocyclic antidepressants in children and adolescents. *Journal of Child and Adolescent Psychopharmacology, 1*, 21–31.

Safer, D. J., & Allen R. D. (1976). *Hyperactive children: Diagnosis and management*. Baltimore: University Park Press.

Shapiro, S. K., & Herod, L. A. (1994) Combining visual and auditory tasks in the assessment of attention deficit disorder. In D. K. Routh (Ed.), *Disruptive behavior disorders of childhood* (pp. 87–108). New York: Plenum Press.

Shaywitz, S. E., & Shaywitz, B. E. (1988). Attention deficit disorder: Current perspectives. In J. F. Kavanagh & T. J. Truss, Jr. (Eds.), *Learning disabilities: Proceedings of the national conference* (pp. 369–546). Parkton, MD: York Press, Inc.

Shroyer, C., & Zentall, S. S. (1986). Effects of rate, non-relevant information and repetition on the listening comprehension of hyperactive children. *Journal of Special Education, 20*, 231–239.

Shum, D. H., McFarland, K. A., & Bain, J. D. (1990). Construct validity of eight tests of attention: Comparison of normal and closed head injured samples. *Clinical Neuropsychologist, 4*, 151–162.

Silver, L. B. (1981). The relationship between learning disabilities, hyperactivity, distractability and behavior problems. A clinical analysis. *Journal of the American Academy of Child Psychiatry, 20*, 285–397.

Simeon, J. G., Ferguson, H. B., & Van Wyck Fleet, J. (1986). Buproprion effects in attention deficit and conduct disorders. *Canadian Journal of Psychiatry, 31*, 581–585.

Sleator, E. K., & Ullmann, R. L. (1981). Can the physician diagnose hyperactivity in the office? *Pediatrics, 67*, 13–17.

Slomka, G. T., & Tarter, R. E. (1993). Neuropsychological assessment. In T. H. Ollendick & M. Hersen (Eds.),

Handbook of child and adolescent assessment (pp. 208–223). Boston: Allyn & Bacon.

Stewart, M. A., Pitts, F. N., Craig, A. G., & Dieruf, W. (1966). The hyperactive child syndrome. *American Journal of Orthopsychiatry, 36*, 861–867.

Taylor, H. G., & Fletcher, J. M. (1990). In M. Hersen & G. Goldstein (Eds.), *Handbook of psychological assessment* (2nd ed., pp. 228–255). New York: Pergamon Press.

Trites, R. L. (1979). *Hyperactivity in children: Etiology, measurement, and treatment implications.* Baltimore: University Park Press.

Weiss, G., & Hechtman, L. (1986). *Hyperactive children grown up.* New York: Guilford Press.

Werry, J. S., & Wollersheim, J. P. (1989). Behavior therapy with children and adolescents: A twenty year overview. *Journal of the American Academy of Child and Adolescent Psychiatry, 28*, 1, 1–18.

Wielkiewicz, R. M. (1990). Interpreting low scores on the WISC-R third factor: It's more than distractibility. *Psychological Assessment: A Journal of Consulting and Clinical Psychology, 2*, 91–97.

Wikler, A., Dixon, J. F., & Parker, L. (1970). Brain function in problem children and controls: Psychometric, neuro-logical, and encephalographic comparisons. *American Journal of Psychiatry, 127*, 634–645.

Wirt, R. D, Lachar, D., Klinedinst, J. K., & Seat, P. D. (1984). *Multi-dimensional description of child personality.* Los Angeles, CA: Western Psychological Services.

Zametkin, A., Rapoport, J. L., Murphy, D. L., Linnoila, M., & Ismond, D. (1985). Treatment of hyperactive children with monoamine oxidase inhibitors. I. Clinical efficacy. *Archives of General Psychiatry, 42*, 962–966.

Zametkin, A. J., & Rappoport, J. L. (1987). Neurobiology of attention deficit disorder with hyperactivity: Where have we come in 50 years? *Journal of the American Academy of Child and Adolescent Psychiatry, 26*, 676–686.

Zametkin, A. J., Nordaha, T. E., Gross, M., King, A. C., Sempk, W. E., Rumsey, J., Hamburger, S., & Cohen, R. M. (1990). Cerebral glucose metabolism in adults with hyperactivity of childhood onset. *New England Journal of Medicine, 323*, 1361–1366.

Zentall, S. S., & Gohs, D. E. (1984). Hyperactive and comparison children's response to detailed vs. global cues in communication tasks. *Learning Disability Quarterly, 7*, 77–87.

CHAPTER 12

ANXIETY DISORDERS

Richard Livingston
John Jolly

DESCRIPTION OF DISORDERS

Fear evokes the familiar "fight or flight" repertoire of psychophysiological responses in people of all ages: anticipatory vigilance, emotional unease, and the release of adrenaline. When these physiologic and emotional responses occur in the absence of a current object of fear, the individual suffers from anxiety. Anxiety is ubiquitous; it is familiar in everyday life and certainly present in people with a wide range of emotional and behavioral disorders. When the primary presenting symptoms are anxiety symptoms and the distress or dysfunction they cause is significant, an anxiety disorder is diagnosed.

Physical, psychological, and social symptoms and signs of anxiety can be present. Physical symptoms and signs may be nonspecific—such as restlessness and motor activity increased beyond what is usual for the individual—or specific symptoms of increased autonomic arousal. Psychological symptoms of an emotional nature include fear and uneasiness, while cognitive symptoms range from distorted thinking (such as catastrophic interpretation of benign events) to the shutdown of reasoning that accompanies overwhelming strong emotions. Social discomfort is common in many of these conditions, and some degree of social withdrawal may be present when an individual experiences separation anxiety, social anxiety, or agoraphobia.

The current classification system in the *Diagnostic and Statistical Manual of Mental Disorders*, Fourth edition (DSM-IV) identifies only one anxiety disorder—*separation anxiety disorder*—among the conditions of infancy, childhood, and adolescence (American Psychiatric Association, 1994). As one would expect, the cardinal sign of this disorder is distress—ranging from uneasiness to full panic—caused by separating from a parent or even when anticipating such a separation. Nightmares, somatic complaints (especially headaches and stomachaches), and reluctance or refusal to go to school are symptoms that may lead a parent to seek medical attention for the child with separation anxiety.

Panic disorder, specific and social phobias, generalized anxiety disorder and *adjustment disorder with anxious mood* can all be diagnosed in children, adolescents, and adults (American Psychiatric Association, 1994). *Panic disorder* is diagnosed when an individual has repeated attacks of feeling intense fear or discomfort accompanied by some combination of physical symptoms, such as palpitations, shortness of breath, dizziness, numbness or tingling in the perioral region or the extremities, sweating, nausea, and chest pain. Psychological symptoms such as a sense of impending disaster and a fear of imminent death, or the feeling of "going crazy" are usually present, but it is often the physical symptoms and thoughts of their possible catastrophic meanings that bring the panicky individual to medical attention.

Specific phobia is a particular irrational fear associated with avoidance behavior; *social phobia* is similar but the stimulus is a social situation such as meeting someone new or speaking before a group. "Stage fright" is a special case of social phobia.

Generalized anxiety disorder is the category that now subsumes the more pervasive and mixed symptom picture that was previously called "overanxious disorder." Generalized uneasiness, anticipatory anxiety, excessive worrying, and various signs and symptoms of autonomic overactivity (e.g., diarrhea, motor agitation, or sweating) may be present. Headache and abdominal pain are common. Tremulousness is usually present in children only in the fearful states. Performance anxiety regarding academics, athletics, or the arts often presents with these generalized symptoms, taking them well beyond the boundaries of a specific phobia.

Adjustment disorder with anxious mood is the pertinent diagnosis when a person has anxiety symptoms temporarily, after experiencing some stressful life event. This diagnosis usually should not be used when the symptom picture meets criteria for another disorder, even when the temporal relationship of stressors to onset of symptoms is clear, to avoid perception of the illness as trivial and to avoid oversimplification in thinking about etiology.

Acute stress disorder (ASD) and *post-traumatic stress disorder (PTSD)*, although not characterized only by anxiety symptoms, are classified as anxiety disorders in the DSM-IV (American Psychiatric Association, 1994). These disorders differ from *adjustment disorder* in several respects. While both kinds of disorders are reactions to stressors, the symptoms and the nature of the precipitant stresses are less extreme in adjustment disorders. Adjustment disorders are associated with stressors that are significant but not outside the usual range of experience—moving, parental divorce, illness, or the family's falling on hard times, for example.

In contrast, acute and post-traumatic stress disorders develop following an experience with stressors that are extraordinary, outside the usual realm of experience, such as physical or sexual abuse, being kidnapped, being intubated while conscious, or witnessing violence. When symptoms develop immediately following the experience, ASD is diagnosed; PTSD may be characterized by more persistent symptoms, delayed onset of symptoms, or both. Re-experiencing the trauma in dreams, cued memories, or the more vivid and dissociative experiences called "flashbacks," may lead to phobic avoidance of situations or places that could precipitate the experiences. Nervous vigilance, tension, preoccupations, over-reactions, and lability may be evident. Terr

(1990) has also described post-traumatic play and superstitious behaviors among traumatized children, as well as certain characterologic changes in children who were repeatedly traumatized.

Obsessive-compulsive disorder (OCD) is the diagnosis when the primary symptoms are either repeated, intrusive, and unwanted thoughts (obsessions) or repeated behaviors that must be performed to relieve or avoid tension (compulsions), causing significant distress or dysfunction (American Psychiatric Association, 1994). Obsessions may include images or musical sequences as well as words or phrases. Common compulsions involve checking, counting, touching, and arranging things in ritualized ways. Both kinds of symptoms may be covert, and only revealed if specific inquiry is made about them. Children and adolescents with OCD may present in medical settings with hypochondriacal fears of an obsessional nature, excoriated skin from compulsive washing, or seemingly bizarre preoccupations or fears related to eating.

Finally, it should be noted that anxiety symptoms are very common in young people with other psychiatric disorders. Regardless of the principal diagnosis, anxiety symptoms associated with significant distress or dysfunction should be identified and treated aggressively.

EPIDEMIOLOGY

Modern epidemiological research has clearly established that anxiety disorders are among the most common psychiatric problems of childhood (see Bernstein & Borchardt, 1991 for review). Developmental epidemiologic studies of anxiety are lacking; however, distribution by age is partially established. Younger children are more likely to have specific phobias. Relatively mild separation anxiety, manifested in reluctance to go to school, is very common during the first weeks of kindergarten and first grade. Full-blown panic attacks are relatively rare among younger children, at least in the form we recognize in adults; panic disorder as such is more likely to begin during adolescence or after. Overt social phobia is rare in the early school grades, becoming more prevalent as increasing age brings increasing social awareness and concern.

Girls and boys have similar prevalence of anxiety disorders before puberty; after puberty, girls are probably more likely than boys to suffer from internalizing or emotional disorders. Cultural, social, and economic determinants of prevalence and incidence have yet to be established for anxiety disorders in youth. Comorbidity of anxiety disorders with depression and attention-deficit/hyperactivity disorder is well established (Anderson, Williams, McGee, & Silva, 1987; Bernstein, 1991).

ASSESSMENT APPROACHES

Medical Issues

Occasionally, the history and examination show the anxiety symptoms to have a medical cause. Probably the anxiety produced by too much caffeine (or another stimulant) is the most common in this category; numerous other medical conditions can produce anxiety symptoms, but side effects of medication (e.g., decongestants, antidepressants, asthma drugs, and steroids), hyperthyroidism, mitral valve prolapse, hypoglycemia in diabetics, and pheochromocytoma are the medical conditions most relevant in young people (see Table 12.1).

Interview and History

Adults are often superior informants regarding observable behavior, especially in children school-aged and younger. Children and adolescents must be interviewed as well, however, because they may not have shared private feelings and thoughts with parents or teachers and children may be superior reporters of internalizing symptoms such as anxiety (Achenbach, McConaughy, & Howell, 1987). Anxiety symptoms may be more consistently reported by children than by parents about their children. Additionally, adults' own emotional states may color their perceptions of children's emotions. Teacher input is important (with appropriate consent, of course), not only for their observations of the child's affect and behaviors, but also to help determine the extent to which reported symptoms are undermining academic performance and social functioning.

It is advisable to inquire about anxiety and fears as part of any overall history, and it is imperative to do so in detail when the presenting problems or known history include any of the following: school refusal or refusal to sleep alone; abdominal pain, headache, dizziness, or other somatic symptoms for which no medical cause is apparent; palpitations, chest pain, and other cardiovascular complaints that are not usual in childhood or adolescence.

The history regarding anxiety should elicit the nature and onset of pertinent symptoms and their relationship to external events or situations. For example, symptoms associated with separation anxiety sometimes occur on Sunday night or Monday morning, or following a long

Table 12.1. Points in the Medical Differential Diagnosis of Anxiety in Children or Adolescents

A. Ingestion of Anxiogenic Substances
1. Caffeine: coffee, tea, sodas, headache pills with caffeine, over-the-counter "energy" pills.
2. Drugs of Abuse: cocaine, methamphetamine, marijuana, LSD, phencyclidine, other hallucinogenics.
3. Prescription and nonprescription medications:
   a. pseudoephedrine, phenylpropanolamine, other decongestants
   b. methylphenidate, dextroamphetamine, pemoline, fenfluramine
   c. fluoxetine, protryptiline, bupropion, other antidepressants
   d. theophylline, ephedrine, other asthma preparations
   e. less frequently: steroidal and nonsteroidal anti-inflammatories, antiarrhythmics, antihypertensives, cancer chemotherapy agents.

B. Primary Medical Conditions in Which Comorbid Anxiety is Common (anticipatory anxiety, phobic avoidance, panic states)
1. Pregnancy or fear of pregnancy
2. Sexually transmitted diseases
3. Life-threatening systemic illness
4. Chronic illnesses, especially insulin-dependent diabetes, asthma
5. Disorders with episodic pain, such as sickle cell anemia
6. Disorders requiring repeated painful procedures
7. Migraine

C. Primary Medical Conditions That Cause Anxiety-like Symptoms
1. Hypoxia, hypoperfusion
2. Hypoglycemia
3. Hyperthyroidism, hyperadrenalism, hypoparathyroidism
4. Pheochromocytoma
5. Mitral prolapse, dysrhythmias
6. Encephalitis, encephalopathies, neurodegenerative diseases
7. Hepatitis, porphyria, Wilson's Disease

break from school. Furthermore, parental anxiety is often notable when a child has separation anxiety, and anxiety can be contagious within a family. Other patterns suggestive of primary medical illness may also emerge in the history. Heat intolerance is associated with hyperthyroidism, exercise intolerance may precede other symptoms in mitral prolapse, and a relationship of symptoms to meals may suggest hypoglycemia.

Finally, it is especially important to ask in detail about what other diagnostic and therapeutic services have been sought. "Doctor shopping" may reflect nothing more than parents' or patients' strong need to find answers to baffling and disturbing symptoms, but when multiple clinicians have been consulted, other parent or child psychiatric problems such as anxiety, somatoform, and factitious disorders must be considered as well. Furthermore, obtaining prior records will prevent unnecessary duplication of procedures.

Regular communication between primary care and mental health professionals is an essential part of the care of anxious young people, whether the anxiety is primary, comorbid with a medical disorder, or caused by a medical condition.

In addition to the environmental impact of parental psychopathology, whether anxiety contagion or otherwise, a genetic contribution must be considered, and an adequate history will include the family history for anxiety disorders, depression, alcoholism, and other psychiatric conditions (Livingston, Nugent, Rader, & Smith, 1985).

Once the nature of the symptoms has been established, the pertinent questions for medical differential diagnosis can be pursued. Laboratory tests and other medical diagnostic procedures should be ordered only to the extent necessary to pursue conditions suggested by specifics of history or findings on physical examination.

For recurrent headache or abdominal pain that does not appear to have a typical physical cause, after history, examinations, and basic laboratory or imaging studies are completed, it is generally wise to avoid invasive and expensive diagnostic procedures unless there is a specific reason compelling the study.

Physical Examination of the Anxious Child

First, it must be understood that an anxious child is likely to be nervous about being examined, and may be even more likely than other children to have preconceived ideas that the exam will be painful or that a painful procedure of some kind is forthcoming. "Talking through" the exam may be helpful. With younger children, various distractors can be of help. Of course, those portions of the physical examination that children typically dislike—such as examinations of the ears and throat—can be left until the end.

The actual exam should emphasize a search for signs of cardiac, pulmonary, endocrine, metabolic, and neurological disorders that can produce symptoms of adrenergic and autonomic overactivity. If the presenting problem was a physical complaint, the examination will address the medical conditions that most often cause the presenting symptom. Invasive procedures and exhaustive work-up should be limited in most cases to situations in which there are objective signs of physical disease.

Psychological and Psychiatric Issues

Psychological assessment of childhood and adolescent anxiety is best accomplished with a multi-method, multi-perspective evaluation (Achenbach, 1993; Achenbach & McConaughy, 1987; Klein, 1991) that includes both dimensional (i.e., severity) and categorical (i.e., diagnostic) information. In addition to clinical interviews, certain more formal measures may be specifically useful for a particular disorder or problem area. Such comprehensive evaluations consist of self-reports, clinician ratings, diagnostic interviews, and parent and teacher reports. The purpose of this section is to discuss assessment methods that are particularly useful in clinical settings. For comprehensive reviews of anxiety assessment, see the excellent reviews by Finch and McIntosh (1990) and Barrios and Hartman (1988).

Self-Report Measures

The revised Children's Manifest Anxiety Scale (RCMAS; Reynolds & Richmond, 1978) is a 37-item self-report measure of anxiety and general distress. The RCMAS demonstrates good internal consistency and test-retest reliability (Finch & Rogers, 1984), as well as content, concurrent, construct, and predictive validity (Hughes, 1988; Strauss, 1988). Although the RCMAS can discriminate disturbed from non-disturbed children, it demonstrates poor discriminant validity with measures of depression (Finch, Lipovsky, & Casat, 1989).

The State-Trait Anxiety Inventory for Children (STAIC; Spielberger, 1983) is a 40-item self-report measure of anxiety. As the name implies, the STAIC is intended to assess both the current state of the child ("at this very moment"), as well as how the child "usually" feels. The STAIC demonstrates adequate reliability and concurrent and construct validity, but the assessment of two time periods in a single measure can be confusing to younger or severely disturbed children (Finch & McIntosh, 1990).

The Revised Fear Survey Schedule (FSSC-R; Ollendick, 1983) is an 80-item measure of specific fears that demonstrates adequate internal consistency, test-retest reliability, and concurrent and discriminant validity. To date, the FSSC-R is the only measure that has demonstrated (in one study) the capability of discriminating among subtypes of childhood anxiety disorders by the pattern of children's intense fears (Last, Francis, & Strauss, 1989). However, Perrin and Last (1992) demonstrated that the RCMAS, FSSC-R, and a modified STAIC (STAIC-M; Fox & Houston, 1983) lacked the capability of discriminating between anxiety and attention-deficit disorders; in fact, the FSSC-R was unable to differentiate anxious subjects from community controls (Perrin & Last, 1992).

The Beck Anxiety Inventory (BAI; Beck, Brown, Epstein, & Steer, 1988) is a 21-item, adult self-report measure of general anxiety that may have significant potential use in younger populations. The BAI was developed to assess the distinctive features of anxiety. Beck et al. (1988) found that the BAI demonstrated excellent reliability and validity with adults. Jolly, Aruffo, Wherry, and Livingston (1993) reported an internal consistency estimate of .94, acceptable (item-total) score correlations and concurrent and discriminant validity with self and clinical ratings of anxiety and depression, respectively, in a sample of adolescent in-patients. Anxiety-disordered adolescents scored significantly higher than those with depressive disorders.

There are self-report measures for specific problem areas. For example, the Social Anxiety Scale for Children-Revised (SASCR; La Greca, Dandes, Wick, Shaw, & Stone, 1988), for children from second to sixth grades, was developed to address the gap in the subjective assessment of social anxiety in children.

Clinician Ratings

The Hamilton Anxiety Rating Scale (HARS; Hamilton, 1959) is a 14-item (Guy, 1976) clinician rating scale of general anxiety symptoms. Clark and Donovan (1984) demonstrated inter-rater reliability and internal consistency estimates of .92 and .86, respectively, and concurrent validity with the anxiety self-reports. The HARS discriminated adults with anxiety disorder diagnoses from psychiatric and normal controls (Clark & Donovan, 1984). Although the HARS has been used with children (Kane & Kendall, 1989), psychometric data were not presented.

Eason, Finch, Brasted, and Saylor (1985) developed two anxiety rating scales for children, the Children's Anxiety Rating Scale (CARS) and the Anxiety Rating Scale for Children (ARSC); both scales were designed to assess general anxiety. Although concurrent validity was demonstrated for both scales with self-report anxiety, discriminant validity with depression self and clinician ratings was not demonstrated.

Specific anxiety syndromes also are assessed with clinical rating scales. The Yale-Brown Obsessive Compulsive Scale (Y-BOCS; Goodman et al., 1989) is considered the clinical rating scale of choice for children and adolescents with Obsessive-Compulsive Disorder (Wolff & Wolff, 1991). The Y-BOCS is useful to assess core and associated features of OCD, as well as global severity of symptoms, improvement ratings, and reliability of informant.

Differential Diagnosis

In addition to the medical conditions noted previously, the psychiatric differential diagnosis includes other mental disorders. Anxiety is quite common in young people with depressive disorders, attention deficit disorder, somatoform disorders and disruptive behavior disorders. Comorbidity with other psychiatric disorders is exceptionally common. For example, anxiety disorder is 3 to 4 times as likely to be diagnosed in children with depressive disorders, 2 to 3 times as often in children with oppositional or conduct disorders, and 3 times as often in children with tic disorders.

In general, these increased frequencies of comorbid anxiety are nonspecific; few specific associations have been established. One notable exception is the well-known overlap of Tourette's Disorder with OCD. Indeed, it is sometimes difficult to decide whether a behavior is a complex tic or a compulsion per se. In adults and presumably in children as well, obsessions in the form of negative ruminations are common experiences in depressive illness.

A particular kind of abrupt, poorly verbalized state suggestive of terror, usually referred to as "sudden catastrophic anxiety," is sometimes seen in children who are psychotic or who have pervasive developmental disorders; this was a criterion symptom for the DSM-III diagnosis of "childhood onset pervasive developmental disorder" (American Psychiatric Association, 1980).

Performance anxiety is probably fairly common among children and adolescents with attention deficit disorder and learning disabilities. Clinically important anxiety symptoms may also be present in young people with oppositional-defiant or conduct disorders, and may be ignored because the noxious disruptive behaviors seem to be primary.

Anecdotal evidence suggests that the combination of multiple fears and oppositional behaviors is not rare. Barcai and Rosenthal (1974) describe this as a "fears and tyranny" syndrome, hypothesizing that having too much power or control within the family causes anxiety in a child, and that establishment or re-establishment of parental control alleviates the fears.

Diagnostic uncertainty should be acknowledged when present. The parenthetical term "provisional diagnosis" is useful for this purpose and is preferable to the prefix "rule out." When more than one diagnosis is evident, all appropriate diagnoses should be made. If one diagnosis is clearly causing the most distress or disability, it should be labeled the *principal diagnosis*.

Standardized Diagnostic Interviews

For comprehensive reviews of structured and semi-structured interviews for anxiety disorders, see Silverman (1991), Hodges (1993), and Hodges and Cools (1990). Two interviews which have particular utility with anxiety-disordered children and adolescents include the Anxiety Disorders Interview Schedule for Children (ADIS-C/P; Silverman & Nelles, 1988) and the modified Schedule for Affective Disorders and Schizophrenia in School-Aged Children (modified K-SADS; Last, 1986).

The ADIS-C/P has two versions: the ADIS-C, which is administered to the child, and the ADIS-P, which is administered to the parents. The ADIS-C/P is designed for and limited to assessing childhood anxiety disorders. Excellent Kappa estimates of .84, .83, and .78 were found over-all for the ADIS-C, ADIS-P, and composite diagnosis between clinicians (Silverman & Nelles, 1988). Composite Kappa statistics ranged from 1.00 for school and simple phobia to .54 for overanxious disorder (Silverman & Nelles, 1988); a second study revealed excellent to good agreement between raters, with Kappas of .84, .73, and .64 for simple phobias, social phobia, and overanxious disorder, respectively. Rapee, Barrett, Dadds, and Evans (1994) found composite principal diagnosis Kappas for the ADIS-C/P that ranged from .82 for social phobia to .63 for overanxious disorders and simple phobias.

Last (1986) modified the original present-episode K-SADS (Chambers, Puig-Antich, & Tabrizi, 1978) to more comprehensively assess childhood anxiety disorders and past psychiatric history. Last (1992) reported high levels of inter-rater reliability for childhood anxiety disorders (as well as other disorders). For a sample of 155 anxiety-disordered children, Kappa statistics were .95, .93, .74, .90, and .88 for separation anxiety disorder, overanxious disorder, avoidant disorder, phobic disorder, and panic disorder, respectively.

Parent and Teacher Ratings

Although there are a number of global behavior rating scales for parents and teachers, few specific anxiety measures exist. For reviews of parent rating scales in the assessment of anxiety, see Klein and Last (1989).

The Child Behavior Checklist (CBCL; Achenbach & Edelbrock, 1979) for parents, and its companion form for teachers, the CBCL-Teacher Report Form (CBCL-TRF; Achenbach & Edelbrock, 1986) are particularly useful for the global assessment of childhood symptoms and syndromes. The CBCL and CBCL-TRF are the most frequently used scales for childhood psychopathology and have well established psychometric properties. The CBCL and CBCL-TRF permit the clinician to compare parent and teacher perceptions of the child across a broad spectrum of behaviors and symptoms.

The Child Symptom Inventory (Gadow & Sprafkin, 1994) is a promising newer screening instrument, keyed to the DSM-IV. The Louisville Fear Survey (Miller, Barrett, Hampe, & Noble, 1972a) is an anxiety-specific parent rating scale with adequate psychometric properties, yet it is not widely used (Klein & Last, 1989). We have found that asking parents to complete the Beck Anxiety Inventory (Beck et al., 1988), based upon their observations of their children, to be clinically useful, though psychometric evaluation of this approach has yet to be completed; this type of approach has demonstrated validity with other self-report measures (Wierzbicki, 1987).

Several parent and teacher rating scales assess specific syndromes of anxiety. The School Refusal Assessment Scale (SRAS; Kearney & Silverman, 1993), with parent, teacher, and self-report versions, identifies the maintaining variables of school refusal behavior; this information points to prescriptive treatment approaches. The Parent Anxiety Rating Scale-Separation (Doris, McIntyre, Kelsey, & Lehman, 1971) and the Teacher's Separation Anxiety Scale (Doris et al., 1971) are brief measures of separation distress.

Formulation and Treatment Planning

Seldom is diagnosis alone an adequate basis for treatment planning. The circumstances and vulnerabilities that gave rise to the disorder must be described, the individual's distress and dysfunction outlined, and potential or known obstacles to resolution noted. This is the *formulation* of the case. Biological, psychological, and social factors that predispose the person to have problems, precipitate symptoms, or tend to perpetuate difficulties should be described, as well as protective factors and strengths of the patient or family.

Specific goals and objectives of treatment should be identified. We think it wise to operationalize these goals and objectives whenever possible, in order to allow the clinician, the patient, and the family to recognize what has been achieved. General goals of treatment include reduction of symptoms, prevention of complications, achievement of the best possible functioning in the "real world," and reduction of risk for recurrence or exacerbation.

A treatment plan must address each significant problem identified and should be based upon what is known about efficacy rather than upon the clinician's philosophy.

TREATMENT OF CHILDHOOD ANXIETY DISORDERS

Space restrictions do not allow an exhaustive discussion of all treatment modalities. We will therefore limit our attention first to a discussion of psychosocial treatments for specific anxiety disorders, and then to a discussion of pharmacologic treatment for anxiety disorders in general.

Psychosocial Treatments

Specific Phobia (Simple Phobia)

The behavioral treatment of specific phobias has a long history of demonstrated efficacy. However, similar to the treatment literature of other child anxiety disorders, limited experimental findings exist. For comprehensive views, see Barrios and O'Dell (1989), King (1993), and Ollendick and Francis (1988). King (1993) noted that many phobia treatment studies lack clinically referred subjects with severe phobias, lack multi-method evaluation of phobias, lack long-term follow up analyses, and do not adequately assess the effects of the individual program components. Ollendick and Francis (1988) suggested the need for additional attention paid to developmental issues. Despite these limitations, the treatment of childhood phobias is the most well-researched area of anxiety treatment in children and adolescents. Frequently used interventions include systematic desensitization, flooding, modeling, reinforcement procedures, and cognitive methods. However, the most effective and durable programs use more than one of these techniques simultaneously (Ollendick & Francis, 1988). For a comprehensive discussion concerning the selection of behavioral techniques for specific syndromes, see Barrios and Hartman (1988). In general, all methods of treatment that involve prolonged exposure of the child to the feared situation appear effective (Marks, 1972).

Systematic desensitization is the most frequently researched technique for childhood anxiety disorders (Barrios & O'Dell, 1989). Systematic desensitization involves three main strategies. First, a hierarchy is developed from most to least feared situations or stimuli. Second, the child is taught relaxation (Ollendick & Cerny, 1981). Third, the steps (from least to most fearful situations) in the hierarchy are alternated with relaxation. In a review of 41 studies with over 587 children and adolescents, Barrios and O'Dell (1989) found that systematic desensitization and its variants were highly effective in reducing childhood fears. King (1993) and Ollendick and Francis (1988) have reported that younger children have difficulties with relaxation and generating the images needed for standard systematic desensitization. In vivo desensitization (desensitization with the actual feared stimulus or situation) and emotive imagery (Lazarus & Abramovitz, 1962) are most effective for young children. Emotive imagery entails the child gradually coping with a fear hierarchy with the assistance of an imagined superhero, such as Batman (Jackson & King, 1981; King, Cranstoun, & Josephs, 1989).

In vitro or imaginal flooding involves the child imagining each step in the fear hierarchy until anxiety is no longer experienced. *In vivo flooding* entails the presenting of the actual feared situation until anxiety is reduced. Few clinical studies have been reported with in vivo flooding, possibly due to ethical concerns. Controlled studies of prolonged exposure therapies are severely lacking (Ollendick, 1986; Ollendick & Francis, 1988).

Modeling methods require the child to observe another person coping with the feared stimulus or situation. While a variety of modeling techniques have been examined, those in which the child directly interacts with the feared stimulus with guidance after observing a model successfully cope with the stimulus ("participant" modeling) appear the most effective (King, 1993; Ollendick, 1979). Other characteristics of the model (e.g., similarity to the patient) and of the patient (e.g., defensiveness) influence the efficacy of this approach (Barrios & O'Dell, 1989; King, 1993; Ollendick & Francis, 1988). Barrios and O'Dell (1989) reviewed 30 studies with over 1100 children and found that virtually all treatments were effective, especially with older children. However, the majority of modeling studies have been completed with children with mild or non-clinical fears; as a result, more research with clinical populations is needed (King, 1993; Ollendick, 1979).

Operant and *cognitive-behavioral programs* are also used in the treatment of childhood phobias. Operant methods or contingency management techniques include the use of rewards and/or their withdrawal for approach and avoidance of the feared stimulus, respectively. Such procedures are best used when the fear is clearly observable, and when the child has low motivation for treatment. Cognitive-behavioral programs add the modification of anxious thoughts that are assumed to mediate anxiety symptoms. However, since the majority of these programs have combined cognitive with behavioral methods, it is difficult to determine what cognitive methods actually add to the efficacy of phobia treatment (King, 1993). In those programs that have examined the components of treatment separately, cognitive procedures add little to the program's efficacy (Fox & Houston, 1981; Ollendick, Hagopian, & Huntzinger, 1991; Sheslow, Bondy, & Nelson, 1983). For example, Sheslow et al. (1983) examined coping skills and exposure methods in the treatment of fears of the dark; they found that only the in vivo exposure procedure demonstrated efficacy. Primarily cognitive techniques for treating phobias, such as verbal self-instruction (Graziano & Mooney, 1980, 1982), are most effective with brighter and older children, and are less effective with those who are defensive and lacking in self-control (Barrios & O'Dell, 1989). Further research, using other cognitive approaches to anxiety (e.g., the cognitive restructuring techniques of Beck & Emery, 1985), needs to be completed with children.

Generalized Anxiety Disorder (Overanxious Disorder)

Although a number of clinical researchers have suggested that a compound treatment program consisting of cognitive and behavioral techniques is needed for the reduction of the broad range of symptoms associated with overanxious disorder (Kendall, 1993, 1994; Kendall et al., 1991; Klein & Last, 1989; Last, 1992; Strauss, 1987, 1988), only recently have several outcome studies been completed. Kendall (1994) noted that the lack of empirical investigation is surprising, given that generalized anxiety disorder is one of the most prevalent childhood anxiety disorders, especially in adolescence (Kashani & Orvaschel, 1988, 1990). Strauss (1988) suggested that a program designed to target generalized anxiety should model itself after successful adult programs,(e.g., Barlow, Rapee, & Brown, 1992; Beck & Emery, 1985; Borkovec & Costello, 1993). Citing the lack of treatment research, she proposed a program that included relaxation and visual imagery, positive self-statements, a home-based reward program to encourage skill development, and cognitive coping strategies. Kendall and his associates (1991) reported that important strategies

of intervention include skill development and exposure to fearful situations. Specific techniques include relaxation training, identifying and modifying anxious feelings, bodily responses, and danger thoughts in specific anxiety-provoking situations, and self-evaluation of coping performance. The development of problem-solving skills and contingency management for skill development are also considered important (Kendall et al., 1991).

Kendall (1994) provided the only randomized clinical trial of a psychosocial treatment program for anxiety-disordered children. Forty-seven children, 30 of whom met criteria for overanxious disorder, were successfully treated with a cognitive-behavioral treatment program. The 16-session program consisted of two phases. Eight skill-oriented sessions included training in identifying feelings, constructing a hierarchy of anxiety-provoking situations, relaxation training, identifying and modifying negative self-talk, and self-evaluation and self-reward. The remaining eight sessions provided both in vitro and in vivo exposure to anxiety situations. Clinically significant treatment gains were demonstrated for two-thirds of the treatment subjects across each of the assessment methods utilized. Results were maintained at one year follow-up. Kane and Kendall (1989) also used a multiple baseline design to demonstrate efficacy with overanxious disorder.

Separation Anxiety Disorder

Experimental evidence for the treatment of separation anxiety disorder in children is almost nonexistent (Thyer & Sowers-Hoag, 1988), with only two comparative studies (Blagg & Yule, 1984; Miller, Barrett, Hampe, & Noble, 1972b); the remaining studies have been either single subjects or case studies (Thyer & Sower-Hoag, 1988).

Graduated in vivo exposure (gradual desensitization with the actual feared situation) and in vivo flooding (or "rapid real life exposure") are the primary approaches to treatment of separation anxiety (Klein & Last, 1989; Last, 1992; Thyer & Sower-Hoag, 1988). Rapid real life exposure entails a rapid forced reentry into school. Klein and Last (1989) and Last (1992) reported that while flooding is quicker, premature dropouts are fewer with the more staged approach of graduated exposure. Strauss (1987) suggested that given ethical concerns about forced exposure techniques, flooding should be considered only after other techniques have been attempted without success.

Typical for a behavioral treatment program, Blagg and Yule (1984) treated 30 children with school refusal, though it was unclear how many of the children suffered specifically from separation anxiety. The program consisted of having a trained escort accompany the child to school and to encourage the child to stay at school. Additional program components included providing parents and teachers education concerning the nature of the problem and treatment, reinforcing the child for school attendance, and withdrawal of attention for somatic complaints and distress. Blagg and Yule (1984) reported 93.3 percent of the behavioral treatment group met criteria for success (i.e., returning to school with only minor attendance problems), compared to 37.5 percent and 10 percent for hospitalized and home-tutored groups, respectively. They concluded that behavior therapy was the treatment of choice for school refusal, as well as the most cost effective.

Recent studies have included a combination of techniques. Hagopian and Silfer (1993) used a changing criterion design and successfully treated a six-year-old girl with separation anxiety who additionally experienced school avoidance. Treatment entailed graduated exposure to separation from her mother with reinforcement for appropriate independent behavior. Ollendick and associates (1991) examined combination therapies in the treatment of two children with primarily separation anxiety. The self-control package included techniques common to compound cognitive-behavioral programs, while reinforcement was targeted for independent behaviors (e.g., sleeping alone). Utilizing a multiple baseline design across subjects, both girls demonstrated significant increases in time spent asleep in their own rooms; results were maintained at one- and two-year follow up assessments. Mansdorf and Lukens (1987) successfully treated two separation anxious children with cognitive coping self-statements, cognitive restructuring of the parents' distorted cognitions, and parental contingency management. Both children returned to school within four weeks; attendance continued at three-month follow-up.

Obsessions and Compulsions

Despite the demonstrated efficacy of behavioral treatments for adult obsessive-compulsive disorder, there are no well-controlled experimental studies examining the impact of such behavioral treatment for obsessive thoughts or compulsive behaviors in children. The most frequently used and efficacious intervention approach with children is exposure with response prevention (Berg, Rapoport, & Wolff, 1989; Bernstein & Borchardt, 1991; Johnston & March, 1992; March, Mulle, & Herbel 1994; Swedo, Leonard, & Rapoport,

1992; Wolff & Rapoport, 1988; Wolff & Wolff, 1991). Within-child case studies suggest that graduated and prolonged exposure to the feared stimuli, with prevention of the compulsive behavior, leads to a habituation of the autonomic response to the stimuli, as well as a reduction in the expectation of harm (Foa & Kozac, 1986; Piacentini, Gitow, Jaffer, Graae, & Whitaker, 1994). It is important to note, however, that the majority of studies completed have used compound cognitive-behavioral treatments and family intervention (e.g., see Bolton, Collins, & Steinberg, 1983), and, as a result, have not examined the isolated impact of exposure and response prevention (Berg et al., 1989; Wolff & Rapoport, 1988). Participant modeling, contingency management, and thought stopping are often components of a multi-method treatment package (Berg et al., 1989). Francis and Pinto (1993) suggested that social skills training may also be beneficial. Recent adult treatments for obsessions (see Salkovskis, 1985) have not been examined in younger populations.

Two recent studies have used standardized treatment programs with children suffering from obsessive-compulsive disorder. March et al. (1994) completed an open trial of a compound cognitive-behavioral treatment program for 15 children and adolescents with OCD. Although not all subjects received identical interventions, all received anxiety management training, graduated exposure and response prevention, and some form of family intervention (primarily psychoeducational). Subjects averaged 10 sessions over eight months. Six subjects were asymptomatic at termination, and nine were considered asymptomatic at follow-up, approximately seven months later. Ten subjects achieved a 50 percent or greater reduction in their obsessive-compulsive symptoms. Although the authors concluded that exposure and response prevention were the treatments of choice for childhood obsessive-compulsive disorder, it is important to note that 14 of the 15 patients received concurrent treatments, such as SSRIs or individual psychotherapy. In a second demonstration of a standardized treatment package, Piacentini et al. (1994) completed treatment with three outpatient children for 10 two-hour sessions. Treatment consisted of exposure plus response prevention, the development of coping skills, contingency management, and concurrent family treatment. Treatment was facilitated by graphic presentations of self-reported distress, homework, and home visits. Two of the three children demonstrated clinically significant reductions in obsessive-compulsive symptoms on a variety of measures at termination and one-year follow-up. The remaining child demonstrated minimal to moderate levels of improvement; his lack of progress was attributed to severe emotional disturbance with concurrent family psychopathology. The authors concluded that family intervention, consisting of behavior management, psychoeducational issues, and cognitive restructuring, was particularly important in the treatment of childhood obsessions and compulsions.

Symptoms Associated with Specific Traumas or Stressors

There are no randomized experimental studies examining the usefulness of standardized treatment programs with children suffering from post-traumatic stress disorder (Lipovsky, 1991; Saigh, 1992). However, a series of single-subject design studies (Saigh, 1986, 1987a, 1987b) and one group study (Deblinger, McLeer, & Henry, 1990) reported that the behavioral treatment of post-traumatic stress disorder symptoms involves five basic sequential steps: (a) education of the child and parent concerning the disorder and treatment, (b) development of the child's fear-evoking images, (c) relaxation training, (d) successive presentation of each of the traumatic images, and (e) a period of "debriefing." In addition to these strategies, Lipovsky (1991) suggested that the affective catharsis, the development of coping skills and distraction techniques, and cognitive restructuring were particularly important, and reported that early intervention helps prevent the development of more severe post-traumatic stress disorder symptoms.

In a case example, Saigh (1987a) successfully treated a 14-year-old boy with post-traumatic stress disorder using in vitro flooding. He had been abducted by the Lebanese militia for a period of 48 hours, and subsequently developed avoidance behaviors, depression, and temper problems. A multiple baseline design across traumatic scenes demonstrated that a program of relaxation training and 60-minute sessions of exposure to imagined scenes of the abduction led to a significant reduction in symptoms post-treatment and at four-month follow-up.

In the first clinical trial of a therapy program for sexually-abused children who met criteria for post-traumatic stress disorder, Deblinger et al. (1990) treated 19 females with a 12-session, structured cognitive-behavioral program that consisted of both individual and non-offending parent components. The child intervention consisted of modeled coping skills training, imaginal exposure to abuse-related memories, and education concerning prevention of future abuse. The parent component consisted of educational material, cognitive re-

structuring, the development of communication skills with the child, and behavior modification skills. Based upon multi-method assessment, children demonstrated significant reductions in specific post-traumatic stress disorder symptoms, as well as internalizing and externalizing symptoms at post-treatment.

Social Phobia and Avoidant Social Behaviors

There are no empirical treatment studies of avoidant disorder or social phobia in children or adolescents (Last, 1992). Although it is generally assumed that the clinical picture of social phobia in adults is similar to that of children (Beidel & Randall, 1993), this assumption lacks empirical validation (Clark et al., 1994). As with other childhood disorders, a successful adult program could provide a good model for treatment of social phobia. Heimberg and Juster (1994) describe an adult cognitive-behavioral group treatment program and present supporting evidence for its efficacy. This program has goals of reducing anxiety in social situations, and modifying beliefs contributing to social anxiety. Specific components of the program include (a) a cognitive-behavioral rationale, (b) training in cognitive restructuring, (c) exposure to simulated social situations, (d) using cognitive restructuring in simulated social situations, (e) homework assignments for in vivo exposure, and (f) cognitive restructuring of in vivo experiences. In noting that some socially phobic children suffer from a lack of social skills, while others primarily suffer from social anxiety, Last (1992) reported that a social skills training approach seems to be effective with both problem areas; social skills training simultaneously teaches skills and exposes children to their social fears.

Panic Disorder

As in the case with social phobia in children and adolescents, there are apparently no empirical studies that examine psychosocial treatments of panic disorder in children and adolescents. Nelles and Barlow (1988) theorized that children may not have the "cognitive capacity" to develop panic disorder. However, it is clear that adolescents suffer from adult-like panic disorder (Moreau & Weissman, 1992). Adult approaches to panic (McNally, 1990), such as those described by Clark (1986) and Barlow and his colleagues (Barlow, Craske, Cerny, & Klosko, 1989) appear particularly promising. For example, Clark focuses on modifying the catastrophic misinterpretations of the bodily sensations associated with panic through behavioral exercises and cognitive restructuring.

Pharmacological Treatments

Rigorous, well-designed studies of the safety and effectiveness of medications used to reduce anxiety in children and adolescents are few. The decision to use medication for these disorders, therefore, must be based upon a careful assessment of potential risks versus potential benefits, given the limited amount of information available. Specific goals or target symptoms should be identified and documented, and the child and family should give consent after an explanation that includes goals, risks, and the limitations of current knowledge. When medication is prescribed, the choice of medication should be appropriate to target symptoms. Regarding the drug information that follows, the reader is encouraged to consult the product information sheet and other comprehensive references on psychopharmacology for dosage information and contraindications for any drug considered for administration, as the following is not intended to serve as a treatment manual for pediatric psychopharmocology. For a review of the pediatric psychopharmacology of anxiety, please see Allen, Leonard, & Swedo (1995) and Kutcher, Reiter, & Gardner (1995).

Buspirone may decrease generalized anxiety after several weeks of treatment with doses ranging from 5 to 10 mg three or four times a day (Simeon et al., 1994). Limited clinical experience suggests that adverse effects are unusual, generally consisting of transient nausea, headaches, or mild sedation, but therapeutic benefit has not been unequivocally established.

Benzodiazepines may reduce generalized anxiety and anticipatory anxiety. Their action may be more rapid than buspirone, but ill effects are not rare and range from oversedation to agitation, and both psychological and physiologic dependence are possible. Diazepam is typical of longer-acting benzodiazepines; alprazolam is an example of a member of this class with a shorter half-life. Shorter half-life is probably associated with a greater risk for withdrawal symptoms among young people, as it is with adults. Diazepam doses range from 2 to 5 mg (up to 10 mg in older adolescents) per dose, three or four times a day. Alprazolam is given in doses of 0.5 to 2 mg per day, in divided doses three or four times per day, and has been reported beneficial for childhood anxiety in some cases (Simeon et al., 1992). Lorazepam (0.5 to 2 mg two to three times a day) has been used to reduce preoperative anxiety, agitation in intensive care settings, and as a preanesthetic; its use for primary anx-

iety has not been thoroughly evaluated. Recommended dosing of clonazepam ranges from 0.25 to 1 mg per day, in divided doses.

Imipramine and other *tricyclic antidepressants* have been utilized to reduce the frequency and intensity of panic-type symptoms in separation anxiety and panic disorder. Results from the one controlled study of patients similar to typical primary care school refusers were positive (Gittleman-Klein & Klein, 1971). A decision to use imipramine might take impetus from severity of symptoms or associated impairment, or from the presence of comorbid enuresis or attention deficit disorder, conditions that also may be improved by imipramine. Adverse effects generally are limited to mild anticholinergic effects (dry mouth, constipation, blurred vision, and orthostatic hypotension), but the potential to precipitate mania is present (especially if the individual or a relative has been manic) and the possibility of cardiotoxicity must be considered (Spencer, Wilens, & Biederman, 1995). Desipramine, a secondary amine tricyclic and a metabolite of imipramine, is available for prescription but its use in children is particularly controversial due to four cases of sudden unexplained death in children taking relatively low doses (Riddle et al., 1991). Because of this and its not having been demonstrated to be effective in child or adolescent anxiety disorders, its use in these disorders cannot be recommended.

Before beginning treatment of anxiety with imipramine or other tricyclic compounds, a baseline electrocardiogram is advisable. The electrocardiogram should be repeated when a stable dose is reached or when the dose exceeds 3 mg/kg of body weight for imipramine, and periodically thereafter. Parent and child must be warned about the dangers of overdose. Starting dose of imipramine may be as little as 10 mg per day in a younger child, or as much as 50 mg in a large adolescent. For adults, a single bedtime dose often suffices; children, with their relatively larger and more efficient livers, may require divided doses to sustain adequate blood levels. The amount and timing of dose increases depend upon the child's tolerance of the medicine, severity of symptoms, and responses to the previous dose. Caution and careful monitoring of vital signs and electrocardiogram are especially important if doses exceed 3.5 mg/kg/day (Spencer et al., 1995).

Amitriptyline and its metabolite nortriptyline have also been prescribed, often for target symptoms such as panic attacks and insomnia, although their efficacy and safety for children with these conditions has not been established. If their use is elected, safety guidelines like those for imipramine should be followed. Amitriptyline is a tertiary amine like imipramine, and similar doses are probably appropriate; nortriptyline is more potent and is usually prescribed at about half to two-thirds the dose.

Finally, clomipramine has demonstrated efficacy for OCD in children and adolescents (e.g., Leonard et al., 1989). Symptom control may be achieved in days or only after several weeks of treatment; effective doses in young people range from 50–150 mg/day, in divided doses. This medication is moderately sedating and anticholinergic, can precipitate seizures, and should be presumed to have potential for cardiotoxicity similar to that of the other tricyclics discussed above.

The antihypertensive *propranolol* may have a place in treatment of panic attacks, and with "stage fright" and other forms of performance anxiety, especially in adolescents. It should be avoided in young people with asthma and used cautiously in those with other severe allergic symptoms. Dizziness and sedation are common side effects; 10 to 80 mg three or four times a day is the usual dose range.

Monoamine oxidase inhibitors (MAOIs) have been used successfully to reduce panic attacks in adults, but their routine use in children or adolescents is not recommended. Tyramine-rich foods, including aged cheeses, organ meats, red wine and dark beers, must be avoided to prevent hypertensive crisis; these dietary restrictions may be objectionable and difficult to enforce in young people. Furthermore, drug interactions are common and must also be guarded against. In carefully selected cases, their use by a physician with experience in the use of MAOIs in teenagers may be appropriate.

Serotonin-specific reuptake inhibitors (SSRIs) are widely prescribed for depression and obsessive-compulsive disorder in adults. Preliminary studies suggest that SSRIs may effectively reduce obsessions or compulsions in young people, as well (Riddle et al., 1992). The SSRIs can cause agitation, anorexia, GI symptoms such as nausea, and irritability. Adults on SSRIs commonly complain of sexual side effects such as anorgasmia, impotence, and reduced libido; these may be problematic for adolescents even if they are not sexually active. SSRIs also require careful consideration of potential drug interactions, including increased clearance and altered blood levels of antipsychotics, tricyclics, and anticonvulsants. Restlessness, akathisia, and worsening anxiety are also possible. Concurrent use of SSRIs with MAOIs is contraindicated due to potentially life-threatening interactions.

Many clinicians are nevertheless more comfortable with SSRIs than tricyclics, because the SSRIs appear to have less cardiotoxicity and are less likely to be lethal in overdose. Case reports and small series suggest some children and adolescents with anxiety disorders may benefit from SSRIs (Birmaher et al., 1994). Fluoxetine has a very long half-life—measurable in days—and doses may have to be adjusted accordingly. Starting doses of 10–20 mg are common; lower doses can be given by using the liquid preparation. The usual starting dose for sertraline is 25 or 50 mg/day. Generally beginning with low doses and gradually increasing to therapeutic levels may be especially important in anxious children and adolescents, who may be particularly prone to early side effects of restlessness and an increase in anxiety (Kutcher et al., 1995).

Antihistamines such as diphenhydramine and hydroxyzine have historically been prescribed fairly often for childhood anxiety and other symptoms requiring calmatives. Children generally tolerate antihistamines well, but anticholinergic effects are frequent and occasionally a paradoxical agitation is seen. If these medicines have any benefit to the anxious child, it is probably directly attributable to their sedative properties. When these antihistamines are used as temporary anxiolytics, 10–50 mg per day usually suffices, either at bedtime (for sleeplessness or other nighttime symptoms) or in divided doses.

Other sedating medications that have been used by many practitioners historically include *neuroleptics* such as thioridazine. We do not recommend their use for uncomplicated anxiety, since their effectiveness as anxiolytics is not established and the potential for drug-induced movement disorders is present.

CASE ILLUSTRATION

Clinical Presentation

Ten-year-old William came to the child psychiatrist's office after his school counselor and school psychological examiner were unable to account for his worsening school performance. During the first quarter of his fourth grade year, he made his usual "B" average, then incomplete work assignments and poor test grades became usual in all subjects.

Assessment Findings

Intelligence testing and academic achievement tests were not suggestive of learning or attention deficit disorders, but the psychological examiner noted an unusually restricted affect and wondered if the child was depressed. William's mother agreed that he seemed preoccupied and less often happy during the past six weeks or so, but said he had not been able or willing to tell his parents about anything that was especially bothering him. She had asked if anyone had "done anything bad" to him, and he said no. She noted only one other change in his behavior: his previous broad range of play activities had narrowed to a single martial-arts-type video game, which he played over and over, becoming very adept. He still played with his friends, but tried to get them to play that particular game with him. His mother also thought he was more easily startled than he had been previously. Because William was not very forthcoming on direct questioning, weekly sessions were scheduled to continue the assessment. The psychiatrist suspected post-traumatic stress disorder because of the startle response and the altered play pattern, but felt the patient would not reveal any trauma until some trust was achieved.

In the middle of a checkers game during the third visit, William revealed he had a "terrible secret" he had been wanting to tell someone, but was afraid. About three months before, walking home through a local park, along the outfield fence of the baseball field, he heard a gunshot in the bleachers behind home plate; when he looked, he saw a man fall down and saw two other men running away. The distance was such that he could not even see the skin color of the men, but he ran home and had since been scared they would think he could identify them.

The scene replayed frequently in William's mind, and he avoided walking anywhere near the park in question. He denied nightmares or insomnia, and was surprised when the psychiatrist mentioned a possible connection between his recent preoccupation with the one video game and the event witnessed. He acknowledged being worried the gunmen might pursue him but said that the main thing bothering him was "seeing it over and over," no matter where he was.

Treatment Selection and Course

First, William was persuaded to reveal his experience to his parents. With his and his parents' consent, the psychiatrist contacted the police, who confirmed that the shooting had taken place. The victim was wounded but not killed, and had identified the perpetrators. One was in custody; the police believed the other had fled the state. Although William and his parents had hoped that his symptoms would stop when he could be assured he was not in danger, this was not the case. His frustration at the continuing symptoms began to result in temper outbursts,

which he had not had since he was a toddler. Medical, psychotherapeutic, and combined treatment options were discussed with the child and parents; the parents preferred to try psychotherapy alone first.

Twice-weekly sessions began with relaxation training sessions of twenty minutes followed by video-game play as reinforcement for participation. After three sessions William was achieving deep relaxation in less than ten minutes, and *in vivo* exposure began. William's father provided a photo of the baseball field, and William, once relaxed, was asked to look at the photo. He tolerated this well and gradual desensitization proceeded over four sessions to visualization of the shooting. The final session was a "field trip" to the baseball field, with William doing his relaxation exercise in the car on the way. This was well tolerated. Thus, *in vivo* exposure to the site was accomplished in eight sessions (four weeks). During this time his school performance gradually improved and his affect became less blunted and more positive. He still had intrusive visual memories at times, but they had much less impact. The martial arts video game continued to be a favorite play activity, but not the only play activity.

Termination and Follow-Up

William showed several classical symptoms of post traumatic stress disorder: intrusive visual memories, being easily startled, avoidance of the site of the trauma, and poor concentration. His nearly-obsessive play pattern with the martial video game can be understood as post-traumatic play, allowing him to have vicarious control and gain mastery of a violent and threatening situation, even if the game situation did not closely parallel the real-life events.

The traumatic memory was treated as if it were a phobic stimulus. The goal then was to reduce the memory's power to cause distress and dysfunction (poor concentration leading to poor schoolwork.) This approach to treatment resulted in significant improvement. A trial of medication would not have been inherently unreasonable; in fact, fluoxetine (to decrease the frequency of intrusive thoughts, as if they were obsessions) or buspirone (to reduce the generalized tension and hypervigilance) were considered and discussed.

If William had been given the combination of medical and psychological treatment and had improved as he did with psychological treatment alone, the psychiatrist would have had to make some surmise as to what helped, and to make decisions about how long to continue medication. If medicine had been prescribed and treatment resources were in short supply relative to demand, the temptation to defer psychological treatment or to schedule it less often would be real and might be a disservice to this patient. For these reasons, we suggest that psychosocial treatments will usually be the most appropriate first-line modalities when distress and impairment are in the mild to moderate range—although we believe patients and parents are entitled to a thorough discussion of all treatment options.

Combined medical and psychosocial modalities should definitely be considered when impairment or distress are severe, or when an adequate trial of appropriately specific psychosocial treatment has not had the desired result. Only in the most unusual circumstances will we recommend medication alone.

Three months following completion of treatment, William remained improved, with more positive affect, less restricted play, diminished intrusive visual memories, and improved school performance, with his grades returning to above average.

SUMMARY

Anxiety symptoms and disorders are prevalent in childhood and adolescence and frequently cause significant distress or impairment. They are common in medical settings, where they may present with somatic symptoms and illness worry, as well as frequent school absences. Following a thorough medical and psychological assessment, a diagnosis, formulation, and treatment plan can be devised. Pharmacotherapy may be helpful in some cases, and for many of these disorders, there is considerable evidence for the effectiveness of behavioral and cognitive treatments.

REFERENCES

Achenbach, T. M. (1993). Implications of multiaxial empirically based assessment for behavior therapy with children. *Behavior Therapy, 24*, 91–116.

Achenbach, T. M., & Edelbrock, C. S. (1979). The Child Behavior Profile: 1. Boys aged 6-11. *Journal of Consulting and Clinical Psychology, 46*, 478–488.

Achenbach, T. M., & Edelbrock, C. S. (1986). *Manual for the Teacher's Report Form and the teacher version of the Child Behavior Profile*. Burlington: U. Vermont Dept. Psychiatry.

Achenbach, T. M., & McConaughy, S. H. (1987). *Empirically based assessment of child and adolescent psychopathology: Practical applications*. Newbury Park, CA: Sage Publications, Inc.

Achenbach, T. M., McConaughy, S. H., & Howell, C. T. (1987). Child/adolescent behavioral and emotional problems: Implications of cross-informant correlations for situational specificity. *Psychological Bulletin, 101*, 213–232.

Allen, A. J., Leonard, H., & Swedo, S. E. (1995). Current knowledge of medications for the treatment of childhood anxiety disorders. *Journal of the American Academy of Child and Adolescent Psychiatry, 34*, 976–986.

American Psychiatric Association. (1994). *Diagnostic and statistical manual of mental disorders (4th ed.)*. Washington, DC: Author.

American Psychiatric Association. (1980). *Diagnostic and statistical manual of mental disorders (3rd ed.)*. Washington, DC: Author.

Anderson, J. C., Williams, S., McGee, R., & Silva, P. A. (1987). DSM-III disorders in pre-adolescent children: Prevalence in a large sample from the general population. *Archives of General Psychiatry, 44*, 69–76.

Barcai, A., & Rosenthal, M. K. (1974). Fears and tyranny. *Archives of General Psychiatry, 30*, 392–395.

Barlow, D. H., Craske, M. G., Cerny, J. A., & Klosko, J. (1989). Behavioral treatment of panic disorder. *Behavior Therapy, 20*, 261–282.

Barlow, D. H., Rapee, R. M., & Brown, T. A. (1992). Behavioral treatment of generalized anxiety disorder. *Behavioral Therapy, 23*, 551–570.

Barrios, B. A., & Hartmann, D. P. (1988). Fears and anxieties. In E. J. Mash & L. G. Terdal (Eds.), *Behavioral assessment of childhood disorders, 2nd ed.* Guilford Press: New York.

Barrios, B. A., & O'Dell, S. L. (1989). Fears and anxieties. In E. J. Mash & R. A. Barkley (Eds.), *Treatment of childhood disorders*. New York: Guilford Press.

Beck, A. T., Brown, G., Epstein, N., & Steer, R. A. (1988). An inventory for measuring clinical anxiety: Psychometric properties. *Journal of Consulting and Clinical Psychology, 56*, 893–897.

Beck, A. T., & Emery, G. (1985). *Anxiety disorders and phobias: A cognitive perspective*. New York: Basic Books.

Beidel, D. C., & Randall, J. (1993). Social phobia. In T. Ollendick & M. Hersen (Eds.), *Handbook of child and adolescent assessment*. Boston: Allyn & Bacon.

Berg, C. Z., Rapoport, J. L., & Wolff, R. P. (1989). *Behavioral treatment for obsessive-compulsive disorder in children and adolescents*. Washington, DC: American Psychiatric Press.

Bernstein, G. A. (1991). Comorbidity and severity of anxiety and depressive disorders in a clinic sample. *Journal of the American Academy of Child and Adolescent Psychiatry, 30*, 43–50.

Bernstein, G. A., & Borchardt, C. M. (1991). Anxiety disorders of childhood and adolescence: A critical review. *Journal of the American Academy of Child and Adolescent Psychiatry, 30*, 519–532.

Birmaher, B., Waterman, G. S., Ryan, N., Cully, M., Balach, L., Ingram, J., & Brodsky, M. (1994). Fluoxetine for childhood and anxiety disorders. *Journal of the American Academy of Child and Adolescent Psychiatry, 33*, 993–999.

Blagg, N. R., & Yule, W. (1984). The behavioral treatment of school refusal: A comparative study. *Behavioral Research and Therapy, 22*, 119–127.

Bolton, D., Collings, S., & Steinberg, D. (1983). The treatment of obsessive-compulsive disorder in adolescence: A report of fifteen cases. *British Journal of Psychiatry, 142*, 456–464.

Borkovec, T. D., & Costello, E. (1993). Efficacy of applied relaxation and cognitive-behavioral therapy in the treatment of generalized anxiety disorder. *Journal of Consulting and Clinical Psychology, 61*, 611–619.

Chambers, W. J., Puig-Antich, J., & Tabrizi, M. A. (1978). *The ongoing treatment of the Kiddie-SADS.* Paper presented at the annual meeting of the American Academy of Child Psychiatry, San Diego.

Clark, D. B., & Donovan, J. E. (1984). Reliability and validity of the Hamilton Anxiety Rating Scale in an adolescent sample. *Journal of the American Academy of Child and Adolescent Psychiatry, 33*, 354–360.

Clark, D. B., Smith, M. G., Neighbors, B. D., Skerlec, L. M., & Randall, J. (1994). Anxiety disorders in adolescence: Characteristics, prevalence, and comorbidities. *Clinical Psychology Review, 14*, 113–137.

Deblinger, E., McLeer, S. V., & Henry, D. (1990). Cognitive behavioral treatment of sexually abused children suffering posttraumatic stress: Preliminary findings. *Journal of the American Academy of Child and Adolescent Psychiatry, 29*, 747–752.

Doris, J., McIntyre, A., Kelsey, C., & Lehman, E. (1971). Separation anxiety in nursery school children. *Proceedings of the 79th Annual Convention of the American Psychological Association, 79*, 145–146.

Eason, L. J., Finch, A. J., Brasted, W., & Saylor, C. F. (1985). The assessment of depression and anxiety in hospitalized pediatric patients. *Child Psychiatry and Human Development, 16*, 57–64.

Finch, A. J., Lipovsky, J. A., & Casat, C. D. (1989). Anxiety and depression in children and adolescents: Negative affectivity or separate constructs? In P. C. Kendall & D. Watson (Eds.), *Anxiety and depression: Distinctive and overlapping features* (pp. 172–202). New York: Academic Press.

Finch, A. J., & McIntosh, J. A. (1990). Assessment of fears and anxieties in children. In A. M. La Greca (Ed.), *Through the eyes of the child: Obtaining self-reports from children and adolescents.* Boston: Allyn & Bacon.

Finch, A. J., & Rogers, T. (1984). Self-report instruments. In T. Ollendick & M. Hersen (Eds.), *Child behavioral assessment: Principles and procedures.* New York: Pergamon Press.

Foa, E., & Kozac, M. (1986). Emotional processing of fear: Exposure to corrective information. *Psychological Bulletin, 99*, 450–472.

Fox, J. E. & Houston, B. K. (1981). Efficacy of self-instructional training for reducing children's anxiety in an evaluative situation. *Behavior Research and Therapy, 19*, 509–515.

Fox, J. E., & Houston, B. K. (1983). Distinguishing between cognitive and somatic trait and state anxiety in children. *Journal of Personality and Social Psychology, 45*, 862–870.

Francis, G., & Pinto, A. (1993). Obsessive-compulsive disorder. In R. T. Ammerman, C. G. Last, & M. Hersen (Eds.), *Handbook of prescriptive treatments for children and adolescents.* Boston: Allyn & Bacon.

Gadow, K., & Sprafkin, J. (1994): *The Child Symptom Inventory.* Checkmate Plus, Box 696, Stony Brook, N.Y.

Gittleman-Klein, R., & Klein, D. (1971). Controlled imipramine treatment of school phobia. *Archives of General Psychiatry, 25*, 204–207.

Goodman, W. K., Price, L. H., Rasmussen, S. A., Masure, C., Fleischmann, R. L., Hill, C. L., Henninger, G. R., & Charney, D. S. (1989). The Yale-Brown obsessive compulsive scale, I: Development, use, and reliability. *Archives of General Psychiatry, 46*, 1006–1011.

Graziano, A. M., & Mooney, K. C. (1980). Family self-control instruction for children's nighttime fear reduction. *Journal of Consulting and Clinical Psychology, 48*, 206–13.

Graziano, A. M., & Mooney, K. C. (1982). Behavioral treatment of "nightfears" in children: Maintenance of improvement at 2½ to 3-year follow up. *Journal of Consulting and Clinical Psychology, 50*, 598–599.

Guy, W. (1976). *ECDEU assessment manual for psychopharmacology.* Washington, DC: U.S. Department of Health, Education, and Welfare.

Hagopian, L. P., & Slifer, K. J. (1993). Treatment of separation anxiety disorder with graduated exposure and reinforcement targeting school attendance: A controlled case study. *Journal of Anxiety Disorders, 7*, 271–280.

Hamilton, M. (1959). The assessment of anxiety states by rating. *British Journal of Medical Psychology, 32*, 50–55.

Heimberg, R. G., & Juster, H. R. (1994). Treatment of social phobia in cognitive-behavioral groups. *Journal of Clinical Psychiatry, 55*, 38–46.

Hodges, K. (1993). Structured interviews for assessing children. *Journal of Child Psychology and Psychiatry, 34*, 49–68.

Hodges, K., & Cools, J. N. (1990). Structured diagnostic interviews. In A. M. La Greca (Ed.), *Through the eyes of the child: Obtaining self-reports from children and adolescents.* Boston: Allyn & Bacon.

Hughes, J. N. (1988). *Cognitive behavior therapy with children in the schools.* New York: Pergamon Press.

Jackson, H. J. E., & King, N. J. (1981). The emotive imagery treatment of a child's trauma-induced phobia. *Journal of Behavior Therapy and Experimental Psychiatry, 12*, 325–328.

Johnston, H. F., & March, J. S. (1992). Obsessive compulsive disorder in children and adolescents. In W. M. Reynolds (Ed.), *Internalizing disorders in children and adolescents.* New York: John Wiley and Sons, Inc.

Jolly, J. B., Aruffo, J. F., Wherry, J. N., & Livingston, R. L. (1993). The utility of the Beck Anxiety Inventory with inpatient adolescents. *Journal of Anxiety Disorder, 7*, 95–106.

Kane, M. T., & Kendall, P. C. (1989). Anxiety disorders in children: A multiple-baseline evaluation of a cognitive-behavioral treatment. *Behavior Therapy, 20*, 499–508.

Kashani, J. H., & Orvaschel, H. (1988). Anxiety disorders in mid-adolescence: A community sample. *American Journal of Psychiatry, 145*, 960–964.

Kashani, J. H., & Orvaschel, H. (1990). A community study of anxiety in children and adolescents. *American Journal of Psychiatry, 147*, 313–318.

Kearney, C. A., & Silverman, W. K. (1993). Measuring the function of school refusal behavior: The School Refusal Assessment Scale. *Journal of Clinical Child Psychology, 22*, 85–96.

Kendall, P. C. (1993). Cognitive-behavioral therapies with youth: Guiding theory, current status, and emerging developments. *Journal of Consulting and Clinical Psychology, 61*, 235–247.

Kendall, P. C. (1994). Treating anxiety disorders in children: Results of a randomized clinical trial. *Journal of Consulting and Clinical Psychology, 62*, 100–110.

Kendall, P. C., Chansky, T. W., Freidman, M., Kim, R., Kortlander, E., Sessa, F. M., & Siqueland, L. (1991). Treating anxiety disorders in children and adolescents. In P. C. Kendall (Ed.), *Child & adolescent therapy: Cognitive-behavioral procedures.* New York: Guilford Press.

King, N. J. (1993). Simple and social phobias. In T. H. Ollendick & R. J. Prinz (Eds.), *Advances in clinical child psychology.* New York: Plenum Press.

King, N. J., Cranstoun, F., & Josephs, A. (1989). Emotive imagery and children's nighttime fears: A multiple baseline design evaluation. *Journal of Behavior Therapy and Experimental Psychiatry, 20*, 125–135.

Klein, R. G. (1991). Parent-child agreement in clinical assessment of anxiety and other psychopathology: A review. *Journal of Anxiety Disorder*, 187–198.

Klein, R. G., & Last, C. G. (1989). *Anxiety disorders in children.* Newbury Park, CA: Sage Publications, Inc.

Kutcher, S., Reiter, S., & Gardner, D. (1995). Pharmacotherapy: Approaches and applications. In J. S. March (Ed.), *Anxiety disorders in children and adolescents* (pp. 341–385). New York: Guilford Press.

La Greca, A. M., Dandes, S. K., Wick, P., Shaw, K., & Stone, W. L. (1988). Development of the Social Anxiety Scale for Children: Reliability and concurrent validity. *Journal of Clinical Child Psychology, 17*, 84–91.

Last, C. G. (1986). *Modification of the Schedule for Affective Disorders and Schizophrenia for School-Aged Children (Present Episode) (K-SADS).* Unpublished manuscript.

Last, C. G. (1992). Anxiety disorders in childhood and adolescence. In W. M. Reynolds (Ed.), *Internalizing disorders in children and adolescents.* New York: John Wiley and Sons, Inc.

Last, C. G., Francis, G., & Strauss, C. C. (1989). Assessing fears in anxiety-disordered children with the Revised Fear Survey Schedule for Children (FSSC-R). *Journal of Clinical Child Psychology, 18*, 137–141.

Lazarus, A. A., & Abramovitz, A. (1962). The use of "emotive imagery" in the treatment of children's phobias. *Journal of Mental Science, 1989*, 1991–1995.

Leonard, H. L., Swedo, S. E., Rapoport, J. L., Koby, E. V., Lenane, M. C., Cheslow, D. L., & Hamburger, S. D. (1989). Treatment of obsessive compulsive disorder with clomipramine and desipramine in children and adolescents. *Archives of General Psychiatry, 46*, 1088–1092.

Lipovsky, J. A. (1991). Posttraumatic stress disorder in children. *Family and Community Health, 14*, 42–51.

Livingston, R., Nugent, H., Rader, L., & Smith, G. R. (1985). Family histories of depressed and severely anxious children. *American Journal of Psychiatry, 142*, 1497–1499.

Mansdorf, I. J., & Lukens, E. (1987). Cognitive-behavioral psychotherapy for separating anxious children exhibiting school phobia. *Journal of the American Academy of Child and Adolescent Psychiatry, 26*, 222–225.

March, J. S., Mulle, K., & Herbel, B. (1994). Behavioral psychotherapy for children and adolescents with obsessive compulsive disorder: An open trail of a new protocol-driven treatment package. *Journal of the American Academy of Child and Adolescent Psychiatry, 33*, 333–341.

Marks, I. A. (1972). Flooding (implosion) and allied treatments. In S. Agras (Ed.), *Behavior modification: Principles and clinical applications*. Boston: Little, Brown.

McNally, R. J. (1990). Psychological approaches to panic disorder: A review. *Psychological Bulletin, 108*, 403–419.

Miller, L. C., Barrett, C. L., Hampe, E., & Noble, H. (1972a). Factor structure of childhood fears. *Journal of Consulting and Clinical Psychology, 39*, 264–268.

Miller, L. C., Barrett, C. L., Hampe, E., & Noble, H. (1972b). Comparison of reciprocal inhibition, psychotherapy, and waiting list control for phobic children. *Journal of Abnormal Psychology, 79*, 269–279.

Moreau, D., & Weissman, M. M. (1992). Panic disorder in children and adolescents: A review. *American Journal of Psychiatry, 149*, 1306–1314.

Nelles, W. B., & Barlow, D. H. (1988). Do children panic? *Clinical Psychology Review, 8*, 359–372.

Ollendick, T. H. (1979). Fear reduction techniques with children. In M. Hersen, R. M. Eisler, & P. M. Miller (Eds.), *Progress in behavior modification*. New York: Academic Press.

Ollendick, T. H. (1983). Reliability and validity of the Revised Fear Survey Schedule for Children (FSSC-R). *Behavior Research and Therapy, 21*, 685–692.

Ollendick, T. H. (1986). Behavior therapy with children and adolescents. In S. L. Garfield & A. E. Bergin (Eds.), *Handbook of psychotherapy and behavior change (3rd ed.)* New York: John Wiley and Sons, Inc.

Ollendick, T. H., & Cerny, J. A. (1981). *Clinical behavior therapy with children*. New York: Plenum Press.

Ollendick, T. H., & Francis, G. (1988). Behavioral assessment and treatment of childhood phobias. *Behavior Modification, 12*, 165–204.

Ollendick, T. H., Hagopian, L. P., & Huntzinger, R. M. (1991). Cognitive-behavioral therapy with nighttime fearful children. *Journal of Behavioral Therapy and Experimental Psychiatry, 22*, 113–121.

Perrin, S., & Last, C. G. (1992). Do childhood anxiety measures measure anxiety? *Journal of Abnormal Child Psychology, 20*, 567–578.

Piacentini, J., Gitow, A., Jaffer, M., Graae, F., & Whitaker, A. (1994). Outpatient behavioral treatment of child and adolescent obsessive compulsive disorder. *Journal of Anxiety Disorders, 8*, 277–289.

Rapee, R. M., Barrett, P. M., Dadds, M. R., & Evans, L. (1994). Reliability of the DSM-III-R childhood anxiety disorders using structured interview: Inter-rater and parent-child agreement. *Journal of the American Academy of Child and Adolescent Psychiatry, 33*, 984–992.

Reynolds, C. R., & Richmond, B. O. (1978). What I think and feel: A revised measure of children's manifest anxiety. *Journal of Abnormal Child Psychology, 6*, 278–280.

Riddle, M. A., Scahill, L., King, R. A., Hardin, M. T., Anderson, G. M., Ort, S. I., Smith, J. C., Leckman, J. F., & Cohen, D. J. (1992). Double-blind, crossover trial of fluoxetine and placebo in children and adolescents with obsessive compulsive disorder. *Journal of the American Academy of Child and Adolescent Psychiatry, 31:6*, 1062–1069.

Riddle, M. A., Nelson, J. C., Kleinman, C. S., Rasmusson, A., Leckman, J. F., King, R. A., & Cohen, D. J. (1991). Sudden death in children receiving norpramin: A review of three reported cases and commentary. *Journal of the American Academy of Child and Adolescent Psychiatry, 30*, 104–108.

Russo, M. F., & Beidel, D. C. (1994). Comorbidity of childhood anxiety and externalizing disorders: Prevalence, associated characteristics, and validation issues. *Clinical Psychology Review, 14*, 199–221.

Saigh, P. A. (1986). In vitro flooding of a 6 yr-old boy's posttraumatic stress disorder. *Behaviour Research and Therapy, 24*, 685–688.

Saigh, P.A. (1987a). In vitro flooding of an adolescent's posttraumatic stress disorder. *Journal of Clinical Child Psychology, 16*, 147–150.

Saigh, P. A. (1987b). In vitro flooding of childhood posttraumatic stress disorder. A systematic replication. *Professional School Psychology, 2*, 133–145.

Saigh, P. A. (1992). The behavioral treatment of child and adolescent posttraumatic stress disorder. *Advances in Behavioral Treatment and Research, 14*, 247–275.

Salkovskis, P. M. (1985). Obsessional-compulsive problems: A cognitive-behavioral analysis. *Behaviour Research and Therapy, 23*, 571–583.

Sheslow, D. V., Bondy, A. S., & Nelson, R. O. (1982). A comparison of graduated exposure, verbal coping skills, and their combination in the treatment of children's fear of the dark. *Child and Family Behavior Therapy, 4*, 33–45.

Silverman, W. K. (1991). Diagnostic reliability of anxiety disorders in children using structured interviews. *Journal of Anxiety Disorders, 5*, 105–124.

Silverman, W. K., & Nelles, W. B. (1988). The Anxiety Disorders Interview Schedule for Children. *Journal of the American Academy of Child and Adolescent Psychiatry, 27*, 772–778.

Simeon, J. G., Ferguson, H. B., Knott, V., et al. (1992). Clinical, cognitive and neuropsychological effects of alprazolam in children and adolescents with overanxious and avoidant disorders. *Journal of the American Academy of Child and Adolescent Psychiatry, 31*, 29–33.

Simeon, J. G., Knott, V. J., Dubois, C., et al. (1994). Buspirone therapy of mixed anxiety disorders in childhood and adolescence: A pilot study. *Journal of Child and Adolescent Psychopharmacology, 4,* 159–170.

Spencer, T., Wilens, T., & Biederman, J. (1995). Psychotropic medication for children and adolescents. *Child and Adolescent Psychiatric Clinics of North America, 4,* 97–121.

Spielberger, C. D. (1983). *Manual for the State-Trait Anxiety Inventory (Form Y).* Palo Alto, CA: Consulting Psychologists Press.

Strauss, C. C. (1987). Anxiety. In M. Hersen & V. B. Van Hasselt (Eds.), *Behavioral therapy with children and adolescents: A clinical approach.* New York: Pergamon Press.

Strauss, C. C. (1988). Behavioral assessment and treatment of overanxious disorder. *Behavior Modification, 12,* 234–251.

Swedo, S. E., Leonard, H. L., & Rapoport, J. L. (1992). Childhood-onset obsessive compulsive disorder. *Pediatric Clinics of North America, 15,* 767–775.

Terr, L. (1990). *Too scared to cry.* New York: Harper & Row.

Thyer, B. A., & Sowers-Hoag, K. M. (1988). Behavior therapy of separation anxiety disorder. *Behavior Modification, 12,* 205–233.

Wierzbicki, M. (1987). A parent form of the Children's Depression Inventory: Reliability and validity in nonclinical populations. *Journal of Clinical Psychology, 43,* 390–397.

Wolff, R., & Rapoport, J. L. (1988). Behavioral treatment of childhood obsessive compulsive disorder. *Behavior Modification, 12,* 252–256.

Wolff, R. P., & Wolff, L. S. (1991). Assessment and treatment of obsessive compulsive disorder in children. *Behavior Modification, 15,* 372–393.

CHAPTER 13

AFFECTIVE DISORDERS

Marla Y. Hooks
Elizabeth McCauley

DESCRIPTION OF DISORDERS

Over the last decade studies of affective disturbance in young people have burgeoned, leading to increased acceptance and understanding of mood disorders in this population. This chapter provides an overview of affective disorders in youth, with particular focus on major depression and bipolar disorder. Affective disorders include those psychological disturbances which have as the core symptom difficulties maintaining a positive and productive mood state. Depressive disorders are most common but some young people, particularly during middle to late adolescence, are troubled by marked mood swings, with periods of hypomanic or even frank manic behaviors suggestive of a bipolar affective disorder.

Depressive Disorders

Clinical Presentation

Young people are not as able as adults to label and describe their feelings, making it sometimes difficult to identify depression. Also there is considerable individual variation in how depression is expressed among young people.

Diagnosis of a major depression requires the presence of at least one of two core features—persistent depressed or irritable mood or marked loss of interest or pleasure. These symptoms must reflect a change in usual functioning and must have been present for at least two weeks. At least four associated symptoms are also required, including a sense of worthlessness, sleep disturbance, appetite disturbance, fatigue, decreased concentration, psychomotor retardation or agitation, and thoughts of death and/or suicide. Dysthymia in children and adolescents requires predominant depressed or irritable mood for at least one year, along with at least two of the following symptoms: abnormal appetite, sleep disturbance, decreased energy, low self-esteem, decreased concentration, and hopelessness. Adjustment disorder may be diagnosed when depression is in response to a specific environmental stressor.

Developmental Differences

Although the diagnostic criteria are the same across ages, young people typically present with a somewhat different symptom cluster than adults. Young people are more likely than adults to present with somatic com-

---

This chapter is dedicated to the memory of Dr. Hooks, who was killed in an automobile accident while vacationing with her family in the summer of 1995. Even though her life was cut far too short, she made a tremendous and lasting contribution to her community and profession.

plaints and marked irritability, as well as increased guilt and low self-esteem (Mitchell, McCauley, Burke, & Moss, 1988; Ryan et al., 1987). Suicide gestures are also much more common among young people than adults (Mitchell et al., 1988; Ryan et al., 1987). Adults, on the other hand, are more likely than youth to report vegetative symptoms of depression such as weight loss and early morning awakening (Mitchell et al., 1988; Ryan et al., 1987). Thus young people frequently present symptoms suggestive of an atypical rather than endogenous type of depression.

Children also differ from adolescents in the profile of depressive symptoms they are most likely to present. Depressed prepubertal children report more separation anxiety and somatic complaints than adolescents and are more frequently rated as having a depressed appearance (Mitchell et al., 1988; Ryan et al., 1987). Adolescents, on the other hand, more frequently report cognitive signs of depression such as hopelessness. Frequency of suicidal attempts or ideation does not differentiate children from adolescents but suicide attempts among adolescents tend to have greater medical lethality, and completed suicide is much more common among adolescents than preadolescent youth (Hoberman & Garfinkel, 1988).

Co-morbidity and Differential Diagnosis

The diagnosis of depression in young people is also complicated by the high rate of comorbid psychiatric diagnoses found in depressed youth. Anxiety, conduct, and dysthymic disorders are frequently found in youth with major depressive disorder. Separation anxiety co-occurs in 33 percent to 59 percent of cases while conduct disorders have been reported in 7 percent to 59 percent of depressed youth (Kovacs, Feinberg, Crouse-Novack, Paulauskas, & Finkelstein, 1984; Kovacs, Gastsonis, Paulauskas, & Richards, 1989; Mitchell et al., 1988; Ryan et al., 1987). Although anxiety disorders are common among depressed adults, separation anxiety and antisocial behaviors are not. Co-morbidity between symptoms associated with attention-deficit/hyperactivity disorder, such as impulsivity and inattention, and major depression has also been reported (Anderson, Williams, McGee, & Silva, 1987; McGee & Williams, 1988).

Comorbid depression and dysthymia, or "double depression," also affects young people. Seventeen percent to 38 percent of youth with a major depression report experiencing either a co-occurring or predisposing dysthymic disorder (Kovacs et al., 1984a, 1984b; Kovacs et al., 1988; Kovacs et al., 1989; Mitchell et al.; 1988; Ryan

et al., 1987). Many youth with a major depression describe a prodromal period of dysthymia and subsyndromal symptoms of depression have been reported in a substantial subset of youth after the resolution of a major depression (McCauley et al., 1993; Rohde, Lewinsohn, & Seeley, 1994). There is, however, supportive evidence that major depression and dysthymia are distinct syndromes. Kovacs, Akiskal, Gatsonis, and Parrone (1994) found that dysthymic disorder differed from major depression in symptom pattern and age of onset. The mean age of onset for children presenting with dysthymic disorder was 8.7 years, which was significantly younger than children who presented with major depression. Dysthymic children were also less likely to show symptoms such as anhedonia (5.65 percent vs. 71.1 percent), social withdrawal (8.3 percent vs. 53.3 percent), and reduced appetite (5.65 percent vs. 46.7 percent) than children with major depression. Rates of suicidal ideation and attempts are similar in individuals with major depression, dysthymia or both (Pfeffer et al., 1991).

Finally, the differential diagnosis can be muddied by the complex role environmental factors play in the expression of depressive symptomatology. More and more children with histories of abuse, neglect, homelessness, and poverty are coming to clinical attention. These youth frequently present with depressive symptoms within the context of a post-traumatic stress disorder or in concert with conduct problems. Many neglected youth may not have symptoms of a full-blown clinical depression, but appear "demoralized" with a profound sense of futility. Too narrow a focus on diagnostic criteria may allow us to overlook this high-risk group.

Clinical Course

Longitudinal studies of depressed youth yield a consistent picture of depression as both a persistent and recurrent problem for young people (see review by McCauley & Myers, 1992). Recovery from an episode of major depression can take weeks to months. The mean length of a depressive episode is about 8 months, with a range from weeks to over a year, and some youth develop a more chronic clinical course (Kovacs et al., 1984a, 1984b; McCauley et al., 1993). Recurrence rates of 35 percent to 72 percent have been reported for samples of depressed youth, with higher rates of recurrence reflecting longer follow-up periods (Kovacs et al., 1984b; McCauley et al., 1993; Strober, 1991). Double depression was associated with increased risk for recurrence (Kovacs et al., 1984b).

There is growing evidence to suggest that an episode of depression impacts the young person even after clinical symptoms resolve. Longitudinal studies of depressed youth document problems in maintaining relationships with parents and in establishing intimate relationships with partners (Fleming, Boyle, & Offord, 1991; Kandel & Davies, 1986). Rohde and colleagues (Lewinsohn, Clarke, Seeley, & Rohde, 1994; Lewinsohn, Hops, Roberts, Seeley, & Andrews, 1993; Rohde et al., 1994) have recent data suggesting that an early episode of depression leaves a "scar" that could compromise subsequent development. Following resolution of the initial episode of major depression, the adolescents in their sample reported more stressful life events, emotional reliance on others, cigarette smoking, and subsyndromal symptoms of depression than before their depression. However, outcome as measured by psychosocial competence is varied and some data suggest that family environment may modulate the overall impact of depression in children and adolescents (McCauley et al., 1993).

Bipolar Disorder

Clinical Presentation

Bipolar disorders are less common than unipolar depression in young people and even more difficult to diagnose. Bowring and Kovacs (1992) outlined four factors that contribute to the difficulty in making this diagnosis in young people: low frequency, variable presentation, overlap with other childhood disorders, and developmental changes in symptom presentation.

The diagnosis of bipolar disorder in children and adolescents is based on the same criteria as for adults. The cardinal feature is presence of a manic episode, which the DSM-IV describes as a distinct period of abnormally and persistently elevated, expansive, and/or irritable mood, which represents a change from the person's normal behavioral pattern, and has persisted for at least one week. Three (four if only irritable mood) associated symptoms are required from the following list: grandiosity, decreased sleep, pressured speech, racing thoughts, distractibility, increased goal-directed activity, and/or excessive involvement in reckless activities. Finally, substantial impairment in functioning is required, and symptoms may not be primarily caused by substance use/abuse or an underlying medical condition. Diagnosis of mixed episode involves the presence of both major depression and mania. Hypomania refers to the presence of symptoms of mania that are less severe and shorter (4 days) than required for mania. Both mixed episodes

and hypomania may be diagnosed in young people as well as adults.

Developmental Differences

Although the same criteria are used to diagnose bipolar disorder in children, adolescents, and adults, there are developmental differences in clinical presentation. Children frequently have labile rather than persistent changes in mood and activity level. Irritability and belligerence are more common than euphoric mood, as is a mixed manic-depressive presentation (Bowring & Kovacs, 1992). Reckless or driven behavior takes the form of typical childhood behavior problems, including difficulties in school, fighting with peers, dangerous play, and sexual acting out, making it difficult at times to differentiate a manic process from sequelae of attention deficit hyperactivity disorder, oppositional defiant disorder, or the residual of maltreatment. Hallmark symptoms of mania such as grandiosity can also be difficult to distinguish from the typical fantasies and imaginary play of childhood.

In adolescence, bipolar disorder typically presents with severe deterioration in the youth's behavior, including greater physical assaultiveness and conflicts with the law than found in adults (McGlashan, 1988). Adolescents also present more frequently with psychotic symptoms. Because of significant psychotic symptoms, many have been given an initial diagnosis of schizophrenia or schizoaffective disorder, with the bipolar diagnosis being made only after closer observation of their clinical symptoms and course (Carlson, Fennig, & Bromet, 1994). This trend reflected the beliefs that schizophrenia was the most common psychotic illness among young people, and that bipolar disorder was an adult disorder. Recent studies suggest that as many as 20 percent of bipolar patients had their first manic episode during middle to late adolescence (ages 15 to 19) (Joyce, 1984) and that bipolar psychosis may be as common as schizophrenia in the adolescent population (Carlson et al., 1994). Suicide is a significant risk, especially among young bipolar males, and when the symptom constellation of very impulsive, aggressive behavior, thought disorder, and substance abuse is present.

Co-Morbidity and Differential Diagnosis

Many young people who develop bipolar disorder first present with a depressive episode. Longitudinal studies of depressed youth suggest that 6 percent to 31.7

percent develop a bipolar disorder (Geller, 1994; Mc-Cauley et al., 1993; Strober & Carlson, 1982). The higher rates of bipolar disorder were found in more severely depressed samples of youth—20 percent in adolescents followed after psychiatric hospitalization (Strober & Carlson, 1982); 28 percent in adolescents with psychotic features (Strober, Lampert, Schmidt, & Morrell, 1993); 31.7 percent in prepubescent youth entered into a medication study because of severe and very persistent depression (Geller, Fox, & Clark, 1994). Lower rates are found in outpatient samples which included both children and adolescents (McCauley et al., 1993). Strober and Carlson (1982) identified three features that predicted bipolarity in their sample: rapid onset of depression accompanied by psychomotor retardation and psychotic features; strong family history of affective disorders, particularly bipolar disorder; and hypomanic features in response to antidepressant medication. However, these factors did not predict bipolar disorder in the other two investigations.

The symptoms of attention-deficit/hyperactivity disorder (ADHD) and conduct disorder are similar to those found in bipolar disorder. And, as with depression, children typically present with multiple problems, so the bipolar child may have a predisposing or co-existing depression, ADHD, or conduct disorder that obfuscates diagnosis and treatment planning. Rates of co-existing diagnoses are not yet established for youth with bipolar disorder, but ADHD and conduct disorder are most commonly considered to co-occur with, or complicate the bipolar diagnostic picture. These problems are so common in children that it can be difficult to recognize the bipolar child. Careful attention to age of onset and clinical course help to make the differential diagnosis of bipolar disorder or to sort out bipolar presentation in a child with a history of ADHD or conduct disorder (Carlson & Weintraub, 1993). Histories of episodic conduct problems are found in some cases of early-onset bipolar disorder (Kovacs & Pollock, 1995). Substance abuse is the other major problem associated with bipolar disorder (Carlson, 1990; McClellan, Werry, & Ham, 1993).

Clinical Course

In the longest follow-up study to date, McGlashan (1988) evaluated 26 adolescent-onset bipolar youth approximately 15 years after initial diagnosis. He found that bipolar youth tend to have longer initial episodes than adults with a more refractory response to treatment. Since many young people present with both psychotic symptoms and histories of comorbid problems with conduct and/or substance abuse, initial treatment may be difficult because of the severity of their prob-

lems. However, in McGlashan's sample psychosocial functioning at follow-up was more positive for the adolescent-onset group than the adult-onset group. Other longitudinal studies suggest that early-onset bipolar disorders follow an episodic course similar to that seen in adults (Werry, McClellan, & Chard, 1991; McClellan et al., 1993). Functional impairment in school performance and social relationships persists beyond resolution of the acute episode in about 50 percent of cases (McClellan et al., 1993).

EPIDEMIOLOGY

Only a handful of studies have investigated the prevalence of depressive disorders among young people, but large-scale epidemiologic studies are currently underway. The available studies report rates of clinical depression between 0.4 and 9.6 percent among adolescents in the general population (Fleming & Offord, 1990; Lewinsohn et al., 1993). Lewinsohn and colleagues (1993) interviewed 1508 randomly selected high schoolers and found that 9.6 percent met criteria for current depression while 20 percent reported at least one episode of depression during their lifetime. Rates among clinical samples of youth vary from 13 to 34 percent (Kashani & Simonds, 1979), with greater frequency reported in the studies that included samples from inpatient units and adolescents.

Although depression has been identified even in some preschool children, the prevalence among preadolescents is low, with a marked increase during early adolescence (Klerman, 1988; Lewinsohn et al., 1993). On surveys of high schoolers, adolescents list depression as one of their most common problems and some reports suggest that up to 65 percent of high school students report subclinical feelings of depression and/or demoralization (Clarke, 1991).

The ratio of girls to boys in depressed samples is fairly equal until adolescence, when girls begin to outnumber boys. Adolescent girls are twice as likely as boys to experience a clinical depression (Allgood-Merton, Lewinsohn, & Hops, 1990). Furthermore, adolescent girls experience longer, more severe depressions than boys, with greater risk for recurrence (Lewinsohn et al., 1993; McCauley et al., 1993). During adulthood, females continued to be at greater risk for depression than males (Kandel & Davies, 1986; Weissman, 1987; Klerman & Weissman, 1989).

Studies of adults suggest that women are socialized in ways that make expression of depression more acceptable, but also might increase risk for depression. This includes the tendency to experience more stress by taking on the stressors of spouses, children, and friends, as well as learning less effective ways of coping. Women tend to ruminate or focus on their depressive symptoms or circumstances while men are better able to use action or distraction coping techniques that facilitate the resolution of depressive symptoms (Nolen-Hoeksema & Girgus, 1994). These issues have not been as fully researched in adolescents, but preliminary data suggest that girls report more stressors during the adolescent years (Petersen, Sarigiani, & Kennedy, 1991) and also perceive events as more stressful than boys (Compas, 1987). Others suggest that adolescent boys express their continuing depressed affect in the form of more antisocial behavior and therefore may be under-reported in rates of depressed youth (McGee & Williams, 1988).

Since bipolar disorder is relatively rare in childhood, few studies have focused on establishing its prevalence. Case reports of bipolar disorder in prepubescent children have been reported (Sylvester, Burke, McCauley, & Clark, 1984), but there is general agreement that the prevalence increases after puberty. The rates among adolescents have been estimated at 0.6 percent to 13.3 percent, with the more conservative rates reflecting studies where the more stringent criteria regarding duration and severity reflected in the DSM-IV were applied (Carlson & Kashani, 1988). Boys are at somewhat greater risk of early-onset bipolar disorder than girls.

A final note about prevalence of affective disorders among young people is indicated. There is considerable documentation of an age cohort effect such that people born since 1940 have a higher lifetime prevalence of mood disorders and suicide than those born earlier. Furthermore, onset of mood disorders appears to be occurring at younger ages than previously documented (Gershon, Hamovit, Guroff, & Nurnberger, 1987; Ryan et al., 1992). This trend is most noticeable in relation to depressive disorders but is also reflected in some increase in reports of bipolar disorders as well. These changes have happened too rapidly to be explained by genetics, and are thought to reflect changes in social systems such as increased mobility, disintegration of the family, and increased violence.

ASSESSMENT APPROACHES

Medical Issues

Evaluation of affective disorders includes a thorough physical assessment to exclude medical conditions that may have a similar presentation. Medical conditions most commonly associated with affective symptoms include endocrine disorders, chronic inflammatory diseases, chronic infectious states, and neurological conditions affecting the central nervous system. Abnormal affective states may also be induced by medications, substance abuse, and withdrawal from substances.

Screening laboratory assessment commonly includes a complete blood count, and assessment of liver, renal and thyroid functions. Other laboratory evaluation may be necessary if specific medical etiologies are suggested by history or physical exam. Prior to initiation of pharmacological treatment, baseline laboratory assessment is indicated (see below).

There are no specific biological markers for depressive disorders in children and adolescents. Studies of biological markers have varied results, probably due to heterogeneity within each of the diagnostic categories. In adults, a positive dexamethasone suppression test (DST), indicated by failure of administration of dexamethasone to suppress normal release of cortisol, has been found to be a marker of a depressed state, particularly melancholia, and to possibly predict response to antidepressant medication (Arana, Baldessarini, & Ornsteen, 1985). The DST was positive in 59 percent of adults with major depression (Howland & Thase, 1991), but can be positive in other non-affective psychiatric conditions (Stein, Szumowski, Ravitz, Frey, & Leventhal, 1994).

In adolescents, the DST is conducted using the same dose, dexamethasone 1 mg, as adults. Studies in adolescents show a positive DST to have a sensitivity (true positive) ranging from 40 to 70 percent and specificity (true negative) ranging from 68 to 100 percent (Casat, Arana, & Powell 1989; Yaylayan, Weller, & Weller, 1991). The predictive value of the DST (likelihood that an individual with a positive test is actually depressed) ranged from 28 to 100 percent.

In prepubertal children, the dexamethasone test typically utilizes a 0.5 mg dose. Studies have yielded a sensitivity ranging from 10 to 86 percent, specificity ranging from 37 to 100 percent, and predictive value ranging from 29 to 89 percent (Birmaher et al., 1992; Casat et al., 1989; Yaylayan et al., 1991).

The above studies generally find greater nonsuppression on the DST in in-patient samples than out-patients. The predictive value is low because the DST can also be positive in other conditions, affecting the number of "false positives." The study finding the lowest predictive value included children with separation anxiety disorder, for whom the DST had a sensitivity of 60 percent (Livingston, Reis, & Ringdahl, 1984). Stress can produce DST nonsuppression and may explain the higher DST nonsuppression rate in in-patients vs. out-patients due to the relationship between stress and hospitalization (Birmaher et al., 1992).

Yaylayan and colleagues (1991) reviewed two studies examining the relationship between suicidality and DST nonsuppression. In one, a higher proportion of adolescents with positive DST made serious suicide attempts, but both studies found that approximately 80 percent of adolescents who attempt suicide have negative DSTs. Studies of suicidality and DST in prepubertal children have not been reported. Overall, the studies of the DST do not support current use in the clinical management of depressed children for diagnostic purposes or assessment of treatment response.

Hyposecretion of growth hormone (GH) has been reported in depressed prepubertal children, in response to insulin-induced hypoglycemia (Ryan et al., 1994), and clonidine challenge (Jensen & Garfinkel, 1990). Postpubertal boys did not have hyposecretion of GH following clonidine challenge. Depressed adolescents have been found to have hypersecretion of GH during sleep, although this may be more specific to suicidality rather than depression per se (Dahl et al., 1992; Kutcher et al., 1988). Mixed results suggest that neurochemical markers, if present, may vary with age and pubertal status.

There are no biochemical markers for bipolar disorder. Organic conditions that may mimic manic behavior include hyperthyroidism, central nervous system infection or tumors, head trauma, seizures, multiple sclerosis, stroke, Wilson's disease, illicit drug intoxication, and various medications including steroids, isoniazid, and sympathomimetics.

There is well-replicated evidence for a major genetic component in bipolar disorder based upon twin, adoptee, and family studies (Merikangas, 1993; Rutter et al., 1990). Specific genetic sites suggested by earlier linkage studies have not been replicated in other samples (Rutter et al., 1990). The extent of genetic mediation in depressive disorders is less clearly defined. Although relative risk of depression is greater with increased familial loading (Rutter et al., 1990), the relative contribution of environmental and genetic factors has yet to be delineated.

Several neurotransmitters have been implicated in major depression and dysthymia in children and are well reviewed by Rogeness, Javors, and Pliszka (1992). There is evidence supporting noradrenergic and serotonergic dysfunction, but not abnormalities in the dopaminergic system.

Psychological and Psychiatric Issues

Overall Approach

Assessment of affective disorders should include careful interviews, preferably utilizing multiple sources including the child/adolescent, parents, and school; and the medical evaluation as noted above. Interviews should elicit information regarding current and past symptomatology, academic and social performance, medical and developmental status, family history, stressors and available supports. Current and past suicidality should always be assessed. Assessment should include evaluation for a broad range of disorders since affective disorders are frequently comorbid with other psychiatric disorders (deMesquita & Gilliam, 1994).

Interview of the child is essential. Children often report more symptoms than their parents (Renouf & Kovacs, 1994; Weissman et al., 1987); are more knowledgeable regarding internal symptoms (including affective symptoms, suicidal ideation/attempts, and psychotic symptoms) and substance abuse; and may have a different perspective on the relative effect of stressors. Ideally, they should be interviewed independently of their parents. Parents are often unaware of the child or adolescent's suicidal ideation or attempts (Walker, Moreau, & Weissman, 1990). The impact of parental psychiatric symptoms on the accuracy of their report of the child's difficulties has been debated (Richters, 1992) and it is best to collect and combine information from both sources.

Bipolar disorder requires some special considerations in addition to the clinical interview issues just outlined. Repeated assessments may be necessary to discern a pattern of affective symptoms in cases early in their course or in the absence of a reliable history. Problems in assessment occur at both ends of the spectrum. It may be difficult to differentiate normal emotional lability or disruptive behavior disorders from hypomania and mania. Concomitant substance use can make diagnosis difficult (Akiksal et al., 1985).

Attention-deficit/hyperactivity disorder can generally be differentiated from bipolar disorder by earlier age of onset prior to age six and more consistently chronic course. Those with externalizing difficulties and bipolar disorder have a greater likelihood for episodic symptoms, affective symptoms (Carlson & Weintraub, 1993) and familial affective disorder (Carlson, 1990; Bowring & Kovacs, 1992), particularly bipolar disorder in a first degree relative (Strober et al., 1988).

Manic adolescents presenting with reckless or episodic destructive behaviors may appear to have conduct difficulties. Psychotic symptoms may make it difficult to differentiate mania from schizophrenia. This appears to be less of a problem as careful attention to the presence of affective symptoms, mood congruent psychotic symptoms, and more rigorous attention to diagnostic criteria improves, but it is still difficult if concurrent substance abuse is present (Carlson et al., 1994).

Structured Interviews

There are five structured interviews for use by clinicians or lay interviewers, most commonly used in research settings, but generally applicable to clinical settings. These interviews provide information regarding affective disorders as well as most other DSM Axis I psychiatric diagnoses. All have been extensively studied for validity and reliability; and most have undergone recent revisions as diagnostic schema change. Most require 60 to 90 minutes per informant to administer, utilizing separate interviews for child and parent. A review of the structured interviews (Gutterman, O'Brien, & Young, 1987) supports their use for depressive disorders, but use for bipolar disorder in childhood has not been extensively studied.

The DICA (Diagnostic Interview for Children and Adolescents) was the first structured interview for children, and was developed by Herjanic and colleagues at Washington University (Welner et al., 1987). It has child and adolescent versions, each with associated parent versions. The DICA provides current and past diagnoses, and can be utilized by most clinicians, with additional training required for less experienced interviewers. It remains in extensive use, and provides good coverage of a broad range of diagnoses.

The Kiddie-SADS (Schedule for Affective Disorders and Schizophrenia; K-SADS) is a semi-structured interview originally developed by Puig-Antich and Chambers at New York State Psychiatric Institute (Chambers et al., 1985). It has clinical and epidemiological versions. The K-SADS provides current and past diagnoses, depending on the version used. It has been widely used in research on affective disorders.

Two other interviews that have as much general use are the CAS (Child Assessment Schedule), a structured interview developed by Hodges and colleagues at the University of Missouri, and the ISC (Interview Schedule for Children), a semistructured interview developed by Kovacs and colleagues at the University of Pittsburgh (Hodges, 1993; Hodges, Cools, & McKnew, 1989).

The DISC (Diagnostic Interview Schedule for Children) is the most recently developed instrument. Principally, it is a highly structured interview that can be administered by lay interviewers or clinicians. It was originally developed under contract with NIMH by Herjanic, Puig-Antich, Conners, and NIMH staff, although it has undergone several revisions, most recently by Shaffer and colleagues at Columbia (Shaffer et al., 1993). It provides current and past year diagnoses. It is being used extensively and computer algorithms are available.

Depression Scales

Questionnaires assessing depression have been developed to screen for depressive symptoms and measure change in symptom level to quantify treatment response. Selection of a screening instrument will depend upon the information desired and the situation. Criteria for choosing an appropriate instrument is well reviewed and critiqued by Costello and Angold (1988). The following are some of the more commonly used self-report scales designed to specifically assess depression.

The Children's Depression Inventory (CDI; Kovacs, 1985), a 27-item self-report questionnaire for ages 7–17 years, is the most widely used and studied. It discriminates between children with and without psychopathology, but has questionable ability to differentiate depression from other diagnostic categories, possibly due to comorbid depression in children with other primary diagnoses. It may be useful in assessing severity of depression (Reynolds 1992).

The Reynolds Child Depression Scale (RCDS) is a 30-item self-report measure designed for use with children ages 8–13 years. The Reynolds Adolescent Depression Scale (RADS) is a 30-item self-report measure for ages 12–18 years. Both instruments are best reviewed by Reynolds (1992), who also developed them. There is high agreement between scores on this scale and the CDI. The instruments are easy to administer and deserve more widespread use. The Reynolds scales are well suited for use in nonclinical (i.e, school) settings.

The Children's Depression Scale (CDS; Lang & Tisher, 1978), a 66-item self-report questionnaire with parent/teacher versions (Moretti, Fine, Haley, & Marriage, 1985) for ages 7–11 years, provides detailed information about depressive symptomatology. It is longer and better for documentation of severity of episode rather than screening.

The Mood and Feelings Questionnaire has 32 items with self-report and parent versions for children ages 8–17 years designed to reflect DSM-III-R criteria for depressive disorders (Costello & Angold, 1988). There is an 11-item short form. It has not been used extensively.

Center for Epidemiological Studies Depression Scale for Children (CES-D; Weissman, Orvaschel, & Padian, 1980) is a 20-item self-report and parent report measure originally designed for adults. Several limitations weigh against its use with children (Costello & Angold, 1988; Reynolds, 1992).

There are several clinician rated scales. For prepubertal children, the most commonly used scale is the Children's Depression Rating Scale—Revised (CDRS-R; Poznanski, Freeman, & Mokros, 1985). It has 17 like scaled items and is fairly easy to administer. The Children's Affective Rating Scales (CARS; McKnew, Cytryn, Efron, Gerson, & Bunney, 1979), which has three items on a 10-point scale, is sometimes used.

The Child Behavior Checklist (CBCL) is widely used in multiple settings as a screening instrument for childhood disorders including affective disorders. It is important to remember that the CBCL's internalizing scale is correlated with both depressive and anxiety disorders, and that both major depression and dysthymia are also significantly correlated to parental ratings on the externalizing scale (Edelbrock & Costello, 1988). Therefore, neither scale specifically differentiates affective disorders from other difficulties.

Mania Scales

Screening instruments have been studied in the assessment of mania in children and adolescents. The Mania Rating Scale (MRS), an 11 item clinical rating scale, has been shown to differentiate prepubertal children with mania from those with attention deficit hyperactivity disorder, while the Conners Parent and Teacher rating scales did not (Fristad, Weller, & Weller, 1992). The Personality Inventory for Children, which includes 600 true-false items and a 16-item clinical scale, correctly identified boys with mania, although 20 percent of boys with ADHD were incorrectly identified as manic (Neiman & Delong, 1987).

TREATMENT

Psychological and Behavioral Treatments

Depressive Disorders

Cognitive behavioral and interpersonal psychotherapeutic approaches have been shown to be effective strategies for treating depressed adults, but such conclusive evidence is not yet available for children or adolescents. Efforts have been made to modify these therapeutic approaches for work with younger samples (Mufson et al., 1994), but research on the efficacy of these approaches is still preliminary. The literature on systematic, controlled studies of individual or family therapy interventions is very limited. Finally, interpersonal therapy has been adapted for use with adolescents, and results of an open trial with 14 are promising. All subjects had remitted by the last week of a 12-week course of treatment, but further follow-up is not yet available (Mufson et al., 1994).

There is a small but substantial set of group therapy studies. Most of these studies have involved time-limited, school-based interventions utilizing cognitive and behavioral techniques, including training in social skills, problem solving, and relaxation (Butler, Miezitis, Friedman, & Cole, 1980; Kahn, Kehle, Jenson, & Clark, 1990; Reynolds & Coats, 1986; Stark, Reynolds, & Kaslow, 1987). All of these skills-oriented interventions had a positive effect on self-reported mood with no clear advantage to one approach over another. The efficacy of these interventions may in part reflect the fact that the children who participated were drawn from school samples. Diagnostic criteria were not used to identify high-risk youth and therefore the youth who participated may be far different from the young person who presents in a medical or psychiatric clinic seeking help for depressive symptoms.

Two studies have used group approaches with clinical populations of depressed youth. Fine and colleagues (1987) contrasted social skills training and a less structured support group approach. About half of the participants showed significant clinical improvement, improvement which persisted at the 9 month follow-up. The youth in the support group showed greatest gains at the end of the 12-week treatment program, while by the 9 month follow-up evaluation youth from both groups appeared equal in terms of social functioning and remission of depressive symptoms. In the other study, depressed students were screened using structured diagnostic interviews; only those who met criteria for a depressive disorder with no co-occurring diagnoses were included. Lewinsohn and colleagues (1990) compared two versions of their Coping with Depression Course for Adolescents with a wait-list control group. This is a psychoeducational approach that teaches skills in the areas of relaxation, pleasant event scheduling, constructive thinking, social skills, communication, negotiation, and problem solving. One group included parental involvement, the other did not. There was improvement in both treatment groups in contrast to the wait-list controls, with a trend toward greater gains in the group with parent involvement. However, again, these findings do not easily generalize to clinical practice, since youth with co-morbidity were not included.

In sum, the psychotherapy treatment data available to date suggest the efficacy of structured cognitive, behavioral skills building, and interpersonal interventions in youth with mild to moderate levels of depression. No clear guidelines exist for psychotherapeutic treatment of more severely depressed youth or youth with complex diagnostic pictures. However, the techniques used in these groups provide a jumping off point for individual and family therapy approaches. Also, as with adults, in youth with marked vegetative signs of depression, such as severe problems with sleep disturbance, consideration of a combination of psychotherapy and pharmacotherapy may be helpful.

Bipolar Disorders

Treatment for bipolar disorders relies much more heavily on pharmacotherapy, as reviewed below. However, treatment requires a comprehensive approach to address the child's symptoms, as well as to help the child, family, and in some cases, school personnel understand the nature of bipolar disorder, prevent recurrence, and facilitate the child's ongoing development. Geller (1994) recently reported on preliminary trials of an adaptation of interpersonal therapy developed for children with bipolar major depressive disorder and their families which holds promise as an intervention strategy. Educating family members about bipolar disorder, as well as providing support, appear to be important adjuncts to therapy in the case of bipolar adults and certainly is indicated when a child or adolescent is the presenting patient (Clarkin et al., 1990). Similarly, techniques to minimize stress and avoid schedule disruptions that are effective with adults also have relevance for work with bipolar youth and their families.

Pharmacological Treatments

Despite the widespread use of antidepressants, there is little evidence to support their efficacy in the pediatric age range, particularly in adolescents. Use of medications for treatment of affective disorders in children has been based upon the pharmacological treatment of affective disorders in adult populations, where there is proven efficacy (Baldessarini, 1989). Popper (1992) suggests that their use in the pediatric population, despite the lack of verification from the research sector, is due to their clinical efficacy, which, because of methodology, research studies fail to confirm. Medications, if used, should be considered one facet of the therapeutic intervention. The use of antidepressants continues to be recommended if there is poor response to nonpharmacological interventions and clear evidence of continuing dysfunction (Ambrosini, Bianchi, Rabinovich, & Elia, 1993). Given that clinicians are continuing to prescribe antidepressants, it appears prudent to be aware of available research.

Tricyclic Antidepressants

Studies of treatment response to tricyclic antidepressants in children and adolescents have been contradictory. Studies utilizing blinded administration of medication have failed to demonstrate superiority over placebo. The difficulty verifying the generally more positive results of open medication trials in prepubertal children and the positive relationship between response and plasma levels of medication (Geller, Cooper, Chestnut, Anker & Schluchter, 1986) suggest caution in interpreting these results.

In a 5-week double blind placebo study of imipramine in 38 prepubertal children (22 placebo; 16 imipramine) there was no difference in response, with 9/16 (56 percent) responding to imipramine and 15/22 (68 percent) to placebo (Puig-Antich et al., 1987). Neither group received psychotherapy during the study. Responders had higher plasma levels than nonresponders. Children with low levels had a worse outcome (22 percent improved) than placebo.

Imipramine was found to be superior to placebo in 22 prepubertal psychiatric inpatients (Preskorn et al., 1987), with response also related to plasma imipramine levels. Following an initial placebo period, children were randomized to continue on placebo or imipramine, the dose was adjusted to provide imipramine/desipramine plasma levels of 125–250 ng/ml. Findings were reported as percent change from baseline, utilizing three rating scales. Scores on two scales were significantly better in the imipramine group, but no different on the third scale. Both groups improved, but on the two scales showing sustained improvement in the imipramine group, there was greater improvement in the initial 3 weeks on medication, and similar rates of change thereafter. The third scale showed a pattern of initial improvement which declined to placebo levels by the sixth week. Improvement with imipramine was greatest in dexamethasone nonsuppressors.

A fixed dose double blind crossover study of amitriptyline, the precursor of nortriptyline, in nine prepubertal in-patients statistically failed to find superiority over placebo ($p < 0.09$) although 6/9 improved on medication (Kashani, Shekim, & Reid, 1984). A double blind placebo study of nortriptyline in 50 prepubertal outpatients failed to show superiority over placebo, or a positive relationship between response and plasma level in those who did respond (Geller et al., 1992). Nortriptyline was administered to yield mean blood levels of 80 ng/ml (mean therapeutic range) following an initial placebo washout period. Differential response rate was not statistically significant with 30.8 percent of those being actively treated showing a response versus 16.9 percent on placebo. There were no differences between responders and nonresponders.

The same study done with 31 adolescent outpatients (Geller, Cooper, Graham, Marsteller, & Bryan, 1990) had only 1 of 12 adolescents respond during the 8-week trial of medication. Higher plasma levels were associated with a worsening of symptoms. The one responder went on to have a bipolar course. Neither group experienced anticholinergic side effects. An earlier study of amitriptyline also failed to find superiority over placebo in adolescents (Kramer & Feiguine, 1981). In an open trial of imipramine in 34 adolescents, 44 percent responded over a 6-week trial, with no differences between responders and nonresponders (Ryan et al., 1986). There were trends for those with comorbid separation anxiety or higher levels to do worse on medication.

Given the small sample sizes, the few studies available, and conflicting results, evidence for efficacy of tricyclic antidepressants in the treatment of depression for children and adolescents awaits further investigation. There is more evidence for efficacy in prepubertal children, with possibly a positive relationship between plasma level and response. In adolescents, there is little if any evidence of efficacy, no evidence of a positive relationship between response and plasma levels, and the suggestion that higher plasma levels may in fact be detrimental.

The four most commonly used tricyclic antidepressants for depression are imipramine (Tofranil), desip-

ramine (Norpramin, Pertofrane), nortriptyline (Pamelor, Aventyl) and amitriptyline (Elavil, Endep, and others). Their mechanism of action is felt to be through the noradrenergic and/or serotonergic systems. Imipramine has been studied the most extensively. It has anticholinergic and antihistaminic effects, and may lower the seizure threshold. Potential side effects include sedation, dry mouth, dizziness upon standing, dry eyes, blurry vision, constipation, delayed micturition, weight gain, shaking or "jitters," headaches, stomachaches, tachycardia, and cardiac arrhythmias. The above applies equally to amitriptyline. Potential cardiac effects are by far the most serious and include tachycardia, hypertension, and arrhythmias, including heart block. Desipramine, the chief metabolite of imipramine, has fewer minor side effects, but has been associated with sudden death in four pediatric patients (Riddle, Geller, & Ryan, 1993) and potential cardiotoxic effects need to be considered prior to use. Imipramine, desipramine, and amitriptyline are used in gradually increasing doses up to a typical dose of 1–3 mg/kg (max 5 mg/kg/day) based upon presence of clinical response, side effects, and blood levels. Older, larger adolescents should be dosed similar to adults rather than on a mg/kg basis. Due to individual differences in metabolism of tricyclic antidepressants, levels achieved using mg/kg dosing may be well above the therapeutic range even in the absence of significant ECG changes (Fetner & Geller, 1992). Reported ECG guidelines are resting heart rate less than 130 beats per minute, widening of the QRS interval by no more than 30 percent of baseline, and PR interval no greater than 0.21 seconds (Fetner & Geller, 1992).

Nortriptyline has fewer anticholinergic and antihistaminic side effects, is more expensive, and is available in elixir form. Nortriptyline is twice as potent; therefore typical doses are 0.5–1.5 mg/kg (max 2.5 mg/kg). Though not associated with sudden death, the same general principles apply.

Although the tricyclics have a long half-life, children and adolescents generally require dosing two to three times a day to prevent anticholinergic rebound due to the fact that youth generally metabolized these medications more rapidly than adults (Rosenberg, Holttum, & Gershon, 1994). Anticholinergic rebound effects include stomachaches, anxiety, excessive dreaming, insomnia, and behavioral activation.

Tricyclic antidepressants may cause activation of mania (Akiskal & Mallya, 1987) and a greater propensity toward rapid cycling in depressed prepubertal children with family histories of bipolar disorder. In the presence of a family history of bipolar disorder, clinicians should be cautious prior to the initiation of tricyclic antidepressants, consider discontinuance if mania or hypomania develops, or initially use alternate medications such as lithium to treat depressive episodes (Akiskal & Mallya, 1987).

Selective Serotonin Re-Uptake Inhibitors (SSRIs)

The selective serotonin reuptake inhibitors including fluoxetine (Prozac), paroxetine (Paxil), sertraline (Zoloft), and most recently fluvoxamine (Luvox), have not been sufficiently studied to provide any positive statement about their use in children and adolescents with depressive disorder. In the one placebo double blind study available, fluoxetine fared no better than the tricyclic antidepressants (Simeon, Dinicola, Ferguson, & Copping, 1990). Of 40 adolescents, two-thirds of the patients in both the fluoxetine and placebo groups improved. There was no statistical difference between groups, except that fluoxetine group had slightly greater improvement in sleep.

The SSRIs have been preferred by some clinicians due to the absence of cardiac side effects; though their efficacy has not been documented, they may be safer, both at therapeutic doses and certainly in overdose. In a chart review of fluoxetine use in 31 patients ages 9–18 years, 74 percent improved, and in 28 percent fluoxetine had to be discontinued due to side effects (Jain, Birmaher, Garcia, Al-Shabbout, & Ryan 1992). Side effects were experienced in 59 percent, including hypomanic symptoms, irritability, insomnia, and gastrointestinal upset. All four depressed bipolar patients had hypomanic symptoms. There were no cardiac side effects. Another report of behavioral activation associated with fluoxetine usage in a small sample of prepubertal children with varying diagnoses found that behavioral activation was not transitory, but continued for two to eight weeks until the fluoxetine was either reduced or discontinued (Riddle et al., 1990/91). Following reduction or discontinuance, activation resolved in one to two weeks. Withdrawal side effects are generally not a problem due to the long half-life of fluoxetine (2–3 days) and the even longer half-life (7–9 days) of the active metabolite norfluoxetine.

Monoamine Oxidase Inhibitors

Double blind studies of monoamine oxidase inhibitors (MAOIs) in children and adolescents have not been published, and potentially serious side effects mitigate against their use. A retrospective chart review of the use of MAOIs in 23 adolescents, some treated concurrently with tricyclic antidepressants, showed 57 percent to have a "good to fair" response and able to be compliant with dietary restrictions (Ryan et al., 1988). Side effects noted on MAOIs were increased headaches, insomnia, and hypertensive episodes. Twenty percent of the adolescents had to discontinue use due to dietary non-compliance. One patient was purposefully non-compliant in a suicide attempt. Their recommendation against use of MAOIs in adolescents at risk for impulsive or unreliable behavior, or with histories of drug abuse, places extreme limitations on their use.

Lithium

The use of lithium for affective disorders in the pediatric age group is generally confined to treatment of bipolar disorder and to a lesser extent the treatment of depression.

Pharmacological treatment of bipolar disorder in children and adolescents is based on more extensive experience and research regarding treatment of adults with bipolar disorder (Prien & Potter, 1990), where 70 to 80 percent with acute mania respond to lithium. Lithium is an appropriate treatment for children and adolescents with bipolar disorder, and it is approved for use in children older than age 12.

Only two double blind studies of the use of lithium in prepubertal children were identified in a recent review (Alessi, Naylor, Ghaziuddin, & Zubieta, 1994). In an early double blind crossover study of six children, the two children with clear-cut symptoms of cyclothymia responded, whereas the others did not (McKnew et al., 1981). DeLong and Aldershof (1987), using a combination of double blind and open trials reported that 66 percent of 48 children younger than 14 years old and identified with bipolar disorder responded to lithium, and 63 percent of 11 children over 14 years of age responded to lithium. This is in contrast to an open trial (Strober et al., 1988) that found 40 percent of prepubertal children versus 80 percent of adolescents to be lithium responsive, leading to the common notion that prepubertal children were lithium resistant. Another open trial (Varanka, Weller, Weller, & Fristad, 1988) reported that all 10 prepubertal children with mania and psychotic features responded to lithium alone, though the study excluded 4 additional children taking neuroleptics concurrently, which could conceivably lower the rate to 71 percent. This report recommends using the same serum levels as in adults (0.8 to 1.2 mEq/L) for therapeutic trials of lithium in children.

Responsivity of adolescents generally parallels experience in adults (Alessi et al., 1994). There are reports that adolescents with mixed mania are less responsive to lithium (Himmelhoch & Garfinkel, 1986).

Lithium may be useful in preventing future affective episodes. A follow-up study of 37 lithium-responsive 13- to 17-year-old adolescents found that twelve (92.3 percent) of the 13 lithium non-compliant adolescents relapsed versus 9 (37.5 percent) of 24 compliant adolescents (Strober, Morrell, Lampert, & Burroughs, 1990). Those who relapsed while on lithium still had significantly fewer episodes than prior to taking lithium. Risk of relapse on lithium was not predicted by age, sex, number of previous episodes, serum lithium level, or use of other medication.

The mechanism by which lithium impacts bipolar disorder is unknown. Lithium affects a number of neurochemical systems including ion-channels, neurotransmitters, and second messenger systems (Alessi et al., 1994).

Prior to the initiation of lithium, children must be screened for abnormalities in renal function (urinalysis, blood urea nitrogen, and creatinine), thyroid function and calcium metabolism (calcium and phosphate); laboratory studies should be repeated at least at six-month intervals during treatment (Biederman 1991). Lithium levels are usually monitored with dose changes, and monthly thereafter. The most common side effects in children are weight gain, gastrointestinal complaints, headache, and tremor; younger children have a greater incidence of side effects (Campbell et al., 1991).

Anti-psychotics may be used in conjunction with lithium to control agitation or reduce psychotic symptoms (Strober et al., 1988). Therapy refractory patients may respond to lithium in combination with carbamazepine, antipsychotics, benzodiazapines, or clonidine (Biederman, 1991).

Lithium may be useful in augmenting the effect of antidepressants in depressed individuals. There have been no placebo double blind trials, but two open trials of lithium to augment treatment effects in adolescents refractory to tricyclic antidepressants show possible benefit in a small subset of patients. In a retrospective chart review of 14 adolescents in which lithium was added after inadequate response to tricyclic antidepressants alone, 43 percent improved, 21 percent had intermediate change, and 36 percent were unchanged. Responders tended to show gradual improvement over a month period (Ryan, Meyer, Dachille, Mazzie, & Puig-Antich, 1988). An additional study found that ten (42 percent) of 24 adolescents nonresponsive to a 6-week trial of imipramine improved following the addition of lithium, with 2 (9 percent) showing marked response, and 8 (33 percent) partial response (Strober, Freeman, Rigali, Schmidt,

& Diamond, 1992). Both studies reported minimal side effects. Neither study was able to identify characteristics predicting response.

Carbamazepine and Valproic Acid

Both of these medications are used primarily as anticonvulsants. Their use for affective disorders in the pediatric age range is inadequately studied and best considered anecdotal. Double blind studies of the short-term management of mania in adults with bipolar disorder have shown carbamazepine to be equivalent to lithium, and valproate to be equivalent or slightly less effective than lithium (Prien & Potter 1990). Similar studies have not been published regarding their use in children. In practice, carbamazepine and valproic acid are considered in bipolar disorder if an individual is intolerant or resistant to lithium.

Carbamazepine is thought to possibly operate through GABA mechanisms and to be a partial agonist of adenosine receptors. Hepatic metabolism and renal clearance occur more rapidly in younger children, declining to adult levels by late adolescence. Dosages are gradually adjusted upward to 10–50mg/kg/day administered in divided doses two to three times a day to achieve therapeutic serum levels of 4–12 ug/ml (Trimble, 1990). Side effects include sedation, allergic rashes, movement disorders, hyponatremia, and gastrointestinal symptoms. Although rare, a range of hematological disorders can occur, including aplastic anemia and agranulocytosis. During treatment, regular monitoring of blood counts, renal and liver function is indicated.

Valproic acid is started at 15 mg/kg/day, and increased weekly to 30–60 mg/kg/day, with a standard therapeutic range for children of 50–100ug/ml, although some individuals respond at lower levels (Trimble, 1990). Common side effects are nausea, vomiting, gastrointestinal discomfort, sedation, weight gain, and tremor. Less common but more serious side effects are hematological disturbances, hepatotoxicity ranging from chemical hepatitis to fatal liver failure, alopecia, pancreatitis, and delirium.

CASE ILLUSTRATIONS

Mood disorders cannot be accurately reflected in one "typical" case example. Clinical presentation varies dramatically, depending on the characteristics of the child, such as developmental level and life circumstances, as well as on the nature of the mood disorder itself. The following cases provide a glimpse at how mood disorders can present.

Case of D.

Clinical Presentation

D. presented as a very attractive, casually dressed girl. D's mother brought her to the clinic because of growing concerns about possible depression. D. was almost 14, and had just begun the 8th grade. Mother described her as depressed or irritable almost all the time with no interest in anything other than watching TV. Over the summer, she had begun staying up late and sleeping during the day. She was now missing school frequently because of feeling sick or simply tired. She was behind in homework, but couldn't get herself to do the work—it seemed too complicated for her and she could not focus on the material. She expressed a desire to spend time with friends but felt very uncomfortable and unsure of herself in social situations, so much so that she was making excuses to avoid friends.

Assessment Findings

Parents participated in an in-depth interview process that covered family, developmental, school, and social history as well as a structured review of symptoms, timing of presentation, and duration. The family was seen together to assess communication styles and D. was seen individually to review symptoms and obtain her perspective on school, social, and family functioning. The school counselor was contacted for collateral data and one of D.'s teachers completed the Teacher Behavior Checklist. Mother completed the Child Behavior Checklist and D. completed the Children's Depression Inventory. D. saw her family physician for a medical work-up and routine laboratory testing to rule out any medical concerns; all findings were within normal limits.

The following information was obtained. D. is the second of two daughters in an intact family. Both parents are employed as professionals. The older sister works hard to do well in school and is socially outgoing. She and D. get along fairly well with typical sibling struggles. Parents describe her as more easy going than D., not as sensitive or "temperamental."

D. had been a relatively happy and well-adjusted child through the 6th grade. She had a difficult transition to Middle School, complaining of feeling overwhelmed by all the changes and demands, but had settled in and had a good 6th grade year. Seventh grade had started off well, but in the second semester her grades had fallen and she had begun to talk about struggles with friends, feeling left out or criticized by other children. The following summer she was unwilling to sign up for any classes or youth programs and was home alone a great deal.

On the CBCL, mother's rating of D. placed her in the normal range on the Social Competency scales but at the low end for both social participation and school performance. On the Behavior Problems subscales, the rating placed D. in the clinically significant range (98th percentile) on the Anxious/Depressed scale and at the 93rd percentile for the Withdrawn and Somatic Complaints subscales. The teacher rated D. as below average on the School Performance and Happy subscales of the section on Adaptive Functioning and within the clinically significant range on the Anxious/Depressed and Withdrawn behavioral subscales.

During her interview, D. wept as she spoke about how unhappy and hopeless she felt. She described feeling easily irritated, especially with her parents, but also felt that they, especially her mother, were her best allies. She talked of wanting to do well in school and to get back into social activities, but felt too self-conscious to speak up in class or talk comfortably with her friends. She laid in bed at night worrying about what she said and did that day and what she would face the next. She could not force herself to do homework and used the TV as a distraction. Appetite was variable but her weight was stable. She frequently felt she would be better off dead, and thought about suicide, but had made no attempts and had no plan. D. had no history of substance abuse and no history of physical or sexual abuse. She saw her father as a highly critical person and as someone she could never please. He was described as having a quick temper and at times being very sarcastic and cutting in his comments.

D.'s CDI revealed a summary score of 21, suggestive of considerable distress. Both parents and D. reported that symptoms had developed gradually over the last 6 to 8 months. A diagnosis of Major Depression, with moderate severity was made.

Treatment Selection and Course

D. and her family agreed to participate in a combination of individual and family treatment. In individual treatment the focus was initially on educating D. about depression and introducing some basic cognitive behavioral principles. She was responsive but drew the line at behavioral attempts to have her structure more positive activities. She complained that when she talked about feeling depressed her parents responded in ways that made her feel unheard—things like "just get your homework done, you'll feel better," "all kids get teased," "let's get you signed up for an art class, that will get you going again." Family sessions allowed time to work with D. and her parents about communication skills so that both sides felt heard and acknowledged. Parents were also coached on ways to respond to D., who made both parents feel very anxious and angry. As D. felt more acknowledged, she gradually engaged in talking about ways to beat her depression. After a period of improvement, a problem arose with a friend at school and D. had a setback. Her rumination increased, accompanied by a resurgence of insomnia and a return of hopelessness; she also had suicidal ideation but no plan. She rebounded from this difficult period and was able to work on ways to decrease her rumination in therapy.

Over the next two months part of each therapy session was set aside to allow her to talk about her feelings, while the other part focused on skill building. She became more comfortable with friends and willing to work with a tutor for her school work. By spring, frequency of therapy sessions was cut back to twice a month. She then initiated a number of plans for the summer and decided with her therapist to take a break from therapy over the summer vacation.

Termination and Follow-Up

D. returned to therapy in the fall as she settled into high school. Her depressive symptoms continued to be greatly improved at this time, but she was worried about becoming depressed again with the start of a new school and school year. Therapy focused on relapse recognition and prevention but also served as a place for D. to problem solve the stresses she felt with the increased academic and social demands of high school. D. and her therapist met every other week for the first two months of high school, then monthly until the end of the first semester, at which time both agreed that she had made an excellent adjustment and therapy was ended.

Case M. K.

Clinical Presentation

M. K. presented at 14 years of age for evaluation regarding depression, suicidal ideation, and reinstitution of antidepressant medication. M. reported that five months earlier he had been started on desipramine for depression and that he had taken it for two to three months. He then discontinued taking it when his family moved to a new

area. M. felt the medication had helped and that he had been more depressed since stopping the medication. Over the past two months, he had had intermittent suicidal ideation but had made no attempts. M. seemed somewhat odd, but acknowledged no other symptoms.

Assessment Findings

It was decided to obtain a thorough history and see M. again before reinstituting medication. A complex history was obtained from M. and his father; consistent reports were obtained from each in individual interviews. M. had an unremarkable history until age 11 when he was hospitalized for three weeks on a psychiatric unit following a suicide attempt. At that time, his parents were divorced and M. lived with his father. He had regular visits with his mother, who was diagnosed with bipolar disorder. His academic performance had declined, but no other stressors or difficulties had been noted. He was treated with psychotherapy and, following his release, did well until age 13 with no treatment.

At 13 years, M. was caught shoplifting and was referred to a psychologist. M. was doing well at school academically, but had been in fights and was more argumentative at home. He denied depression and suicidality, but had increasing difficulty controlling his temper. His mood, thought processes, and behavior were felt to be appropriate. M. was diagnosed with an impulse control disorder and referred to anger management and outpatient counselling.

Four months later, M. reported feelings of "confusion" and "detachment from others" to his outpatient therapist. His anger was increasingly difficult to control, and his motivation, energy, and concentration had decreased. Appetite and sleep were variable. M. reported low to moderate use of alcohol. Mood and affect were depressed and irritable. M. denied suicidal ideation. M. reported that he had experienced an auditory hallucination two years earlier when under a lot of stress but denied current psychotic symptoms. M. denied feelings of anxiety, panic, or dissociative symptoms. M. was diagnosed with major depression and referred to a psychiatrist for consideration of medication to supplement counselling. The psychiatrist initiated the desipramine after obtaining baseline EKG and blood testing, working up to a dose of 150 mg per day. Two months after starting on the medication the family moved.

After obtaining the history, M. was seen again four days later. M.'s father stated that M. had been increasingly hostile, and out of control. M. expressed increasing feelings of depression and suicidal ideation. His affect was labile, rapidly shifting from dysphoric/tearful to angry/irritable. Speech was pressured and circumstantial. His thoughts were disorganized. He felt others were controlling him and altering reality. M. denied drug use. Concerns regarding possible bipolar disorder were raised and M. was referred for an in-patient psychiatric assessment, given the level of his disorganization.

Treatment Selection and Course

M. was admitted to a psychiatric hospital. Medication treatment was initiated with 300 mg of lithium and an antipsychotic, trilafon, at a dosage of 16 mg per day. The lithium was gradually increased until a blood level in the .7 to 1.0 range was obtained. M. improved but was felt to have significant residual difficulties after two months in the hospital; he was referred to a longer-stay facility and treated with group, family, and individual treatment.

M. showed gradual improvement and was tapered off the antipsychotic; it was felt that he was responding well to the lithium, which was continued. Three months later, M. was discharged. Back at home, M. became noncompliant with his lithium and rapidly deteriorated, becoming withdrawn, mute, and internally preoccupied. He was restarted on medication, and improved, but had not regained his discharge status.

Termination and Follow-Up

Over the following 6 months M. has had an unstable course, running away from home for brief periods. He has difficulty participating in an alternative school setting. His mood remains labile and irritable. He is not psychotic. His psychiatrist, case manager, and in-home counselor are continuing to work with M. and his father around M.'s running away behavior and medication compliance in an attempt to avoid rehospitalization. The psychiatrist would like to consider other medications (e.g., Tegretol, Valproate) and is working with M. regarding these options.

SUMMARY

Affective disorders include a range of disturbances in which a person's mood state interferes with their functional ability. While affective disorders occur in younger children, incidence is greater in older children, particularly during middle to late adolescence. Developmental differences in the presentation of symptoms previously led to debate about the occurrence of affective disorders in childhood, and continues to hinder diagnosis.

A spectrum of disorders exists, ranging from relatively brief difficulties in response to specific stressors to persistent and recurrent problems that may follow a more chronic course. Diagnostic criteria for affective disorders have been generated and directly applied from schema developed for adults, but accurate assessment of specific symptoms requires an understanding of the impact of developmental level, comorbid conditions, and individual differences in the expression of difficulties. Within the group of affective disorders, depressive disorders are more common, more extensively studied, and better understood than bipolar affective disorder.

Assessment of the child or adolescent requires a comprehensive multi-faceted approach that takes into account the relative contribution of psychological, environmental, and biological influences. A variety of instruments have been designed as adjuncts to clinical assessment, particularly in reference to depressive symptoms. Although various interventions are used in clinical practice, the research base regarding their efficacy is still being developed. Ideally, interventions should address each of the factors related to causation or maintenance of the individual's difficulties. Many individuals nonetheless continue to have residual difficulties, possibly due to only partial response to available treatments, the impact of affective symptoms on the developmental process, or a combination of both.

Investigations substantiating the efficacy of therapeutic interventions are still in a preliminary phase. Available data suggest that structured cognitive behavioral skills building and interpersonal psychotherapeutic interventions are helpful in youth with mild to moderate levels of depression. It is unclear whether more severely depressed youth or youth with complex diagnostic pictures would experience equal benefit. While psychopharmacological interventions are being used more frequently in clinical practice and are recommended in individuals with severe difficulties or inadequate response to psychotherapeutic approaches, their efficacy has yet to be convincingly demonstrated in rigorous research studies. Many of the same issues that hampered the identification of affective disorders interfere with efforts to test the usefulness of therapeutic techniques. In addition, most individuals with serious difficulty will undoubtedly require a combination of approaches in order to optimize their clinical improvement. Efforts to both better understand and treat these complex youth will continue to challenge both researchers and clinicians.

REFERENCES

Akiskal, H. S., Downs, J., Jordan, P., Watson, S., Daugherty, D., & Pruitt, D. B. (1985). Affective disorders in referred children and younger siblings of manic depressives. *Archives of General Psychiatry, 42,* 996–1003.

Akiskal, H. S., & Mallya, G. (1987). Criteria for the "soft" bipolar spectrum: Treatment implications. *Psychopharmacology Bulletin, 23,* 68–73.

Alessi, N., Naylor, M. W., Ghaziuddin, M., & Zubieta, J. K. (1994). Update on lithium carbonate therapy in children and adolescents. *Journal of the American Academy of Child and Adolescent Psychiatry, 33,* 291–304.

Allgood-Merton, B., Lewinsohn, P., & Hops, H. (1990). Sex differences and adolescent depression. *Journal of Abnormal Psychology, 99,* 55–63.

Ambrosini, P. J., Bianchi, M. D., Rabinovich, H., & Elia, J. (1993). Antidepressant treatments in children and adolescents I. Affective disorders. *Journal of the American Academy of Child and Adolescent Psychiatry, 32,* 1–6.

Anderson, J., Williams, S., McGee, R., & Silva, P. A. (1987). The prevalence of DSM-III disorders in a large sample of preadolescent children from the general population. *Archives of General Psychiatry, 44,* 69–76.

Arana, G. W., Baldessarini, R. J., & Ornsteen, M. (1985). The dexamethasone suppression test for diagnosis and prognosis in psychiatry. *Archives of General Psychiatry, 42,* 1193–1204.

Baldessarini, R. J. (1989). Current status of antidepressants: Clinical pharmacology and therapy. *Journal of Clinical Psychiatry, 50,* 117–126.

Biederman, J. (1991). Psychopharmacology. In J. M. Wiener (Ed.), *Textbook of child and adolescent psychiatry* (pp. 545–570). Washington, DC: American Psychiatric Press.

Birmaher, B., Ryan, N. D., Dahl, R., Rabinovich, H., Ambrosini, M. D., Williamson, D. E., Novacenko, H., Nelson, B., Lo, S. E., & Puig-Antich, K. (1992). Dexamethasone suppression test in children with major depressive disorder. *Journal of the American Academy of Child and Adolescent Psychiatry, 31,* 291–297.

Bowring, M. A., & Kovacs, M. (1992). Difficulties in diagnosing manic disorders in children and adolescents. *Journal of the American Academy of Child and Adolescent Psychiatry, 31,* 611–614.

Butler, L., Miezitis, S., Friedman, R., & Cole, E. (1980). The affect of two school-based intervention programs on depressive symptoms on preadolescents. *American Educational Research Journal, 17,* 111–119.

Campbell, M., Silva, R. R., Kafantaris, V., Locascio, J. J., Gonzalez, N. M., Lee, D., & Lynch, N. S. (1991). Predictors of side effects associated with lithium administration in children. *Psychopharmacology Bulletin, 27,* 373–380.

Carlson, G. A. (1990). Child and adolescent mania: Diagnostic considerations. *Journal of Child Psychology and Psychiatry, 31,* 331–342.

Carlson, G. A., Fennig, S., & Bromet, E. J. (1994). The confusion between bipolar disorder and schizophrenia in youth: Where does it stand in the 1990's. *Journal of the American Academy of Child and Adolescent Psychiatry, 48,* 453–460.

Carlson, G. A., & Kashani, J. H. (1988). Phenomenology of major depression from childhood through adulthood: Analysis of three studies. *American Journal of Psychiatry, 145,* 1222–1225.

Carlson, G. A., & Weintraub, S. (1993). Childhood behavior problems and bipolar disorder—Relationship or coincidence. *Journal of Affective Disorders, 28,* 143–153.

Casat, C. D., Arana, G. W., & Powell, K. P. (1989). The DST in children and adolescents with major depressive disorder. *American Journal of Psychiatry, 146,* 503–507.

Chambers, W. J., Puig-Antich, J., Hirsch, M., Paez, P., Ambrosini, P. J., Tabrizi, M. A., & Davies, M. (1985). The assessment of depression in children and adolescents using a semistructured interview. Test-retest reliability of the schedule for affective disorders and schizophrenia for school-aged children, present episode version. *Archives of General Psychiatry, 42,* 696–702.

Clarke, G. N. (1991). Treatment of depression in adolescents. Workshop Presentation. Portland, Oregon.

Clarkin, J. F., Glick, I. D., Haas, G. L., Spencer, J. H., Lewis, A. B., Peyser, J., DeMane, N., Good-Ellis, M., Harris, E., & Lestelle, V. (1990). A randomized clinical trial of inpatient family intervention. V. Results for affective disorder. *Journal of Affective Disorders, 18,* 17–28.

Compas, B. (1987). Stress and life events during childhood and adolescence. *Clinical Psychology Review, 7,* 275–302.

Costello, E. J., & Angold, A. (1988). Scales to assess child and adolescent depression: Checklist, screens, and nets. *Journal of the American Academy of Child and Adolescent Psychiatry, 27,* 726–737.

Dahl, R. E., Ryan, N. D., Williamson, D. E., Ambrosini, P. J., Rabinovich, H., Novacenko, H., Nelson, B., & Puig-Antich, J. (1992). Regulation of sleep and growth hormone in adolescent depression. *Journal of the American Academy of Child and Adolescent Psychiatry, 31,* 615–621.

Delong, G. R., & Aldershof, A. L. (1987). Long-term experience with lithium treatment in childhood: Correlation with clinical diagnosis. *Journal of the American Academy of Child and Adolescent Psychiatry, 26,* 389–394.

deMesquita, P. B., & Gilliam, W. S. (1994). Differential diagnosis of childhood depression: Using comorbidity and symptom overlap to generate multiple hypotheses. *Child Psychiatry and Human Development, 24,* 157–172.

Edelbrock, C., & Costello, A. J. (1988). Convergence between statistically derived behavior problem syndromes and child psychiatric diagnoses. *Journal of Abnormal Child Psychiatry, 16,* 219–231.

Fetner, H. H., & Geller, B. (1992). Lithium and tricyclic antidepressants. *Psychiatric Clinics of North America, 15,* 223–241.

Fine, S., Forth, A., Gilbert, M., & Haley, G. (1991). Group therapy for adolescent depressive disorder: A comparison of social skills and therapeutic support. *Journal of the American Academy of Child and Adolescent Psychiatry, 30,* 79–85.

Fleming, J. E., Boyle, M., & Offord, D. (1991). *Four-year outcome of depressed adolescents: Ontario child health study.* Paper presented at the 38th Annual Meeting of the American Academy of Child and Adolescent Psychiatry, San Francisco.

Fleming, J. E., & Offord, D. R. (1990). Epidemiology of childhood depressive disorders. *Journal of the American Academy of Child and Adolescent Psychiatry, 29,* 571–576.

Fristad, M. A., Weller, E. B., & Weller, R. A. (1992). The mania rating scale: Can it be used in children? A preliminary report. *Journal of the American Academy of Child and Adolescent Psychiatry, 31,* 252–257.

Geller, B. (1994). Advancement from drug to psychotherapy research for bipolar depression in children. The Nathan Cummings Foundation Award Address, Meeting of the American Academy of Child and Adolescent Psychiatry, New York, October 19–21, 1994.

Geller, B., Cooper, T. B., Chestnut, E. C., Anker, J. A., & Schluchter, M.D. (1986). Preliminary data on the relationship between nortriptyline plasma level and response in depressed children. *American Journal of Psychiatry, 143,* 1283–1286.

Geller, B., Cooper, T. B., Graham, D. L., Fetner, H. H., Marsteller, F. A., & Wells, J. M. (1992). Pharmacokinetically designed double-blind placebo-controlled study of nortriptyline in 6- to 12-year-olds with major depressive disorder. *Journal of the American Academy of Child & Adolescent Psychiatry, 31,* 34–44.

Geller, B., Cooper, T. B., Graham, D. L., Marsteller, F. A., & Bryan, D. M. (1992). Double-blind placebo-controlled study of nortriptyline in depressed adolescents using a "fixed plasma level" design. *Psychopharmacology Bulletin, 26,* 85–90.

Geller, B., Fox, L. W., & Clark, K. A. (1994). Rate and predictors of prepuberal bipolarity during follow-up of 6- to 12-year-old depressed children. *Journal of the American Academy of Child and Adolescent Psychiatry, 33,* 461–468.

Gershon, E. S., Hamovit, J. H., Guroff, J. J., & Nurnberger, J. I. (1987). Birth-cohort changes in manic and depressive disorders in relatives of bipolar and schizoaffective patients. *Archives of General Psychiatry, 44,* 314–319.

Gutterman, E. M., O'Brien, J. D., & Young, J. G. (1987). Structured diagnostic interviews for children and adolescents: Current status and future directions. *Journal of the American Academy of Child and Adolescent Psychiatry, 26,* 621–630.

Himmelhoch, J. M., & Garfinkel, M. E. (1986). Mixed mania: Diagnosis and treatment. *Psychopharmacology Bulletin, 22,* 613–620.

Hoberman, H. M., & Garfinkel, B. D. (1988). Completed suicide in children and adolescents. *Journal of the American Academy of Child and Adolescent Psychiatry, 27,* 689–695.

Hodges, K. (1993). Structured interviews for assessing children. *Journal of Child Psychology and Psychiatry and Allied Disciplines, 34,* 49–68.

Hodges, K., Cools, J., & McKnew, D. (1989). Test-retest reliability of a clinical research interview for children: The Child Assessment Scale. *Psychological Assessment, 1,* 317–322.

Howland, R. H., & Thase, M. E. (1991). Biological studies of dysthymia. *Biological Psychiatry, 30,* 283–304.

Jain, J., Birmaher, B., Garcia, M., Al-Shabbout, M., & Ryan, N. (1993). Fluoxetine in children and adolescents with mood disorders: A chart review of efficacy and adverse effects. *Journal of Child and Adolescent Psychopharmacology, 2,* 259–265.

Jensen, J. B., & Garfinkel, B. D. (1990). Growth hormone dysregulation in children with major depressive disorder. *Journal of the American Academy of Child and Adolescent Psychiatry, 29,* 295–301.

Joyce, P. R. (1984). Age of onset in bipolar affective disorder and misdiagnosis as schizophrenia. *Psychological Medicine, 14,* 145–149.

Kahn, J. S., Kehle, T. J., Jenson, W. R., & Clark, E. (1990). Comparison of cognitive-behavioral, relaxation and self modeling interventions for depression among middle-school students. *School Psychology Review, 19,* 196–211.

Kandel, D. B., & Davies, M. (1986). Adult sequelae of adolescent depressive symptoms. *Archives of General Psychiatry, 43*, 255–262.

Kashani, J. H., Shekim, W.O., & Reid, J. C. (1984). Amitriptyline in children with major depressive disorder: A double-blind cross-over pilot study. *Journal American Academy of Child and Adolescent Psychiatry, 23*, 348–351.

Kashani, J. H., & Simonds, J. F. (1979). The incidence of depression in children. *American Journal of Psychiatry, 136*, 1203–1207.

Klerman, G. L. (1988). The current age of youthful melancholia: Evidence for increase in depression among adolescents and young adults. *British Journal of Psychiatry, 152*, 4–14.

Klerman, G. L., & Weissman, M. M. (1989). Increasing rates of depression. *Journal of the American Medical Association, 261*, 2229–2235.

Kovacs, M. (1985). The Children's Depression Inventory (CDI). *Psychopharmacology Bulletin, 21*, 995–998.

Kovacs, M., Akiskal, H. S., Gatsonis, C., & Parrone, P. L. (1994). Childhood onset dysthymic disorder. Clinical features and prospective naturalistic outcome. *Archives of General Psychiatry, 51*, 365–375.

Kovacs, M., Feinberg, T. L., Crouse-Novak, M., Paulauskas, S. L., & Finkelstein, R. (1984a). Depressive disorders in childhood I: A longitudinal prospective study of characteristics and recovery. *Archives of General Psychiatry, 41*, 229–237.

Kovacs, M., Feinberg, T. L., Crouse-Novak, M., Paulauskas, S. L., Pollack, M., & Finkelstein, R. (1984b). Depressive disorders in childhood II: A longitudinal study of the risk for a subsequent major depression. *Archives of General Psychiatry, 41*, 643–649.

Kovacs, M., Gatsonis, C., Paulauskas, S. L., & Richards, C. (1989). Depressive disorders in childhood IV: A longitudinal study of comorbidity with and risk for anxiety disorders. *Archives of General Psychiatry, 46*, 776–782.

Kovacs, M., Paulauskas, S., & Richards, C. (1988). Depressive disorders in childhood III: A longitudinal study of comorbidity with and risk for conduct disorders. *Journal of Affective Disorders, 15*, 205–217.

Kovacs, M., & Pollock, M. (1995). Bipolar disorder and comorbid conduct disorder in childhood and adolescence. *Journal of the American Academy of Child and Adolescent Psychiatry, 34*, 715–723.

Kramer, A. D., & Feiguine, R. J. (1981). Clinical effects of amitriptyline in adolescent depression. A pilot study. *Journal of the American Academy of Child and Adolescent Psychiatry, 20*, 636–644.

Kutcher, S. P., Williamson, P., Silverberg, J., Marton, P., Malkin, D., & Malkin, A. (1988). Nocturnal growth hormone secretion in depressed older adolescents. *Journal of the American Academy of Child and Adolescent Psychiatry, 27*, 751–754.

Lang, M., & Tisher, M. (1978). Children's Depression Scale. Australian Council for Educational Research, Victoria, Australia.

Lewinsohn, P. M., Clarke, G. N., Seeley, J. R., & Rohde, P. (1994). Major depression in community adolescents: Age at onset, episode duration, time to recurrence. *Journal of the American Academy of Child and Adolescent Psychiatry, 33*, 809–818.

Lewinsohn, P. M., Hops, H., Roberts, R. E., Seeley, J. R., & Andrews, J. A. (1993). Adolescent psychopathology: I. Prevalence and incidence of depression and other DSM-III-R disorders in high school students. *Journal of Abnormal Psychology, 102*, 133–144.

Livingston, R., Reise, C. J., & Ringdahl, I. C. (1984). Abnormal dexamethasone suppression test results in depressed and nondepressed children. *American Journal of Psychiatry, 141*, 106–108.

McCauley, E., & Myers, K. (1992). The longitudinal clinical course of depression in children and adolescents. *Child and Adolescent Psychiatric Clinics of North America, 1*, 183–196.

McCauley, E., Myers, K. M., Mitchell, J., Calderon, R., Schloredt, K., & Treder, R. (1993). Depression in young people: Initial presentation and clinical course. *Journal of the American Academy of Child and Adolescent Psychiatry, 32*, 714–722.

McClellan, J. M. & Werry, J. S. (1995, October) *Practice parameters for the assessment and treatment of children and adolescents with bipolar disorder*. Paper presented at the American Academy of Child and Adolescent Psychiatry, New Orleans.

McClellan, J., Werry, J. S., & Ham, M. (1993). A follow-up study of early onset psychosis: Comparison between outcome diagnoses of schizophrenia, mood disorders, and personality disorders. *Journal of Autism and Developmental Disorders, 23*, 243–262.

McGee, R., & Williams, S. (1988). A longitudinal study of depression in nine-year-old children. *Journal of the American Academy of Child and Adolescent Psychiatry, 27*, 342–348.

McGlashan, T. H. (1988). Adolescent versus adult onset of mania. *American Journal of Psychiatry, 145*, 221–223.

McKnew, D. H., Cytryn, L., Buchsbaum, M. S., Hamovit, J., Lamour, M., Rapoport, J. L., & Gershon, E. S. (1981). Lithium in children of lithium-responding parents. *Psychiatry Research, 4*, 171–180.

McKnew, D. H., Cytryn, L., Efron, A. M., Gerson, E. S., & Bunney, W. E. (1979). Offspring of patients with affective disorders. *British Journal of Psychiatry, 134,* 148–152.

Merikangas, K. R. (1993). Genetic epidemiological studies of affective disorders in childhood and adolescents. *European Archives of Psychiatry and Clinical Neuroscience, 243,* 121–130.

Mitchell, J., McCauley, E., Burke, P. M., & Moss, S. (1988). Phenomenology of depression in children and adolescents. *Journal of the American Academy of Child and Adolescent Psychiatry, 27,* 12–20.

Moretti, M. M., Fine, S., Haley, G., & Marriage, K. (1985). Child and adolescent depression: Child-report versus parent-report information. *Journal of the American Academy of Child and Adolescent Psychiatry, 24,* 298–302.

Mufson, L., Moreau, D., Weissman, M. M., Wickramatne, P., Martin, J., & Samoilov, A. (1994). Modification of interpersonal psychotherapy with depressed adolescents. (IPT-A): Phase I and II studies. *Journal of the American Academy of Child and Adolescent Psychiatry, 33,* 695–705.

Neiman, G. W., & Delong, R. (1987). Use of the personality inventory for children as an aid in differentiating children with mania from children with attention deficit disorder with hyperactivity. *Journal of the American Academy of Child and Adolescent Psychiatry, 26,* 381–388.

Nolen-Hoeksema, S., & Girgus, J. S. (1994). The emergence of gender differences in depression during adolescence. *Psychological Bulletin, 115,* 424–443.

Petersen, A. C., Sarigiani, P. A., & Kennedy, R. E. (1991). Adolescent depression: Why more girls? *Journal of Youth and Adolescence, 18,* 617–626.

Pfeffer, C. R., Klerman, G. L., Hurt, S. W., Lesser, M., Peskin, J. R., & Siefker, C. A. (1991). Suicidal children grow up: Demographic and clinical use factors for adolescent suicide attempts. *Journal of the American Academy of Child and Adolescent Psychiatry, 30,* 609–616.

Popper, C. (1992). Are clinicians ahead of researchers in finding a treatment for adolescent depression? *Journal of Child and Adolescent Psychopharmacology, 2,* 1–3.

Poznanski, E. O., Freeman, L. N., & Mokros, H. B. (1985). Children's depression rating scale-revised. *Psychopharmacology Bulletin, 21,* 979–989.

Preskorn, S. H., Weller, E. B., Hughes, C. W., Weller, R. A., & Bolte, K. (1987). Depression in prepubertal children: Dexamethasone nonsuppression predicts differential response to imipramine vs. placebo. *Psychopharmacology Bulletin, 23,* 128–133.

Prien, R. F., & Potter, W. Z. (1990). NIMH workshop report on treatment of bipolar disorder. *Psychopharmacology Bulletin, 26,* 409–427.

Puig-Antich, J., Perel, J. M., Lupatkin, W., Chambers, W. J., Tabrizi, M. A., King, J., Goetz, R., Davies, M., & Stiller, R. L. (1987). Imipramine in prepubertal major depressive disorders. *Archives of General Psychiatry, 44,* 81–89.

Renouf, A. G., & Kovacs, M. (1994). Concordance between mother's reports and children's self reports of depressive symptoms: A longitudinal study. *Journal of the American Academy of Child and Adolescent Psychiatry, 33,* 208–216.

Reynolds, W. M. (1992). Depression in children and adolescents. In Reynolds, W. M. (Ed.), *Internalizing disorders in children and adolescents* (149–254). New York: John Wiley & Sons.

Reynolds, W. M., & Coats, K. I. (1986). A comparison of cognitive-behavioral therapy and relaxation training for the treatment of depression in adolescents. *Journal of Clinical and Consulting Psychology, 54,* 653–660.

Richters, J. E. (1992). Depressed mothers as informants about their children: A critical review of the evidence for distortion. *Psychological Bulletin, 112,* 485–499.

Riddle, M. A., Geller, B., & Ryan, N. (1993). Another sudden death in a child treated with desipramine. *Journal of the American Academy of Child and Adolescent Psychiatry, 32,* 792–797.

Riddle, M. A., King, R. A., Hardin, M. T., Scahill, L., Ort, S. I., Chappell, P., Rasmusson, A., & Leckman, J. F. (1990/1991). Behavioral side effects of fluoxetine in children and adolescents. *Journal of Child and Adolescent Psychopharmacology, 1,* 193–198.

Rogeness, G. A., Javors, M. A., & Pliszka, S. R. (1992). Neurochemistry and child and adolescent psychiatry. *Journal of the American Academy of Child and Adolescent Psychiatry, 31,* 765–781.

Rohed, P., Lewinsohn, P. M., & Seeley, J. R. (1994). Are adolescents changed by an episode of major depression? *Journal of the American Academy of Child and Adolescent Psychiatry, 33,* 1289–1298.

Rosenberg, D. R., Holttum, J., & Gershon, S. (1994). Tricyclic antidepressants. In D. R. Rosenberg, J. Holttum, & S. Gershon (Eds.), *Textbook of pharmacotherapy for child and adolescent psychiatric disorders* (pp. 55–103). New York: Brunner/Mazel, Inc.

Rutter, M., MacDonald, H., Couteur, A. L., Harrington, R., Bolton, P., & Bailey, A. (1990). Genetic factors in child psychiatric disorder II. Empirical findings. *Journal of Child Psychology and Psychiatry, 31,* 39–83.

Ryan, N. D., Dahl, R. E., Birmaher, B., Williamson, D. E., Iyengar, S., Nelson, B., Puig-Antich, J., & Perel, J. M. (1994). Stimulatory test of growth hormone secretion in prepubertal major depression: Depressed versus normal children. *Journal of the American Academy of Child and Adolescent Psychiatry, 33*, 824–833.

Ryan, N. D., Meyer, V., Dachille, S., Mazzie, D., & Puig-Antich, J. (1988). Lithium antidepressant augmentation in TCA-refractory depression in adolescents. *Journal of the American Academy of Child and Adolescent Psychiatry, 27*, 371–376.

Ryan, N. D., Puig-Antich, J., Cooper, T., Rabinovich, H., Ambrosini, P., Davies, M., King, J., Torres, D., & Fried, J. (1986). Imipramine in adolescent major depression: Plasma level and clinical response. *Acta Psychiatrica Scandinavia, 73*, 273–288.

Ryan, N. D., Puig-Antich, J., Ambrosini, P., Rabinovich, H., Robinson, D., Nelson, B., Iyengar, S., & Twomey, J. (1987). The clinical picture of major depression in children and adolescents. *Archives of General Psychiatry, 44*, 854–861.

Ryan, N. D., Williamson, D. E., Iyengar, J., Orvaschel, H., Reich, T., Dahl, R. E., & Puig-Antich, J. (1992). A secular increase in child and adolescent onset affective disorder. *Journal of the American Academy of Child and Adolescent Psychiatry, 31*, 600–605.

Shaffer, D., Schwab-Stone, M., Fisher, P. W., Cohen, P., Piacenini, J., Davies, M., Conners, C. K., & Regier, D. (1993). The Diagnostic Interview Schedule for Children—Revised version (DISCR): I. Preparation, field testing, interrater reliability and acceptance. *Journal of the American Academy of Child and Adolescent Psychiatry, 32*, 643–650.

Simeon, J. G., Dinicola, V. F., Ferguson, H. B., & Copping, W. (1990). Adolescent depression: A placebo-controlled fluoxetine treatment study and follow-up. *Progress Neuro-Psychopharmacology and Biologic Psychiatry, 14*, 791–795.

Stark, K. D., Reynolds, W. M., & Kaslow, N. J. (1987). A comparison of the self-central therapy and a behavioral problem-solving therapy for depression in children. *Journal of Abnormal Child Psychology, 15*, 91–113.

Stein, M. A., Szumowski, E., Ravitz, A. J., Frey, M. J., & Leventhal, B. L. (1994). Dexamethasone suppression and childhood depression: Association with categorical and dimensional measures. *Journal of Child and Adolescent Psychopharmacology, 4*, 43–52.

Strober, M. (1991). *The prospective, naturalistic course of depressive illness during adolescence.* Paper presented at the 38th Annual Meeting of the American Academy of Child and Adolescent Psychiatry, San Francisco.

Strober, M., & Carlson, G. (1982). Bipolar illness in adolescents with major depression: Clinical, genetic, and psychopharmacological predictors in a three- to four-year prospective follow-up investigation. *Archives of General Psychiatry, 39*, 549–555.

Strober, M., Freeman, R., Rigali, J., Schmidt, S., & Diamond, R. (1992). The pharmacotherapy of depressive illness in adolescence: II. Effects of lithium augmentation in nonresponders to imipramine. *Journal of the American Academy of Child and Adolescent Psychiatry, 31*, 16–20.

Strober, M., Lampert, C., Schmidt, S., & Morrell, W. (1993). The course of major depressive disorder in adolescents: I. Recovery and risk of manic switching in a follow-up of psychotic and non-psychotic subtypes. *Journal of the American Academy of Child and Adolescent Psychiatry, 32*, 34–42.

Strober, M., Morrell, W., Burroughs, J., Lampert, C., Danfort, H., & Freeman, R. (1988). A family study of bipolar I disorder in adolescence: Early onset of symptoms linked to increased familial loading and lithium resistance. *Journal of Affective Disorders, 15*, 255–268.

Strober, M., Morrell, W., Lampert, C., & Burroughs, J. (1990). Relapse following discontinuation of lithium maintenance therapy in adolescents with bipolar I illness: A naturalistic study. *American Journal of Psychiatry, 147*, 457–461.

Sylvester, C., Burke, P. M., McCauley, E., & Clark, C. J. (1994). Manic psychosis in childhood: Report of two cases. *Journal of Nervous and Mental Disease, 172*, 12–15.

Trimble, M. R. (1990). Anticonvulsants in children and adolescents. *Journal of Child and Adolescent Psychopharmacology, 1*, 107–124.

Varanka, T. M., Weller, R. A., Weller, E. B., & Fristad, M. A. (1988). Lithium treatment of manic episodes with psychotic features in prepubertal children. *American Journal of Psychiatry, 145*, 1557–1559.

Walker, M., Moreau, D., & Weissman, M. M. (1990). Parents' awareness of children's suicide attempts. *American Journal of Psychiatry, 147*, 1364–1366.

Weissman, M. M. (1987). Advances in psychiatric epidemiology: Rates and risks for major depression. *Journal of Public Health, 77*, 445–451.

Weissman, M. M., Orvaschel, H., & Padian, N. (1980). Children's symptoms and social functioning self report scales. *Journal of Nervous and Mental Disorders, 168*, 736–740.

Weissman, M. M., Wickramaratne, P., Warner, V., John, K., Prusoff, B. A., Merikangas, K. R., & Gammon, G. D. (1987). Assessing psychiatric disorders in children. *Archives of General Psychiatry, 44*, 747–753.

Welner, Z., Reich, W., Herjanic, B., Jung, K. G., & Amado, H. (1987). Reliability, validity and parent-child agreement studies of the Diagnostic Interview for Children and Adolescents (DICA). *Journal of the American Academy of Child and Adolescent Psychiatry, 26,* 649–653.

Werry, J. S., McClellan, J., & Chard, L. (1991). Childhood and adolescent schizophrenia, bipolar and schizoaffective disorders: A clinical and outcome study. *Journal of*

the American Academy of Child and Adolescent Psychiatry, 30,* 457–465.

Yaylayan, S. A., Weller, E. B., & Weller, R. (1991). Biology of depression in children and adolescents. *Journal of Child and Adolescent Psychopharmacology, 1,* 215–225.

CHAPTER 14

EATING DISORDERS

Mary J. Sanders
Cynthia J. Kapphahn
Hans Steiner

DESCRIPTION OF DISORDERS

Differential Diagnosis

As the *Diagnostic and Statistical Manual, Fourth Edition* (American Psychiatric Association, 1994) describes, the core diagnostic feature of patients with either anorexia or bulimia is that they are unduly influenced by body weight. For anorexia, the diagnosis includes refusal to maintain adequate weight. This is not a necessary criterion for the diagnosis of bulimia. Bulimia is further characterized by binge eating, involving both the consumption of a large quantity of food and the feeling of being "out of control." Currently, both diagnoses include the possibility of compensatory behaviors. These may include activities such as over-exercise, vomiting, or diuretic or laxative use. A diagnosis of "eating disorder, not otherwise specified" refers to subthreshold situations in which eating problems are identified, but not all of the diagnostic criteria for either anorexia or bulimia are met. This diagnostic category may be particularly relevant for pediatric or adolescent populations, as ideally many of these patients would be identified and begin treatment at relatively early stages of the disorder.

Distorted Body Image in Children and Adolescents

Adolescence is the peak age period for onset of eating disorders (Bruch, 1974). Weight concerns are quite common in this age group. Over 70 percent of girls 15 years and older have been found to desire weight loss or engage in dieting (Wadden, Foster, Stunkard, & Linowitz, 1989). About 30 percent to 40 percent of junior high girls (Childress, Brewerton, Hodges, & Jarrell, 1993; Richards, Casper, & Larson, 1990) and school-age children (Maloney, McGuire, Daniels, & Specker, 1989) also admit to concerns about weight.

Current media messages urging women to achieve not just a slender, but a slender-tight and muscular body may promote behaviors that are risky, such as over-exercising and extreme dieting. Adolescents are vulnerable to this "ideal" as they struggle for an identity during this developmental stage, and may be influenced significantly by the media during this search (White, 1992a).

Development of Eating Disorders in Adolescents

There are many theories regarding the underlying problems that manifest themselves through eating disorders in adolescents. One formulation that has gained wide acceptance involves inner conflict over developmental issues. As preadolescents move toward puberty, they may experience cultural pressures to be ineffective and have difficulty interpreting physical and emotional sensations associated with pubertal growth and development (Crisp, 1980). This may lead to fears about sexuality or problems with identity issues. In addition, conflict may develop around the tasks of individuation and separation. In an effort to gain a sense of mastery, patients may attempt to control their bodies, perhaps avoiding physical development (and, therefore, further individuation or sexual development) through weight loss (Crisp, 1980; White, 1992b).

EPIDEMIOLOGY

Most data regarding the incidence and prevalence of eating disorders are based on cases referred to specialty treatment clinics. Comparison of these findings is difficult, owing to differences in case definition, populations compared (i.e., community vs. school-based), age groups compared (some include adult groups), methods of gathering data (questionnaire vs. a two-stage process of questionnaire combined with interview), and diagnostic criteria used to determine inclusion (i.e., DSM-III v. DSM-IV). Fairburn and Beglin's (1990) review of epidemiology reveals that the more methodologically sophisticated studies may not necessarily be more accurate, as there is evidence that some portion of nonresponders did, in fact, have eating disorders. The authors comment that it may be impossible to obtain a precise estimate of prevalence due to all of the sampling limitations.

Anorexia Nervosa

In the United States, about 1 percent to 2 percent of females aged 14 to 40 have been estimated to meet DSM-III-R criteria for anorexia nervosa, and 5 percent to 15 percent of the college-age population have been estimated to have subthreshold levels of eating disorders (Hsu, 1991). Most studies that draw subjects from clinic referral populations indicate a rise in the incidence and prevalence of anorexia nervosa over the past 40 years (Jones, Fox, Babigian, & Hutton, 1980; Kendell, Hall, Hailey, & Babigian, 1973; Willi & Grossmann, 1983). However, epidemiological studies done by Lucas, Beard, O'Fallon, and Kurland (1991) provide insight into variations in disease incidence over time within a community-based population. They followed the incidence of eating disorders in Rochester, Minnesota over a 50-year period (1935–1984). A "case" was defined as an individual who met the criteria for the DSM-III-R diagnosis of anorexia nervosa. The overall age-adjusted incidence rate was 14.6 for females and 1.8 for males per 100,000. Incidence rates for females went from 16.6 per 100,000 in 1935–1939 to 7 in 1950–1954, and then increased to 26.3 in 1980–1984.

Lucas and colleagues (1991) note that fluctuations in the incidence of anorexia nervosa reflect changing rates in the 15- to 24-year-old group. While incidence rates for older women (24 years old and older) and for males have remained constant, there has been a significant increase in the rate for females 15 to 24 over time. They observe that fluctuations in incidence for the 15-24-year-old group mirrors periods in which the media has focused on portraying thinner models. They suggest that there is a more severe and chronic form of anorexia nervosa with an incidence that has remained constant over time. A milder form of anorexia nervosa may be present in the teenage group that remits quickly and completely in response to treatment, with variations in incidence that reflect adolescents' heightened vulnerability to cultural pressures.

Bulimia

Bulimia has only recently been included in epidemiological studies, so long-term trends cannot be examined. In their review, Fairburn and Beglin (1990) found a prevalence among women and adolescents of approximately 1 percent. A two-stage study combining questionnaire and interview data, using the more strict criteria in the DSM-III-R and sampling a high-school population, found a prevalence rate of 1 percent in a population from the western United States (Lucas, 1992) as well as in a London population (Johnson-Sabine, Wood, Patton, Mann, & Wakeling, 1988).

In comparing two population-based studies, Hoek (1991) found an incidence rate of 9.9/100,000 in the Netherlands from 1985 to 1986 as compared to Cullberg and Engstrom-Lindberg (1988), who found an incidence of 3.9/100,000. Both studies accessed case material from a number of sources, sampled a large age range (10 to 35 years), and used DSM-III criteria. Both studies found the highest incidence of bulimia was in the older-adolescent, young-adult population, approximately 16–24 years of age.

Incidence of Eating Disorders by Gender

Current data suggest that the incidence of anorexia nervosa is 8 times greater for females than for males (Anderson, 1988; Lucas et al., 1991; Rastam, Gillberg, & Garton, 1989). Girls desire a thin body while, generally, boys do not (Nylander, 1971). It has been suggested that the western cultural ideal of thinness for women may serve as a substitute for areas in their lives in which they feel they have little control (Steiner-Adair, 1986). Perhaps the changing of women's roles in society over the past few decades has contributed to an emphasis on achieving success in all areas, including control of the body.

Within the small population of males who are treated for eating disorders, approximately 30 percent may be homosexual (Herzog, Bradburn, & Newman, 1990). Burns and Crisp (1984) found that outcomes for the male population they studied did not differ significantly from those expected for female patients. It may be that males are also experiencing cultural pressures and transitions of role, but are less apt to channel these concerns through body control.

ASSESSMENT APPROACHES

A comprehensive multidisciplinary assessment includes a medical, nutritional, and psychological evaluation of the identified patient, as well as a family interview. The assessment should be considered the beginning of treatment. The clinician should attempt to build a relationship based on respect and recognition of power issues that are fundamentally apparent in doctor-patient relationships. Specific questions regarding eating symptoms should be asked, and the context and meaning of the problem in the lives of these patients should be ascertained.

Medical Issues

In addition to their impact on psychological well-being, eating disorders have a significant deleterious effect on physical health (Comerci, 1990; Palla & Litt, 1988). Medical sequelae can be permanent or even fatal. Pubertal growth and development may be significantly compromised by eating disorders, placing adolescents at particularly high risk for medical complications (Fisher et al., 1995). Evaluation and coordination with a designated medical provider who is experienced in treating patients with eating disorders is essential, to create an environment in which the underlying psychological issues can be safely addressed.

The first phase in which medical input is necessary is in the initial diagnosis. Many illnesses associated with weight loss, amenorrhea, vomiting, and/or changes in appetite share certain common characteristics with eating disorders, and may be missed unless a thorough initial history and physical examination are performed. These include malignancies, infectious diseases such as tuberculosis or acquired immune deficiency syndrome (AIDS), inflammatory bowel disease, celiac sprue, chronic renal failure, substance abuse, Addison's disease, diabetes mellitus, and other endocrine disorders (Wright, Smith, & Mitchell, 1990). A complete medical evaluation to rule out such illnesses is essential before diagnosing an eating disorder.

During the treatment phase, serious medical issues may arise. Patients with eating disorders often develop bradycardia, hypothermia, or orthostatic changes in blood pressure or pulse (Palla & Litt, 1988). The initial refeeding phase is particularly critical because congestive heart failure may occur if refeeding is too rapid. Great caution must be taken to ensure that calories do not exceed the body's metabolic limit, and yet are sufficient to promote recovery.

Life-threatening electrolyte disturbances such as hypokalemia may result from purging or laxative abuse. Cardiac function may become impaired (Kreipe & Harris, 1992; Schocken, Holloway, & Powers, 1989). Heart muscle mass is decreased in malnourished patients (Moodie, 1987; Moodie & Salcedo, 1983) and regional cardiac wall motion abnormalities have been noted (Goldberg, Comerci, & Feldman, 1988; Kahn, Halls, Bianco, & Perlman, 1991) and may contribute to less effective cardiac function. Cardiac arrhythmias can occur and are potentially fatal (Kreipe & Harris, 1992). Syrup of Ipecac is a cardiotoxin, and may cause cardiomyopathy if used for purging (Palmer & Guay, 1986). Other potential medical complications include renal abnormalities. Decreased renal filtration rates, partial diabetes insipidus, hypokalemic nephropathy, and renal calculi may occur (Brotman, Stern, & Brotman, 1986; Fohlin, 1977; Mitchell, Pomeroy, Seppala, & Huber, 1988).

Osteopenia is another significant medical complication of anorexia nervosa and is of particular concern in adolescents (Bachrach, Guido, Katzman, Litt, & Marcus, 1990; Davies et al., 1990). The majority of life-time, adult bone density is acquired during adolescence, so alterations in bone metabolism at this time may result in permanent deficits and potential disability.

In eating disorders, bone loss may be promoted by a number of factors, including low estrogen levels associated with amenorrhea and glucocorticoid excess resulting from chronic physical stress (Biller et al., 1989; Joyce, Warren, Humphries, Smith, & Coon, 1990; Newman & Halmi, 1989). Studies of patients with a history of both restriction and purging suggest that they comprise a group at particularly high risk for osteopenia (Anderson & LaFrance, 1990). Adolescents with osteopenia may be more prone to fractures, at levels of impact that would normally be well tolerated. In the long term, bone density may recover slowly, if at all, potentially resulting in life-long alterations in bone resilience and strength.

Bone mineral density in adolescents with anorexia nervosa correlates with body mass index and age of disease onset (Bachrach et al., 1990). There is a trend toward even lower bone densities in adolescents with primary amenorrhea (Bachrach et al., 1990) when compared to girls who have had menarche. Studies in adults with anorexia nervosa suggest that an earlier age of onset for secondary amenorrhea is associated with greater decreases in bone density. However, this has not yet been substantiated in adolescent populations (Biller et al., 1989). While research into factors contributing to outcome in adolescents with osteopenia continues, it is clear that the duration of the malnourished state is significant in determining whether bone density will recover (Bachrach et al., 1990; Bachrach, Katzman, Litt, Guido, & Marcus, 1991). Weight rehabilitation is associated with improvements in bone density, even before menses return in adolescents (Bachrach et al., 1991).

Alterations in bone growth during starvation can affect height, particularly in young adolescents. Having anorexia nervosa during adolescence is associated with shorter adult stature (Kreipe, Churchill, & Strauss, 1989a; Nussbaum, Baird, Sonnenblick, Cowan, & Shenker, 1985).

Pubertal delay is also common in adolescents with eating disorders. In most adolescents, weight rehabilitation results in a normalization of hormonal function. However, many experience delays of a year or more before return of menses, and a portion may never regain normal hormonal function and fertility (Herzog, Keller, & Lavori, 1988; Kreipe, Churchill, & Strauss, 1989b; Nussbaum, Shenker, Baird, & Saraway, 1985; Steinhausen, Rauss-Mason, & Seidel, 1991).

In addition, anorexia and bulimia are associated with alterations in brain structure and function. CT and MRI scans of patients with anorexia nervosa and bulimia nervosa reveal enlarged external cerebrospinal fluid spaces and ventricular dilatation (Krieg, Backmund, & Pirke, 1987; Krieg, Lauer, & Pirke, 1989; Nussbaum, Shenker, Marc, & Klein, 1980). There are differences in the type of positron emission tomography (PET) scan abnormalities observed in patients with anorexia and with bulimia (Herholz et al., 1987; Wu et al., 1990). An organic brain syndrome secondary to malnutrition may develop in patients with an eating disorder, thereby interfering with psychotherapy until nutritional rehabilitation is well underway. Seizures and baseline electroencephalography (EEG) abnormalities may occur if there is prolonged cachexia or alterations in electrolytes (Crisp, Fenton, & Scotton, 1968).

The Neurochemistry of Eating Disorders

Starvation is thought to cause the vast majority of neurochemical abnormalities found in anorexia nervosa (Yates, 1989). The neurotransmitter amines, norepinephrine and serotonin, modulate feeding, mood, and neuroendocrine function (Kaye & Weltzin, 1991; Liebowitz, 1983). Abnormalities in the function or distribution of these amines are thought to cause many of the symptoms noted in eating disorders. Serotonin deficiency is associated with carbohydrate craving, a frequent complaint seen in patients with bulimia. Serotonin deficiency is also associated with compulsive behavior, which is common among patients with eating disorders. These neurotransmitters are affected by the availability of certain nutrients, such as tryptophan in the case of serotonin (Clippen et al., 1976), and thus abnormalities may be perpetuated by continued starvation.

Abnormalities in cholecystokinin (CCK) have also been noted in patients with bulimia (Geracioti & Liddle, 1988). CCK is a peptide that is secreted by the gastrointestinal tract when food is ingested. It induces a sense of satiety via stimulation of vagal afferents to the brain. Lower CCK levels have been noted in patients who purge. However, it is unclear whether this biochemical abnormality precedes the onset of bulimia or whether it reflects CCK supply depletion from repeated binges (Yates, 1992).

Abnormalities in central nervous system endorphins also may play a role in eating disorders. Starvation results in increased opioid release. Higher levels of opioids have been found in the plasma and cerebrospinal fluid of malnourished patients with anorexia nervosa than in patients who are weight-restored (Kaye, Pickar, Naber, &

Ebert, 1982), or in healthy controls (Tepper, Weizman, Apter, Tyano, & Beyth, 1992). Higher levels of plasma beta-endorphin have also been noted in patients with bulimia who vomit, compared both to those who do not vomit and control subjects (Fullerton, Swift, Getto, & Carlson, 1986; Fullerton, Swift, Getto, Carlson, & Gutzmann 1988). Starvation or purge-induced endorphin elevation may reinforce these behaviors in patients who have eating disorders (Yates, 1992).

Another neurochemical abnormality observed in patients with anorexia nervosa and bulimia is a disturbance in the pattern of arginine vasopressin release (Demitrack et al., 1992; Gold, Kaye, Robertson, & Ebert, 1983). This CNS peptide is responsible for water balance, and may also be involved in memory consolidation (DeWied, 1971).

Pediatric/Medical Evaluation

The first step in the medical evaluation should be to assess initial vital signs and percentage of body mass index (BMI) or ideal body weight (IBW) (see section on Achieving Healthy Weight) to determine if immediate hospitalization is necessary for severe malnutrition or vital sign instability. Guidelines recently issued by the Society for Adolescent Medicine (Fisher et al., 1995) indicate that any of the conditions listed in Table 14.1 would justify admission for an adolescent with an eating disorder.

Initial blood pressure and pulse should be checked after the patient has been prone for 5 minutes. Blood pressure and pulse should be rechecked after 2 minutes standing, to assess for orthostatic changes. Oral temperature should also be obtained. When assessing for medical instability, the following vital sign limits are suggested:

1. Hypothermia: oral temperature = 36.3°C during the day or = 36.0°C at night.
2. Bradycardia: heart rate = 45/min.
3. Orthostasis: drop in systolic blood pressure of greater than 10 mmHg or increase in pulse by more than 35 beats/min.

For patients taking medications (such as tricyclic antidepressants) that would be expected to alter vasomotor stability, expanded orthostatic limits are suggested. In this case, a patient would be considered orthostatic if he or she experienced a drop of greater than 15 in systolic blood pressure, or a rise of more that 45 beats/minute in pulse. If no aspect of the initial vital sign assessment re-

Table 14.1. Society for Adolescent Medicine Guidelines: Indications for Hospitalization

Any one or more of these criteria would justify hospitalization:

1. Severe malnutrition
   Weight less than 75 percent ideal body weight
2. Dehydration
3. Electrolyte disturbances
4. Cardiac dysrhythmia
5. Physiological instability
   Severe bradycardia
   Hypotension
   Hypothermia
   Orthostatic changes
6. Arrested growth and development
7. Failure of outpatient treatment
8. Acute food refusal
9. Uncontrollable bingeing and purging
10. Acute medical complications of malnutrition (e.g., syncope, seizures, cardiac failure, pancreatitis, etc.)
11. Acute psychiatric emergencies (e.g., suicidal ideation, acute psychosis)
12. Comorbid diagnosis that interferes with the treatment of the eating disorder (e.g., severe depression, obsessive-compulsive disorder, severe family dysfunction)

Source: From "Eating Disorders in Adolescents: A Background Paper," by Fischer et al., (1995), *Journal of Adolescent Health, 16*, p. 429. Reprinted with permission.

quires urgent intervention, a thorough history should be taken. For details about the eating history, see the section devoted to that subject below.

In addition, a review of systems is important. It should cover symptoms suggestive of vasomotor instability, such as dizziness or fainting, and other symptoms related to malnutrition or depression, such as fatigue, weakness, and difficulty concentrating. Patients who abuse laxatives may experience diarrhea, hematochezia, steatorrhea, or laxative dependence with extreme constipation (Mitchell & Boutacoff, 1986). Constipation is also seen in patients with restricted food intake. Other common gastrointestinal complaints in patients with eating disorders include nonfocal abdominal pain and a bloated sensation.

In patients with bulimia, it is important to inquire about hematemesis, as it may indicate more severe gastrointestinal pathology requiring intervention. If there is a long history of purging or rumination, reflex regurgitation may result from decreased esophageal sphincter tone. Scarring can develop from repeated trauma to the lower esophagus, leading to strictures and difficulty swallowing.

Determining if menstrual irregularities or amenorrhea are present and the date of the last menstrual period (if any) may provide insight into the duration of illness. Sleep patterns and changes in appetite may be associated with the eating disorder itself, or can suggest comorbid depression.

In addition, inquiries should be made regarding symptoms that suggest other etiologies for weight loss or vomiting. These include visual changes or headaches (intracranial mass), polydypsia and polyuria (diabetes mellitus), skin hyperpigmentation (Addison disease), breast tenderness or fullness (pregnancy), diarrhea (inflammatory bowel disease or chronic infection), and fever or night sweats (autoimmune disorders or infection).

Confidential inquiry about sexual activity is essential. A history of sexual abuse may be obtained by inquiring about whether the adolescent has ever been touched in a way that he or she felt was inappropriate. Regardless of response, a pregnancy test is warranted in any adolescent with a history of recurrent vomiting or amenorrhea, as adolescents may not feel comfortable disclosing information about pregnancy risk factors during their evaluation. Use of substances, such as illicit drugs, cigarettes, or alcohol, should also be assessed, as these agents may alter appetite or promote weight loss.

The physical examination may also provide useful clues to diagnosis. Signs suggestive of an eating disorder include those listed in Table 14.2.

Table 14.2. Medical Complications and Physical Findings in Anorexia and Bulimia

Head, eyes, ears, nose, throat:

Pathophysiology: Acid exposure and increased intrathoracic pressure associated with purging.

Complications: Gingivitis, eroded tooth enamel (particularly on lingual surface of the upper teeth) (Cuellar & Van Thiel, 1986; Levin, Falko, Dixon, Gallup, & Saunders, 1980; Mitchell, Hatsukami, Eckert, & Pyle, 1985), parotid gland irritation and overstimulation, conjunctival hemorrhage.

Physical findings: Parotid enlargement (generally bilateral and painless) (Levin et al., 1980), loss of tooth enamel, dental caries, prominent dental fillings, gingival erosions, erythema or petechiae of soft palate, conjunctival hemorrhage.

Cardiac:

Pathophysiology: Malnutrition, dehydration, electrolyte imbalances, ingestion of stimulants in diet pills or cardiotoxins such as ipecac.

Complications: Congestive heart failure, mitral valve prolapse (Johnson, Humphries, Shirley, Mazzoleni, & Noonan, 1986), cardiac muscle atrophy, cardiomyopathy, arrhythmias (Kreipe & Harris, 1992).

Physical findings: Alterations in cardiac rhythm, murmurs, faint heart sounds, displaced point of maximal impulse.

Vasomotor:

Pathophysiology: Down-regulation of the autonomic nervous system from malnutrition; dehydration from inadequate intake or laxative or diuretic abuse; abuse of stimulants.

Complications: Hypotension, orthostasis, hypertension.

Physical findings: Alterations in blood pressure or pulse.

Pulmonary:

Pathophysiology: Aspiration or increased intrathoracic pressure associated with purging; congestive heart failure associated with malnutrition or toxins.

Complications: Pulmonary edema, aspiration pneumonia, pneumomediastinum.

Physical findings: Rales; decreased, absent or asymmetric breath sounds.

Abdominal:

Pathophysiology: Malnutrition and purging.

Complications: Hepatic congestion, fatty liver infiltrate, gastritis, esophagitis, ulcers, gastric or esophageal dilatation (Mitchell, Pyle, & Miner, 1982), Mallory-Weiss tear of the lower esophagus, perforated viscus (Schechter, Altemus, & Greenfeld, 1986), pancreatitis (Cox, Cannon, Ament, Phillips, & Schaffer, 1983; Gavish et al., 1987), decreased gastrointestinal motility (Lautenbaucher, Galfe, Hoelzl, & Pirke, 1989) with associated delay in gastric emptying, postprandial fullness, bloating, early satiety, and constipation.

Physical findings: Hepatomegaly, abdominal tenderness, distention, altered bowel sounds.

Neurologic:

Pathophysiology: Malnutrition.

Complications: Cortical atrophy, organic brain syndrome.

Physical findings: Hyporeflexia, cognitive deficits.

Extremities:

Pathophysiology: Hypoalbuminemia or congestive heart failure associated with malnutrition; chronic dehydration and associated increase in aldosterone secretion from purging or laxative/diuretic abuse (Mitchell, Pomeroy, Seppala, & Huber, 1988).

Complications: Poor perfusion, fluid retention.

Physical findings: Cool to touch cyanosis, edema.

Skin:

Pathophysiology: Malnutrition, purging.

Complications: Capillary rupture, skin erosions or lacerations.

Physical findings: Dry skin, dull or brittle hair, alopecia, lanugo, skin erosion along spine from excessive exercise and sit-ups, petechia on the soft palate or face, lacerations, scarred knuckles, or skin hypopigmentation over the dorsum of the dominant hand from self-induced vomiting (Williams, Friedman, & Steiner, 1986).

Weights should be taken with patients in gown only, after voiding. Clinicians need to be attuned to the fact that patients may try various means to alter recorded weight. Patients with eating disorders may be so desperate to avoid weight gain that they may try to give the impression of higher body weights by drinking large amounts of fluids or hiding weights in clothes or on their body prior to being weighed. Both height and weight should be plotted on growth charts to compare with standard age and sex norms and with weight-for-height growth curves. Alternatively, the BMI may be used (see the section on Achieving Healthy Weight).

Pubic hair and breast or genital development should be compared to standards for Tanner staging to assess pubertal development. Nutritional assessment should include an assessment of percent body fat. Measuring triceps skin-fold thickness can be helpful in this assessment.

Physical examination can also be useful in ruling out other possible diagnoses. Papilledema or cranial nerve abnormalities suggest an intracranial mass. Focal neurologic findings should not be present in anorexia nervosa or bulimia and suggest an underlying organic diagnosis. Skin hyperpigmentation may be associated with Addison disease, and striae and changes in body fat distribution may suggest cortisol excess in Cushing disease. Adolescents with a history of substance abuse may have an ulcerated nasal septum from inhalation of powdered drugs, conjunctival injection from marijuana use, or skin lesions at injection sites. Lymphadenopathy or splenomegaly suggest an infectious etiology or malignancy. Abnormalities on palpation of the thyroid gland may suggest an underlying thyroid disorder.

Laboratory assessment varies, depending on clinical circumstances. While electrolyte abnormalities may be striking in patients who have a long history of purging, patients who only restrict caloric intake may have laboratory data that look deceptively benign. For these patients, laboratory studies are primarily used to rule out other potential diagnoses. For recommended laboratory studies, see Table 14.3. For common laboratory abnormalities seen in patients with eating disorders, refer to Table 14.4.

Routine urinalysis is a useful screening test for renal abnormalities and for diabetes mellitus. Measuring urine specific gravity is also helpful in assessing hydration status. Normal values are between 1.010 and 1.020. Lower values suggest excessive fluid intake or "water-loading" by the patient to increase fluid weight and give an impression of true body weight gain. Higher specific gravities may indicate dehydration. In severely malnourished patients, consistently low urine specific gravities may indicate nephrogenic diabetes insipidus. Urine Ph is an-

Table 14.3. Recommended Laboratory Evaluation for Eating Disorders by Clinical Presentation

1. Weight loss: Complete blood count, erythrocyte sedimentation rate (ESR), blood urea nitrogen (BUN)/creatinine levels, thyroid studies, electrolytes.

Additional studies if severely malnourished: Liver function tests, calcium, phosphorous, magnesium.

2. Purging or laxative abuse suspected: Electrolytes, amylase, blood urea nitrogen (BUN), creatinine.

Additional studies, as indicated: Stool phenolphthalein to screen for laxatives, serum emetine to screen for Syrup of Ipecac. Cardiac enzyme (creatinine phosphokinase) levels if Ipecac abuse is suspected.

3. Amenorrhea or menstrual irregularities: Pregnancy test, thyroid studies, LH/FSH, prolactin.

Table 14.4. Common Laboratory Abnormalities in Patients with Eating Disorders

Hematologic (Mant & Faragher, 1972; Palla & Litt, 1988):

1. Erthroctye sedimentation rate: Low.
2. Platelets: Mild thrombocytopenia.
3. Red blood cells: Mild anemia (usually normochromic and normocytic).
4. White blood cells: Slight decrease.

Serum chemistry (Casper, Kirchner, Sandstead, Jacob, & Davis, 1980; Waldholz & Anderson, 1988; Warren & Vande Wiele, 1973):

1. Amylase: Possible elevation if purging.
2. Bicarbonate: Metabolic alkalosis if purging or using diuretics, metabolic acidosis if abusing laxatives.
3. Blood urea nitrogen: Elevated if dehydrated.
4. Cholesterol: Elevated.
5. Creatinine: Elevated if dehydrated.
6. Glucose: Decreased.
7. Liver function tests: Mild elevation in ALT, AST.
8. Phosphate: Low in starvation or rapid refeeding.
9. Potassium: Decreased if purging or using laxatives/diuretics.
10. Zinc: Decreased.

Endocrine studies (Kaplan & Garfinkel, 1988):

1. Estrogen (females), testosterone (males): Decreased.
2. FSH & LH: Decreased.
3. Thyroid studies: Normal or low TSH, low normal T4, decreased T3, elevated reverse T3 levels.

other useful screening test, as elevations greater than 7.0 suggest possible vomiting.

Urine drug screening tests may reveal phenylpropanolamine if over-the-counter diet pills are being used. Occasionally, amphetamines are used for weight loss and may also be detected by a urine screen. Obtain stool to screen for phenolphthalein (Mitchell & Boutacoff, 1986) if laxative use is suspected, as certain laxatives result in a positive test. Debate continues about when it is appropriate to screen adolescents for other illicit drug use (Schonberg, 1988). Weight loss is fairly common in adolescents with substance abuse problems, due to alterations in appetite and/or changes in lifestyle and self-care behaviors. In addition, there is a high prevalence of substance abuse among patients with bulimia (Hatsukami, Eckert, Mitchell, & Pyle, 1984; Hudson, Pope, Yurgelun-Todd, Jonas, & Frankenburg, 1987; Laessle, Wittchen, Fichter, & Pirke, 1989; Mitchell, Hatsukami, Eckert, & Pyle, 1985). Substance abuse can complicate the diagnosis of an eating disorder. These considerations may be sufficient to warrant routine urine drug screening for patients who present with a possible eating disorder, although there is no consensus on this issue.

An EKG should be performed to rule out arrhythmias, heart block, or ischemia in patients with significant bradycardia (pulse less than or equal to 45), an irregular pulse, extreme cachexia, or a history of ipecac use. A general decrease in voltage is a common finding in malnourished patients, owing to loss of cardiac muscle mass. A prolonged QTc (QT/sq. root of R-R interval) has been associated with ventricular tachycardia and is presumed to be a major cause of sudden death in anorexia (Isner, Roberts, Heymsfield, & Yager, 1985).

It is helpful to obtain a bone density study (dual proton absorptiometry of whole body and vertebral bodies) shortly after initial diagnosis and at yearly intervals while weight rehabilitation is in progress. Bone density studies can determine whether a significant degree of osteopenia is present. This information is useful in determining whether high-impact physical activities should be curtailed. In addition, it may also identify patients for whom a more urgent weight rehabilitation schedule is required.

Other imaging studies, such as MRI or CT scans, are not part of a routine evaluation. They should be done only if the physical examination or history suggest underlying neurological disease.

While physical signs and laboratory values that suggest malnutrition or purging are helpful in confirming a diagnosis, many of these signs and symptoms may not be present even when extensive weight loss or purging has occurred. Therefore, a normal examination may belie the seriousness of a patient's illness, and in addition would miss potential long-term complications such as osteopenia. Normal physical findings should therefore be regarded solely as evidence that immediate life-threatening complications are not present, not that the patient is healthy or in a medically safe state.

Psychological and Psychiatric Issues

History of Eating Issues

Assessment includes gathering information regarding weight history, including highest, lowest, and "desired" weight described by the patient. Knowing when the patient began attempting to lose weight and any factors that influenced the decision to lose weight, may provide clues to underlying psychological issues and may also clarify the duration of acute illness. Inquiring about weight loss goals and the patient's perception of the need to lose more weight can highlight body image distortions. Feelings and thoughts regarding present weight and attitude toward weight gain should be explored.

Food preferences (such as low calorie and/or low fat foods), range of food selection, food restrictions, and history of bingeing should be assessed. It is important to note whether the patient counts calories, as this gives an indication of the amount of time and energy given to regulation of his or her body.

If the patient reports bingeing, details about the activity should be sought. Essential information includes the amount of food consumed, triggers for restriction of calories or bingeing, frequency, and whether the patient feels in control of behavior during the binge.

The patient should also be assessed for compensatory behaviors promoting weight loss or calorie utilization. These include activities such as exercise or vomiting, and the use of medications such as laxatives, diuretics, diet pills, ipecac, and in rare cases thyroid medication or insulin. For each behavior, it is important to quantify the activity, determine the frequency, and explore the associated thoughts and feelings.

Psychometric Measures

Even though patients may under- or over-estimate their involvement in weight-loss behaviors, self-report instruments can be a useful way to gather baseline data before beginning treatment. Two popular evaluation tools include the Eating Disorder Inventory (EDI; Garner, Olmstead, & Polivy, 1983) and the Eating Attitudes Test (EAT; Garner, Olmstead, Bohr, & Garfinkel, 1982). The EDI has normative data for ages 14 years and older. One potential limitation of the EAT is that results may be influenced by social class (Eisler & Szmukler, 1985) and cultural background (King & Bhugra, 1989).

Patient's Experience of the Problem

Many times, patients report feeling "labeled" by doctors and feel that their specific experiences are not acknowledged. These patients may have difficulty expressing their experiences (Bruch, 1962). If so, it may be helpful for clinicians to give some examples of what other patients have told them about their experiences, and encourage patients to compare the examples with their own perception of the problem and its effect on their lives.

The overwhelming theme expressed by most patients is the fear of fat or weight gain. Patients with a diagnosis of anorexia nervosa tend to report feeling extremely powerful and even superior as a result of their ability to lose weight. They frequently report that they do not wish to give up their restricting behaviors. While patients with bulimia also voice a desire to lose weight, they tend to express more dissatisfaction regarding their binge and purge activities.

Effects on Relationships and Activities

The clinician should assess how the eating problem affects patients' thoughts and feelings about themselves and their bodies. Patients often report that the desire to lose weight and the fear of weight gain is so compelling that the thought of weight gain leads to self-destructive thoughts. For many, concerns regarding food and body image are constantly present.

The clinician should assess how the patient's experience of the problem has interrupted life activities, such as school, hobbies, and socialization. Many patients report a desire to perform extremely well, especially in schoolwork and sports. Sometimes they report having intensely competitive feelings toward others, especially siblings. Losing weight often becomes an activity in which they feel they can excel.

Of utmost importance is the effect of the problem on the patient's relationships with others. Many patients report that they avoid social activities so that they do not have to eat with others and experience the scrutiny they feel they receive while eating. They also report that they feel compelled to decline social invitations, to reserve time to exercise or engage in other weight loss activities.

Psychiatric Co-Morbidity

As Shaw and Garfinkel (1990) note, most eating disorder patients included in research projects come from specialized eating disorder clinics where there may be an overrepresentation of more seriously compromised individuals. If this is the case, the incidence of psychiatric co-morbidity may be greater in this population than in individuals from the community.

Frequently, eating disordered patients carry a dual diagnosis of an affective disorder (Halmi et al., 1991; Hsu, 1990), an obsessive-compulsive disorder (Kasvikis, Tsakiris, Marks, Basogul, & Noshirvani, 1986), alcohol and drug abuse (Bulik, 1987; Katz, 1990), or a personality disorder (Gartner, Marcus, Halmi, & Loranger, 1989; Piran, Lerner, Garfinkel, Kennedy, & Brouillette, 1988). However, other researchers have found insufficient evidence linking eating disorders and depression (Laessle, Wittchen, Fichter, & Pirke, 1989; Levy, Dixon, & Stern, 1989; Mitchell, Specker, & de Zwaan, 1991). Certainly when present, co-morbidity can influence treatment decisions. It is also an important variable to consider when designing or interpreting research in eating disorders.

When taking a patient's history it is important to assess the presence of other problems such as depression, anxiety, suicidality, drug or alcohol use, obsessive and compulsive behaviors, and relationship difficulties. The patient's thoughts about the severity and effect of these problems on their life should be ascertained. In addition, it is important to explore their views regarding the effect of these problems on their eating difficulties, and vice versa. The patients' perception of whether the eating issues are primary or are secondary to another diagnosis, such as depression, may help influence treatment decisions.

Family Assessment

The effect of eating disorders on family relationships must also be ascertained. Often parents are quite concerned and frightened regarding the health of their child. Sometimes they have engaged in self-blame and are also blaming the child for the problem. This may result in feelings of anger, frustration, and helplessness.

Family history should include information on weight problems in other family members (obesity, anorexia nervosa, bulimia, or malnutrition resulting from chronic illness), psychiatric problems, substance abuse, and endocrine disorders. These may indicate either a genetic predisposition to eating disorders or familial experiences that have influenced eating problems. Changes in the patient's social and academic functioning can be assessed by asking parents about their child's recent grades in school, interactions with friends, and extracurricular activities.

Previous Treatments and Motivations for Treatment

Previous medical and psychiatric/psychological treatments should be assessed. This includes obtaining information regarding the type and length of previous treatment attempts, as well as soliciting opinions about whether the interventions were helpful. Asking the patient and family what they hope will occur as a result of the current evaluation may be quite informative when developing treatment plans.

Diagnosis, Information, and Treatment Recommendations

Sometimes the diagnosis of an eating disorder evolves over time. Certain patients may report that they see themselves as underweight and want to gain weight, but find it is difficult to do anything to gain weight. These patients may initially appear to have an atypical eating disorder, but may later meet criteria for a diagnosis of anorexia nervosa or bulimia. Also, a patient initially diagnosed with anorexia may later develop binge/purge behaviors, qualifying them for a diagnosis of bulimia.

The patient and family should be provided with the results of the evaluation, as well as information regarding current and potential effects of the problem on physical health. Effort should be made to give this information in a helpful and respectful manner. Many patients report that they are expecting to be reprimanded for their problem and "punished." Sometimes they perceive the information as "scare tactics" and become more resistant to treatment.

Treatment recommendations should be a collaborative effort between the patient, family, and treatment team. Members of the treatment team should act as consultants to the family, helping to inform families about treatment options.

TREATMENT STRATEGIES

Psychological and Behavioral Treatments

Treatment Outcome Research

As highlighted by Shaw and Garfinkel (1990), outcome studies are difficult to compare, owing to differences in diagnostic criteria used, number of years post-onset for follow-up studies, and measures of success. Not only is it difficult to compare outcomes in treatment research, but even when a successful treatment is identified, the mechanisms of treatment contributing to the success are usually not determined. In addition, particular combinations of treatment approach and level of intensity may vary in effectiveness, depending on the patient population.

Many different types of therapy have been found to be effective. However, no ideal specific treatment exists. Treatment usually focuses initially on weight restoration, followed by individual and family intervention (Anderson, 1985; Morgan & Russell, 1975). However, no treatment has been demonstrated to promote long-term recovery in all patients. It has been suggested that until one treatment approach can be consistently identified as superior in outcome studies, it would be useful to identify components of treatment that are beneficial and to develop new treatment components (Agras & Kraemer, 1984).

Anorexia nervosa. Hsu's (1988) review of outcome studies indicate five factors associated with poor outcome: lower weights, longer illness duration, reported social and personality difficulties prior to illness, and family problems. Psychotherapy (Hall & Crisp, 1987) has been used more often than drug therapies for anorexia nervosa. Patients dealing with anorexia nervosa tend to deny or minimize symptoms (Crisp, 1967) making treatment difficult and long. Hospitalization may be required intermittently for treatment of medical complications related to malnutrition, or for failure to progress with weight gain, physical growth, or pubertal development.

More recent reviews of treatment outcome and follow-up studies (American Psychiatric Association, 1993) report that the prognosis for those afflicted with anorexia nervosa indicate that approximately 44 percent of patients followed at least 4 years post-onset have a "good" outcome, defined as reaching a weight within 15 percent of ideal weight. Twenty-four percent had a "poor" outcome, defined as never reaching 15 percent of ideal weight, and 28 percent experienced an "intermediate outcome," between these two extremes. Fewer than 5 percent of patients died of the disorder.

Bulimia nervosa. Overall, hospitalization is less likely for patients with bulimia. However, certain patients may require medical hospitalization to correct fluid or electrolyte imbalance or address gastrointestinal complications. Psychiatric hospitalization may be necessary for suicidal patients.

Many therapeutic approaches have been found to be useful in treating bulimia. One of the most studied is cognitive-behavior therapy. A number of investigators have found this approach effective (Agras, Schneider, Arnow, Raeburn, & Telch, 1989; Fairburn et al., 1991; Tobin & Johnson, 1991) in the treatment of bulimia nervosa, while others report equivocal results (Channon, De Silva, Hemsley, & Perkins, 1989). Blouin et al. (1994) found cognitive change to be an important but not necessary factor in promoting behavioral changes, such as binge-purge reduction. They found that patients most likely to evidence both cognitive and behavioral changes were those who perceived their families to be less controlling, were at lower weights, and were less likely to use laxatives or diuretics.

Exposure and response prevention is based on the model that purging provides relief from anxiety and that preventing this mode of release decreases bingeing as well as vomiting (Rosen & Leitenberg, 1982). This treatment requires that the patient eat feared foods in front of the therapist without the option of purging later. There are conflicting reports as to whether this method is more or less effective than other cognitive behavioral approaches (Agras et al., 1989).

Psychodynamic therapies have also been found useful in selected cases (Schwartz, 1990). However both Bruch (1978) and Steiner-Adair (1991) report the need for therapists to challenge the bounds of psychodynamic approaches, providing a "real" relationship by being open and responsive.

Outcomes for those suffering with bulimia indicate that 27 percent of previously hospitalized patients have a "good" outcome, defined as binge/purge events occurring less than once a month. Thirty-three percent indicate a "poor" outcome, defined as daily binge/purge events and 40 percent indicate an "intermediate" outcome (between these two) (American Psychiatric Association, 1993). Those patients dealing with both anorexia nervosa and bulimia tend to have very poor outcomes (Russell, 1979).

Family Therapy

Russell, Szmukler, Dare, and Eisler (1987) found family therapy for adolescents dealing with anorexia nervosa or bulimia to be more effective than individual therapy. This is in contrast to older patients, with whom individual therapy appears to be more effective than family therapy.

Minuchin, Rosman, and Baker (1978) and others (Selvini-Palazzoli, 1974) base their therapeutic approach on the premise that individuals in families dealing with anorexia nervosa and bulimia tend to engage family members in somewhat destructive interactions, leading to problems with separation and individuation. Minuchin et al. used therapeutic interventions based on these interactions in working with intact nuclear families of adolescents with recent onset (less than 6 months) of anorexia nervosa, and found an 88 percent cure rate based on self-report. However, there is a dearth of empirical studies assessing the presence of these interactional styles and the research that has been done indicate differing results. Two of the interactive styles described by Minuchin et al. were "enmeshment" and "overprotectiveness." Dare, Le Grange, Eisler, and Rutherford (1994) found that while families appeared "close" (or enmeshed) to the outside observer, they did not perceive themselves to be as close as they would like. Also, Dare et al. found families to be supportive but not "overprotective." Further research is needed to evaluate how these families perceive their interactive styles and to assess the effect of the eating problem on these interactions.

Humphrey (1989) analyzed videotapes of families of girls with eating disorders. They found that parents of girls diagnosed with anorexia nervosa communicated a combination of nurturance and neglect of their daughter's needs to express feelings. In these families, daughters appeared ambivalent about disclosing their feelings. In contrast, parents of the girls diagnosed with bulimia appeared to be enmeshed in a hostile pattern. They undermined their daughter's self-assertion and attempts to "separate."

It is unclear whether dysfunctional family interactions precede onset of the disorders or whether they evolve as a response to stressors related to anorexia nervosa and bulimia and associated treatment. Unfortunately the cost of a longitudinal study to assess family interactions prior to the onset of eating disorders appears prohibitive at this time. However, we conducted a cross-sectional study in an attempt to determine if the family's perceptions of their functioning changes in response to the stress of the problem. Galante, Sanders, and Steiner (1994) administered several self-report measures to families of teenage daughters diagnosed with anorexia nervosa, bulimia, or both disorders, at different phases of their experience. They found that independent of diagnosis, families perceive themselves as more cohesive and adaptable in the beginning than they do later on. Therefore, family interactions may appear different at various stages of the struggle with the problem and may indicate that the eating disorder invites negative interactions rather than the family interactions creating the eating disorder.

Treatment of Physical Problems

While effective psychological intervention is the key to recovery, ensuring physical safety is essential. *All patients should be co-managed with a physician experienced in the treatment of medical problems associated with eating disorders.* Team management with a medical physician and nutritionist allows the therapist to focus on the psychological underpinnings of the eating disorder, clearly defining her or his role as separate from food or weight issues. It also helps ensure that the patient is in the best possible physical state, so that response to psychotherapy can be enhanced and physical complications minimized.

The medical care physician contributes to the ongoing management of a patient with eating disorders in several ways. The first is by using objective data to monitor progress toward weight goals. At each office visit, weight should be recorded with the patient in gown only, after voiding. Urine specific gravity should be checked to screen for water-loading, and pH should be measured to assess purging.

In addition, the medical care physician should determine when the patient is medically unstable and requires hospitalization (see Table 14.1). The physician should monitor for the development of medical complications, such as loss of bone density in patients with anorexia or gastro-esophageal reflux and gastrointestinal bleeding in patients with bulimia. For patients who vomit or use laxatives, the physician should provide ongoing monitoring of serum potassium levels, treating chronic hypokalemia with oral potassium supplements or administering intravenous therapy when necessary.

Constipation is common in patients with eating disorders or a history of laxative abuse. In general, treating constipation in patients with eating disorders with laxatives should be avoided. Nutritional interventions such as increased fiber or appropriate fluid intake should be encouraged. Nutritional repletion gradually results in the resolution of most gastrointestinal symptoms. In extreme cases, bulk-forming laxatives such as Metamucil may be useful during weaning from purgatives.

Input from other specialists may be required for medical problems related to the eating disorder. In patients who purge, dental complications may require on-going treatment by a dentist (Simmons, Grayden, & Mitchell, 1986). Consultation by a cardiologist may also be necessary if cardiac abnormalities develop. Gastrointestinal bleeding from purging may require evaluation by a gastroenterologist. Chronic hypokalemia can lead to renal damage, requiring consultation with a nephrologist.

Nutritional Repletion

Ongoing management by an experienced nutritionist is an essential component of care. A weight gain of 1/2 to 2 pounds or 0.2 to 0.9 kilograms a week is a reasonable expectation during outpatient treatment. Serial assessment of body fat by measuring triceps skin-fold thickness may determine if actual weight gain and changes in body composition are occurring. While general nutritional depletion is a significant problem in patients with eating disorders, calcium, zinc, and possibly magnesium loss are of particular concern (Birmingham, Goldner, & Bakan, 1994; Casper, Kirchner, Sandstead, Jacob, & Davis, 1980; Hall et al., 1988; Powers, 1982). Daily supplementation with 100 mg zinc and a multivitamin is recommended. Eating disorder patients often eat a diet rich in diary products. If so, supplementation with 400 mg calcium (2 Tums™) is usually sufficient to meet the 1200 mg recommended for daily calcium intake.

In patients who have restricted their intake, the initial phase of nutritional repletion is particularly critical. If intake is excessive during the recovery phase, metabolic demand can surpass cardiac output, leading to congestive heart failure (Powers, 1982). Rapid re-feeding may also precipitate significant hypophosphatemia, with potential for cardiac compromise (Sheridan & Collins, 1983).

Initial calories should generally be less than 500 calories over average recent intake. The initial caloric intake usually recommended is approximately 30–40 kcal/kg per day (1000–1600 kcal/day). However, intake may need to be gradually increased to up to 70–100 kcal/kg per day to achieve adequate weight gain during weight rehabilitation, decreasing to 40–60 kcal/kg per day during the weight maintenance phase (American Psychiatric Association, 1993).

For hospitalized patients, input from an experienced nutritionist to assess recent intake and recommend gradual safe incremental increases is essential. A weight gain of three pounds or 1.4 kilograms a week is a reasonable and safe goal during in-patient treatment. Initial meal selection is best done by the nutritionist, to ensure that adequate calories and balanced nutrients are provided. For in-patients who are medically unstable, an initial diet consisting of only liquid nutritional supplements, such as Ensure™ or Osmolyte™ is recommended. This allows for close monitoring of calories and assurance of balanced vitamin and mineral intake. Nasogastric tube feeding is not generally recommended, even for severely malnourished patients in a hospital setting (American Psychiatric Association, 1993). Closely supervised oral intake is preferred, distributing the recommended calories between 3 meals and several snack periods. A nasogastric tube may be placed to administer any remaining calories, if the patient is unable to complete the recommended caloric intake by the end of the day. Nutritional supplements are continued until medical stability is achieved (vital signs stable and weight greater than 75 percent of ideal body weight), at which time solid food is gradually reintroduced.

On rare occasions, ongoing nasogastric tube feedings or even total parenteral nutrition may be required in life-threatening situations. In these situations, extreme care must be taken to avoid rapid refeeding and associated risks, including fluid retention and cardiac failure.

Achieving Healthy Weight

A series of weight goals may be calculated for each patient and can serve as treatment milestones. Weight goals are best determined by a nutritionist with experience in evaluating patients with eating disorders.

A minimum weight should be established, below which a patient is considered medically unstable based on weight alone. This is generally at 75 percent of their "ideal" weight. Several methods of estimating ideal weight for height and age are available. The most precise estimate is the appropriate body mass index [weight (kg)/height (m)^2]. Healthy ranges for the body mass index by age and gender are listed in available tables (Beumont, Al-Alami, & Touyz, 1988; Hammer, Kraemer, Wilson, Ritter, & Dornbusch, 1991). Another option is to determine a patient's ideal body weight based on published standards of weight for height (National Center for Health Statistics, 1973). Although this is the primary method used in the past, it is generally considered a less accurate measure than body mass index. If growth failure has occurred, an ideal body weight based on expected height for age is a more medically appropriate standard than actual height. If patients fall below 75 percent of their ideal weight, they are considered to be medically unstable and in-patient hospitalization is recommended.

A healthy weight goal for a patient is the target weight. Although usually less than their "ideal" weight, the target weight is that weight at which endocrine function generally normalizes and menses with ovulatory cycles usually resume. Since amenorrhea and anovulatory cycles are associated with bone loss (Prior, Vigna, Schechter, & Burgess, 1990), bone demineralization is likely to stop and often even reverse in patients who are able to maintain their weight at or above the target weight.

Target weights are calculated individually for each patient. A rough estimate in girls is the last weight at which regular menstrual periods occurred. A more precise estimate can be made based on a patient's percent body fat. Menses generally resume when patients are at 17 percent body fat. In general, body fat increases by 1 percent for every kilogram of actual weight gained. Target weight can therefore be estimated by using a patient's initial weight and body fat percentage to predict the weight at which 17 percent body fat is likely to be achieved.

Being at or above target weight does not necessarily imply medical stability. Altered homeostasis and vital sign instability can occur even with weights within the normal range, if there is a history of purging or of rapid weight loss from a higher premorbid weight. Conversely, vital sign stability may occur even with severely low weights and should not be mistaken for homeostatic normality. Even in patients with bulimia who are at a normal weight, metabolic studies reflect a state of biological starvation (Pirke, Pahl, Schweiger, & Warnhoff, 1985).

Guidelines for Safe Exercise

While exercise is not a necessary or even recommended part of treatment, it may be useful to incorporate guidelines for safe exercise into a patient's treatment program. Many patients with eating disorders feel compelled to exercise, and setting guidelines may assist them in recognizing appropriate and safe limits for aerobic activity. Exercise programs should emphasize fitness instead of calorie expenditure.

For patients without any long-term cardiac compromise, it may be helpful to establish a minimum weight above which moderate amounts of aerobic exercise would generally be safe from a cardiovascular perspective. This "exercise weight" generally lies between the target weight and 75 percent of ideal body weight. While no data are available to assess the precise weight that is safe, at the Eating Disorders Program at Lucile Salter Packard Children's Hospital at Stanford an estimate is made empirically, by adding approximately 2–3 kilograms to the highest weight at which vital sign instability occurred. In addition, we require patients to be at least 85 percent of ideal body weight, with body fat of 12–13 percent before allowing participation in aerobic activities (Shih, 1994, personal communication). Patients should also be advised that exercising will increase their caloric requirements.

The range of physical activity that is safe and appropriate depends on a number of factors, including whether bone density is within normal limits. Studies of adult patients with anorexia and of young dancers suggest that adolescents who have low bone densities may be at risk for fractures as a result of osteopenia (Rigotti, Neer, Skates, Herzog, Nussbaum, 1991; Warren, Brooks-Gunn, Hamilton, Warren, & Hamilton, 1986). Therefore, these patients should be advised to avoid activities in which there is a risk of impact, including running on hard surfaces, jumping, high-impact aerobics, skiing, and horseback riding.

Treatment of Psychological Issues

With the pediatric/medical team addressing the patient's medical needs, the therapist is in a position to explore aspects of attaining health that are difficult for the patient. It is helpful to work with the pediatric/medical team to develop a "weight-gain" plan, setting incremental goals to promote slow weight gain over time. In therapy, patients are invited to explore difficult aspects of taking on these weight goals for themselves, and of placing the struggle between the patient and the problem, rather than between the doctors and the problem.

The therapist then begins to help patients explore other aspects of their lives in addition to their eating problems. The initial step in this is to assist patients in identifying goals in other areas of their lives. The therapist then supports the patient in developing strategies for obtaining these life goals and overcoming obstacles that exist. In this way, the patient becomes more aware of other concerns outside of the eating problem and may begin to struggle against the effects of the problem.

In situations in which a multidisciplinary clinic is not available, the therapist should develop liaisons with local medical care physicians and nutritionists in order to create a multidisciplinary team approach. Of utmost importance is the need to maintain open lines of communication to ensure the safety of the patient and promote restoration of health.

Treatment Settings

Outpatient and partial hospitalization. For patients who appear motivated to gain weight and participate in therapy, the least restrictive setting is recommended. If the patient finds it difficult to make progress in an outpatient setting, a partial hospitalization day-treatment setting may offer a more supportive environment. Treatment in these settings still requires the patient to be able to fight the effects of the problem enough to take in adequate calories and decrease purgative behaviors within a less intense structure than that provided by complete hospitalization.

In the out-patient setting, the patient should be seen one to two times a week during the initial acute phase of illness and recovery, by both the therapist and the medical care physician. Frequency of medical visits may decrease once the patient has attained weight goals and progress seems well underway. Ongoing medical follow-up at least monthly is recommended, until target weight is achieved. Frequency of visits for psychotherapy after the acute phase will vary depending on patient needs. However, intensive psychotherapy often continues for a longer period of time than medical intervention.

In-patient setting: Medical management. In-patient treatment is recommended for patients who become medically unstable by any of the criteria outlined previously and/or psychiatrically unstable due to suicidal ideation. If the patient and/or family refuse hospitalization, a decision must be made by the treatment team as to medical necessity and possible need for legal intervention.

Medical care and monitoring should be provided as indicated. Cardiac monitoring should be provided for severely malnourished patients, and for patients in which cardiac complications are suspected for other reasons. Vital signs should be checked frequently, including assessment of orthostatic blood pressure and pulse changes.

The in-patient setting should contain a qualified and well-trained multidisciplinary staff. Because patients with eating disorders may be ambivalent about fighting the effects of the problem, they sometimes engage in practices to alter weight or food intake even when hospitalized. These activities may include hiding food, purging, exercising, and water-loading or wearing concealed weights to indicate higher weight gain than has actually been achieved. A trained staff needs to be available for close monitoring and observation, to help patients avoid these harmful practices and to ensure their medical safety.

Behavioral programs in which health restoration is linked to behavioral privileges have been shown to be associated with shorter hospital stays and be more effective than programs relying on medications alone (Agras, Dorian, Kirkley, Arnow, & Bachman, 1987). Behavioral programs should include decreasing structure and increasing responsibility and privileges, as patients demonstrate ability to take over more control in their struggle with the problem.

Group therapies should include a milieu group in which the patients are able to contribute to the program and work together to support each other in their struggles. Group therapies may include process, skills, and specific problem-focused groups.

Every effort should be made to provide an ongoing school experience for patients in in-patient or partial hospitalization programs. Academic achievement tends to be very important to patients with eating disorders and the opportunity to keep up their schoolwork helps patients remain connected to their "outside" lives. School tends to be more of a problem socially rather than academically for these patients and the hospital school setting may further also provide a supportive social environment.

Daily individual and weekly or bi-weekly family meetings are important throughout the hospital stay. Even when the child is extremely malnourished, the child and family may benefit from involvement with a therapist. The therapist may facilitate transfer of information regarding the physical effects of eating disorders, as well as begin to explore the impact of the problem on their lives. They may also benefit from information from the therapist regarding how other families have experienced these problems. As the child begins to recover physically and is able to take more responsibility for his or her caloric intake, therapy may be especially helpful in exploring how the problem makes it difficult for the child to progress and the effect this has on both the child and family. Throughout the therapy process, the therapist should help the family prepare for discharge from the hospital and plan for continuing progress on an outpatient or day treatment basis.

Our theoretical approach is based on the Narrative Approach described by White and Epston (White, 1986; White & Epston, 1990). The basic tenets of this approach as they relate to eating issues are as follows:

1. *Naming the Problem*   As we mentioned in the assessment portion of the chapter, the patient is invited to explore his or her experience of the problem. The patient is given respect and recognition for his or her expertise in regards to the problem and its effects.

If a patient is severely malnourished and is slowly being refed, the effects of starvation may make it more difficult to make full use of therapy. However, it seems that at this time patients may be aware of the seriousness of their symptoms, and they may be able to gain some insight into the negative and serious effects of their eating problems.

2. *Differentiating the Voice of Anorexia and Own Voice*   Once patients have begun to name the problem they are experiencing, they are encouraged to begin to "externalize" the problem, or recognize that they are separate from and are not defined by the problem. Patients begin to find their own voice, speaking up on their own behalf. This is a difficult task for many patients, as they seem to have problems differentiating themselves from the anorexia and bulimia and believe the "voice" of anorexia to be their own.

3. *Separating Self from the Problem*   Through self-exploration and concurrent exploration of the problem and its effect on their lives, patients begin to see themselves as separate from the problem and "more" than the problem. This allows them to reclaim their own identity separate from what the problem invites them to be.

Although our patients report that they feel they have gained a sense of power as a result of their eating disorders, they find that it becomes a "false power." The problem takes over and takes them from their lives, separates them from their friends, and sometimes threatens their lives. They report that they begin to feel afraid of "crossing" the "voice" of anorexia or bulimia and, despite its tyranny, they report feeling "safer" abiding by its rules.

The Narrative approach attempts to frame the struggle between the individual and the problem, rather than between the individual and the treatment team. In an in-patient unit, this is a tremendous challenge, given the confines of the setting. In such settings, the individual is faced with following a strict medical regime in which almost everything is monitored: intake, output, behaviors, statements, all of which are charted and read by members of the treatment team. Also, as mentioned above, the patients tend to become very "protective" of the eating disorder. Often it seems that everyone is trying to take the eating disorder away from them while the eating disorder may be perceived by the individual as their only friend. We believe that placing the struggle back between the person and the problem is very important, especially toward the end of the hospital stay, so that the patient has some experience confronting their eating disorder before leaving the hospital.

4. *Becoming More Visible*   Not only does anorexia and bulimia invite the patient to disappear physically, but the patient also finds that they disappear from activities, friendships, and sometimes from family. Many times this is the negative effect most identified by patients. By exploring times in which the patient was able to fight these effects and remain visible in their lives, we explore the "alternative story" of visibility and competence. As patients fight the negative effects of the voice of anorexia, they find their own voice and discover their own wants and desires.

5. *Family Therapy* In family therapy, the family is invited to explore their experience of the eating disorder and the effects it has had on their lives. As for the patient, family members are encouraged to work through and overcome the negative effects of the problem. This approach is carried out while avoiding the mistake of blaming mothers and families for the eating disorder.

Pharmacological Treatments

General Principles

Psychopharmacological agents may be of some value in the treatment of eating disorders, but no medication has been shown to be consistently superior to others or to other forms of interventions at this point. This is especially true in the treatment of restrictive anorexia nervosa (American Psychiatric Association, 1993).

All medications should only be used after considerable thought and careful planning, as all of them have side effects and many of these can in fact act synergistically to accentuate the effects of malnutrition and dehydration (Palla & Litt, 1988). In no instance is it reasonable to have medications be the sole intervention for the patient. Medications can be a useful part of a carefully constructed treatment package that takes into account the developmental needs of the patient. Targets for medications vary according to the subcategory of eating disorder present, and will be discussed separately for anorexia and bulimia. Individual doses need to be calculated carefully, according to body weight. Clinicians should expect to encounter unusual reactions and interferences when using medications with patients who have an eating disorder. In anorexia nervosa, medication management may be complicated by the patient's subjective response, as these patients may be highly anxious and monitor their bodily reactions carefully, mindful of intrusion and external control. In addition, their malnourished state and possible rapid fluctuations in hydration status can influence their physical response to medications. Patients with bulimia may also experience problems with medications. This population is more likely than patients with anorexia to abuse medications and illicit drugs. This may lead to substantial interference with medications, produce extraordinary side effects, or even make the primary pathology much worse. One needs to be particularly mindful of dosage scheduling and its overlap with binge/purge cycling, as it is necessary to titrate these medicines to achieve effectiveness.

Anorexia Nervosa

The number of controlled studies evaluating medication treatment of anorexia nervosa is very small. Currently there are no studies available that focus on children and adolescents alone. Of the medications studied so far, there have been some positive findings for amitriptyline and cyproheptadine. However, these results have not been replicated by other groups (Halmi, Eckert, & La Du, 1986). Lithium, clomipramine, and pimozide all have had very unimpressive performances when subjected to empirical evaluation (Gross, Ebert, & Faden, 1981; Lacey & Crisp, 1980; Vandereycken & Pierloot, 1982). There are many uncontrolled studies of a variety of medications, some of which have only a very tenuous theoretical basis, which also have been quite unimpressive. Vitamin treatments, ECT, and hormonal interventions are of dubious value when given as the sole vehicle of change (Garfinkel & Garner, 1982). At the present time there is very little evidence that any of the core features of anorexia nervosa (drive for thinness, body image distortions, weight loss, and inadequate caloric intake) are appreciably and reliably influenced by any medication.

A more reasonable approach to the problem is to select specific targets for intervention, as they become problematic in the course of treatment, and treat them as specifically as possible with suitable medications. The decision about whether to start medications at all should largely depend on the patient's status in regard to weight rehabilitation. If the patient is reasonably stable from a medical standpoint, and anxiety, depression, and compulsive thinking are not improving as weight gain proceeds, it may be time to consider medications. As a general rule, in the Lucile Salter Packard Children's Hospital at Stanford (LPCH) Eating Disorders Program we allow at least three weeks to elapse from the beginning of weight rehabilitation and/or the attainment of approximately 80 percent of ideal body weight, before assessing for persistent excessive anxiety, compulsiveness, or depression that may suggest a need for medication. It is important to consider the impact of recommending such a step on the patient and the family, as the implicit message is that certain elements of the illness are out of control for the patient. This may or may not be advantageous in treatment, depending on the patient's status concerning compliance. In a patient who is having extreme difficulty recognizing the negative effects of the problem, such a message may set up a series of control struggles around medicine. In a desperate and demoralized patient who has been trying to comply, but finds himself or herself unable to meet even the most modest goals of weight gain, such a message may come as a salvation. One also needs to consider the long-term implications of such a message, as the abdication of responsibility for weight control may profoundly influence the patients' views that they are victims, passive partners in the fight for health.

To target depression, a trial of the serotonin reuptake inhibitors (SSRIs) is usually first recommended. These tend to have a better side effect profile, and produce fewer problems for undernourished patients in terms of heart rate and blood pressure regulation. One needs to carefully monitor appetite and weight gain, as these medications can occasionally cause significant reductions in appetite and in fact cause weight loss at higher doses (Gwirtsman, Guze, Yager, & Gainsley, 1990; Kaye, Weltzin, Hsu, & Bulik, 1991). Should these medications fail, a trial of tricyclic antidepressants is usually recommended. Patients on tricyclic antidepressants need to be carefully monitored for vital signs instability and for carbohydrate hunger, which is induced by these medications in some patients [about 10 percent in the (LPCH) Eating Disorders Program] and may lead to vomiting or even bulimia. SSRIs may also be used to specifically target excessive obsessionality and compulsions regarding food intake, although in our patients the effects have only been quite modest. Behavioral interventions have no physical side effects and can be as effective as medications in the treatment of obsessions and compulsions. If anticipatory anxiety prior to meals is the primary target, antianxiety agents should be considered. Caution is needed here as well, as some of the side effects of antianxiety agents are highly undesirable. These include withdrawal anxiety, addiction potential in short-acting diazepam-related medications, and seizure induction with buproprion. The neuroleptics are potent inducers of vital sign instability and may accentuate the effects of malnutrition on vasomotor dysfunction. In addition, neuroleptics have induced binge/purge episodes in some patients (Garfinkel & Garner, 1982, 1987; Wells & Logan, 1987). At times the choice of a tricyclic antidepressant (TCA) may be the best compromise. While TCAs may be used to target depression and anticipatory anxiety, beneficial effects are usually slow to develop and are tied to a therapeutic blood level, requiring prolonged commitment to taking the medication.

Bulimia Nervosa

The evidence supporting use of medications in the treatment of bulimia nervosa is much stronger than in the case of anorexia nervosa. Efficacy seems to be independent of a concurrent mood disorder. Imipramine (Pope, Hudson, Jonas, & Yurgelun-Todd, 1983; Agras et al., 1987), desipramine (Hughes, Wells, Cunningham, & Ilstrup, 1986), trazodone (Pope, Keck, McElroy, & Hudson, 1989), and fluoxetine (Fluoxetine Bulimia Nervosa Collaborative Study Group, 1992; Freeman, Morris, Cheshire, Davies, & Hamson, 1988) were all found to be effective in controlled studies, although not appreciably different in their success rates. There appears to be a dose effect with desipramine (Hughes et al., 1986). Monoamine-oxidase inhibitors (MAO) appear to be equally effective (Kennedy et al., 1988; Walsh, Stewart, Roose, Gladis, & Glassman, 1984), but the fact that one deals with highly impulsive patients who must avoid high dietary intake of tyramine (or other vasopressive substances often found in illicit drugs) to avoid sometimes lethal hypertensive crises, makes them unsuitable for use in adolescents with bulimia, especially since there are so many other equally effective medications available that carry no such risk. Medications that are effective in treating bulimia appear to influence the desire to binge, which then secondarily reduces purging. This theory is supported by the finding that these medications appear to work as well in non-purging forms of bulimia (McCann & Agras, 1990). The exact mechanism of action is not known, although it is thought that the effects could be mediated via the brain-gut-peptide systems, especially cholecystokinin (Geracioti & Liddle, 1988).

When psychotherapy and medications are compared, however, it once again becomes clear that medications are no more effective than interventions such as group therapy (Agras et al., 1992; Mitchell et al., 1990) in reducing binge/purging. In addition, all methods of intervention at the present time have a very high relapse rate at one year prospective follow up, once intervention has ceased.

The following approach is recommended in cases of bulimia nervosa, based on current knowledge and our experience through the Stanford Eating Disorders Clinic. Having ascertained repeatedly that the patient's symptoms are not due to drug abuse alone, and that the patient is medically stable, chronicity of symptoms is assessed. If the bulimic symptoms have persisted for over six months and/or the frequency of symptoms is more than two binge/purge episodes per day, the use of medications is recommended. In cases that do not meet these criteria, psychosocial/nutritional interventions are initiated. After three to six weeks, their impact is reassessed prior to considering medications. As a first line drug, we tend to use fluoxetine, again for its relatively uncomplicated side effect profile. However, we switch to the more potent tricyclics after about 6 weeks of treatment, if there is not adequate improvement. MAO inhibitors are reserved only for a few select patients, in whom we also have indications of excellent compliance and possibly evidence of atypical forms of depression. Neuroleptics are not recommended for these patients, nor do we prescribe medications with high addiction potential. Lithium, carbamazepine, clonidine, and other medications have no established efficacy, and are rarely prescribed.

CASE ILLUSTRATION

Clinical Presentation

Maude is a 17-year-old Caucasian female who presented to our clinic when she was age 15, at 55 percent of her ideal body weight and 0 percent body fat measured by the triceps caliper. She reported a maximum weight of 106 lb. She had been amenorrheic for the past five months. She stated that six months ago she had changed to a vegetarian diet and was trying to eat "healthier." Her diet consisted of very low fat foods and she was eating a very limited variety of foods. She denied diuretics, laxatives, purging or over-exercising, although she did engage in aerobics.

Maude's parents had become concerned about her weight seven months prior to her admission, and had taken her to see a pediatrician. Her weight at that time was 106 pounds. They began family therapy at the pediatrician's suggestion. Maude's therapist asked her to keep a diary of her food intake and weights, and requested that the parents not be involved with food or weight issues. The pediatrician suggested the family return if any medical problems occurred, but did not arrange for ongoing follow-up.

After months of therapy, with weight monitoring only through the food weight diary Maude kept, she finally disclosed to her mother that she had been entering false data and had not actually been weighing herself. They arranged a follow-up visit with her pediatrician, where Maude was found to weigh only 55 percent of ideal body weight. She was referred for further evaluation and care.

Assessment Findings

Medically, Maude's temperature upon admission was 35.9°C and she was orthostatic with a change in

pulse from 62 to 104 beats per minute with standing. Blood pressure was 126/73 lying and 137/87 with standing. Physical examination revealed a very cachectic girl. Tanner staging was IV for breasts and pubic hair. Mucous membranes were slightly dry. The physical examination was otherwise unremarkable.

Her electrolytes were within normal limits. Liver function tests revealed a slightly elevated aspartate aminotransferase (AST) of 39 U/L, and alanine aminotransferase (ALT) of 48 U/L. Her complete blood cell count was remarkable for a white blood cell count of 4.1, and the hematocrit was within normal limits. Her erythrocyte sedimentation rate (ESR) was 4. Thyroid function tests were within normal limits.

Psychiatrically, on admission Maude appeared appropriately dressed and groomed. She stated feeling confused about being admitted to the hospital and placed on a heart monitor, saying, "I just walked all over town today, I'm fine." Maude was oriented and her thoughts were linear and goal-directed. Cognitively, she was intact, but appeared a bit slowed in her responses. She denied suicidal or homicidal ideation. Her affect appeared a bit blunted and she seemed to be genuinely surprised that she was admitted to the hospital. However, over a few days time, she seemed to gain an understanding of the seriousness of her condition.

In the initial family interview, Maude's parents stated that they were also shocked at the seriousness of Maude's condition. They had taken her to the pediatrician and therapist and were surprised that her condition had deteriorated to this extent. Historically, the parents reported normal milestones. Maude has done quite well academically and socially throughout her life. The current problem is the first time that they could recall that Maude had ever experienced any significant difficulty in her life.

Treatment Selection and Course

Given her low body weight and medical instability, Maude was hospitalized. She was initially placed on strict medical bedrest with continuous cardiac monitoring, remaining on her bed with use of the bedside commode until her weight began to improve. Gradual nutritional repletion began with the use of Ensure™ by mouth, with close observation by staff during feeds. A nasogastric tube was available as back-up if Maude was unable to meet the daily calorie limits specified, but it was not needed. Initial caloric intake was set at a level no greater than 500 kcal more than what Maude had been eating prior to her admission. Calories were increased by increments of 100–200 Kcal/day, whenever daily weight gain fell below 0.2 kg. A fluid maximum near maintenance requirements was established, to avoid fluid overload. She continued to be medically unstable despite nutrition repletion with 100 percent Ensure™ for several weeks. When her vital signs eventually stabilized and she reached 75 percent of ideal body weight, she was gradually advanced to a solid food diet, increasing solid food intake by 25 percent a day while decreasing Ensure™ to maintain equivalent calories. Frequently her specific gravity was low (below 1.010). This likely reflected mild nephrogenic diabetes insipidus related to malnutrition, rather than fluid loading, in this patient. The following criteria were established for discharge: attain 75 percent of Ideal Body Weight; advance to solid food; gain 0.2 kg for 2 consecutive days without staff supervising intake.

Therapy consisted of daily individual and group therapy and weekly family meetings. In our work, we identified what we referred to as "food focus," which Maude described as similar to "tunnel vision" in which she became more aware of foods and less aware of other aspects of her life. This included feeling somewhat unaware of the extent of the weight she was losing. She was able to externalize the problem and explore the negative effects of the problem on her life, including the fact that it may have come close to taking her life. During her hospital stay, she had a bone density test and results indicated she had severe bone loss. While she appeared quite concerned about her health, she continued to find weight gain to be extremely difficult.

Maude identified feeling caught in the middle between "food focus" and the treatment team. She described the desire to hold onto the problem and fight the treatment team's attempts to "take it from her." This struggle may be seen in the following quote taken from a therapy session:

> "It is harder to work with clinic rather than against it. It is easier to just be mad at clinic for having to gain weight and to try to cheat clinic rather than realize the only way you will ever get healthy (especially with bone density) is to gain the weight because you can't really cheat your body."

Termination and Follow-Up

Maude was discharged (after 2 months) on 100 percent food, medically stable at 75 percent of ideal body weight. She was to attend the outpatient clinic 2x/wk to work on weight gain and to explore (and fight) the effects of "food focus" on her life. Maude found weight gain to be an extremely difficult task and despite her efforts to add foods to her diet and increase caloric intake, she lost weight and was rehospitalized briefly on two occasions.

On an out-patient basis, Maude is working successfully on slow weight gain in clinic according to a behavioral program that she created with the clinic. Her goal is to gain slowly to a weight in which she is expected to resume menses. A "weight gain line" was drawn so that she can monitor her goal of staying above the line on clinic visits. The treatment team agreed that if she is able to stay above the line, she can decrease her frequency of clinic visits.

In out-patient treatment, Maude is taking back power in her life and working toward exploring goals for herself. She plans to attend college and is adding "friends" back into her life according to her desire to socialize.

Maude is still finding it quite difficult to feel motivated to do things and experiences "feeling empty" at times. She reports that she began to experience feeling "depressed" when she first entered treatment. She described feeling something of a "high" when she was losing weight and has experienced depression while attempting to regain weight. She reports that she does not wish to try antidepressants due to a fear of being "dependent" and her concern that the medication will change her in some way. While she has been assured that the medications will not change her core personality, she continues to wish to proceed without medications. She is also working with her family to negotiate their involvement in her life.

SUMMARY

Eating disorders represent prototypical psychosomatic illnesses and require a multidisciplinary team approach to assessment and treatment. Adolescents are especially at risk for developing eating problems. The development of anorexia nervosa or bulimia in a child or adolescent places the child at risk for serious medical, psychological, and developmental sequelae.

A complete pediatric medical assessment includes a physical examination to assess for acute complications of the eating disorder and also to ensure that there is no underlying organic etiology for the weight loss or vomiting. Evaluation includes specific assessment of nutritional status. Nutritional repletion should be done cautiously, under the supervision of an experienced nutritionist. Psychologically, assessment includes a basic psychological/psychiatric battery as well as specific evaluation of eating problems and the effects of these problems on current functioning and relationships.

In order to ensure adequate ongoing treatment, the medical care physician and therapist must work together in tandem. The medical care physician should monitor weight and vital signs and assess physical functioning as the therapist assists the patient in his or her struggle to reclaim physical and psychosocial health.

REFERENCES

Agras, W. S., Dorian, B., Kirkley, B. G., Arnow, B., & Bachman, J. (1987). Imipramine in the treatment of bulimia: A double-blind controlled study. *International Journal of Eating Disorders, 6*, 29–38.

Agras, W. S., & Kraemer, H. C. (1984). The treatment of anorexia nervosa: Do different treatments have different outcomes? In A. J. Stunkard & E. Stellar (Eds.), *Eating and it's disorders* (pp. 193–207). New York: Raven Press.

Agras, W. S., Rossiter, E. M., Arnow, B., Schneider, J. A., Telch, C. F., Raeburn, S. D., Bruce, B., Perl, M., & Koran, L. M. (1992). Pharmacologic and cognitive-behavioral treatment for bulimia nervosa: A controlled comparison. *American Journal of Psychiatry, 149*, 82–87.

Agras, W. S., Schneider, J. A., Arnow, B., Raeburn, S. D., & Telch, C. F. (1989). Cognitive-behavioral and response-prevention treatments for bulimia nervosa. *Journal of Consulting and Clinical Psychology, 57*, 215–221.

American Psychiatric Association. (1993). Practice guideline for eating disorders. *American Journal of Psychiatry, 150*, 212–228.

American Psychiatric Association. (1994). *Diagnostic and statistical manual of mental disorder.* (4th ed.). Washington, DC: Author.

Anderson, A. E. (1988). Anorexia nervosa and bulimia nervosa in males. In P. E. Garfinkel & D. M. Garner (Eds.), *Diagnostic issues in anorexia nervosa and bulimia nervosa* (pp. 166–207). New York: Brunner/Mazel.

Anderson, A. E. (1985). *Practical comprehensive treatment of anorexia nervosa and bulimia.* Baltimore: Johns Hopkins.

Anderson, A. E., & LaFrance, N. (1990). *Persisting osteoporosis in bulimia nervosa patients with past anorexia nervosa.* Paper presented at Fourth International Conference on Eating Disorders, New York.

Bachrach, L. K., Guido, D., Katzman, D., Litt, I. F., & Marcus, R. (1990). Decreased bone density in adolescent girls with anorexia nervosa. *Pediatrics, 86*, 440–447.

Bachrach, L. K., Katzman, D. K., Litt, I. F., Guido, D., & Marcus, R. (1991). Recovery from osteopenia in adolescent girls with anorexia nervosa. *Journal of Clinical Endocrinology and Metabolism, 72*, 602–606.

Beumont, P., Al-Alami, M., & Touyz, S. (1988). Relevance of a standard measurement of undernutrition to the diagnosis of anorexia nervosa: Use of Quetelet's Body Mass Index (BMI). *International Journal of Eating Disorders, 7*, 399–405.

Biller, B. M. K., Saxe V., Herzog, D. B., Rosenthal, D. I., Holzman, S., & Klibanski, A. (1989). Mechanisms of osteoporosis in adult and adolescent women with anorexia nervosa. *Journal of Clinical Endocrinology and Metabolism, 68*, 548–554.

Birmingham, C. L., Goldner, E. M., & Bakan, R. (1994). Controlled trial of zinc supplementation in anorexia nervosa. *International Journal of Eating Disorders, 15*, 251–255.

Blouin, J. H., Carter, J., Blouin, A. G., Tener, L., Schnare-Hayes, K., Zuro, C., Barlow, J., & Perez, E. (1994). Prognostic indicators in bulimia nervosa treated with cognitive-behavioral group therapy. *International Journal of Eating Disorders, 15*, 113–123.

Brotman, A. W., Stern, T. A., & Brotman, D. L. (1986). Renal disease and dysfunction in two patients with anorexia nervosa. *Journal of Clinical Psychiatry, 47*, 433–434.

Bruch, H. (1974). *Eating disorders.* New York: Basic Books.

Bruch, H. (1978). *The golden cage: The enigma of anorexia nervosa.* London: Open Books.

Bruch, H. (1962). Perceptual and conceptual disturbances in anorexia nervosa. *Psychosomatic Medicine, 24*, 187–194.

Bulik, C. M. (1987). Drug and alcohol abuse by bulimic women and their families. *American Journal of Psychiatry, 144*, 1604–1606.

Casper, R. C., Kirchner, B., Sandstead, H. H., Jacob, R. A., & Davis, J. M. (1980). An evaluation of trace metals, vitamins, and taste function in anorexia nervosa. *American Journal of Clinical Nutrition, 33*, 1801–1808.

Channon, S., De Silva, P., Hemsley, D., & Perkins, R. (1989). A controlled trial of cognitive behavioural and behavioural treatment of anorexia nervosa. *Behaviour Research and Therapy, 27*, 529–535.

Childress, A., Brewerton, T., Hodges, E., & Jarrell, M.

(1993). The kids eating disorder survey (KEDS): A study of middle school students. *Journal of the American Academy of Child and Adolescent Psychiatry, 32*, 843–850.

Clippen, A. V., Gupta, R. K., Eccleston, E. G., Wood, K. M., Wakeling, A., & deSousa, V. F. (1976). Plasma tryptophan in anorexia nervosa. *Lancet, 1*, 962.

Comerci, G. D. (1990). Medical complications of anorexia nervosa and bulimia nervosa. *Medical Clinics of North America, 74*, 1293–1310.

Cox, K. L., Cannon, R. A., Ament, M. E., Phillips, H. E., & Schaffer, C. B. (1983). Biochemical and ultrasonic abnormalities of the pancreas in anorexia nervosa. *Digestive Diseases & Sciences, 28*, 225–229.

Crisp, A. H. (1980). *Anorexia nervosa: Let me be*. London: Academic Press.

Crisp, A. H. (1967). The possible significance of some behavioural correlates of weight and carbohydrate intake. *Journal of Psychosomatic Research, 11*, 117–131.

Crisp, A. H., Fenton, G. W., & Scotton, L. (1968). A controlled study of the EEG in anorexia nervosa. *British Journal of Psychiatry, 114*, 1149–1160.

Cuellar, R. E., & Van Thiel, D. H. (1986). Gastrointestinal complications of the eating disorders: Anorexia nervosa and bulimia nervosa. *American Journal of Gastroenterology, 81*, 1113–1124.

Cullberg, J., & Engstrom-Lindberg, M. (1988). Prevalence and incidence of eating disorders in a suburban area. *Acta Psychiatrica Scandinavica, 78*, 314–319.

Dare, C., Le Grange, D., Eisler, I., & Rutherford, J. (1994). Redefining the psychosomatic family: Family process of 26 eating disorder families. *International Journal of Eating Disorders, 16*, 211–226.

Davies, K. M., Pearson, P. H., Huseman, C. A., Greger, N. G., Kimmel, D. K., & Recker, R. R. (1990). Reduced bone mineral in patients with eating disorders. *Bone, 11*, 143–147.

Demitrack, M. A., Kalogeras, K. T., Altemus, M., Pigott, T. A., Listwak, S. J., & Gold, P. W. (1992). Plasma and cerebrospinal fluid measures of arginine vasopressin secretion in patients with bulimia nervosa and in healthy subjects. *Journal of Clinical Endocrinology and Metabolism, 74*, 1277–1283.

DeWied, D. (1971). Long term effect of vasopressin on the maintenance of a conditioned avoidance response in rats. *Nature, 232*, 58–60.

Eisler, I. & Szmukler, G. (1985). Social class as a confounding variable in the Eating Attitudes Test. *Journal of Psychiatric Research, 19*, 171–176.

Fairburn, C. G., & Beglin, S. J. (1990). Studies of the epidemiology of bulimia nervosa. *The American Journal of Psychiatry, 147*, 401–408.

Fairburn, C. G., Jones, R., Peveler, R. C., Carr, S. J., Solomon, R. A., O'Connor, M. E., Burton, J., & Hope, R. A. (1991). Three psychological treatments for bulimia nervosa. *Archives of General Psychiatry, 48*, 463–469.

Fisher, M., Golden, N. H., Katzman, D. K., Kreipe, R. E., Rees, J., Schebendach, J., Sigman, G., Ammerman, S., & Hoberman, H. M. (1995). Eating disorders in adolescents: A background paper. *Journal of Adolescent Health, 16*, 420–437.

Fluoxetine Bulimia Nervosa Collaborative Study Group. (1992). Fluoxetine in the treatment of bulimia nervosa: A multicenter, placebo-controlled, double-blind trial. *Archives of General Psychiatry, 49*, 139–147.

Fohlin, L. (1977). Body composition, cardiovascular and renal function in adolescent patients with anorexia nervosa. *Acta Paediatrica Scandinavica, 268 (supplement)*, 1–20.

Freeman, D. P., Morris, J. E., Cheshire, K. E., Davies, F., & Hamson, M. (1988). A doubled-blind controlled trial of fluoxetine versus placebo for bulimia nervosa. *Proceedings of the Third International Conference on Eating Disorders*. New York.

Fullerton, D. T., Swift, W. J., Getto, C. J., & Carlson, I. H. (1986). Plasma immunoreactive beta-endorphin in bulimics. *Psychological Medicine, 16*, 59–63.

Fullerton, D. T., Swift, W. J., Getto, C. J., Carlson, I. H., & Gutzmann, L. D. (1988). Differences in plasma beta-endorphin levels of bulimics. *International Journal of Eating Disorders, 7*, 191–200.

Galante, D., Sanders, M. J., & Steiner, H. (1994, October). *Characteristics of families of daughters with anorexia or bulimia: A study of treatment phases*. Paper presented at the meeting of the American Academy of Child and Adolescent Psychiatry, New York.

Garfinkel, P. E., & Garner, D. M. (Eds.). (1987). *The role of drug treatments for eating disorders*. New York: Brunner/Mazel.

Garfinkel, P. E., & Garner, D. M. (1982). *Anorexia nervosa: A multidimensional perspective*. New York, Brunner/Mazel.

Garner, D. M., Olmsted, M. P., Bohr, Y., & Garfinkel, P. E. (1982). The Eating Attitudes Test: Psychometric features and clinical correlates. *Psychological Medicine, 12*, 871–878.

Garner, D. M., Olmsted, M. P., & Polivy, J. (1983). Development and validation of a multidimensional eating disorder inventory for anorexia and bulimia. *International Journal of Eating Disorders, 2*, 15–34.

Gartner, A. F., Marcus, R. N., Halmi, K., & Loranger, A. W. (1989). DSM-III-R personality disorders in patients with eating disorders. *American Journal of Psychiatry, 146*, 1585–1591.

Gavish, D., Eisenberg, S., Berry, E. M., Kleinman, Y., Witztum, E., Norman, J., Nutr, D., & Leitersdorf, E. (1987). Bulimia: An underlying behavioral disorder in hyperlipidemic pancreatitis: A prospective multidisciplinary approach. *Archives of Internal Medicine, 147*, 705–708.

Geracioti, T. D., & Liddle, R. A. (1988). Impaired cholecystokinin secretion in bulimia nervosa. *New England Journal of Medicine, 319*, 683–688.

Gold, P. W., Kaye, W., Robertson, G. L., & Ebert, M. E. (1983). Abnormalities in plasma and cerebrospinal-fluid argenine vasopressin in patients with anorexia nervosa. *New England Journal of Medicine, 308*, 1117–1123.

Goldberg, S. J., Comerci, G. D., & Feldman L. (1988). Cardiac output and regional myocardial contraction in anorexia nervosa. *Journal of Adolescent Health, 9*, 15–21.

Gross, H. A., Ebert, M. H., & Faden, V. B. (1981). A doubled-blind controlled study of lithium carbonate in primary anorexia nervosa. *Journal of Clinical Psychopharmacology, 1*, 376–381.

Gwirtsman, H. E., Guze, B. H., Yager, J., & Gainsley, B. (1990). Fluoxetine treatment of anorexia nervosa: An open clinical trial. *Journal of Clinical Psychiatry, 51*, 378–382.

Hall, A., & Crisp, A. H. (1987). Brief psychotherapy in the treatment of anorexia nervosa: Outcome at one year. *British Journal of Psychiatry, 151*, 185–191.

Hall, R. C. W., Hoffman, R. S., Beresford, T. P., Wooley, B., Tice, L., & Hall, A. K. (1988). Hypomagnesemia in patients with eating disorders. *Psychosomatics, 29*, 264–272.

Halmi, K. A., Eckert, E., & LaDu, T. J. (1986). Anorexia nervosa: Treatment efficacy of cyproheptadine and amitriptyline. *Archives of General Psychiatry, 43*, 177–181.

Halmi, K. A., Eckert, E., Marchi, P., Sampugnaro, V., Apple, R., & Cohen, J. (1991). Comorbidity of psychiatric diagnoses in anorexia nervosa. *Archives of General Psychiatry, 48*, 712–718.

Hammer, L. D., Kraemer H. C., Wilson, D. M., Ritter P. L., & Dornbusch, S. M. (1991). Standardized percentile curves of body-mass index for children and adolescents. *American Journal of Diseases of Children, 145*, 259–263.

Hatsukami, D., Eckert, E., Mitchell, J., & Pyle, R. (1984). Affective disorder and substance abuse in women with bulimia. *Psychological Medicine, 14*, 701–704.

Herholz, K., Krieg, J. C., Emrich, H. M., Pawlik, G., Beil,

C., Pirke, K. M., Pahl, J. J., Wagner, R., Weinhard, K., Ploog, D., & Heiss, W. D. (1987). Regional cerebral glucose metabolism in anorexia nervosa measured by positron emission tomography. *Biological Psychiatry, 22*, 43–51.

Herzog, D. B., Bradburn, I. S., & Newman, K. (1990). Sexuality in males with eating disorders. In A. E. Anderson (Ed.), *Males with eating disorders* (pp. 40–53). New York: Brunner/Mazel.

Herzog, D. B., Keller, M. B., & Lavori, P. W. (1988). Outcome in anorexia nervosa and bulimia nervosa. *Journal of Nervous and Mental Disease, 176*, 131–143.

Hoek, W. (1991). The incidence and prevalence of anorexia nervosa and bulimia nervosa in primary care. *Psychological Medicine, 21*, 455–460.

Hsu, L. K. C. (1990). *Eating disorders*. New York: Guilford.

Hsu, L. K. C. (1991). Outcome studies in patients with eating disorders. In S. M. Mirin, J. T. Gossett & M. C. Grob (Eds.), *Psychiatric treatment: Advances in outcome research* (pp. 159–180). Washington, DC.: American Psychiatric Press.

Hsu, L. K. C. (1988). The outcome on anorexia nervosa: A reappraisal. *Psychological Medicine, 18*, 807–812.

Hudson, J. I., Pope, H. G., Yurgelun-Todd, D., Jonas, J. M., & Frankenburg, F. R. (1987). A controlled study of lifetime prevalence of affective and other psychiatric disorders in bulimic outpatients. *American Journal of Psychiatry, 144*, 1283–1287.

Hughes, P. L., Wells, L. A., Cunningham, C. J., & Ilstrup, D. M. (1986). Treating bulimia with desipramine: A double-blind placebo-controlled study. *Archives of General Psychiatry, 43*, 182–186.

Humphrey, L. L. (1989). Observed family interactions among subtypes of eating disorders using structural analysis of social behavior. *Journal of Consulting and Clinical Psychology, 57*, 206–214.

Isner J. M., Roberts, W. C., Heymsfield, S. B., & Yager, J. (1985). Anorexia nervosa and sudden death. *Annals of Internal Medicine, 102*, 49–52.

Johnson, G. L., Humphries, L. L., Shirley, P. B., Mazzoleni, A., & Noonan, J. A. (1986). Mitral valve prolapse in patients with anorexia nervosa and bulimia. *Archives of Internal Medicine, 146*, 1525–1529.

Johnson-Sabine, E., Wood, K., Patton, G., Mann, A., & Wakeling, A. (1988). Abnormal eating attitudes in London school girls—A prospective epidemiological study: Factors associated with abnormal responses on screening questionnaires. *Psychological Medicine, 18*, 615–622.

Jones, D., Fox, M., Babigan, H., & Hutton, H. (1980). Epidemiology of anorexia nervosa in Monroe County,

New York: 1960–1976. *Psychosomatic Medicine, 42,* 551–558.

Joyce, J. M., Warren, D. L., Humphries, L. L., Smith, A. J., & Coon, J. S. (1990). Osteoporosis in women with eating disorders: Comparison of physical parameters, exercise, and menstrual status with SPA and DPA evaluation. *Journal of Nuclear Medicine, 31,* 325–331.

Kahn, D., Halls, J., Bianco, J. A., & Perlman, S. B. (1991). Radionuclide ventriculography in severely under-weight anorexia nervosa patients before and during refeeding therapy. *Journal of Adolescent Health, 12,* 301–306.

Kaplan, A. S., & Garfinkel, P. E. (1988). Neuroendocrinology of anorexia nervosa. In R. Collu, G. Brown, & R. Van Loon (Eds.), *Clinical neuroendocrinology* (pp. 105–122). Boston: Blackwell Scientific Publications.

Kasvikis, Y. G., Tsakiris, F., Marks, I. M., Basogul, M., & Noshirvani, H. F. (1986). Past history of anorexia nervosa in women with obsessive compulsive disorder. *International Journal of Eating Disorders, 5,* 1969–1976.

Katz, J. L. (1990). Eating disorders: A primer for the substance abuse special: 1. Clinical features. *Journal of Substance Abuse Treatment, 7,* 143–149.

Kaye, W. H., Pickar, D., Naber, D., & Ebert, M. H. (1982). Cerebrospinal fluid opioid activity in anorexia nervosa. *American Journal of Psychiatry, 139,* 643–645.

Kaye, W. H., & Weltzin, T. E. (1991). Neurochemistry of bulimia nervosa. *Journal of Clinical Psychiatry, 52 (supplement),* 21–28.

Kaye, W. H., Weltzin, T. E., Hsu, L. K., & Bulik, C. M. (1991). An open trial of fluoxetine in patients with anorexia nervosa. *Journal of Clinical Psychiatry, 52,* 464–471.

Kendell, R. E., Hall, D. J., Hailey, A., & Babigian, H. M. (1973). The epidemiology of anorexia nervosa. *Psychological Medicine, 3,* 200–203.

Kennedy, S. H., Piran, N., Warsh, J. J., Prendergast, P., Mainprize, E., Whynot, C., & Garfinkel, P. E. (1988). A trial of isocarboxazid in the treatment of bulimia nervosa. *Journal of Clinical Psychopharmacology, 8,* 391–396.

King, M. B., & Bhugra, D. (1989). Eating disorders: Lessons from a cross-cultural study. *Psychological Medicine, 19,* 955–958.

Kreipe, R. E., Churchill B. H., & Strauss, J. (1989a). Short stature in females with anorexia nervosa. *Pediatric Research, 25,* 7A.

Kreipe, R. E., Churchill B. H., & Strauss, J. (1989b). Long-term outcome of adolescents with anorexia nervosa. *American Journal of Diseases of Children, 143,* 1322–1327.

Kreipe, R. E., & Harris J. P. (1992). Myocardial impairment resulting from eating disorders. *Pediatric Annals, 21,* 760–768.

Krieg, J. C., Backmund, H., & Pirke, K. M. (1987). Cranial computed tomography findings in bulimia. *Acta Psychiatrica Scandinavica, 75,* 144–149.

Krieg, J. C., Lauer, C., & Pirke, K. M. (1989). Structural brain abnormalities in patients with bulimia nervosa. *Psychiatry Research, 27,* 39–48.

Lacey, J. H., & Crisp, A. H. (1980). Hunger, food intake and weight: The impact of clomipramine on a refeeding anorexia nervosa population. *Postgraduate Medicine Journal 56,* 79–85.

Laessle, R. G., Wittchen, H. U., Fichter, M. M., & Pirke, K. M. (1989). The significance of subgroups of bulimia and anorexia nervosa: Lifetime frequency of psychiatric disorders. *International Journal of Eating Disorders, 8,* 569–574.

Lautenbaucher, S., Galfe, G., Hoelzl R., & Pirke, K. M. (1989). Gastrointestinal transit is delayed in patients with bulimia. *International Journal of Eating Disorders, 8,* 203–208.

Levin, P. A., Falko, J. M., Dixon, K., Gallup, E. M., & Saunders, W. (1980). Benign parotid enlargement in bulimia. *Annals of Internal Medicine, 93,* 827–829.

Levy, A. B., Dixon, K. N., & Stern, S. L. (1989). How are depression and bulimia related? *American Journal of Psychiatry, 146,* 162–169.

Liebowitz, S. F. (1983). Hypothalamic catecholamine systems controlling eating behavior: A potential model for anorexia nervosa. In P. L. Darby, P. E. Garfinkel, D. M. Garner, & D. V. Coscina (Eds.), *Anorexia nervosa: Recent developments in research* (pp. 221–229). New York: Alan R. Liss.

Lucas, A. R., Beard, M., O'Fallon, W. M., & Kurland, L. T. (1991). 50-year trends in the incidence of anorexia nervosa in Rochester, Minn.: A population-based study. *American Journal of Psychiatry, 148,* 917–922.

Maloney, M. J., McGuire, J. B., Daniels, S. R., & Specker, B. (1989). Dieting behavior and eating attitudes in children. *Pediatrics, 84,* 482–489.

Mant, M. J., & Faragher, B. S. (1972). The hematology of anorexia nervosa. *British Journal of Haematology, 23,* 737–749.

McCann, U. D., & Agras, W. S. (1990). Successful treatment of nonpurging bulimia nervosa with desipramine: A double-blind, placebo-controlled study. *American Journal of Psychiatry, 147,* 1509–1513.

Minuchin, S., Rosman, B. L., & Baker, L. (1978). *Psychosomatic families*. Cambridge, Mass.: Harvard.

Mitchell, J. E., & Boutacoff, L. I. (1986). Laxative abuse complicating bulimia: Medical and treatment implications. *International Journal of Eating Disorders, 5*, 325–334.

Mitchell, J. E., Hatsukami, D., Eckert, E. D., & Pyle, R. L. (1985). Characteristics of 275 patients with bulimia. *American Journal of Psychiatry, 142*, 482–485.

Mitchell, J. E., Pomeroy, C., Seppala, M., & Huber, M. (1988). Pseudo-Bartter's syndrome, diuretic abuse, idiopathic edema, and eating disorders. *International Journal of Eating Disorders, 7*, 225–237.

Mitchell, J. E., Pyle, R. L., Eckert, E. D., Hatsukami, D., Pomeroy, C., & Zimmerman, R. (1990). A comparison study of antidepressants and structured intensive group psychotherapy in the treatment of bulimia nervosa. *Archives of General Psychiatry, 47*, 149–157.

Mitchell, J. E., Pyle, R. L., & Miner, R. A. (1982). Gastric dilatation as a complication of bulimia. *Psychosomatics, 23*, 96–97.

Mitchell, J. E., Specker, S. M., & de Zwaan, M. (1991). Comorbidity and medical complications of bulimia nervosa. *Journal of Clinical Psychiatry, 52*, 13–20.

Moodie, D. S. (1987). Anorexia and the heart. *Postgraduate Medicine, 81*, 46–61.

Moodie, D. S., & Salcedo, E. (1983). Cardiac function in adolescents and young adults with anorexia nervosa. *Journal of Adolescent Health, 4*, 9–14.

Morgan, H. G., & Russell, G. (1975). Value of family back-ground and clinical features as predictors of long-term outcome in anorexia nervosa: Four-year follow-up study of 41 patients. *Psychological Medicine, 5*, 355–371.

National Center for Health Statistics. (1973). Height and weight of youths 12–17 years, United States. *Vital and Health Series 11*, No. 124. Washington, DC: U.S. Government Printing Office.

Newman, M. M., & Halmi, K. A. (1989). Relationship of bone density to estradiol and cortisol in anorexia nervosa and bulimia. *Psychiatry Research, 29*, 105–112.

Nussbaum, M., Baird, D., Sonnenblick, M., Cowan, K., & Shenker, I. R. (1985). Short stature in anorexia nervosa patients. *Journal of Adolescent Health, 6*, 453–455.

Nussbaum, M., Shenker, I. R., Baird, D., & Saraway, S. (1985). Follow-up investigation of patients with anorexia nervosa. *Journal of Pediatrics, 106*, 835–840.

Nussbaum, M., Shenker, I. R., Marc, J., & Klein, M. (1980). Cerebral atrophy in anorexia nervosa. *Journal of Pediatrics, 96*, 867–869.

Nylander, I. (1971). The feeling of being fat and dieting in a school population: An epidemiologic interview investigation. *Acta Sociomedica Scandinavica, 3*, 17–26.

Palla, B., & Litt, I. F. (1988). Medical complications of eating disorders in adolescents. *Pediatrics, 81*, 613–623.

Palmer, E. P., & Guay, A. T. (1986). Reversible myopathy secondary to abuse of ipecac in patients with major eating disorders. *New England Journal of Medicine, 313*, 1457–1459.

Piran N., Lerner, P., Garfinkel, P. E., Kennedy, S., & Brouillette, C. (1988). Personality disorders in restricting and bulimic forms of anorexia nervosa. *International Journal of Eating Disorders, 7*, 589–599.

Pirke, K. M., Pahl, J., Schweiger, U., & Warnhoff, M. (1985). Metabolic and endocrine indices of starvation in bulimia: A comparison with anorexia nervosa. *Psychiatry Research, 15*, 33–39.

Pope, H. G., Jr., Hudson, J. I., Jonas, J. M., & Yurgelun-Todd, D. (1983). Bulimia treated with imipramine: A placebo-controlled, double-blind study. *American Journal of Psychiatry, 140*, 554–558.

Pope, H. G., Jr., Keck, P. E., Jr., McElroy, S. L., & Hudson, J. I. (1989). A placebo-controlled study of trazodone in bulimia nervosa. *Journal of Clinical Psychopharmacology, 9*, 254–259.

Powers, P. S. (1982). Heart failure during treatment of anorexia nervosa. *American Journal of Psychiatry, 139*, 1167–1170.

Prior, J. C., Vigna, Y. M., Schechter, M. T., & Burgess, A. E. (1990). Spinal bone loss and ovulatory disturbance. *New England Journal of Medicine, 323*, 1221–1227.

Rastam, M., Gillberg, C., & Garton, M. (1989). Anorexia nervosa in a Swedish urban region: A population-based study. *British Journal of Psychiatry, 155*, 642–646.

Richards, M. H., Casper, R. C., & Larson, R. (1990). Weight and eating concerns among pre- and young adolescent boys and girls. *Journal of Adolescent Health Care, 11*, 203–209.

Rigotti, N. A., Neer, R. M., Skates, S. J., Herzog, D. B., & Nussbaum, S. R. (1991). The clinical course of osteoporosis in anorexia nervosa: A longitudinal study of cortical bone mass. *Journal of the American Medical Association, 265*, 1133–1138.

Rosen, J. C., & Leitenberg, H., (1982). Bulimia nervosa: Treatment with exposure and response prevention. *Behavior Therapy, 13*, 117–124.

Russell, G. F. M. (1979). Bulimia nervosa: An ominous variant of anorexia nervosa. *Psychological Medicine, 9*, 429–448.

Russell, G., Szmukler, G., Dare, C., & Eisler, I. (1987). An evaluation of family therapy in anorexia nervosa and bulimia nervosa. *Archives of General Psychiatry, 44,* 1047–1056.

Schechter, J. O., Altemus, M., & Greenfeld, D. G. (1986). Food bingeing and esophageal perforation in anorexia nervosa. *Hospital & Community Psychiatry, 37,* 507–508.

Schocken, D. D., Holloway, D., & Powers, P. (1989). Weight loss and the heart: Effects of anorexia nervosa and starvation. *Archives of Internal Medicine, 149,* 877–881.

Schonberg, S. K. (Ed.) (1988). *Substance abuse: A guide for health professionals.* Elk Grove Village, IL: American Academy of Pediatrics.

Schwartz, H. J. (1990). *Bulimia: Psychoanalytic treatment and theory* (2nd ed.). Madison, CT: International Universities Press.

Selvini-Palazzoli, M. P. (1974). *Self-starvation: From individual to family therapy in the treatment of anorexia nervosa.* New York: Jason Aronson.

Shaw, B. F., & Garfinkel, P. E. (1990). Research problems in the eating disorders. *International Journal of Eating Disorders, 9,* 545–555.

Sheridan, P. H., & Collins, M. (1983). Potentially life-threatening hypophosphatemia in anorexia nervosa. *Journal of Adolescent Health Care, 4,* 44–46.

Simmons, M. S., Grayden, S. K., & Mitchell, J. E. (1986). The need for psychiatric-dental liaison in the treatment of bulimia. *American Journal of Psychiatry, 143,* 783–784.

Steiner-Adair, C. (1986). The body politic: Normal female adolescent development and the development of eating disorders. *Journal of the American Academy of Psychoanalysis, 14,* 95–114.

Steiner-Adair, C. (1991). When the body speaks: Girls, eating disorders and psychotherapy. In C. Gilligan, A. Rogers, & D. Tolman (Eds.), *Women, girls & psychotherapy: Reframing resistance* (pp. 253–266). Boston: Haworth Press.

Steinhausen, H. C., Rauss-Mason, C., & Seidel, R. (1991). Follow-up studies of anorexia nervosa: A review of four decades of outcome research. *Psychological Medicine, 21,* 447–454.

Tepper, R., Weizman, A., Apter, A., Tyano, S., & Beyth, Y. (1992). Elevated plasma immunoreactive beta-endorphin in anorexia nervosa. *Clinical Neuropharmacology, 15,* 387–391.

Tobin, D. L., & Johnson, C. L. (1991). The integration of psychodynamic and behavior therapy in the treatment of eating disorders: Clinical issues versus theoretical mystique. In C. L. Johnson (Ed.), *Psychodynamic treatment of anorexia nervosa and bulimia* (pp. 374–397). New York: Guilford.

Vandereycken, W., & Pierloot, R. (1982). Pimozide combined with behavior therapy in the short-term treatment of anorexia nervosa: A double-blind placebo-controlled cross-over study. *Acta Psychiatrica Scandinavia, 66,* 445–450.

Wadden, T. A., Foster, G. D., Stunkard, A. J., & Linowitz, J. R. (1989). Dissatisfaction with weight and figure in obese girls: Discontent but not depression. *International Journal of Obesity, 13,* 89–97.

Waldholtz, B. D., & Anderson, A. E. (1988). Hypophosphatemia during starvation in anorexia nervosa. *International Journal of Eating Disorders, 7,* 551–555.

Walsh, B. T., Stewart, J. W., Roose, S. P., Gladis, M., & Glassman, A. H. (1984). Treatment of bulimia with phenelzine: A double-blind, placebo-controlled study. *Archives of General Psychiatry, 41,* 1105–1109.

Warren, M. P., Brooks-Gunn, J., Hamilton, L. H., Warren, L. F., & Hamilton, W. G. (1986). Scoliosis and fractures in young ballet dancers. *The New England Journal of Medicine, 314,* 1348–1353.

Warren, M. P., & VandeWiele, R. L. (1973). Clinical and metabolic features of anorexia nervosa. *American Journal of Obstetrics and Gynecology, 117,* 435–449.

Wells, L. A., & Logan, K. M. (1987). Pharmacologic treatment of eating disorders: A review of selected literature and recommendations. *Psychosomatics, 28,* 470–479.

White, J. H. (1992a). Women and eating disorders, part I: Significance and sociocultural risk factors. *Health Care for Women International, 13,* 351–362.

White, J. H. (1992b). Women and eating disorders part II: Developmental, familial, and biological risk factors. *Health Care for Women International, 13,* 363–373.

White, M. (1986). Anorexia nervosa: A cybernetic perspective. In J. Elka-Harkaway (Ed.), *Eating disorders* (pp. 117–129). New York: Aspen.

White, M., & Epston, D. (1990). *Narrative means to a therapeutic end.* New York: Norton.

Willi, J., & Grossman, S. (1983). Epidemiology of anorexia nervosa in a defined region of Switzerland. *American Journal of Psychiatry, 140,* 564–567.

Williams, J. F., Friedman, I. M., & Steiner, H. (1986). Hand lesions characteristic of bulimia. *American Journal of Diseases of Children, 140,* 28–29.

Wright K., Smith, M. S., & Mitchell, J. (1990). Organic diseases mimicking atypical eating disorders. *Clinical Pediatrics, 29,* 325–328.

Wu, C. J., Hagman, J., Buchsbaum, M. S., Blinder, B., Derrfler, M., Tai, W. Y., Hazlett, E., & Sicotte, N. (1990). Greater left cerebral hemispheric metabolism in bulimia assessed by positron emission tomography. *American Journal of Psychiatry, 147,* 309–312.

Yates, A. (1989). Current perspectives on the eating disorders: History, psychological and biological aspects. *Journal of the American Academy of Child and Adolescent Psychiatry, 28*, 813–828.

Yates, A. (1992). Biologic considerations in the etiology of eating disorders. *Pediatric Annals, 21*, 739–744.

CHAPTER 15

SUBSTANCE USE AND ABUSE

Eric F. Wagner
Yifrah Kaminer

DESCRIPTION OF DISORDERS

Substance Use versus Substance Abuse

Newcomb and Bentler (1988) have suggested the following conceptualization of adolescent substance use: ". . . experimental use of various drugs, both licit and illicit, may be considered a normative behavior among United States teenagers in terms of prevalence, and from a developmental task perspective" (p. 214). This quote captures two important considerations in thinking about adolescent substance use. First, most teens will try licit and/or illicit substances at some point during their adolescent years. For example, 87 percent of the 1993 high school graduating class reported using alcohol, 51 percent admitted alcohol use within the last 30 days, 35 percent reported using marijuana, and 15 percent admitted marijuana use within the last 30 days (Johnston, O'Malley, & Bachman, 1994). Second, teen substance use can be usefully conceptualized from a developmental standpoint. Many adolescents experiment with substance use much the same way as they experiment with clothing styles and political views. Substance use is one way of engaging in independent, adult-like behavior and can serve as a vehicle for testing the limits of adult rules for teen behavior and establishing one's own definition of appropriate behavior. In short, substance use among some adolescents can be thought of as part of normal development (see Shedler & Block, 1990).

Despite the prevalence and developmental importance of substance use among adolescents, a sizable minority of teens will demonstrate substance-related problems. For example, a recent epidemiological study found that 4 percent of randomly selected high school students can be expected to meet DSM-III-R diagnostic criteria for substance abuse during the course of a single year (Lewinsohn, Hops, Roberts, Seeley, & Andrews, 1993). Among more highly selected adolescent samples (e.g., emotionally disturbed adolescents, juvenile offenders), much higher rates of substance abuse have been documented (Greenbaum, Prange, Friedman, & Silver, 1991; Kaminer, Wagner, Plummer, & Seifer, 1993; Milin, Halikas, Meller, & Morse, 1991; Winters, 1991).

The use of substances among teens lies on a continuum, ranging from nonuse to addiction (Steinberg & Levine, 1990). *Nonusers* are adolescents who have never tried alcohol and other drugs and have no intention to do so. *Experimenters* are teens who try substances (typically alcohol or marijuana) once or twice but decide they do not like the effects. *Recreational users* use alcohol and/or other drugs on an occasional basis but generally can take or leave substance use. *Regular users* are adolescents who actively seek alcohol and/or other drugs and use substances on a regular basis. Such teens tend to prefer friends and activities associated with getting high yet still care about their reputations and parents' approval. *Abusers* are frequent substance users who tend to use alcohol and other drugs in multiple situations. These adolescents lose interest in the non-substance-related activities they used to enjoy and begin to demonstrate declines and/or problems in areas such as school performance and relations with parents. Finally, *alcoholics/addicts* are chronic and heavy substance users who use alcohol and other drugs compulsively. Addicted adolescents start seeking drugs and routes of administration with the most immediate effects (e.g., high proof alcohol, smoking crack cocaine, shooting up).

Most adolescents fall in the experimenter-regular user range. Such adolescents rarely come into contact with treatment professionals in the absence of some acute provoking event (e.g., an intoxication-related accident). The types of substance using teens more typically seen in treatment settings are the abusers and addicts, with the abusers outnumbering the addicts simply because very few adolescents have a long enough substance use history to develop the combination of symptoms that define addiction (e.g., physical dependence on a substance, medical complications related to the use of a substance).

Current Assessment and Treatment Practice

Despite widespread recognition that a significant minority of adolescents use substances in a manner that places them at high risk for experiencing serious negative consequences, current literature concerning the assessment and treatment of substance abuse among youth is meager. For example, Donovan and Marlatt's (1988) influential book, *Assessment of Addictive Behaviors*, includes only *one paragraph* pertaining to the assessment of substance abuse among adolescents. With some recent exceptions (e.g., Center for Substance Abuse Treatment, 1993; Kaminer, 1994a; Wagner, Myers, & Brown, 1994), a similar state of affairs exists in the adolescent substance abuse treatment literature.

One of the worst consequences of this scarcity of knowledge is a lack of standardized and widely accepted diagnostic criteria and treatment procedures for adolescent substance abuse. To date, most attempts to assess and treat substance use problems among teens have been disparate and atheoretical (Harrell & Wirtz, 1989; Win-

ters, 1990). As a result, most adolescent substance abuse treatment programs base their services primarily on their own specific philosophical orientation (e.g., multidimensional vs. unitary etiology of substance abuse; disease model vs. self-control model of substance abuse), using procedures extrapolated from adult substance abuse treatment models (Blum, 1987).

These philosophical differences across adolescent substance abuse treatment programs result in wide variation among treatment settings in (a) who gets diagnosed as substance abusing, (b) what events need to occur to address substance use problems, and (c) what outcomes indicate successful treatment. For example, Minnesota Model treatment programs (see Cook, 1988a, 1988b; Laudergan, 1982) are likely to diagnose teens with more chronic substance-related problems as substance abusing and to assume a large degree of etiological homogeneity among substance abusing teens based on the belief that they share in common the "disease" of substance abuse. Furthermore, Minnesota Model programs typically involve an intensive residential treatment process during which adolescents are encouraged to adopt a 12-step ideological framework for understanding and addressing their substance use problems (see Kassel & Wagner, 1993). Finally, the ideal treatment outcome, according to the Minnesota Model, is life-long abstinence from all mood-altering chemicals. In contrast, a cognitive-behavioral coping skills approach to adolescent substance abuse treatment (for an example, see Wagner, Myers, & Brown, 1994) is likely to consider a wide range of substance use problems as appropriate for intervention and to assume a large degree of etiological heterogeneity among substance abusing teens. A continuum of treatment intensities is endorsed, ranging from a single session to long-term residential programs, and the focus throughout treatment is on the role of environmental influences and learned beliefs and behaviors in determining alcohol and drug use behaviors. Finally, the definition of successful treatment outcome may be expanded to include limited continued use of substances if significant reductions in prior problematic use patterns can be achieved and maintained. While it is currently premature to conclude which of the variety of treatment approaches available to substance abusing adolescents is most effective, it is important to realize that adolescents' experiences in treatment will vary greatly on the basis of where they present for treatment.

The problem with using adult-derived procedures is that adolescents and adults with substance use problems differ significantly. Symptoms such as the progressive nature of the disorder, medical complications, and physical dependence are less clearly associated with adolescent substance abuse than with adult substance abuse (Blum, 1987; Kaminer, 1991; White & Labouvie, 1989). Teens who use alcohol and/or other drugs tend to use chemicals less frequently but in larger amounts than adult substance users. This usage pattern increases the risks for adolescent substance users to suffer from the acute effects (e.g., blackouts and hangovers) and display the behavioral concomitants (e.g., belligerence) of intoxication (White & Labouvie, 1989). Furthermore, many adolescents with substance use problems will mature and leave behind their problem use patterns by early adulthood without exposure to formal intervention or treatment (Blum, 1987; Winters & Henly, 1988).

DSM-IV Diagnostic Criteria Applied to Adolescents

The substance-related disorder diagnostic criteria most commonly used in psychiatric and substance abuse treatment settings across the country are those from the DSM-IV (American Psychiatric Association, 1994). While often used with adolescents, DSM-IV does not distinguish between adult and adolescent presentations of substance use problems, despite the fact that many of the adult diagnostic criteria are inappropriate for teens. For example, the diagnosis of substance dependence is based primarily on clinical manifestations of tolerance and withdrawal, the progressive nature of the disorder, medical complications, and other chronic symptoms. However, substance abusing adolescents are unlikely to meet such criteria, given the relatively brief histories of their substance use problems.

Teens with substance use problems are much more likely to meet substance abuse diagnostic criteria, which involve "a maladaptive pattern of substance use leading to clinically significant impairment or distress." In order to meet DSM-IV diagnostic criteria for substance abuse, one or more of the following is required to have occurred during a twelve-month period: (1) recurrent substance use resulting in a failure to fulfill major role obligations, (2) recurrent substance use in situations in which it is physically dangerous, (3) recurrent substance-related legal problems, or (4) continued substance use despite having persistent or recurrent social problems caused by or exacerbated by the effects of the substance. Adolescents are also likely to meet DSM-IV diagnostic criteria for substance intoxication, which involves clinically significant yet reversible behavioral or psychological changes due to the recent ingestion of alcohol and/or other drugs.

EPIDEMIOLOGY

Substance Use Rates

The Monitoring the Future Survey (Johnston, O'Malley, & Bachman, 1994) is conducted annually to assess the extent of alcohol and other drug use among American teens in the eighth, tenth, and twelfth grades. This survey is administered to a large and representative sample of adolescents and provides valuable data concerning substance use and related behaviors. However, the survey is limited to students who attend school on the day the survey is administered. Thus, data are not obtained from high school dropouts (approximately 20 percent of all adolescents) or absentees, subgroups of adolescents whose substance use rates are likely to be higher on average than teens participating in the Monitoring the Future Survey. Moreover, the survey, while anonymous, is self-report in nature, raising questions as to the validity of the responses since substance use by adolescents is a proscribed behavior. Despite these limitations, the Monitoring the Future Survey provides the best available estimate of substance use rates among teens.

The 1993 results of the Monitoring the Future Survey indicate an upswing in the use of substances among American teens (Johnston, O'Malley, & Bachman, 1994). The investigators reported a rise in marijuana use throughout the country at all three grade levels, as well as increases in the use of cigarettes, stimulants, LSD, and inhalants. These findings signify a reversal of the general downward trend in the prevalence of adolescent substance use which characterized the period between 1985 and 1991. This change in use patterns was accompanied by shifts in attitudes and beliefs about drugs thought to be influential in deterring use. Specifically, decreases in (a) the perceived dangers associated with substance use and (b) personal disapproval of substance use were observed across all three grades.

Alcohol, tobacco, and marijuana continue to be the substances used most widely by adolescents. Alcohol consumption during the past year (1992–1993) was reported by 52 percent of 8th graders, 69 percent of 10th graders, and 76 percent of 12th graders. In regard to binge drinking, 14 percent of 8th graders, 23 percent of 10th graders, and 28 percent of 12th graders admitted to binge drinking during the two weeks prior to the survey. Daily cigarette smoking was reported by 8 percent of 8th graders, 14 percent of 10th graders, and 19 percent of seniors at the time of the 1993 survey. In contrast to most other substances used by adolescents in the last ten years, daily cigarette use rates among females have been slightly higher than among males. Finally, the proportion of students who reported using marijuana during the past year was 9 percent for 8th graders, 19 percent for 10th graders, and 26 percent for 12th graders.

Substance Abuse Rates

The above-noted substance use rates serve at best as a periodic "snapshot" of adolescent drug use. It has not been reported how many of the students included in the Monitoring the Future Survey were polysubstance users. Such data are important given that polysubstance use increases the risk for developing substance use problems in adolescence (Brown, 1993). Furthermore, the clinical significance of the Monitoring the Future data is unclear. A very cautious generalization is that adolescents identified as daily users are at a very high risk for developing substance use problems. More alarming are the data suggesting recent increases in the use of several substances including cigarettes, marijuana, and LSD, especially among younger students. Indeed, Graham, Collins, Wugalter, Chung, and Hansen (1991) have found that junior high school students who have tried tobacco are on an accelerated trajectory toward heavy use of other drugs compared with agemates who have not tried tobacco. Such results suggest that the increased prevalence of tobacco use in eighth graders may lead to an increased prevalence of substance use problems later in adolescence.

One recent study has examined the rates of substance use problems among a community sample of high school students. Using the relatively stringent substance abuse diagnostic criteria of the Schedule for Affective Disorders for School-Age Children–Epidemiological Version (Orvaschel, Puig-Antich, Chambers, Tabrizi, & Johnson, 1982), Lewinsohn and colleagues (1993) found a lifetime substance abuse prevalence of 8 percent among randomly selected high school students. The point prevalence was estimated at 2 percent, and the annual incidence rate for the disorder was 4 percent. Projected onto a high school of 1,000 students, these data indicated that 40 new or relapsed cases of substance abuse can be expected to be identified in a one-year period.

ASSESSMENT APPROACHES

Given our current state of knowledge, substance use problems are best conceptualized as resulting from interactions among biological, psychological, and social factors (see Donovan & Marlatt, 1988). However, the degree to which each of these factors influences adolescent substance use behavior varies from individual to individual (Farrell & Strang, 1991). Teens with substance use problems differ markedly from one another in the type and frequency of substances used, the actual and anticipated effects and consequences resulting from that use, the contexts and motivations in which use occurs, and the factors which have contributed to or accompany substance use involvement (Henly & Winters, 1989).

Given the varied and multidimensional nature of substance use problems among adolescents, Tarter, Ott, and Mezzich (1991) have suggested that the ideal adolescent substance abuse assessment should include evaluation of each of the following domains: (1) substance use behavior itself; (2) type and severity of psychiatric morbidity that may be present and whether it preceded or developed after the substance use disorder; (3) cognition, with specific attention to neuropsychological functioning; (4) family organization and interactional patterns; (5) social skills; (6) vocational adjustment; (7) recreation and leisure activities; (8) personality; (9) school adjustment; (10) peer affiliation; (11) legal status; and, (12) physical health.

Medical Issues

Adolescents with apparent or possible substance use problems should be medically examined in the same systematic manner as is routinely employed in pediatrics and adolescent medicine. A medical history should be taken and a physical examination should be performed in a methodical fashion. Adherence to routine throughout the medical examination is important to avoid omission, duplication, and lack of clarity. Despite obvious findings related to the recent or chronic use of psychoactive substances, other areas must be evaluated.

Emergency Medical Evaluation

Emergency medical evaluation of a substance abusing adolescent should be differentiated from elective medical evaluation. According to Felter, Izsak, and Lawrence (1987), the most common reasons for emergency-related adolescent substance abuse admissions are (1) accidental or intentional overdose of one or more psychoactive substances; (2) associated trauma, motor vehicle accidents, falls, and near drowning; (3) intoxication, idiosyncratic (pathological) intoxication, "bad trip," or panic reactions; (4) drug-seeking behavior; and (5) parents wanting their child checked for "drug use."

The first priority in the emergency treatment of overdose or severe intoxication, particularly when the teen is unconscious, is to follow the ABC mnemonic: assure that the Airway is unobstructed, Breathing (ventilation) is adequate and regular, and Circulatory system-related vital signs, such as pulse and blood pressure, are sufficient for life support. Differential diagnoses for the comatose adolescent need also to be considered (e.g., hypoglycemia, ketoacidosis).

Subsequently, a thorough physical examination is essential to identify signs and symptoms of trauma. Indeed, clues for the psychoactive substance(s) responsible for a toxic state and a possible trauma may be found by meticulous assessment of the eyes, pupils, and skin. Odors and a search of the adolescent's clothing can also provide valuable information about the substance(s) responsible for the patient's condition. Examples of substance-specific physical findings include needle marks in heroin or stimulant injection, bullae usually secondary to barbiturate injection, pustular dermatosis or rash around the mouth in chronic solvent abuse, odors of hydrocarbons and solvents on the patient's breath in chronic solvent abuse, and signs of paint on the hands or the face indicating the use of spray paint cans for inhalation "bagging."

The patient (if conscious) and accompanying parties can also provide important information concerning the teen's recent substance use, following a comprehensive history. It is noteworthy that street drugs are often misrepresented, and what adolescents think they bought, took, or smoked may be altogether different from what they actually ingested. A list of locally-used street names of drugs can help improve communication with the patient and accompanying parties and increase the likelihood of accurate identification of the abused agents.

There is no perfect laboratory panel that should be covered for every substance-related emergency patient. Laboratory work should include an immediate analysis of bodily fluids such as urine, blood, and gastric contents if a gastric lavage has been done. Proper precautions against contamination of clinical personnel by the patient's body fluids must be taken to prevent HIV or hepatitis infection.

The immediately preceding discussion of substance abuse emergency evaluation is necessarily brief, given the scope of the current chapter. Felter et al. (1987) and Schuckit (1989) are two particularly good references for those readers who would like greater detail on the emergency treatment of toxic states related to psychoactive substances.

Elective Medical Evaluation

An elective or a nonemergency-related admission of an adolescent also requires a comprehensive physical evaluation. Laboratory work should include analysis of urine for psychoactive substances, a breathalyzer test for alcohol, and a broad-spectrum blood laboratory panel (e.g., SMAC 24) as a routine baseline. Hepatitis B and HIV tests should be considered for patients who are either IV substance users and/or who have had high-risk sexual encounters (e.g., multiple partners, unprotected sex, sex with substance abusers). Inhalant abusers should receive a chest x-ray to rule out chemical pneumonitis, and adolescents who are treated with antidepressants, particularly tricyclics, need an electrocardiogram. Additional tests should be performed on a case-by-case basis.

A detailed and reliable history of substance use, including medical, family, psychiatric, legal, and academic histories should be obtained from the patient and family members. Special emphasis should be given to recent changes in any domain of functioning that might be related to substance use. Such data are essential for understanding the findings from the medical examination and will aid in developing a framework for a treatment plan.

Psychological and Psychiatric Issues

Psychological/psychiatric evaluations of adolescents with apparent or possible substance use problems should be conducted in the same rigorous and systematic manner as is routinely employed in child and adolescent clinical psychology and psychiatry. At a minimum, psychological evaluations of substance abusing teens should include the following four components: (1) a description of the purposes behind the assessment given to adolescents and their family members, (2) an interview with adolescents and their family members about the presenting problem, (3) administration to adolescents of one or more standardized measures of domains of functioning related to the presenting problem, and (4) a feedback session with adolescents and their family members concerning the results of the evaluation. When time permits, evaluation should also include reports from additional significant others (e.g., teachers), direct observation of adolescents' behavior in one or more settings, and neuropsychological and/or biological measures.

Purposes

The purposes behind an adolescent substance abuse evaluation may include the following: (1) to screen for problems; (2) to establish a diagnosis; (3) to establish eligibility and appropriateness for treatment; (4) to understand the individual more comprehensively; (5) to determine which form of treatment, if any, is most appropriate; (6) to provide pretreatment scores that later can be compared with status on these same dimensions after treatment in order to assess and document improvement; and/or (7) to build motivation (i.e., motivation defined as the probability that a person will enter into, continue, and adhere to a specific change strategy) and strengthen commitment for change (Miller & Rollnick 1991; Skinner, 1980). As noted above, it is essential that the purpose(s) behind an assessment be explained to adolescents and their family members prior to initiating the evaluation. By doing so, misunderstandings will be avoided, and compliance with both the assessment itself and subsequent treatment recommendations will be maximized.

Presenting Problem Interview

Actual evaluation should begin with a brief open-ended interview with adolescents and their parents about the presenting problem. Important topics to discuss include adolescents and their family members' perceptions of the chronicity, severity, and origins of the substance use problem. During this interview, the assessing clinician should keep in mind that adolescents and their parents' descriptions of presenting problems can often be contradictory. In such cases, it is usually best to openly acknowledge any contradictions that emerge without siding with the adolescents or their parents. Parents may request to meet with the clinician without their adolescent present, and such a meeting can be pursued if judged by the clinician to be necessary and helpful. However, issues related to confidentiality should be carefully considered and discussed before meeting with parents alone. Adolescents may also request to meet with the clinician without their parents present, and this can be accomplished during the actual testing session. Again, issues related to confidentiality need to be considered prior to initiating such a meeting.

Assessment Administration

Psychological evaluations of substance abuse are likely to involve one of two approaches to assessment (Donovan, 1988). *Sequential evaluation* involves beginning with a substance abuse screen, following with a basic substance use assessment if the screen is positive, and moving on to specialized assessment (e.g., neuropsychological evaluation) if indicated. This approach is de-

sirable when little, prior to the assessment, is known about whether the adolescent has been involved with substances. *Clinical hypothesis testing* involves generating a number of hypotheses about the identified problem that cut across biological, psychological, and social domains, and then examining each in turn. This approach is desirable when it is relatively certain prior to the assessment that the adolescent is experiencing substance-related difficulties.

As noted earlier in this chapter, there is a general lack of research concerning the assessment of adolescent substance abuse. It is important to recognize, however, that a valid and clinically relevant assessment is essential for effective intervention with adolescent substance abusers (Tarter, 1990). Until recently, clinicians have relied mostly on clinical judgment or locally developed procedures to diagnose adolescent substance use problems (Owen & Nyberg, 1983). However, this is gradually changing as standardized and clinically valid instruments are introduced into the literature.

The standardization of assessment practices has become a high priority in the adolescent chemical dependency field, primarily because standardized assessment offers several advantages over more traditional approaches to evaluation (Henly & Winters, 1989). For example, standardized tests provide a benchmark against which clinical decisions can be compared and validated. Furthermore, standardized assessment procedures are not as prone to rater bias and inconsistencies as are more traditional assessment methods. In addition, standardized assessment provides a common language from which improved communication in the field can develop.

Assuming that the reader is convinced of the advantages of standardized assessment procedures, the remainder of this section will provide examples of standardized instruments for screening for adolescent substance abuse and for more comprehensive evaluation of substance abusing teens. Several good screening inventories for sequential evaluation of substance abuse have been developed for use with adolescents. For example, the Personal Experience Screening Questionnaire (PESQ; Winters, 1991) is a 40-item self-report inventory designed to identify adolescents in need of a drug abuse assessment referral. It includes a problem severity scale, two response distortion scales, and a supplemental information section providing data about the respondent's psychosocial status and drug use history. Published psychometric data support the reliability and validity of the PESQ in both nonclinical and clinical populations.

When a more comprehensive assessment is required and a self-report format is preferred, the use of a longer multidimensional substance abuse measure is warranted. For example, the Drug Use Screening Inventory (DUSI; Tarter, 1990) is a self-report measure that profiles substance use involvement in conjunction with the severity of disturbance in nine spheres of everyday functioning (e.g., school adjustment, social skills, family functioning). Unique to the DUSI is an explicit attempt to link assessment findings to treatment; the DUSI produces a needs assessment and diagnostic summary intended to lead directly to the development of a treatment plan. Published psychometric data support the validity and reliability of the instrument. Additional standardization data are currently being collected.

The semi-structured interview is the "gold standard" of psychological assessment methods, and several interview formats have been developed for use with substance abusing adolescents. For example, the Teen Addiction Severity Index (T-ASI; Kaminer, Bukstein, & Tarter, 1991; Kaminer, Wagner, Plummer, & Seifer, 1993) is an adaptation of the Addiction Severity Index (ASI; McLellan, Luborsky, Woody, & O'Brien, 1980), an interview concerning substance use widely used with adults. The T-ASI evaluates seven domains including substance use, school, employment, family, peer/social, legal, and psychiatric disturbance. Initial validity and reliability data support the use of the measure with clinical populations.

The assessment clinician may also choose to cast a wider diagnostic net and use one of the many semi-structured psychiatric diagnostic interviews that have been developed for use with children and adolescents. While not solely intended for the evaluation of substance abuse, many of these interviews include portions that can aid in the diagnosis of substance-related disorders. Furthermore, many have complementary versions that can be administered to parents or other collaterals. One of the more prominent of these instruments is the Diagnostic Interview Schedule for Children (DISC; Costello, Edelbrock, Dulcan, Kalas, & Klaric, 1984, 1987). This structured diagnostic interview for adolescents and children demonstrates high reliability and validity and is appropriate, pending training in its administration, for use by interviewers with little previous experience with such measures (e.g., Costello, Edelbrock, & Costello, 1985; Weinstein, Noam, Grimes, Stone, & Schwab-Stone, 1990).

Feedback

The manner in which feedback about the results of a substance assessment is provided to adolescents and their family members is a critical determinant of their compliance with treatment recommendations. Miller and Rollnick (1991) have described a particularly useful approach to giving substance abuse assessment feedback based on the principles of Motivational Interviewing. The core assumption of their approach is that personalized feedback can be persuasive input for convincing patients that they are not where they ought to be. As applied to adolescents and their families, Miller and Rollnick's strategy has the following characteristics: avoid trying to prove things to adolescents and their families; describe each result, along with information necessary to understand what it means; avoid a scare tactic tone; solicit and reflect adolescents' and their families' own reactions to the assessment information; remain open to feedback from adolescents and their families; be prepared to deal with strong emotional reactions; and conclude with a summary of what has transpired that includes (a) the risks and problems that have emerged from assessment findings, (b) adolescents' and their families' own reactions to the feedback, with an emphasis on statements reflecting a willingness and interest to make positive changes, and (c) an invitation for the patients and families to add to or correct the summary.

TREATMENT STRATEGIES

Psychological and Behavioral Treatments

In the past two decades, multiple psychosocial intervention approaches have been developed for the treatment of adolescent substance abuse. Unfortunately, little is currently known about which of these many approaches is most effective for which individuals. Indeed, certain approaches to treating substance abuse may be effective with some adolescents but not others due to individual differences among teens in the factors that led up to and accompany their substance use problems. However, given the current state of the literature, the strongest conclusions that can be drawn about the effectiveness of different adolescent substance abuse interventions is that some treatment is better than none and that no particular treatment method is superior to any other (Catalano, Hawkins, Wells, Miller, & Brewer, 1990–91).

As there is little research concerning the effectiveness of adolescent substance abuse treatment, Wagner and Kassel (1995) have suggested five rules that should be followed when developing a substance abuse treatment program for teens. First, treatment approaches should embrace empirically validated interventions, even if these interventions need to be adapted from the adult substance abuse literature. Second, treatment needs to take into account the unique developmental issues and problems inherent in adolescence (e.g., ascendancy of the peer group, identity formation issues, propensity toward limit-testing), rather than directly apply unmodified versions of intervention approaches developed for adult substance abusers. Third, active efforts should be made to identify the key curative factors, or mechanisms of change, that underlie positive behavioral change in order to improve our approaches to treating adolescent substance abuse. Fourth, it is important to remember that "the modal adolescent patient in chemical dependency treatment has multiple problems" (Hoffmann, Sonis, & Halikas, 1987, p. 453). Thus, multiple domains of a substance abusing adolescent's life (e.g., comorbid psychopathology, family functioning) should be assessed, and when necessary treated. Finally, interventions should be tailored to meet the individual needs of teen substance abusers. For example, an emphasis on family therapy is likely to be the most effective treatment plan for adolescents whose substance abuse appears to be related to family problems. In contrast, an emphasis on social skills training is likely to be more effective for substance abusing adolescents who have poor peer interaction and drug refusal skills.

Specific Strategies

Despite limitations in the current knowledge base, several psychosocial approaches hold potential for effectively treating adolescent substance abusers. One promising treatment approach consists of teaching substance abusing adolescents to use more adaptive coping skills (e.g., Wagner, Myers, & Brown, 1994). This approach developed from research showing that some adolescents engage in drug use as a way of coping with stress (Wagner, 1993; Wills, 1985). Strategies utilized in coping skills approaches include relaxation training, biofeedback, deep breathing exercises, autogenic training, aerobic exercise, meditation, deep muscle relaxation, coping skill rehearsal, and desensitization. Several controlled trials support the efficacy of these interventions with substance abusing adults (e.g., Lanyon, Primo, Terrell, & Wener, 1972; Murphy, Pagano, & Marlatt, 1986; Rohsenow, Smith, & Johnson, 1985). However, controlled evaluations of the effectiveness of these methods for treating substance abuse among adolescents have yet to be published.

Coping in the face of temptations (craving) to use alcohol and/or other drugs has also been shown to be an important determinant of substance use outcomes among substance abusing adolescents (Brown, Stetson, & Beatty, 1989). It has been demonstrated, for example, that temptation-coping is a highly significant predictor of teen substance use even after taking into account the influence of stress-coping (Wagner & Myers, 1994). Given such research findings, treatment programs, in order to be maximally effective, should include a component that communicates to the adolescent substance abuser the importance of developing and using temptation-coping strategies when confronted with the urge to drink or use drugs.

Social skills training has been used widely for treating a broad range of clinical populations with social skills deficits, including substance dependent individuals (e.g., Chaney, O'Leary, & Marlatt, 1978; Oei & Jackson, 1982; Sanchez-Craig & Walker, 1982). This approach emphasizes the development and rehearsal of more effective interpersonal communication skills, as well as how to cope with negative intrapersonal situations. Social skills training may be particularly important when treating substance abusing adolescents, as chronic drug use during the teenage years appears to interfere with the normal development of social skills (Pentz, 1985; Van Hasselt, Null, Kempton, & Bukstein, 1993). Furthermore, studies of prevention programs have found that social skills training appears to produce decreases in adolescent alcohol and other drug use (Pentz, 1985). However, the effectiveness of social skills training in treating adolescent substance abuse has yet to be examined in a controlled study.

Motivational Interviewing (Miller & Rollnick, 1991) is an approach to treating substance abuse that aims to bolster patients' motivation to modify their own destructive behavior. Strategies employed by Motivational Interviewing include giving advice, removing barriers to change, instilling a sense of choice, decreasing the attractiveness of substance using behavior, establishing external contingencies designed to persuade the patient to seek help, providing personal feedback, setting up goals for change, and expressing optimism and empathy about the patient's situation. This approach can be particularly useful with teens because it appeals to adolescents' desire for personal autonomy (Tober, 1991). However, no controlled outcome trials of motivational interviewing for treating adolescent substance abuse have been conducted to date.

Behavioral self-control training is a treatment strategy developed especially for problem drinkers. This approach utilizes various behavioral techniques (e.g., self-monitoring, self-reward for success, functional analysis of drinking situations) aimed at instilling a sense of personal control over drinking behavior, and it can accommodate both abstinence or moderation drinking outcomes. Moderation drinking outcomes, while controversial, may be particularly appropriate for some substance abusing adolescents because (a) many adolescents in abstinence-oriented treatments subsequently return to drinking anyway (Catalano et al., 1990–91) and (b) many substance abusing adolescents "mature out" of their problematic use patterns without any formal treatment (Blum, 1987; see Peele, 1987). A growing research literature supports the efficacy of behavioral self-control training with adult problem drinkers (e.g., Harris & Miller, 1990; Sanchez-Craig, Annis, Bornet, & MacDonald, 1984). However, the effectiveness of behavioral self-control training has not yet been examined in an adolescent sample.

Family characteristics have repeatedly been found to be highly related to adolescent substance abuse (see Bry, 1988; Bry & Krinsley, 1990). As a result, most teen substance abuse treatment programs include a family therapy component. Furthermore, several recent studies offer support for the effectiveness of family therapy in the treatment of adolescent substance abusers (e.g., Szapocznik, Kurtines, Foote, Perez-Vidal, & Hervis, 1986; Szapocznik et al., 1988). However, additional research needs to be performed to identify (a) the "active ingredients" of family therapy, and (b) those adolescents for whom family therapy will be maximally effective.

Pharmacological Treatments

In contrast to the burgeoning literature and increasing acceptance of pharmacotherapy for adults with DSM-IV substance-related disorders, there has been no systematic research evaluating the efficacy and safety of psychotropic medications in the treatment of adolescents with substance-related disorders. Pharmacotherapy in this population may be viewed as a new subset of pediatric psychopharmacology and has met with similar difficulties in developing and achieving recognition (Biederman, 1992). Differences between the specific pharmacotherapy of adolescents with substance-related disorders (with or without psychiatric comorbidity) and general pediatric psychopharmacology stem mostly from the fact that the pharmacotherapeutic approach used in substance-related disorders is embedded in a treatment model developed for adults and derived from the disease model of addiction. Such a model has dominated the addiction field for almost sixty years but is inadequate for conceptualizing adolescent substance use problems because it lacks a developmental perspective and fails to take into consideration heterogeneity among adolescents who abuse substances (Kaminer, 1994a).

There are four drug-specific pharmacological strategies that are commonly utilized for the treatment of substance-related disorders (Kaminer, 1992): (1) make psychoactive substance administration aversive (e.g., disulfiram for alcohol dependence); (2) provide a less destructive chemical substitute for the abused substance (e.g., methadone for heroin dependence); (3) block the reinforcing effects of the psychoactive substance (e.g., naltrexone for opioid abuse); and, (4) relieve craving/withdrawal symptoms during detoxification attempts (e.g., desipramine for cocaine dependence). The success of each of these approaches depends on two conditions: identifying the appropriate pharmacotherapeutic agent and promoting a feeling of well-being that will encourage the patient to comply with the assigned treatment.

Cigarette Smoking (Nicotine)

Current practice in the pharmacotherapy of nicotine dependence involves a variation on the substitution strategy: provide a less destructive mode of administration of the abused substance and then gradually wean the patient off the substance. Nicotine gum and the nicotine transdermal patch are the modes of nicotine administration most often used in this approach. Research has found that the addition of these agents to traditional smoking cessation interventions can double their success, increasing rates of long-term abstinence from about 15 percent to about 30 percent (West, 1992). Even higher success rates have been found in studies where these pharmacological interventions have been paired with cognitive-behavioral interventions.

The effectiveness of nicotine substitution strategies with adolescents is virtually unknown. An unspecified number of 15 to 18 year olds were included in a study of 612 smokers prescribed nicotine gum, but no special mention was made regarding differential treatment outcome for these younger subjects (Johnson, Stevens, Hollis, & Woodson, 1992). Thus, at present it can be cautiously concluded that there are no specific contraindications for the use of the nicotine gum or patch with nicotine-dependent adolescents. However, the effectiveness of such procedures with adolescents specifically remains unexamined.

Alcohol

The most common unidimensional pharmacotherapy to prevent alcohol consumption is aversive therapy using disulfiram. This antidipsotropic agent produces a sensitivity to alcohol that results in a highly unpleasant reaction (i.e., flushing, throbbing in the head and neck, respiratory difficulty, nausea, hypotension, hyperventilation, tachycardia) when even small amounts of alcohol are ingested. From a behavioral perspective, disulfiram decreases the likelihood of alcohol consumption because drinking behavior is punished by the onset of aversive symptoms.

Support for the effectiveness of disulfiram in the treatment of alcohol dependence in adults has been limited (Alterman, O'Brien, & McLellan, 1991). A recent study of the effectiveness of disulfiram in the treatment of alcohol problems in two adolescent males failed to show positive outcomes (Myers, Donahue, & Goldstein, 1994). Moreover, aversive therapy for the treatment of any behavioral problem demonstrated by children and adolescents has always been controversial, and given little research to support its clinical utility it appears unlikely that disulfiram pharmacotherapy will become a treatment of choice for adolescents with alcohol use problems (American College of Physicians, 1989).

Recently, reinforcement blocking strategies have received increasing interest as a pharmacotherapy for alcohol-related disorders. For example, research by O'Malley and associates (1992) has supported the potential utility of an opioid antagonist such as naltrexone to block the reinforcing properties of alcohol. Such a pharmacotherapeutic strategy holds potential for treating substance-related disorders in adolescents. Also, the serotonergic system appears to play a role in the pathophysiology of alcohol dependence. Research by Naranjo, Kadlec, Sanhueza, Woodley-Remus, and Sellers (1990) has found that fluoxetine, a pharmacological agent that increases the availability of serotonin, significantly reduces alcohol consumption. To the extent that substance abusing adolescents with aggressive behavior and depressive symptomatology share considerable similarity with Type 2 (Cloninger, 1987) or Type B alcoholism (Babor et al., 1992), a reasonable hypothesis is that such adolescents may benefit from pharmacotherapy with serotonin reuptake inhibitors because serotonin is the neuromodulator affecting behavioral inhibition (Cloninger, 1987).

Cocaine

Based on the theory that chronic stimulant use results in a depletion of dopamine and a reduction in dopaminergic activity, it has been hypothesized that craving for cocaine will be reduced by increasing dopaminergic stimulation. To date, there has been little evidence to support this theory. However, the following direct and indirect dopaminergic agents have shown some efficacy for treating cocaine dependence in open trials in adults:

L-dopa, carbidopa, bromocriptine, amantadine, methylphenidate, and mazindol (Meyer, 1992).

A second theory that has received greater empirical support suggests that craving is mediated by supersensitivity of presynaptic inhibiting dopaminergic autoreceptors. Based on this theory, Kaminer (1992) prescribed desipramine to an adolescent cocaine abuser and found that it facilitated long-term cocaine abstinence (Kaminer, 1992). Similar results have been obtained with two additional cocaine dependent adolescents (Kaminer, 1994b).

It is noteworthy that cocaine addicts show more conditioned responses than other drug addicts to cues associated with ingesting their substance of choice. This suggests that a combination of pharmacologic intervention and cognitive-behavioral therapy (e.g., cue exposure) may currently be the optimal treatment strategy for cocaine abuse. Such an approach has potential utility for the treatment of cocaine abuse in adolescents but has not been systematically evaluated in a teenage sample.

Opioids

Methadone maintenance is a common form of opioid substitution therapy. The desired response from methadone maintenance is threefold: (1) to prevent the onset of opioid abstinence syndrome; (2) to eliminate drug hunger or craving; and (3) to block the euphoric effects of any illicitly self-administered opioids. As a general rule, only patients who have been dependent on opioids for at least one year and who have previously failed at attempts at withdrawal are appropriate candidates for methadone maintenance (Jaffe, 1986).

Methadone maintenance, and *not* opioid detoxification, is the treatment of choice for pregnant adolescents who abuse heroin. This pharmacotherapeutic strategy eliminates the danger of contracting AIDS from a contaminated needle and assures a relatively stable plasma level of methadone that reduces the fetus's risk of developing intrauterine distress (Finnegan & Kandall, 1992).

No person under 18 years of age may be admitted to a methadone maintenance treatment program unless an authorized adult signs an official consent form (FDA-2635 consent for methadone maintenance treatment). Patients under the age of 18 are required to have two documented attempts at short-term detoxification or drug-free treatment to be eligible for methadone maintenance. In addition, a one-week waiting period is required after a detoxification attempt before a patient can enter into methadone maintenance. Furthermore, the program physician has to document in the minor's record that the patient continues to be or is again physiologically dependent on narcotic drugs before methadone maintenance treatment can begin (State Methadone Maintenance Treatment Guidelines, 1992).

Dual Diagnosis

Psychiatric comorbidity in the form of dual and triple diagnosis has been found to be common among substance abusing adolescents (Bukstein, Brent, & Kaminer, 1989; Kaminer, 1991). Among teens with substance-related disorders, the most common comorbid psychiatric diagnoses are mood disorders and/or conduct disorder. Other diagnoses frequently reported include anxiety disorders, eating disorders, attention deficit hyperactivity disorder, and schizophrenia. Substance abusing adolescents also sometimes present with personality disorders, especially cluster B of DSM-IV, which includes antisocial, borderline, histrionic, and narcissistic personality disorders (Kaminer, 1994a).

The sequelae of psychoactive substance intoxication and/or withdrawal are often difficult to distinguish from the signs and symptoms of concurrent psychiatric disorders. It is important to emphasize that dual diagnosis is a term limited to the relationship between disorders only and not for symptoms associated with substance-related disorders. These symptoms may serve as indications of the severity of substance-related disorders.

From a treatment perspective, the process of diagnosing comorbid psychiatric disorders and the reliability and stability of such diagnoses are of great significance. A misdiagnosis of comorbidity can result in the precocious introduction of medications that may lead to serious errors and misattributions (e.g., the medication worked) in treatment. This is especially important in the case of depression because 25 percent of all children and adolescents diagnosed as depressed have a spontaneous syndromatic recovery within two weeks (Ambrosini, Bianchi, Rabinovich, & Elia, 1993). Among substance abusing adolescents, one study found that 65 percent of teens diagnosed as depressed at admission will demonstrate a spontaneous syndromatic recovery within three weeks (DeMilio, 1989). Thus, a washout period (from substances of abuse) of at least two weeks and sometimes longer is recommended before initiating pharmacotherapy for comorbid psychiatric conditions.

Specific pharmacotherapies for comorbid psychiatric disorders are beyond the scope of this chapter. In general, the indications for pharmacotherapeutic treatments for comorbid psychiatric conditions in substance abusing teens are quite similar to those in adolescents who are not substance abusing. Though large controlled outcome studies of the effectiveness of pharmacotherapies

for dual-diagnosed substance abusing teens are pending, pilot studies of interventions among dual-diagnosed adult patients have been positive (Kofoed, Kania, Walsh, & Atkwson, 1986).

CASE ILLUSTRATION

Clinical Presentation

David was a 16-year-old Caucasian male with a 9-year history of polysubstance abuse, mainly alcohol, marijuana, and cocaine. He was admitted for treatment in an in-patient program for adolescent substance abusers with comorbid psychiatric disorders. Presenting symptoms included (1) suicidal plan to overdose on cocaine, (2) severe dysphoria that failed to respond to increasing doses of cocaine, and (3) cocaine dependence and alcohol and marijuana abuse.

David's substance abuse history began at age 7 when he was introduced to alcohol and marijuana by his two adopted teenage brothers. By age 14, he had begun to use cocaine intranasally and experimented with heroin intravenously. After six months of cocaine abuse, he was referred to a residential treatment program for adolescent substance abusers where he spent six months. Following residential treatment, he remained substance free for almost a year; however, a parental job opportunity caused him to move with his family to another state, and he soon relapsed to his previous "drug habits." David was once again using alcohol, marijuana, and cocaine in an abusive manner, and he quickly developed cocaine dependence. During the last six months prior to his admission, he used cocaine daily, consuming approximately two grams of cocaine intranasally every week.

Assessment Findings

Upon admission, physical examination was unremarkable. On mental status examination, David appeared to be sad, withdrawn, and tired. Self-esteem was low. He disclosed that he been using cocaine to fight depression during the last few months but that cocaine was becoming less and less effective for mood management (i.e., he demonstrated tolerance). Furthermore, he noted that he had developed early and midnight insomnia. These changes were quite distressing to him, and he admitted to contemplating suicide by overdose. The patient also expressed a wish to get help for his depression and cocaine dependence, and he agreed to contract for safety (i.e., make an antisuicide agreement). Toxicological analysis of urine samples collected upon admission were positive for cocaine and marijuana.

After admission, two child psychiatrists diagnosed the following DSM-III-R Axis I diagnoses: major depressive disorder, cocaine dependence, alcohol and marijuana abuse, and attention deficit hyperactivity disorder. David was also interviewed using the Teen Addiction Severity Index (T-ASI; Kaminer, Bukstein, & Tarter, 1991; Kaminer, Wagner, Plummer, & Seifer, 1993), and the substance-related diagnoses were confirmed. Other noteworthy findings from the T-ASI concerned David's legal, occupational, social, and academic functioning. David had no legal problems, and he supported his cocaine dependence by working a job and by associating with a drug dealer who enabled him to buy cocaine below the market prices. Social functioning and academic performance had gradually deteriorated during the last year prior to his admission.

About a year before his hospitalization and shortly after the family moved, David was diagnosed as having attention deficit hyperactivity disorder. He was treated with dexedrine 20 mg/day. His physician was unaware of his alcohol and marijuana abuse and cocaine dependence, which developed approximately three months after he was started on dexedrine. Family history for medical and psychiatric disorders was unremarkable. However, the two adopted brothers were active substance abusers and had ongoing legal problems related to substance use and distribution. David's birth, developmental, and medical histories were unremarkable.

Treatment Selection and Course

David was started on a regimen of the antidepressant desipramine 50 mg/day, increased by 25 mg every second day. This pharmacotherapeutic intervention was intended both to relieve craving/withdrawal symptoms as David underwent detoxification from cocaine and to address David's depressive symptoms. Orthostatic vital signs were monitored twice per day, while an electrocardiogram was performed at baseline and with each increase of dosage. Blood levels for desipramine and desipramine metabolites were monitored with the aim of reaching a plasma level of at least > 125 ng/ml. During the second through the fourth days of hospitalization, immunological and viral screens (hepatitis and HIV test included) and routine blood and urine examinations were also completed. All were within normal limits. After the second day of hospitalization, David was gradually tapered off dexedrine.

After 24 hours had passed since David consumed his last dose of cocaine, he was instructed to begin to keep a subjective cocaine craving log. He was also administered the Minnesota Cocaine Craving Scale (MCCS; Halikas, Kuhn, Crosby, Carlson, & Crea, 1991) the day following admission. The MCCS is a standardized self-report measure that assesses craving related to acute abstinence from cocaine, with special emphasis on the intensity, frequency, and duration of craving episodes. The MCCS was administered to David on a weekly basis to monitor treatment effects. On the first day of hospitalization, David's subjective craving log contained descriptions of heat flashes, hand tremors, headache, itching of the hands and elbows, tension, and continued difficulty falling asleep. He reported hearing a "buzz" and seeing "stars." On both craving measures, urges for cocaine were very high.

David was also administered two standardized self-report measures of depressive symptoms, the Beck Depression Inventory (BDI; Beck, 1978) and the Hopelessness Scale (Beck, Weissman, Lester, & Trexler, 1974). Scores on both measures were elevated and suggested moderate levels of depressive symptomatology. Along with the MCCS, these instruments were administered on a weekly basis to monitor treatment effects.

David participated in the full curriculum of a progressive, four-level, goal-oriented treatment program for adolescent substance abuse. The six domains addressed in this program correspond to those assessed by the T-ASI: (1) psychoactive substance use, (2) psychiatric status, (3) family functioning, (4) peer-social relationships, (5) school or employment performance, and (6) legal status. The treatment program consisted of the following nine components: (1) individual treatment contracting (according to the above-noted T-ASI domains), (2) individual psychotherapy, (3) family therapy, (4) social skills training and training in relapse prevention techniques, (5) substance abuse education, (6) self-help groups, (7) school work, (8) random urine analyses for psychoactive substances, and (9) medication.

After the first week, desipramine dosage was 100 mg/day with a plasma level of 79 ng/ml. After the second week, the patient was on the highest dosage he could tolerate without developing moderate orthostatic hypotension, 200 mg, plasma level 97 ng/ml. After three weeks, the patient was stabilized at around 130 ng/ml.

During the six weeks that David was hospitalized, he was compliant with treatment, lacked any expression of suicidal ideation, did not demonstrate any behavior consistent with a diagnosis of attention deficit hyperactivity disorder, and experienced diminished craving for cocaine as measured by the MCCS. BDI and Hopelessness

Scale scores also decreased to subclinical levels after two and three weeks, respectively.

Termination and Follow-Up

Discharge diagnoses were identical to the admission diagnoses except for attention deficit hyperactivity disorder, which was not confirmed during hospitalization. The physician who had initially diagnosed attention deficit hyperactivity disorder and prescribed dexedrine failed to recognize David's resumption of polysubstance abuse and cocaine dependence. This added additional liability potential to David's health due to synergistic/cumulative effects of the two stimulants (i.e., dexedrine and cocaine) upon release and reuptake inhibition of catecholamines. It is noteworthy that David did not abuse dexedrine, using it only as prescribed. This supports the rule of thumb that the use of stimulants in a therapeutic context rarely results in abuse. However, David's case illustrates the complexities of pharmacotherapy with adolescent substance abusers with comorbid psychiatric diagnoses.

After six months of weekly follow-up, which included psychotherapy, urine analysis, and ongoing pharmacotherapy, David remained drug free. Mild cocaine cravings were occasionally reported, and mood was mostly euthymic with restricted-appropriate affect except for a period of two weeks when he was depressed and suicidal. David did not report cocaine cravings during this dysthymic period.

SUMMARY

Most adolescents will try alcohol and other drugs by the time they graduate from high school. Some of those teens who try substances will go on to use alcohol and/or other drugs in a manner that places them at high risk for experiencing serious negative consequences. Despite widespread societal concern about adolescents who experience substance use problems, very little is currently known about how best to assess and treat substance abuse among teens. As a result, most adolescent substance abuse treatment programs base their services on their own specific philosophical orientation, using procedures extrapolated from adult substance abuse treatment models. The problem with having philosophical differences across adolescent substance abuse treatment programs is that it results in wide variation among treatment settings in diagnosis, treatment process, and treatment outcome. The problem with using procedures extrapolated from adult treatment is that adolescents and adults with sub-

stance use problems differ in many fundamental ways, including substance use patterns, symptoms associated with substance abuse, and developmental status.

Recent epidemiological studies of alcohol and other drug use by adolescents indicate a rise in marijuana, cigarette, stimulant, LSD, and inhalant use. These findings are in contrast to the general downward trend in the prevalence of adolescent substance use during the period between 1985 and 1991. This change in use patterns was accompanied by a decrease in the perceived dangers associated with substance use and a decrease in personal disapproval of substance use. Overall, tobacco and alcohol are the substances most widely used by adolescents, and marijuana is the illicit substance most widely used by adolescents. Concerning substance abuse, a conservative estimate of the number of adolescents who will demonstrate a new or relapsed case of substance abuse during the course of a single year is 4 percent.

Adolescents with substance use problems should be medically examined in the same systematic manner that is routinely employed in pediatrics and adolescent medicine. Somewhat different procedures should be used when conducting an emergency medical evaluation versus an elective medical evaluation. Psychological/psychiatric evaluations of substance abusing adolescents should be conducted in the same rigorous and systematic manner that is routinely employed in child and adolescent clinical psychology and psychiatry. At a minimum, the process of evaluation should include a description of the purposes behind the assessment, an interview with adolescents and their family members, the administration of standardized measures, and a feedback session concerning the results of the evaluation.

Currently, little is known about which of the many existing psychosocial approaches to the treatment of teen substance abuse is most effective. A review of the literature reveals some promising strategies, including stress-coping skills training, temptation-coping skills training, social skills training, motivational interviewing, behavioral self-control training, and family therapy. Similarly, little is known about the efficacy and safety of pharmacotherapeutic approaches to the treatment of adolescents with substance-related disorders. Substitution strategies, reinforcement blocking strategies, and withdrawal reduction strategies all have potential for treating adolescent substance abuse but none have been systematically examined in teenagers.

Dual diagnosis is common in adolescents who are substance abusers, and mood disorders and/or conduct disorder are especially prevalent comorbid conditions in substance abusing teens. Such adolescents can be difficult to treat because of the complexities of pharmacotherapy of multiple co-occurring psychiatric conditions. However, careful attention to the individual characteristics of dual-diagnosed teens will maximize the chances of positive treatment outcomes for such individuals. The case example presented in this chapter illustrates such a process.

To summarize, the current state of adolescent substance abuse assessment and treatment is far from ideal. However, progress is being made as empirically validated assessment and intervention approaches are gradually being introduced into clinical practice. Currently, it is incumbent on any professional attempting to treat substance abuse among teens to remain current with the literature and to apply the most rigorous scientific standards in evaluating clinical approaches. Only then can we make meaningful advances in addressing the formidable problem of substance abuse among adolescents.

REFERENCES

Alterman, A. I., O'Brien, C. P., & McLellan, A. T. (1991). Differential therapeutics for substance abuse. In R. J. Frances & S. I. Miller (Eds.), *Clinical textbook of addictive disorders* (pp. 369–390). New York: Guilford Press.

Ambrosini, P. J., Bianchi, M. D., Rabinovich, H., & Elia, J. (1993). Antidepressant treatments in children and adolescents: I. Affective disorders. *Journal of the American Academy of Child and Adolescent Psychiatry, 32*, 1–6.

American College of Physicians. (1989). Disulfiram treatment of alcoholism. *Annals of Internal Medicine, 111*, 943–945.

American Psychiatric Association. (1994). *Diagnostic and statistical manual of mental disorders*, 4th edition. Washington, DC: American Psychiatric Association.

Babor, T. F., Hofmann, M., DelBoca, F. K., Hesselbrock, V., Meyer, R. E., Dolinsky, Z. S., & Rounsaville, B. (1992). Types of alcoholics: II. Evidence for an empirically-derived typology based on indicators of vulnerability and severity. *Archives of General Psychiatry, 49*, 599–608.

Beck, A. T. (1978). *Depression inventory*. Philadelphia: Center for Cognitive Therapy.

Beck, A. T., Weissman, A., Lester, D., & Trexler, L. (1974). The measurement of pessimism: The Hopelessness Scale. *Journal of Consulting and Clinical Psychology, 42*, 861–865.

Biederman, J. (1992). New developments in pediatric psychopharmacology. *Journal of the American Academy of Child and Adolescent Psychiatry, 31*, 14–15.

Blum, R. W. (1987). Adolescent substance abuse: Diagnostic and treatment issues. *Pediatric Clinics of North America, 34*, 523–537.

Brown, S. A. (1993). Recovery patterns in adolescent substance abuse. In J. S. Baer, G. A. Marlatt & R. J. McMahon (Eds.), *Addictive behaviors across the life span: Prevention, treatment, and policy issues*. Newbury Park, CA: Sage.

Brown, S. A., Stetson, B. A., & Beatty, P. (1989). Cognitive and behavioral features of adolescent coping in high risk drinking situations. *Addictive Behaviors, 14*, 291–300.

Bry, B. H. (1988). Family-based approaches to reducing adolescent substance use: Theories, techniques, and findings. In E. R. Rahdert & J. Grabowski (Eds.), *Adolescent drug abuse: Analyses of treatment research*. National Institute on Drug Abuse Research Monograph 77 (pp. 39–68). Washington, DC: U.S. Government Printing Office.

Bry, B. H., & Krinsley, K. A. (1990). Adolescent substance abuse. In E. L. Feindler & G. R. Kalfus (Eds.), *Adolescent behavior therapy handbook* (pp. 275–302). New York: Springer.

Bukstein, O. G., Brent, D. A., & Kaminer, Y. (1989). Comorbidity of substance abuse and other psychiatric disorders in adolescents. *American Journal of Psychiatry, 146*, 1131–1141.

Catalano, R. F., Hawkins, J. D., Wells, E. A., Miller, J., & Brewer, D. (1990–91). Evaluation of the effectiveness of adolescent drug abuse treatment, assessment of risks for relapse, and promising approaches for relapse prevention. *The International Journal of the Addictions, 25*, 1085–1140.

Center for Substance Abuse Treatment. (1993). *Guidelines for the treatment of alcohol- and other drug-abusing adolescents*. (Department of Health and Human Services Publication No. SAM 93-2010). Washington, DC: U.S. Government Printing Office.

Chaney, E. F., O'Leary, M. R., & Marlatt, G. A. (1978). Skill training with alcoholics. *Journal of Consulting and Clinical Psychology, 46*, 1092–1104.

Cloninger, C. R. (1987). Neurogenetic adaptive mechanisms in alcoholism. *Science, 236*, 410–416.

Cook, C. C. H. (1988a). The Minnesota model in the management of drug and alcohol dependency: Miracle, method, or myth? Part 1. The philosophy and the programme. *British Journal of Addiction, 83*, 625–634.

Cook, C. C. H. (1988b). The Minnesota model in the management of drug and alcohol dependency: Miracle, method or myth? Part II. Evidence and conclusions. *British Journal of Addiction, 83*, 735–748.

Costello, A. J., Edelbrock, C., Dulcan, M. K., Kalas, R., & Klaric, S. (1984). Development and testing of the NIMH Diagnostic Interview Schedule for Children on a clinical population: Final report. (Contract #RFP-DB-81-0027). Rockville, MD: Center for Epidemiologic Studies, National Institute for Mental Health.

Costello, A. J., Edelbrock, C., Dulcan, M. K., Kalas, R., & Klaric, S. (1987). Diagnostic Interview Schedule for Children (DISC). Pittsburgh, PA: Western Psychiatric Institute and Clinic, School of Medicine, University of Pittsburgh.

Costello, A. J., Edelbrock, C., Dulcan, M. K., Kalas, R., & Klaric, S. (1987). Validity of the NIMH Diagnostic Interview for Children: A comparison between psychiatric and pediatric referrals. *Journal of Abnormal Child Psychology and Psychiatry, 13*, 579–595.

DeMilio, L. (1989). Psychiatric syndromes in adolescent substance abusers. *American Journal of Psychiatry, 146*, 1212–1214.

Donovan, D. M. (1988). Assessment of addictive behaviors: Implications of an emerging biopsychosocial model. In D. M. Donovan & G. A. Marlatt (Eds.), *Assessment of addictive behaviors*. New York: Guilford Press.

Donovan, D. M., & Marlatt, G. A. (1988). *Assessment of addictive behaviors*. New York: Guilford Press.

Farrell, M., & Strang, J. (1991). Substance use and misuse in childhood and adolescence. *Journal of Child Psychology, Psychiatry, and Allied Disciplines, 32*, 109–128.

Felter, R., Izsak, E., & Lawrence, H. S. (1987). Emergency department management of the intoxicated adolescent. *Pediatric Clinics of North America, 34*, 399–421.

Finnegan, L. P., & Kandall, S. R. (1992). Maternal and neonatal effects of alcohol and drugs. In J. H. Lowinson, P. Ruiz, R. B. Millman, & J. G. Langrod (Eds.), *Substance Abuse Comprehensive Textbook*. (pp. 628–656). Baltimore: Williams & Wilkins.

Graham, J. W., Collins, L. M., Wugalter, S. E., Chung, N. K., & Hansen, W. B. (1991). Modeling transitions in latent stage-sequential processes: A substance use prevention example. *Journal of Consulting and Clinical Psychology, 59*, 48–57.

Greenbaum, P. E., Prange, M. E., Friedman, R. M., & Silver, S. E. (1991). Substance abuse prevalence and comorbidity with other psychiatric disorders among adolescents with severe emotional disorders. *Journal of the Academy of Child and Adolescent Psychiatry, 30*, 575–583.

Halikas, J. A., Kuhn, K. L., Crosby, R., Carlson, G., & Crea, F. (1991). The measurement of craving in cocaine patients using the Minnesota Cocaine Craving Scale. *Comprehensive Psychiatry, 32*, 22–27.

Harrell, A. V., & Wirtz, P. W. (1989). Screening for adolescent problem drinking: Validation of a multidimensional instrument for case identification. *Psychological Assessment: A Journal of Consulting and Clinical Psychology, 1*, 61–63.

Harris, K. B., & Miller, W. R. (1990). Behavioral self-control training for problem drinkers: Components of efficacy. *Psychology of Addictive Behaviors, 4*, 82–90.

Henly, G. A., & Winters, K. C. (1989). Development of psychosocial scales for the assessment of adolescents involved with alcohol and drugs. *The International Journal of the Addictions, 24*, 973–1001.

Hoffmann, N. G., Sonis, W. A., & Halikas, J. A. (1987). Issues in the evaluation of chemical dependency treatment programs for adolescents. *Pediatric Clinics of North America, 34*, 449–459.

Jaffe, J. H. (1986). Opioids. In A. I. Frances & R. E. Hales (Eds.), *Annual Review* (pp. 137–159), Vol. 5. Washington, DC: American Psychiatric Press.

Johnson, R. E., Stevens, V. J., Hollis, J. F., & Woodson, G. T. (1992). Nicotine chewing gum use in the outpatient care setting. *Journal of Family Practice, 34*, 61–65.

Johnston, L. D., O'Malley, P. M., & Bachman, J. G. (1994). *Details of annual drug survey*. Ann Arbor: A release by the University of Michigan News and Information Services, January 27.

Kaminer, Y. (1991). Adolescent substance abuse. In R. J. Frances & S. I. Miller (Eds.), *Clinical textbook of addictive disorders*. New York: Guilford.

Kaminer, Y. (1992). Desipramine facilitation of cocaine abstinence in an adolescent. *Journal of the American Academy of Child and Adolescent Psychiatry, 31*, 312–317.

Kaminer, Y. (1994a). Adolescent substance abuse: A comprehensive guide to theory and practice. New York: Plenum Press.

Kaminer, Y. (1994b). Tricyclic antidepressants: Therapeutic use for cocaine craving and potential for abuse. *Journal of the American Academy of Child and Adolescent Psychiatry, 33*, 592.

Kaminer, Y., Bukstein, O. G., & Tarter, R. E. (1991). The Teen Addiction Severity Index (T-ASI): Rationale and reliability. *International Journal of Addictions, 26*, 219–226.

Kaminer, Y., Wagner, E., Plummer, B., & Seifer, R. (1993). Validation of the Teen Addiction Severity Index (T-ASI). *American Journal on Addictions, 2*, 250–254.

Kassel, J. D., & Wagner, E. F. (1993). Processes of change in Alcoholics Anonymous: A review of possible mechanisms. *Psychotherapy, 30*, 222–234.

Kofoed, L., Kania, J., Walsh, T., & Atkwson, R. M. (1986). Outpatient treatment of patients with substance abuse and co-existing psychiatric disorders. *American Journal of Psychiatry, 143*, 867–872.

Lanyon, R. I., Primo, R. V., Terrell, F., & Wener, A. (1972). An aversion-desensitization treatment for alcoholism. *Journal of Consulting and Clinical Psychology, 38*, 394–398.

Laudergan, J. C. (1982). *Easy does it! Alcoholism treatment outcomes, Hazelden and the Minnesota Model.* Center City, MN: Hazelden.

Lewinsohn, P. M., Hops, H., Roberts, R., Seeley, J. R., & Andrews, J. A. (1993). Adolescent psychopathology: I. Prevalence and incidence of depression and other DSM-III-R disorders in high school students. *Journal of Abnormal Psychology, 102*, 133–144.

McLellan, A. T., Luborsky, L., Woody, G. E., & O'Brien, C. P. (1980). An improved diagnostic evaluation instrument for substance abuse patients. *Journal of Nervous and Mental Disease, 40*, 620–625.

Meyer, R. E. (1992). New pharmacotherapies for cocaine dependence revisited. *Archives of General Psychiatry, 49*, 900–904.

Milin, R., Halikas, J. A., Meller, J. E., & Morse, C. (1991). Psychopathology among substance abusing juvenile offenders. *Journal of the American Academy of Child and Adolescent Psychiatry, 30*, 569–574.

Miller, W. R., & Rollnick, S. (1991). *Motivational interviewing: Preparing people to change addictive behavior.* New York: Guilford Press.

Murphy, T. J., Pagano, R. R., & Marlatt, G. A. (1986). Lifestyle modification with heavy alcohol drinkers: Effects of aerobic exercise and meditation. *Addictive Behaviors, 11*, 175–186.

Myers, W. C., Donahue, J. E., & Goldstein, M. R. (1994). Disulfiram for alcohol use disorders in adolescents. *Journal of the American Academy of Child and Adolescent Psychiatry, 33*, 484–489.

Naranjo, C. A., Kadlec, K. E., Sanhueza, P., Woodley-Remus, D., & Sellers, E. M. (1990). Fluoxetine differentially alters alcohol intake and other consummatory behaviors in problem drinkers. *Clinical Pharmacological Therapy, 47*, 490–498.

Newcomb, M., & Bentler, P. (1988). *Consequences of adolescent drug use: Impact on the lives of young adults.* Newbury Park, CA: Sage.

Oei, T. P. S., & Jackson, P. R. (1982). Social skills and cognitive behavioral approaches to the treatment of problem drinking. *Journal of Studies on Alcohol, 43*, 532–547.

O'Malley, S. S., Jaffe, A. J., Chang, G., Schottenfeld, R. S., Meyer, R. E., & Rounsaville, B. (1992). Naltrexone and coping skills therapy for alcohol dependence. *Archives of General Psychiatry, 49*, 881–887.

Orvaschel, H., Puig-Antich, J., Chambers, W., Tabrizi, M. A., & Johnson, R. (1982). Retrospective assessment of prepubertal major depression with the Kiddie-SADS-E. *Journal of the American Academy of Child Psychiatry, 21*, 392–397.

Owen, P., & Nyberg, L. (1983). Assessing alcohol and drug problems among adolescents: Current practice. *Journal of Drug Addiction, 13*, 249–254.

Peele, S. (1987). What can we expect from treatment of adolescent drug and alcohol abuse? *Pediatrician, 14*, 62–69.

Pentz, M. A. (1985). Social competence and self-efficacy as determinants of substance use in adolescence. In S. Shiffman & T. A. Wills (Eds.), *Coping and substance use* (pp. 117–142). New York: Academic Press.

Rohsenow, D. J., Smith, R. E., & Johnson, S. (1985). Stress management training as a prevention program for heavy social drinkers: Cognitive, affect, drinking and individual differences. *Addictive Behaviors, 10*, 45–54.

Sanchez-Craig, M., Annis, H. M., Bornet, A. R., & MacDonald, K. R. (1984). Random assignment to abstinence and controlled drinking: Evaluation of a cognitive-behavioural program for problem drinkers. *Journal of Consulting and Clinical Psychology, 52*, 390–403.

Sanchez-Craig, M., & Walker, K. (1982). Teaching coping skills to chronic alcoholics in a coeducational halfway house: I. Assessment of programme effects. *British Journal of Addiction, 77*, 35–50.

Schuckit, M. A. (1989). *Drug and alcohol abuse: A clinical guide to diagnosis and treatment.* New York: Plenum Press.

Shedler, J., & Block, J. (1990). Adolescent drug use and psychological health. A longitudinal inquiry. *American Psychologist, 45* 612–630.

Skinner, H. (1981). Assessment of alcohol problems. In Y. Israel (Ed.), *Research advances in alcohol and drug problems.* New York: Plenum Press.

State Methadone Maintenance Treatment Guidelines. (1992). A draft compiled by M. W. Parrino. Rockville, MD: U.S. Department of Health and Human Services.

Steinberg, L., & Levine, A. (1990). *You and your adolescent: A parent's guide for ages 10 to 20.* New York: Harper & Row.

Szapocznik, J., Kurtines, W. M., Foote, F. H., Perez-Vidal, A., & Hervis, O. (1986). Conjoint versus one-person family therapy: Further evidence for the effectiveness of conducting family therapy through one person with drug abusing adolescents. *Journal of Consulting and Clinical Psychology, 54*, 395–397.

Szapocznik, J., Perez-Vidal, A., Brickman, A. L., Foote, F. H., Santisteban, D., & Hervis, O. (1988). Engaging adolescent drug abusers and their families in treatment: A strategic structural systems approach. *Journal of Consulting and Clinical Psychology, 56*, 552–557.

Tarter, R. E. (1990). Evaluation and treatment of adolescent substance abuse: A decision tree method. *American Journal of Drug and Alcohol Abuse, 16*, 1–46.

Tarter, R. E., Ott, P. J., & Mezzich, A. C. (1991). Psychometric assessment. In R. J. Frances & S. I. Miller (Eds.), *Clinical textbook of addictive disorders*. New York: Guilford Press.

Tober, G. (1991). Motivational interviewing with young people. In W. R. Miller & S. Rollnick (Eds.), *Motivational interviewing: Preparing people to change addictive behavior* (pp. 248–259). New York: Guilford Press.

Van Hasselt, V. B., Null, J. A., Kempton, T., & Bukstein, O. G. (1993). Social skills and depression in adolescent substance abusers. *Addictive Behaviors, 18*, 9–18.

Wagner, E. F. (1993). Delay of gratification, coping with stress, and substance use in adolescence. *Experimental and Clinical Psychopharmacology, 1*, 27–43.

Wagner, E. F., & Kassel, J. D. (1995). Substance use and abuse. In R. T. Ammerman & M. Hersen (Eds.), *Handbook of child behavior therapy in the psychiatric setting* (pp. 367–388). New York: John Wiley & Sons.

Wagner, E. F., & Myers, M. G. (1994, April). *Stress-coping and temptation-coping as predictors of adolescent substance use*. Paper presented at the Society of Behavioral Medicine Annual Meeting, Boston.

Wagner, E. F., Myers, M. G., & Brown, S. A. (1994). Adolescent substance abuse: Assessment and treatment strategies. In L. VandeCreek (Ed.), *Innovations in clinical practice: A source book*. Sarasota, FL: Professional Resource Press.

Weinstein, S. R., Noam G. G., Grimes, K., Stone, K., & Schwab-Stone, M. (1990). Convergence of DSM-III diagnoses and self-reported symptoms in child and adolescent inpatients. *Journal of the American Academy of Child and Adolescent Psychiatry, 29*, 627–634.

West, R. (1992). The 'nicotine replacement paradox' in smoking cessation: How does nicotine gum really work? *British Journal of Addiction, 87*, 165–167.

White, H. R., & Labouvie, E. W. (1989). Towards the assessment of adolescent problem drinking. *Journal of Studies on Alcohol, 50*, 30–37.

Wills, T. A. (1985). Stress, coping, and tobacco and alcohol use in early adolescence. In S. Shiffman & T. A. Wills (Eds.), *Coping and substance use* (pp. 67–94). New York: Academic Press.

Winters, K. C. (1990). The need for improved assessment of adolescent substance use involvement. *Journal of Drug Issues, 20*, 487–502.

Winters, K. C. (1991). *The personal experience screening questionnaire*. Los Angeles: Western Psychological Services.

Winters, K. C., & Henly, G. A. (1988). Assessing adolescents who abuse chemicals: The Chemical Dependency Assessment Project. *National Institute on Drug Abuse Research Monograph Series, 77*, 4–18.

AUTHOR INDEX

SUBJECT INDEX